Published

RADIOLOGY OF THE PANCREAS AND DUODENUM
S. Boyd Eaton, Jr., M.D., and Joseph T. Ferrucci, Jr., M.D.

THE HAND IN RADIOLOGIC DIAGNOSIS
Andrew K. Poznanski, M.D.

RADIOLOGY OF THE ILEOCECAL AREA
Robert N. Berk, M.D., and Elliott C. Lasser, M.D.

FUNDAMENTALS OF ABDOMINAL AND PELVIC ULTRASONOGRAPHY
George R. Leopold, M.D., and W. Michael Asher, M.D.

RADIOLOGY OF THE ORBIT
G. A. S. Lloyd, B.M., B.Ch. Oxf., F.F.R., D.M.R.D.

SPECIAL PROCEDURES IN CHEST RADIOLOGY
Stuart S. Sagel, M.D.

RADIOLOGY OF RENAL FAILURE
Harry J. Griffiths, M.D.

PEDIATRIC RADIOLOGY OF THE ALIMENTARY TRACT
Edward B. Singleton, M.D., Milton L. Wagner, M.D., and Robert V. Dutton, M.D.

RADIOLOGIC DIAGNOSIS OF RENAL PARENCHYMAL DISEASE
Alan J. Davidson, M.D.

RADIOLOGY OF THE GALLBLADDER AND BILE DUCTS
Robert N. Berk, M.D., and Arthur R. Clemett, M.D.

RADIOLOGY OF THE LIVER
James G. McNulty, M.B., F.R.C.R.

GASTROINTESTINAL ANGIOGRAPHY—2nd Edition
Stewart R. Reuter, M.D., and Helen C. Redman, M.D.

CLINICAL RADIOLOGY OF THE EAR, NOSE AND THROAT—2nd Edition
Eric Samuel, M.D., and G. A. S. Lloyd, B.M., B.Ch. Oxf., F.F.R., D.M.R.D.

PEDIATRIC ORTHOPEDIC RADIOLOGY
M. B. Ozonoff, M.D.

THE RADIOLOGY OF JOINT DISEASE—2nd Edition
D. M. Forrester, M.D., J. C. Brown, M.D., and John W. Nesson, M.D.

THE RADIOLOGY OF VERTEBRAL TRAUMA
John A. Gehweiler, Jr., M.D., Raymond L. Osborne, Jr., M.D., and R. Frederick Becker, Ph.D.

RADIOLOGY OF THE ADRENALS with Sonography and CT
Harold A. Mitty, M.D., and Hsu-Chong Yeh, M.D.

CARDIAC IMAGING IN INFANTS AND CHILDREN
Michael J. Kelley, M.D., C. Carl Jaffe, M.D., and Charles S. Kleinman, M.D.

SELECTED TECHNIQUES IN INTERVENTIONAL RADIOLOGY
Saadoon Kadir, M.D., Stephen Kaufman, M.D., Klemens H. Barth, M.D., and Robert I. White, Jr., M.D.

Volume 20 in the Series

SAUNDERS
MONOGRAPHS
IN CLINICAL
RADIOLOGY

Forthcoming Monographs

KNEE ARTHROGRAPHY
Richard D. Wolfe, M.D.

CARDIAC IMAGING IN ADULTS
C. Carl Jaffe, M.D.

RADIOLOGY OF ORTHOPEDIC PROCEDURES
Martin I. Gelman, M.D.

RADIOLOGY OF HYPERTENSION
Bruce J. Hillman, M.D.

SECOND EDITION

INTENSIVE CARE RADIOLOGY: IMAGING OF THE CRITICALLY ILL

LAWRENCE R. GOODMAN, M.D.

Professor of Radiology
Hahnemann Medical College and Hospital
Philadelphia, Pennsylvania

CHARLES E. PUTMAN, M.D.

Chairman
Department of Radiology
Duke University Medical Center
Durham, North Carolina

1983

W. B. SAUNDERS COMPANY Philadelphia London Toronto
Mexico City Rio de Janeiro Sydney Tokyo

W. B. Saunders Company: West Washington Square
Philadelphia, PA 19105

1 St. Anne's Road
Eastbourne, East Sussex BN21 3UN, England

1 Goldthorne Avenue
Toronto, Ontario M8Z 5T9, Canada

Apartado 26370 – Cedro 512
Mexico 4, D.F., Mexico

Rua Coronel Cabrita, 8
Sao Cristovao Caixa Postal 21176
Rio de Janeiro, Brazil

9 Waltham Street
Artarmon, N.S.W. 2064, Australia

Ichibancho, Central Bldg., 22-1 Ichibancho
Chiyoda-Ku, Tokyo 102, Japan

Library of Congress Cataloging in Publication Data
Main entry under title:

Intensive care radiology. Imaging of the critically ill

Includes bibliographies and index.
1. Critical care medicine. 2. Diagnosis, Radiographic. 3. Critically ill. I. Goodman, Lawrence R., 1943– II. Putman, Charles E., 1941– [DNLM: 1. Critical care. 2. Emergencies. 3. Intensive care units. 4. Radiography. WX 218 I605]
RC86.7.I56 1982 616.07′57 82–47767
ISBN 0-7216-4166-0

Intensive Care Radiology. Imaging of the Critically Ill ISBN 0-7216-4166-0

Last digit is the print number: 9 8 7 6 5 4 3 2 1

To our wives,
Hannah and Mary,
for their patience.
And to our children,
Roy, Julie, Cammie, Shannon, and Garrett.

CONTRIBUTORS

HARVEY J. BERGER, M.D.
Assistant Professor of Diagnostic Radiology and Medicine, Director of Cardiovascular Imaging, Yale University School of Medicine, New Haven, Connecticut.

MORTON G. GLICKMAN, M.D.
Professor of Diagnostic Radiology, and Chief, Vascular and Interventional Radiology, Yale University School of Medicine, New Haven, Connecticut.

DAVID J. GOODENOUGH, Ph.D.
Associate Professor of Radiology, and Director, Division of Radiation Physics, Department of Radiology, George Washington University School of Medicine, Washington, D.C.

LAWRENCE R. GOODMAN, M.D.
Professor of Radiology, Hahnemann Medical College and Hospital, Philadelphia, Pennsylvania.

H. JOEL GORFINKEL, M.D.
Clinical Associate Professor of Medicine, Ohio State University School of Medicine, and Attending Cardiologist, Mt. Carmel Medical Center, Grant Hospital, St. Anthony Hospital, Columbus, Ohio.

ALEXANDER GOTTSCHALK, M.D.
Professor of Diagnostic Radiology, and Vice-Chairman, Department of Diagnostic Radiology, Yale University School of Medicine, New Haven, Connecticut.

R. BROOKE JEFFREY, M.D.
Assistant Professor, Department of Radiology, University of California, San Francisco, and Radiologist, San Francisco General Hospital, San Francisco, California.

GERALD A. MANDELL, M.D., F.A.A.P.
Clinical Associate Professor of Pediatrics and Radiology, Hahnemann Medical College and Hospital, Philadelphia, and Fellow in Nuclear Medicine, University of Pennsylvania Hospital, Philadelphia, Pennsylvania.

HIDEYO MINAGI, M.D.
Professor of Radiology, University of California, San Francisco, and Radiologist, San Francisco General Hospital, San Francisco, California.

ARL V. MOORE, JR., M.D.
Assistant Professor, Duke University Medical Center, Durham, North Carolina.

CHARLES E. PUTMAN, M.D.
Chairman, Department of Radiology, Duke University Medical Center, Durham, North Carolina.

CARL E. RAVIN, M.D.
Professor of Radiology, Department of Radiology, Duke University Medical Center, Durham, North Carolina.

ARTHUR L. RIBA, M.D.
Assistant Professor of Medicine, University of Connecticut Health Science Center, and Chief of Cardiology, Mt. Sinai Hospital, Hartford, Connecticut.

KENNETH E. WEAVER, M.S.
Assistant Professor of Radiology, Department of Radiology, George Washington University School of Medicine, Washington, D.C.

BARRY L. ZARET, M.D.
Professor of Medicine and Diagnostic Radiology, and Chief of Cardiology, Yale University School of Medicine, New Haven, Connecticut.

JACK E. ZIMMERMAN, M.D.
Professor of Anesthesiology, George Washington University School of Medicine, Washington, and Director, Intensive Care Unit, George Washington University Medical Center, Washington, D.C.

PREFACE TO THE SECOND EDITION

Both intensive care medicine and diagnostic imaging have made great strides since the writing of the first edition. The portable radiograph and conventional radiographic techniques remain the mainstay of imaging in the critically ill. However, the armamentarium of the radiologist has been greatly expanded in the last few years with the increasing use of ultrasound, the increasing availability of rapid CT scanning, and the continued progress of nuclear medicine. These new imaging modalities have changed the diagnostic approach to many intrathoracic and intra-abdominal disorders in the seriously ill, and contributed to the development of many percutaneous interventional procedures for the treatment of certain intrathoracic and intra-abdominal conditions. Techniques such as percutaneous drainage of abscesses, percutaneous catheterization of the biliary and urinary tract, balloon dilatation of obstructed vessels and ducts, and the use of directed skinny-needle aspirations of the lung, pleura, and abdomen are especially valuable in the critically ill patient. Although some procedures may be done at the bedside, most require the transporting of the patient to the fluoroscopic or ultrasound suite. Because these procedures often obviate the need for general anesthesia and surgical exploration, a decreased mortality and morbidity is anticipated.

The second edition has also been made more comprehensive with the inclusion of chapters on chest trauma and the postoperative chest radiograph, two areas of frequent concern in the intensive care setting. The special problems of the critically ill newborn are also addressed in detail in this edition.

We would again like to thank the numerous residents and colleagues whose suggestions have been incorporated into the second edition. This book could not have been completed without the excellent photographic support of the Audiovisual Department at George Washington University and the secretarial help provided by Ms. Connie Brennan, Mrs. Mary Cody, and Miss Carol Perry. Special thanks are due to Mr. Michael Brown, who helped expedite this publication.

LAWRENCE R. GOODMAN, M.D.
CHARLES E. PUTMAN, M.D.

CONTENTS

Chapter 1

LIFE SUPPORT TECHNIQUES

by Jack E. Zimmerman

HISTORY AND GROWTH OF INTENSIVE CARE

The intensive care unit (ICU) has evolved from postanesthetic recovery rooms and from experiences during polio epidemics in the early 1950s. The development of arrhythmia monitoring, cardiopulmonary resuscitation, and improved ventilators has provided a further impetus. These advances in methodology, instrumentation, and approach to the critically ill patient created problems for which ICUs have provided practical solutions.

Current ICUs provide for centralization of the expensive and complex equipment and of the large number of highly trained staff required for life support. In some hospitals ICUs have been established according to department or specialty, whereas those in other hospitals are interdepartmental or multidisciplinary (Safar and Grenvik, 1971). Specialized units that have evolved include coronary, respiratory, pediatric, renal, burn, shock/trauma, stroke, and neonatal units. Although they have developed out of necessity, there is ample evidence that ICUs save lives. The mortality for acute myocardial infarction, respiratory failure, and many other conditions has been reduced by treatment in an ICU setting (Petty et al., 1975).

Knowledge of life support techniques and monitoring apparatus involving the cardiovascular and respiratory systems is central to the care and radiographic evaluation of most ICU patients. This chapter emphasizes these techniques and their relationship to radiographic examination.

RESPIRATORY CARE TECHNIQUES

Many patients in the ICU who have respiratory problems are not on ventilators and do not have artificial airways. The care of these individuals is in many ways more challenging and at times more difficult than that of the intubated patient on a respirator. Utilization of a number of noninvasive respiratory care techniques can help to avoid the morbidity and mortality associated with the use of more invasive respiratory care.

Oxygen Therapy and Toxicity

Oxygen therapy is indicated whenever oxygen transport to tissues is, or is likely to become, inadequate. This broad statement compels the physician to evaluate pulmonary as well as cardiovascular, hematologic, and biochemical variables. Table 1–1 lists the most commonly used equipment for increasing inspired oxygen concentration.

Pulmonary oxygen toxicity should rarely be encountered in current practice, since it now is generally recognized that the use of an inspired oxygen concentration of 50 per cent or less is not associated with pulmonary damage (Winter and Smith, 1972). Patients who formerly required toxic oxygen concentrations can currently be managed with nontoxic oxygen concentrations and positive end-expiratory pressure (PEEP) or extracorporeal membrane oxygenation before the complication develops. The relationship of pulmonary oxygen toxicity

TABLE 1–1. Commonly Utilized Methods of Oxygen Administration

Equipment	Flow (liters/min)	O_2 Concentration (%)	Remarks
Nasal catheter	6–8	30–50	Gastric distention, air swallowing, nasal irritation
Nasal prongs	4–6 1–3	30–40 24–32	Best patient tolerance, unreliable O_2 concentration, nasal soreness
Non-rebreathing mask with bag	6 8 8–12	40–50 50–60 70–85	Highest delivered O_2 concentration (danger of O_2 toxicity); hard to fit, possible CO_2 retention at lower flows
Aerosol mask	10 liters via nebulizer	30–60	Uncomfortable wetness, nebulizer; O_2 underdelivered at higher concentration; usual apparatus after extubation
Venturi mask	4–8	24, 28, 35, 40	Precise concentration even with flow variation; used in alveolar hypoventilation
Adult tent	10–15	21–50	Of historical interest but expensive and poor patient tolerance
Face tent	4–8	30–50	Comfortable, fair humidification

to adult respiratory distress syndrome (ARDS) is discussed in Chapter 5.

Humidification and Nebulization

The major indications for adding water to inspired gases are: (1) the prevention and treatment of thickened or obstructing secretions; (2) to provide a substitute for the warming, filtering, and humidifying functions of the upper airway in intubated patients; and (3) to deposit water and drugs in the lower airway. The equipment commonly used to increase the water content of inspired gases is listed in Table 1–2.

There are a number of radiographically apparent hazards associated with the humidification of gases. These include infection (deposition of contaminated water or overheating resulting in mucosal damage) and overhydration. Ultrasonic nebulization therapy is associated with additional unique hazards, including increases in airway resistance, changes in pulmonary surface activity, and a decline in Pa_{O_2} in patients with obstructive lung disease.

TABLE 1–2. Equipment Used to Increase the Water Content of Inspired Gases

Apparatus	Body Humidity (%)
Bubble humidifier	20
Unheated nebulizer	40–75
Heated nebulizer	60–120
Heated mainstream humidifier	60–120
Ultrasonic nebulizer	100–400

Intermittent Positive Pressure Breathing

Intermittent positive pressure breathing (IPPB) treatment refers to the periodic mechanical application of positive airway pressure and should not be confused with continuous mechanical ventilator support.The value of IPPB in respiratory therapy has become very controversial (Gold, 1975). Its purported effectiveness in treating postoperative atelectasis, asthma, and chronic obstructive pulmonary disease (COPD) has not been confirmed by controlled studies (Van de Water et al., 1972). There is general agreement that, if employed in an inexact manner and without supervision, IPPB is worthless if not potentially harmful.

Theoretically, IPPB should equalize gas distribution by increasing pressure in the tracheobronchial tree. As gas distribution is improved, secretion drainage should also improve along with pulmonary function. IPPB is commonly used in conjunction with nebulization of bronchodilator or mucolytic aerosols.

Chest Physiotherapy

The purpose of chest physiotherapy is to achieve satisfactory ventilation of all regions of the lung and to mobilize secretions from the tracheobronchial tree. Chest physiotherapy comprises several techniques, each with definite indications and contraindications. These include breathing exercises, postural drainage, and manual techniques (percussion and vibration). All techniques are accompanied by the encouraging of effective coughing or by nasotracheal suctioning. Most frequently, these techniques are combined as a treatment program designed to drain or re-expand specific areas of infiltration or atelectasis.

The radiologist should occasionally suggest intensive chest physiotherapy, suctioning, or fiberoptic bronchoscopy as a means of differential diagnosis. ICU patients frequently develop single or multiple ill defined densities suggesting either pneumonia or atelectasis (see Chapter 4). Differentiation clinically or on a single film is often impossible. A second radiograph showing dramatic clearing after treatment confirms that secretion plugging rather than pneumonia is the problem.

Cough Stimulation

Patients with adequate ventilatory mechanics frequently cough ineffectively because of obtundation, pain, or lack of cooperation. Passage of a suction catheter through the nose to the larynx or carina is one means of providing mechanical stimulation and secretion mobilization. Suctioning is preceded and followed by reoxygenation to prevent atelectasis and cardiac arrhythmias.

Occasionally, patients require cough stimulation but have anatomic variations or limitations in positioning that make nasotracheal suctioning impossible. In such situations, cough stimulation can be achieved by transcricoid passage of a polyethylene catheter into the trachea (Fig. 1–1). A position slightly above the carina is confirmed radiographically, and saline is instilled periodically to stimulate coughing. The catheter may have to be discontinued because of persistent coughing and irritation or because of displacement into the pharynx.

Fiberoptic Bronchoscopy

The fiberoptic bronchoscope (Fig. 1–2) is an extremely useful new tool in acute respiratory care (Lindholm et al., 1974). Because of its small size and flexibility, the instrument can be utilized even while the patient requires simultaneous ventilator support. Diagnostic uses include detection of aspiration of gastric contents, foreign bodies, and endobronchial lesions; localization of the source of hemoptysis; and evaluation of damage caused by artificial airways. Cultures of aspirate obtained with the fiberoptic bronchoscope are not reliable for diagnosis (Bartlett et al., 1976). Therapeutic uses include aspiration of secretions, segmental and lobar lavage, and precise localization of artificial airways.

TRACHEAL INTUBATION

Indications

Indications for tracheal intubation include the need to establish an airway (for example, in laryngeal obstruction), the need for mechanical ventilation, management of tracheobronchial secretions, and protection of the airway (prevention of aspiration pneumonia). Extubation simply relates to the clinical determination that these indications no longer exist.

Nasal and Oral Intubation

Nasotracheal intubation is the preferred route for long-term ventilatory support because of better patient tolerance and stability in tube fixation. Nasotracheal intubation is associated with complications of nasal necrosis and bleeding, sinus infection, and gastric distention. Orotracheal intubation is preferred under emergency circumstances; when an adequately sized tube cannot be passed transnasally; or when there are contraindications to nasal intubation, such as coagulopathy or sinus infection.

The generous length of most endotracheal tubes together with the operator's feeling of relief as the tube passes through the vocal cords often lead to a little extra shove and accidental right main stem bronchus intubation. Regardless of breath sounds, a chest radiograph is indicated to ensure proper tube positioning. Repeated clinical and radiographic examination

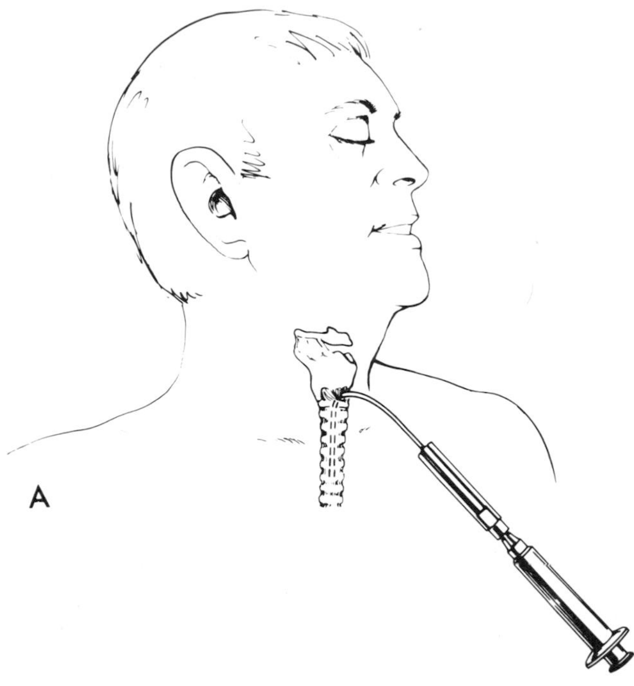

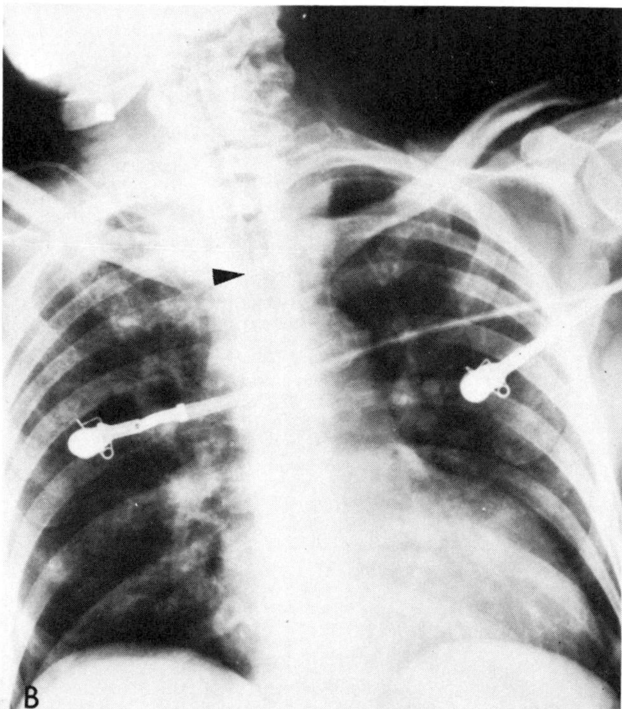

Figure 1–1. *A*, Placement of transcricoid cough stimulator. *B*, Proper position of the catheter tip several centimeters above the carina (*arrowhead*).

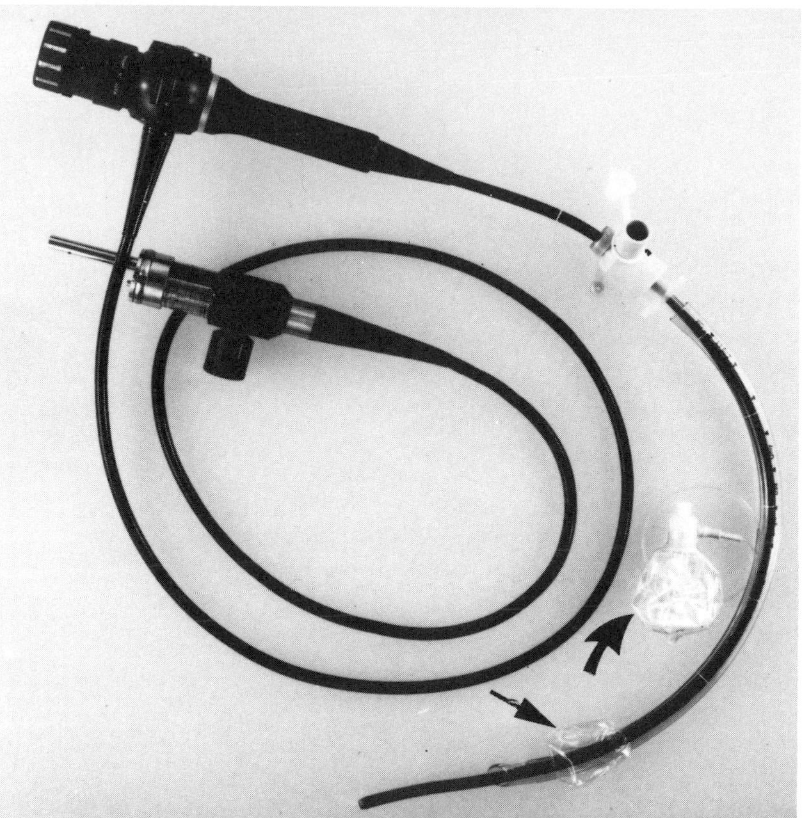

Figure 1–2. Olympus Bronchofiberscope Model BF inserted through an endotracheal tube and adapter for use during ventilator support. Note the high-volume, low-pressure cuff (*arrow*). The external pressure reservoir (*curved arrow*) occasionally projects over the chest radiograph as a "thin-walled cyst" (see Fig. 2–9).

to assess position are needed, since tubes commonly move during retaping and suctioning and through manipulation by the intubated patient.

Tracheostomy

In current practice, tracheostomy is rarely performed as a primary procedure and is almost always preceded by a period of nasotracheal or orotracheal intubation. In general, recent improvements in manufacture, design, and care of endotracheal tubes have led to safer and more prolonged nasotracheal or orotracheal intubation. Periods of three to seven days are common, although periods of 10 to 21 days or longer are utilized under selected circumstances. The complications of endotracheal intubation and tracheostomy are discussed further in Chapter 2.

Recent Advances in Tube Design

A recent improvement common to all tracheal tubes is the substitution of polyvinylchloride for rubber; this makes the tube less tissue reactive and more moldable to the anatomy of the patient's airway. Many ICUs prefer endotracheal tubes with a Murphy tip (end and side outlet holes) to those with a Magill tip (single end outlet hole) (Fig. 1–3), in order to minimize the frequency of atelectasis and consequent hypoxia accompanying right main stem bronchus intubation.

Another improvement common to endotracheal and tracheostomy tubes is the use of high-volume, low-pressure cuffs (Figs. 1–2, 1–3). These cuffs seal the airway during artificial ventilation by virtue of their high residual volume and bulk rather than by exerting a high pressure against the tracheal wall (Carroll,

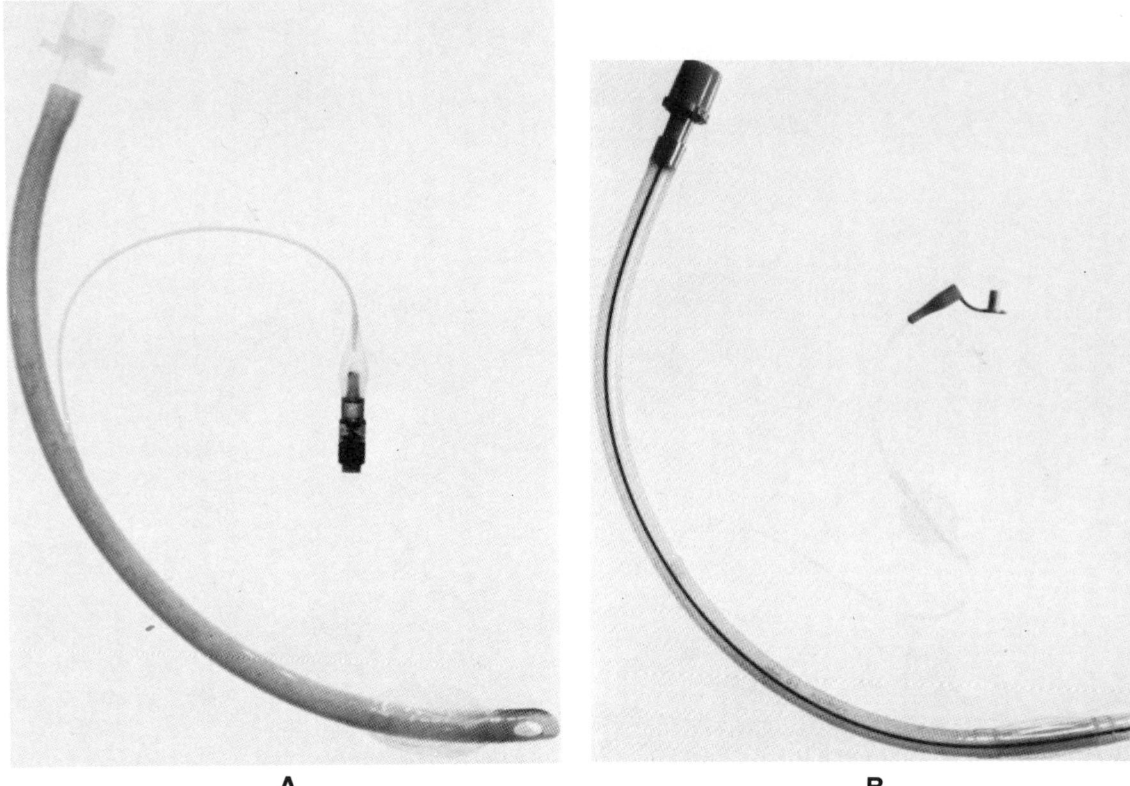

Figure 1–3. Commonly used endotracheal tubes. *A*, National Catheter Corporation endotracheal tube with high-volume, low-pressure cuff and Murphy tip (side hole). *B*, Portex endotracheal tube with low-volume, high-pressure cuff and Magill tip.

1973). By using the minimal amounts of air needed to avoid air leakage, it is possible to ventilate most patients with cuff pressures that are less than normal mucosal capillary perfusion pressure (22 mm Hg), thus reducing the likelihood of tracheal necrosis (Carroll et al., 1974).

In comparison, small-volume cuffs may exert 100 to 400 mm Hg pressure in sealing the airway. Accidental overinflation of high-volume, low-pressure cuffs results in similarly high pressures and larger areas of tracheal necrosis. This can be suspected radiographically if the air-filled cuff is widely dilating the trachea (see Fig. 2–13). Occasionally, tracheal dilatation is seen without overinflation in patients who require very high ventilatory pressures for prolonged periods.

VENTILATORY SUPPORT

Indications

The techniques for treating respiratory failure have improved, and increased emphasis is placed on early diagnosis and treatment of respiratory insufficiency (Pontoppidan et al., 1972). With serial evaluation of clinical, radiographic, and functional indices, proper therapeutic interventions can be initiated before the onset of frank respiratory failure.

Table 1–3 lists guidelines that, together with clinical judgment, have proved most useful in defining appropriate intervention in patients with respiratory diseases of diverse etiology. Although seemingly complex, these measurements constitute the everyday language of acute respiratory care.

The total volume of gas exhaled after maximial inspiration (vital capacity) is the best measurement of mechanical impairment in patients with restrictive lung disease. The amount of pressure generated by an inspiratory effort (inspiratory force) mainly reflects the neuromuscular aspects of respiration. Together, these two measurements provide quantitation of the patient's mechanical reserve available for coughing, for deep breathing, and for performing the work of breathing. The forced expiratory volume in one second (FEV_1) provides a measure

TABLE 1–3. Guidelines for Ventilatory Support in Adults with Acute Respiratory Failure

Physiologic Data (Treatment)	Normal Range (No Treatment)	Moderately Abnormal (Intensive Respiratory Care)	Severely Abnormal (Intubation and Ventilation)
Mechanics			
Respiratory rate (per min)	12–20	25–35	>40
Vital capacity (ml/kg ideal weight)	65–75	15–30	<15
FEV_1 (ml/kg ideal weight)	50–60	15–25	<10
Inspiratory force (cm H_2O)	75–100	25–50	<20
Oxygenation			
Pa_{O_2} (mm Hg)	75–100 air	—	<70 on oxygen mask
$AaDo_2$ (mm Hg) 100% O_2, 20 min)	50–75	200–350	>350
Ventilation			
Pa_{CO_2} (mm Hg)	35–45	45–60	<65, pH < 7.25

of the severity of airway obstruction and is particularly useful in defining appropriate intervention in status asthmaticus.

Arterial blood gas studies including partial pressure of oxygen (Pa_{O_2}) and carbon dioxide (Pa_{CO_2}) must be interpreted with caution. The fall in pH below 7.25 as a result of carbon dioxide retention is more critical than the absolute value for Pa_{CO_2} in the decision to support ventilation. Likewise, relating the Pa_{O_2} to the inspired oxygen concentration is more important than the absolute value.

Placing a patient on 100 per cent oxygen for 20 to 30 minutes allows complete nitrogen washout, so that alveolar oxygen tension (PA_{O_2}) is easily calculated. Measurement of arterial oxygen tension (Pa_{O_2}) under these conditions and calculation of the difference between alveolar and arterial tension (AaD_{O_2}) provide a fair estimation of the severity of intrapulmonary shunting.

Each of these values may occasionally fail as indicators of a patient's need for a respirator. This is particularly true in the patient with COPD. The combination of several indices and the clinical state of the patient constitute the deciding factors in the initiation of ventilatory support.

Mechanical Ventilators

Respirators have become increasingly complex and sophisticated. Volume-limited respirators have largely replaced the older, less powerful, pressure-limited machines. These volume respirators all share a characteristic feature of delivering a prescribed tidal volume regardless of the pressure required. The modes of ventilation have also become more complex. These include controlled (respirator-determined) ventilation, assisted (patient-triggered) ventilation, and a newer mode intermittent mandatory ventilation (IMV). The IMV mode combines a prescribed (mandatory) number of respiratory breaths with the patient's own spontaneous breathing. The advantages of this increasingly used technique have recently been reviewed (Luce et al., 1981).

A number of factors should be kept in mind when interpreting the radiographs of a respirator patient:

1. A patient's tidal volume setting usually ranges from 10 to 15 ml/kg. Since volume delivery is constant despite changes in airway resistance or lung compliance, the depth of inspiration during film exposure should be consistent unless settings are changed.

2. Most respirators are equipped with an automatic hyperinflation ("sigh") system that periodically delivers one and one half to two times the usual tidal volume in order to minimize atelectasis. An automatic sigh coinciding with film exposure will markedly increase the depth of inspiration and may alter the appearance of infiltrates (Fig. 1–4).

3. Patients being ventilated in the IMV mode have two different inspiratory volumes: respirator breaths (usually 700 to 1000 ml); and spontaneous breaths (150 to 400 ml). Technicians must be cautioned to expose films only during respirator breaths.

4. Many respirators have an inflation hold device that will maintain inspiratory volume for 0.2 to one second. Use of this device can ensure more consistent inspiratory volumes during film exposure.

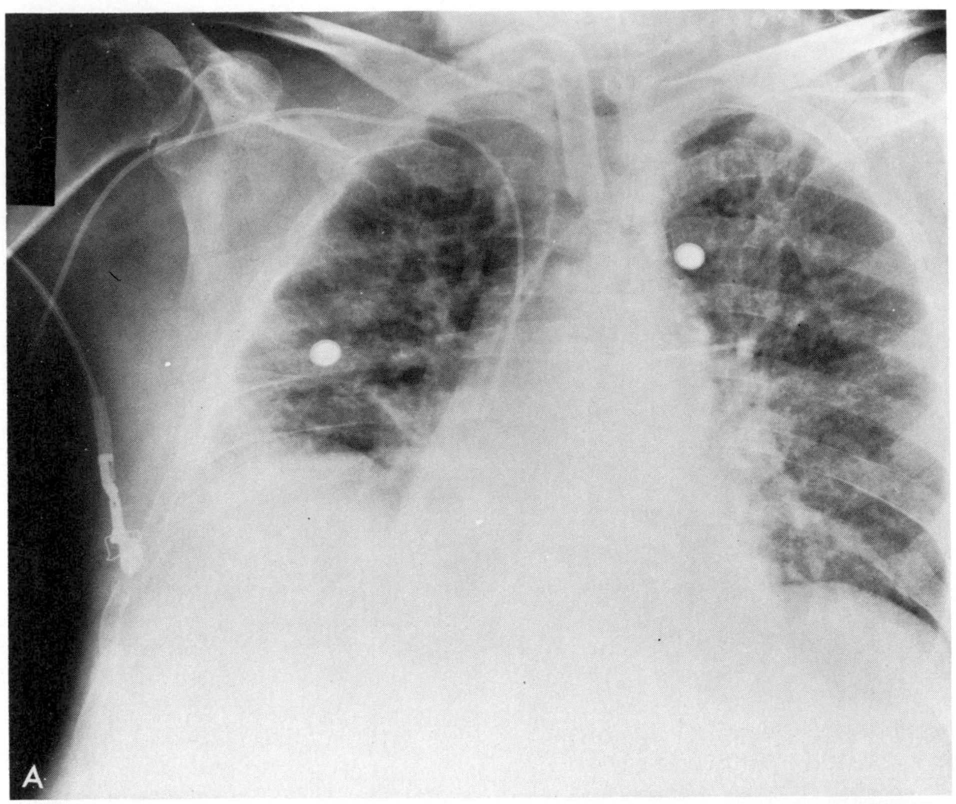
A

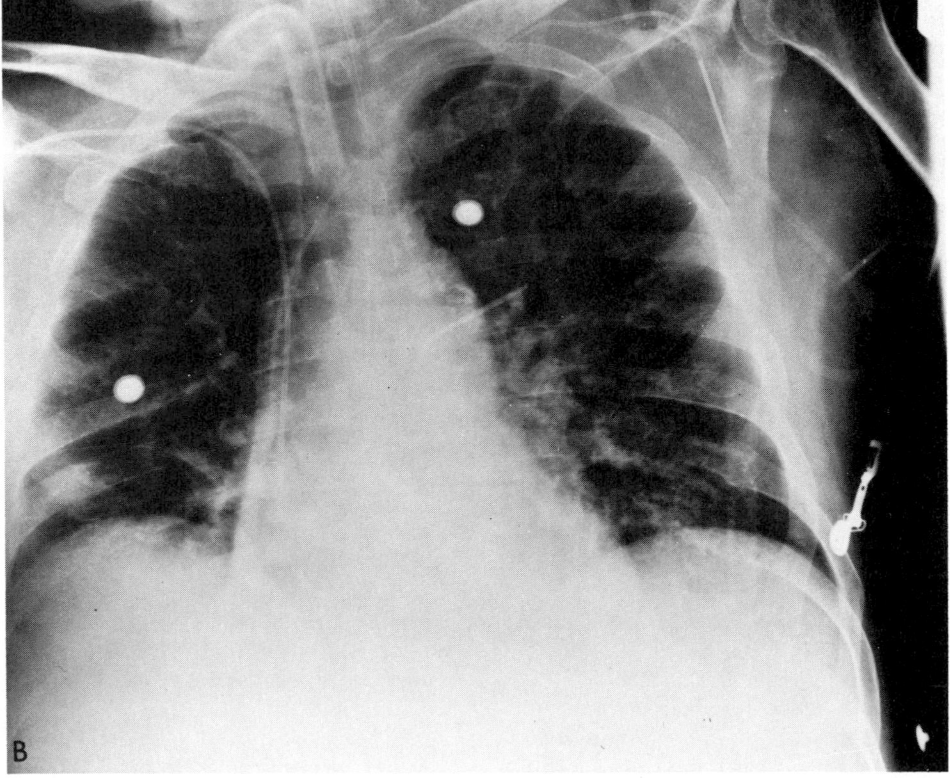
B

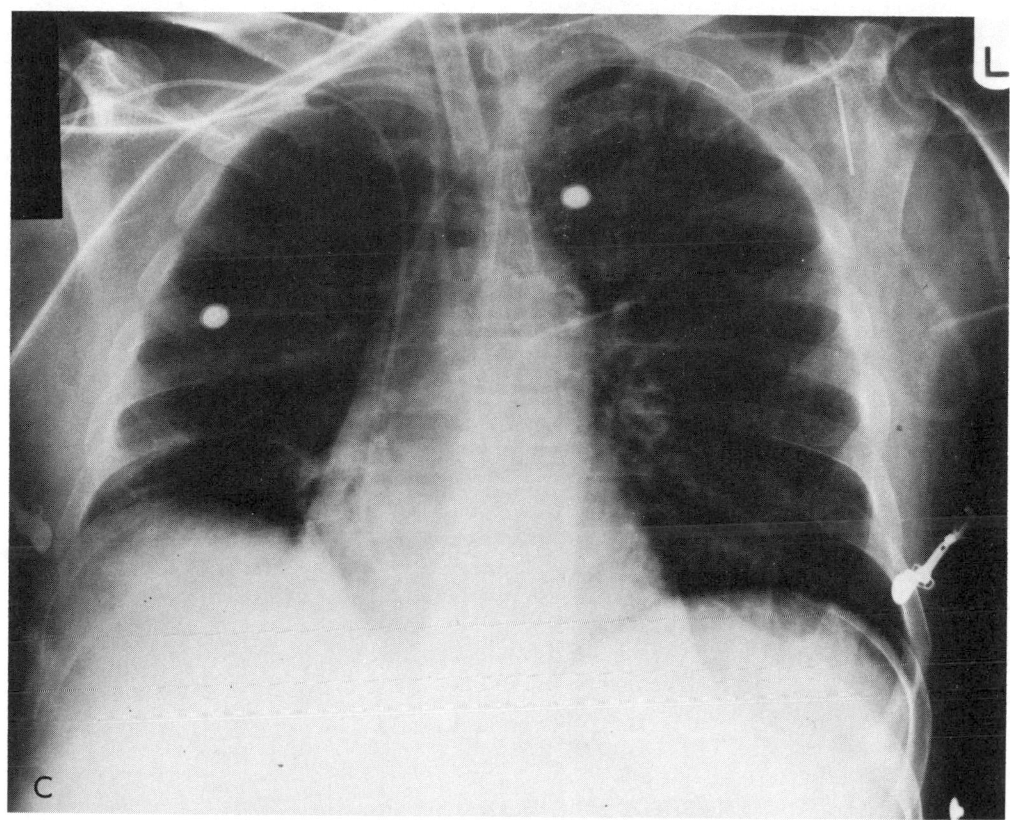

Figure 1–4. Effect of respirator inflation volume and positive end-expiratory pressure (PEEP) on chest radiographs. All films were taken within 15 minutes by the same technician using the same equipment and technical factors. Note that the central venous pressure catheter is coiled in the superior vena cava. *A*, Pulmonary edema in a patient receiving an 800 ml tidal volume without PEEP. *B*, Repeat film with a 1200 ml sigh without PEEP. *C*, Repeat film with an 800 ml tidal volume and 12-cm PEEP.

5. Respirators are quite powerful, most being capable of delivering volume at peak pressures of 80 to 120 cm H_2O. In general, the risk of pneumothorax rises precipitously as pressures increase from 30 to 80 cm H_2O (Nennhaus et al., 1967). The incidence of pulmonary barotrauma during mechanical ventilation (subcutaneous emphysema, pneumomediastinum, and pneumothorax) has been reported to be as high as 15 per cent (Fleming and Bower, 1972).

6. The efficient humidifiers of the modern respirator may not only negate normal insensible respiratory water losses, but also add 300 to 500 ml of insensible water gain per day. These alterations may contribute to pulmonary edema and overhydration in the absence of an appreciably positive fluid balance (Sladen et al., 1968).

7. All volume respirators are equipped to deliver positive end-expiratory pressure (PEEP). PEEP is frequently used in acute restrictive lung disease (for example, pulmonary edema or ARDS) to decrease intrapulmonary shunting. The application of PEEP traps gas in the lung at end-expiration, resulting in increased lung volume (functional residual capacity) and the opening or recruitment of previously unventilated alveoli.

The physiologic effect of PEEP is one of improved oxygenation as a result of decreased intrapulmonary shunting, thus allowing the use of a lower (usually nontoxic) inspired oxygen concentration. The radiographic effect is both immediate and dramatic (Fig. 1–4). The increase in functional residual capacity plus the usual tidal volume results in a marked increase in inspiratory lung volume. The lungs will appear more expanded and infiltrates less prominent (Fig. 2–19). These changes can markedly alter radiographic interpretation (Zimmerman et al., 1979).

Maintenance on Ventilators

The experience in our ICU and in other units has shown that once appropriate ventilator support is initiated, complications are to be expected (Zwillich et al., 1974). Although some complications are attributable to the operation of the ventilator (disconnection, leak, inadequate humidification, and so on), many problems are encountered with intubation or involve medical complications closely associated with mechanical ventilation. Since the problems are well defined, most of them are easily detectable, and many are simply treated. If recognized early, the stage is hopefully set for anticipation or prevention.

Medical Complications Closely Associated with Mechanical Ventilation

- Pulmonary barotrauma
  - Subcutaneous emphysema
  - Pneumomediastinum
  - Pneumothorax
  - Pneumoretroperitoneum
  - Pneumoperitoneum
  - Interstitial emphysema
- Atelectasis
- Bacterial pneumonia
- Aspiration pneumonia
- Pulmonary edema
- Hyperventilation-alkalosis syndrome
- Cardiac arrhythmias
- Pulmonary oxygen toxicity
- Massive gastric distention
- Cecal dilatation or perforation

Daily radiographic examination is indicated in respirator patients in order to detect the medical complications of ventilator support and of tracheal intubation. The clinician evaluating such patients, although equipped with a good deal of clinical and physiologic data, usually needs a chest radiograph to confirm all but the most blatantly obvious pulmonary abnormalities.

Weaning

Weaning is generally begun as early as possible because of complications related to the respirator, intubation, and inactivity of respiratory muscles during ventilatory support. Removal from respirator support is considered when there is clinical, radiographic, and physiologic evidence of reversal of the cause of respiratory failure (Hodgkin et al., 1974). The physiologic criteria that represent indications for ventilator support (Table 1–3) are measured throughout the patient's course, and improvements constitute criteria for weaning. Radiographic improvement frequently lags behind improvement in the patient's clinical and physiologic condition.

The majority of patients are removed from ventilator support quickly and without difficulty. In spite of patient selection based on clinical and physiologic indices, however, there are individuals who should wean but who do not and who appear marginal but who do well. The ability to breathe without assistance, then, constitutes the final test for removal from respirator support.

During spontaneous breathing trials, patients are removed from the ventilator and given a source of oxygen and humidity. While being carefully monitored, patients remain off of the ventilator for progressively longer periods (hours to days) until total independence has been achieved.

Patients who are ventilated with the IMV mode are usually weaned in a different fashion (Downs et al., 1973). The number of respirator breaths per minute is progressively decreased while the patients' own respiratory efforts play an increasing role in maintaining oxygenation and ventilation. When an IMV rate of two per minute is well tolerated, most patients require no further respiratory support.

Radiographically, the weaning period may be an eventful one. Atelectasis is frequent because of the removal of respirator hyperexpansion and a decreased ability to clear pulmonary secretions. Increased central blood volume and decreased alveolar pressure following removal of the ventilator predisposes the patient to pulmonary edema. A major hazard in radiographic interpretation exists because the degree of lung expansion during film exposure is often less than during respirator therapy. Unless the patient is returned to the ventilator or the lungs are hyperinflated during exposure, it is not uncommon to see a "useless expiratory" or apparently deteriorated chest radiograph in a patient who is doing quite well clinically and physiologically.

When tracheostomized patients are weaned, they may still require an artificial airway for removal of tracheobronchial secretions. A tracheal "button" may be substituted for the tracheostomy tube at this time (Fig. 1–5). Such devices allow the patient to speak and cough normally while they continue to provide access to the trachea for suctioning or replacement of a tracheostomy tube.

CARDIOVASCULAR SUPPORT

Monitoring Techniques

Cardiac arrhythmias are both frequent and potentially lethal for ICU patients (Lewis, 1971). Thus, the electrocardiographic (ECG) monitor is a standard piece of equipment in the ICU. Less frequently, patients undergo direct intra-arterial pressure monitoring. Direct mon-

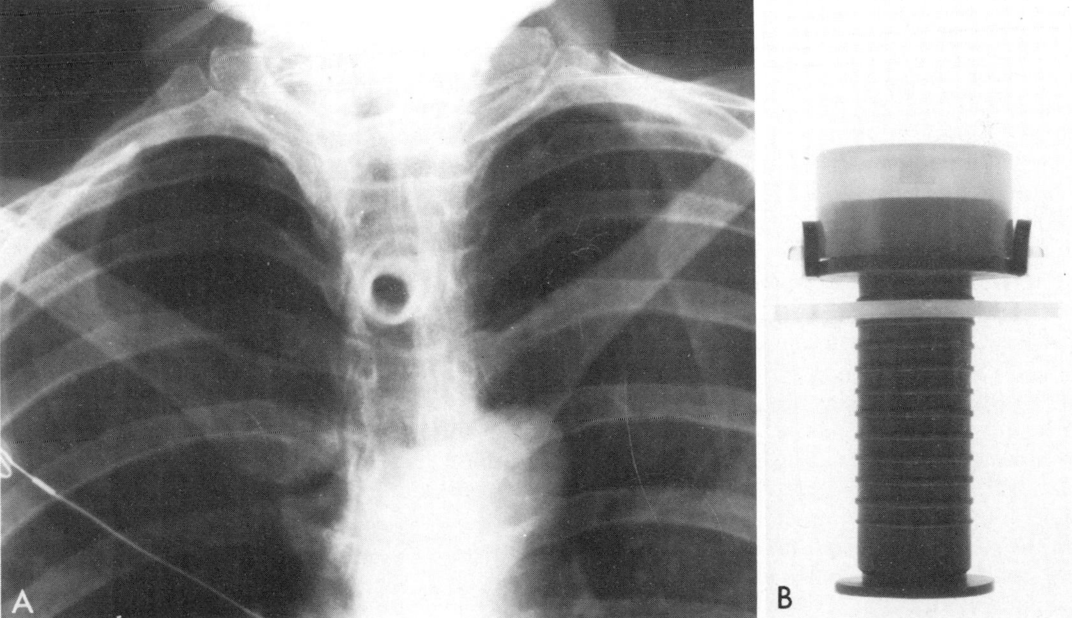

Figure 1–5. *A*, Radiographic and *B*, photographic appearances of Kistner tracheal "button." (Courtesy of Pilling Co., Fort Washington, PA.)

itoring avoids inaccuracies in blood pressure measurement during low flow states (cuff pressure usually falsely low) and allows continuous recording during infusion of vasoactive agents, repeated arterial blood sampling, and cardiac output determination.

More pertinent to the radiography of intensive care are the techniques of hemodynamic monitoring that involve filling pressure measurement. Patients in circulatory failure or shock demonstrate many signs and symptoms indicating the presence and severity of underperfusion. Although clinical and laboratory evaluation will often define the cause, appropriate supportive therapy may not be possible until hemodynamic data are obtained. This is usually accomplished by monitoring right- or left-sided cardiac filling pressure.

Central Venous Pressure

Central venous pressure (CVP) measurement provides a direct reflection of right atrial pressure, which in turn reflects both right and, by inference, left ventricular end-diastolic pressure and volume. High pressures (>15 cm H_2O) and a poor circulation suggest cardiac failure, tamponade, or volume overload, whereas low pressures (0 to 4 cm H_2O) suggest hypovolemia.

Peripheral venous pressure reflects neither right atrial pressure nor blood volume changes. Therefore, it is essential that venous pressure catheters be within the thorax, preferably in the superior vena cava (Fig. 1–6). Techniques of placement include peripheral venipuncture with use of long catheters, internal and external jugular cannulation, and subclavian venipuncture utilizing both supraclavicular and infraclavicular approaches. A host of complications and errors in placement are possible with each of these techniques, and are discussed in Chapter 3.

The ease of placement and clinical success of CVP monitoring make it the most commonly utilized filling pressure measurement. CVP monitoring, however, does have significant shortcomings (James and Myers, 1972). Although CVP does indirectly reflect left-sided cardiac pressures, one cannot assume that right- and left-sided cardiac pressures will always vary in the same magnitude or direction. Predictable discrepancies occur in patients with predominantly right-sided (for example, cor pulmonale) or left-sided (for example, myocardial infarction) heart disease. Discrepancies that are totally unpredictable occur in patients with multiple system failure or injury. During rapid volume expansion, there may be no increase in CVP at a time when left atrial pressure has already risen to dangerous (pulmonary edema) levels. Because of these factors, pulmonary capillary wedge (PCW) pressure is a more precise guide to circulatory diagnosis and treatment.

Pulmonary Capillary Wedge Pressure

The development of a No. 5 French balloon-tipped catheter by Swan and Ganz has made possible effective, safe and widespread application of bedside right-sided cardiac catheterization and repeated determination of pulmonary arterial and PCW pressures (Swan et al., 1970). The PCW pressure provides a direct index of left atrial pressure. High pressures (>20 mm Hg) and a poor circulation reflect left ventricular failure, whereas low pressures (>5 mm Hg) suggest hypovolemia.

With the use of pressure monitoring, these catheters are passed from an antecubital or jugular vein through the right side of the heart into the pulmonary artery without the use of fluoroscopy (Civetta and Gabel, 1972). The balloon tip provides flow guidance and protection from cardiac arrhythmias during insertion. The catheter tip, when optimally placed, is in the right or left pulmonary artery 2 to 3 inches distal to the bifurcation of the main pulmonary artery (Fig. 1–6). From this position, balloon inflation causes the catheter to float distally into the "wedge" position, allowing repeated measurements. When the balloon is deflated, the tip returns to its original position.

Recently developed catheters (No. 7 French) have three lumens (pulmonary artery, right atrium, and balloon) and a thermistor for cardiac output determination by thermodilution technique. Catheters are also available with electrodes for intracavitary ECG monitoring and emergency pacing (Chatterjee et al., 1975).

Catheters placed too far distally may cause gross inaccuracies in thermodilution cardiac output determinations. Distal placement may also cause constant wedging, leading to pulmonary ischemic lesions. The likelihood of such problems is great when proper positioning is not documented radiographically. Even when initial positioning is optimal, catheters have a tendency to migrate distally with blood flow.

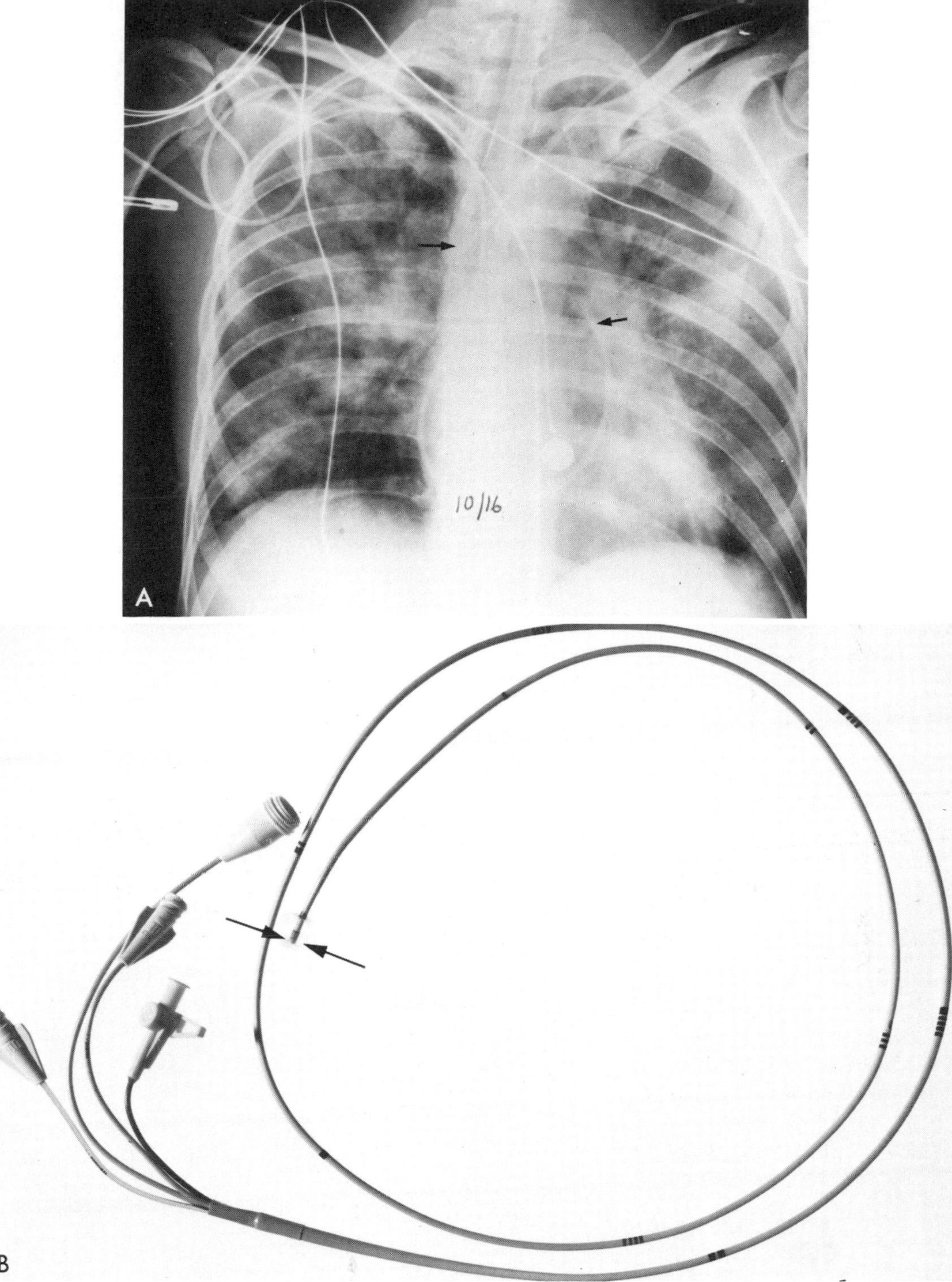

Figure 1–6. A, Chest radiograph showing proper positioning of a Swan-Ganz catheter with its tip in the proximal left pulmonary artery (*lower arrow*). The tip of the left central venous pressure catheter is in the superior vena cava (*upper arrow*). B, No. 7 French thermodilution catheter with the balloon inflated (*arrows*).

Although distal migration is common, optimal maintenance of catheters will minimize complications (Archer and Cobb, 1974). This includes daily radiographic evaluation of catheter position, use of a continuous low-volume flushing device, and balloon inflation only during wedge pressure measurement. These precautions serve to prevent clotting and thromboembolism from the catheter lumen, and provide constant display of the pulmonary arterial tracing so that wedging is immediately obvious at the bedside. A continuous wedge tracing suggests distal migration, and calls for radiographic confirmation followed by catheter withdrawal and repositioning. Radiographic findings of an inflated balloon or a catheter tip more distal than lobar vessels should be brought to the attention of the clinician. Radiology involving Swan-Ganz catheters is discussed in Chapter 3.

Pulmonary capillary wedge pressure monitoring, although primarily utilized as a guide to circulatory resuscitation, is also proving a useful diagnostic tool in patients with acute respiratory failure.

The clinical diagnosis of left ventricular failure in patients with ARDS or COPD may be difficult or impossible. Measurement of a high wedge pressure in such patients may be the only means of detecting left ventricular failure or of demonstrating that pulmonary edema is related, at least in part, to heart failure (Unger et al., 1975).

Pulmonary edema among ICU patients is frequently noncardiac in origin. The mechanisms of pulmonary edema in these patients include altered capillary permeability, decreased oncotic pressure, and mixed or unknown mechanisms (Robin et al., 1973). The demonstration of low or normal PCWs in such patients is an important means of determining that extracardiac factors, rather than left ventricular failure, are the cause of pulmonary edema.

Concepts of Therapy

When filling volume or pressure is related to indices of circulatory competence (stroke work or less direct clinical measurements), a Frank-Starling cardiac function curve is constructed (Fig. 1–7). This curve expresses the fact that increases in filling pressure have the effect of augmenting stroke work, provided that pressures are not excessive. In the failing heart, this response is severely limited but can be im-

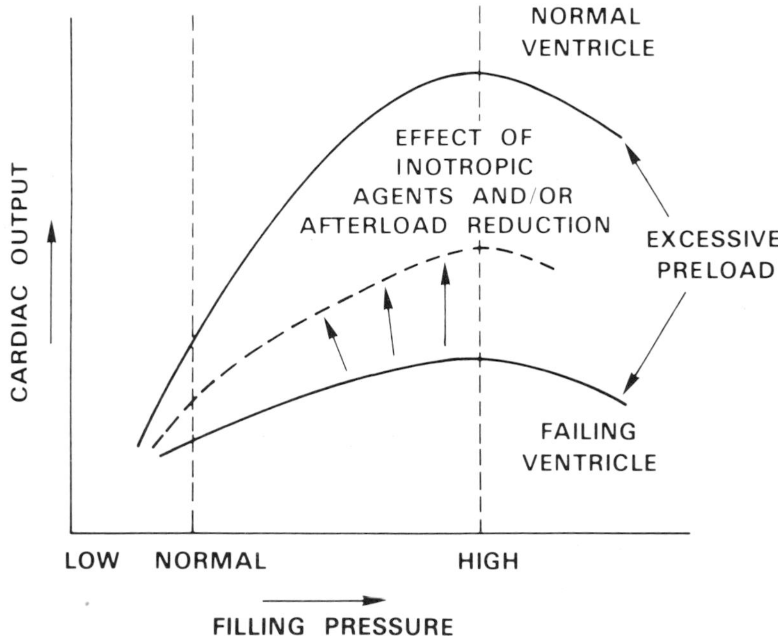

Figure 1–7. Ventricular function curves. Cardiac output, a measure of pumping function, is plotted against filling pressure, a measure of end-diastolic dimension. At each level of filling pressure, performance of the failing ventricle is less than normal. The dotted line indicates improvement in performance resulting from inotropic agents, afterload reduction, or both.

proved through treatment. Filling pressure measurement focuses therapy on correction of hypovolemia, myocardial failure, or both (Winslow et al., 1973). Serial monitoring provides a useful guide during treatment, since filling pressures normalize during optimal therapy, or demonstrate abrupt rises suggesting overinfusion or incipient cardiac failure.

Volume expansion may be accomplished by using blood or blood products, dextran, or crystalloid solutions. Crystalloid solutions must be used with caution to avoid aggravation of pre-existing or complicating pulmonary disease. Past experience has indicated that excessive crystalloid infusion can contribute significantly to the pulmonary insufficiency associated with shock (Petty and Ashbaugh, 1971).

When myocardial failure appears to be of primary hemodynamic significance, a number of approaches are possible (Fig. 1–7). Cardiac performance may be improved directly by using inotropic agents (digitalis, dobutamine, dopamine) or indirectly with preload or afterload reduction. Preload reduction refers to therapy that tends to lower filling pressure (for example, phlebotomy or diuresis). The clinical improvement that follows preload reduction is more likely related to factors such as diminished vascular congestion than a true displacement from a descending limb of the cardiac function curve. Afterload reduction consists of therapy that lowers the resistance to cardiac emptying (for example, nitroprusside infusion), thereby improving cardiac function (Chatterjee et al., 1973). Depending on patient response, these approaches may be used singly or in combination.

In cardiogenic shock, these interventions are initiated pharmacologically but may also be approached mechanically by means of intra-aortic balloon counterpulsation (Scheidt et al., 1973). A dual-chambered balloon catheter is placed surgically through a femoral artery into the descending thoracic aorta (see Chapter 3). The balloon is rapidly inflated with helium or carbon dioxide at the onset of diastole and rapidly deflated just before the onset of systole by means of R-wave synchronization. Systolic pressure (afterload) is decreased by balloon deflation, thus decreasing left ventricular work, and the flow is augmented in diastole, so that perfusion pressure is maintained. Clinical and hemodynamic improvement is common, and mortality from cardiogenic shock is somewhat lowered, but the precise indications for initiation and termination of balloon counterpulsation remain controversial.

MISCELLANEOUS SUPPORT TECHNIQUES

Life support techniques relating to renal and hematologic function and to the central nervous system are of lesser importance in the radiology of intensive care and are not discussed. The radiographic techniques dealing with the diagnosis and treatment of hemorrhage, particularly gastrointestinal, are discussed in Chapter 9. Some aspects of nutritional and metabolic support are of radiographic importance and are discussed here.

The ability to accomplish total parenteral nutritional support has only recently been realized. The intravenous (IV) infusion of hypertonic solutions (1500 to 1800 mOsm/liter) of glucose and amino acids can achieve positive nitrogen balance and weight gain even in critically ill patients (Fischer, 1976; Shils, 1972). This nutritional support can promote wound healing and fistula closure, and provides the substrate for survival in the patient whose gastrointestinal tract is nonfunctional. Such hypertonicity requires infusion into central veins, where high blood flow provides rapid dilution and long-term cannulation is possible. The most commonly used route for such infusions is a superior vena caval catheter placed via a subclavian or internal jugular vein. The complications of placement and solution hypertonicity make radiographic confirmation of catheter placement mandatory (see Chapter 3).

RADIOLOGY AND THE RADIOLOGIST IN INTENSIVE CARE

Critically ill patients defy hospital routines, time schedules, and standard operating procedures; and crisis can be a chronic condition in the ICU. The processes of diagnosis and treatment are necessarily compressed into an abbreviated time span. When radiographic examination is a part of this process, exposure, development, film availability, and interpretation must conform to these constraints. Thus, such innovations as the ICU multiviewer, with continuous availability of films and interpretative consultation, are invaluable in critical care.

On the other hand, overselling the words

crisis and *critical* is somewhat unfair; ICUs have routines and routine days, as do other hospital subdivisions. Routines in our ICU regarding radiographic examination include examination after insertion of any foreign body into the chest, daily examination in acutely ill patients receiving respirator support, and joint review of films by ICU and radiology staff.

Those who would argue against daily radiographic examination should recognize that physical diagnosis of pulmonary abnormalities is difficult in the ventilator patient. One cannot ask a ventilator patient to breathe deeply through his mouth in order to auscultate the chest. The slow, even inspiratory flow that ensures equal distribution of ventilation also tends to diminish sound transmission considerably, so that pneumothorax, atelectasis, pneumonia, and pulmonary edema are not uncommonly missed clinically. Likewise, the use of PEEP commonly obscures the rales that ordinarily would be heard accompanying pulmonary edema.

Patients receiving intensive care and requiring special studies outside the ICU frequently pose a problem. Transport is often difficult (because of the ECG monitor, arterial and Swan-Ganz lines, IV setups, and so on) and at times dangerous (because of such factors as unstable circulation and the need for ventilatory support). Despite the stresses placed on nursing or physician resources, or both, we feel very strongly that patients must receive at least as much coverage (minimally one nurse) during the study as they require in the ICU. Unstable patients should be accompanied by a physician; however, it is as unreasonable to expect a physician to accompany every patient as it is to expect the radiologist to perform the study and simultaneously care for the patient. Special study areas that receive critically ill patients must be equipped with oxygen outlets, suction apparatus, and monitoring and resuscitation equipment (see Chapter 10 and Appendix).

Coordination between the ICU and the department of radiology is vital in order to minimize delays in patient arrival or in the starting of procedures, and to ensure proper life support during examinations. We have safely performed special studies on patients receiving two- and three-organ system support. When problems arise, they are invariably caused by failure to anticipate and communicate. The radiologist is a necessary and welcome part of the multidisciplinary team caring for the critically ill patient.

REFERENCES

Applebaum, E. L., and Bruce, D. L.: Tracheal Intubation. Philadelphia, 1976, W. B. Saunders Co.

Archer, G., and Cobb, L. A.: Long term pulmonary artery monitoring in the management of the critically ill. Ann. Surg. 180:747, 1974.

Bartlett, J. G., Alexander, J., Nadine, J. M., et al.: Should fiberoptic bronchoscopy aspirates be cultured? Am. Rev. Respir. Dis. 114:73, 1976.

Carroll, R. G.: Evaluation of tracheal tube cuff designs. Crit. Care Med. 1:45, 1973.

Carroll, R. G., McGinnis, G. E., and Grenvik, A.: Performance characteristics of tracheal cuffs. Int. Anesthesiol. Clin. 12(3):111, 1974.

Chatterjee, K., Parmley, W. W., Ganz, W., et al.: Hemodynamic and metabolic responses to vasodilator therapy in acute myocardial infarction. Circulation 48:1183, 1973.

Chatterjee, K., Swan, H. J. C., Ganz, W., et al.: Use of a balloon-tipped flotation electrode catheter for cardiac monitoring. Am. J. Cardiol. 36:56, 1975.

Civetta, J. M., and Gabel, J. C.: Flow directed pulmonary artery catheterization in surgical patients; indications and modifications of technic. Ann. Surg. 176:753, 1972.

Downs, J. B., Klein, E. F., Desautels, D., et al.: Intermittent mandatory ventilation; a new approach to weaning patients from mechanical ventilators. Chest 64:331, 1973.

Fischer, J. F.: Total Parenteral Nutrition. Boston, 1976, Little, Brown & Co.

Fleming, W. H., and Bower, J. C.: Early complications of long-term respiratory support. J. Thorac. Cardiovasc. Surg. 64:729, 1972.

Gold, M.: The present status of IPPB therapy. Chest 67:469, 1975.

Hedley-Whyte, J., Burgess, G. E. III, Feeley, T. W., et al.: Applied Physiology of Respiratory Care. Boston, 1976, Little, Brown & Co.

Hodgkin, J. E., Bowser, M. A., and Burton, G. G.: Respirator weaning. Crit. Care Med. 2:96, 1974.

James, P. M., Jr., and Myers, R. T.: Central venous pressure monitoring; misinterpretation, abuses, indications and a new technic. Ann. Surg. 175:693, 1972.

Lewis, F. J.: Monitoring of patients in intensive care units. Surg. Clin. North Am. 51:15, 1971.

Lindholm, C. E., Ollman, B., Snyder, J. V., et al.: Flexible fiberoptic bronchoscopy in critical care medicine. Crit. Care Med. 2:250, 1974.

Luce, J. M., Pierson, D. J., and Hudson, L. D.: Intermittent mandatory ventilation. Chest 79:678, 1981.

Nennhaus, H. P., Javid, H., and Julian, O. C.: Alveolar and pleural rupture; hazards of positive pressure respiration. Arch. Surg. 94:136, 1967.

Petty, T. L., and Ashbaugh, D. G.: The adult respiratory distress syndrome; clinical features, factors influencing prognosis, and principles of management. Chest 60:233, 1971.

Petty, T. L., Lakshminarayan, S., Sahn, S. A., et al.: Intensive respiratory care unit; review of ten years' experience. J.A.M.A. 233:34, 1975.

Pontoppidan, H., Geffin, B., and Lowenstein, E.: Acute respiratory failure in the adult, parts 1–3. N. Engl. J. Med. 287:690, 743, 799, 1972.

Robin, E. D., Cross, C. E., and Zelis, R.: Pulmonary edema, parts 1 and 2. N. Engl. J. Med. 288:239, 292, 1073.

Safar, P., and Grenvik, A.: Critical care medicine; organizing and staffing intensive care units. Chest 59:535, 1971.

Scheidt, S., Wilner, G., Mueller, H., et al.: Intra-aortic balloon counterpulsation in cardiogenic shock. N. Engl. J. Med. 288:979, 1973.

Shils, M. E.: Guidelines for total parenteral nutrition. J.A.M.A. 220:1721, 1972.

Skillman, J. J.: Intensive Care. Boston, 1975, Little, Brown & Co.

Sladen, A., Laver, M. B., and Pontoppidan, H.: Pulmonary complications and water retention in prolonged mechanical ventilation. N. Engl. J. Med. 279:448, 1968.

Swan, J. H. C., Ganz, W., Forrester, J., et al.: Catheterization of the heart in man with use of a flow-directed balloon-tipped catheter. N. Engl. J. Med. 283:447, 1970.

Unger, K. M., Shibel, M. D., and Moser, K. M.: Detection of left ventricular failure in patients with adult respiratory distress syndrome. Chest 67:8, 1975.

Van de Water, J. J., Watring, W. G., Lenton, L. A., et al.: Prevention of postoperative pulmonary complications. Surg. Gynecol. Obstet. 135:229, 1972.

Wayne, K. S.: Positive end expiratory pressure (PEEP) ventilation. J.A.M.A. 236:1394, 1976.

Weil, M. H., and Shubin, H.: Critical Care Medicine Handbook. New York, 1974, John N. Kolen, Inc.

Winslow, E. J., Loeb, H. S., Rahimtoola, S. H., et al.: Hemodynamic studies and results of therapy in 50 patients with bacteremic shock. Am. J. Med. 54:421, 1973.

Winter, P. M., and Smith, G.: The toxicity of oxygen. Anesthesiology 37:210, 1972.

Zimmerman, J. E., Goodman, L. R., and Shahvari, M. B.: Effect of mechanical ventilation and positive end-expiratory pressure on chest radiograph. AJR 133:811, 1979.

Zwillich, C. W., Pierson, D. J., Creagh, C. E., et al.: Complications of assisted ventilation; a prospective study of 354 consecutive episodes. Am. J. Med. 57:161, 1974.

Chapter 2

PULMONARY SUPPORT AND MONITORING APPARATUS

by Lawrence R. Goodman

In the intensive care unit (ICU), various types of catheters, tubes, and support equipment are routinely used. Proper placement of this equipment is essential if it is to achieve its monitoring and support goals. Many potential problems can be recognized on the radiograph and prevented before they occur. Other complications can be diagnosed soon after their occurrence and corrective action taken before further damage is done. This chapter discusses the correct placement of pulmonary support and monitoring equipment and the early identification of complications associated with their use.

ENDOTRACHEAL TUBES

Normal Position and Appearance

Proper positioning of the endotracheal tube (orotracheal or nasotracheal) minimizes complications associated with intubation. Although an improperly situated tube may often be diagnosed through physical examination, the radiograph is frequently the first indicator of malpositioning. Therefore, radiographs should be routinely obtained immediately after each intubation. Frequent radiographs will ensure that the tube has not been inadvertently displaced by the weight of the respirator apparatus, by the patient coughing, or by other unforeseen events (Tisi et al., 1968).

Proper radiographic evaluation of the endotracheal tube position requires an estimate of the position of the tube tip relative to the carina and a knowledge of the position of the head and neck at the time of the radiograph. The carina is most accurately located by following the inferior wall of the left main stem bronchus medially until it joins the right main stem bronchus. If the carina is not visible on a given radiograph, its position may be estimated in one of two ways: (1) from previous portable radiographs, because the carina maintains a relatively constant position relative to the vertebral bodies; (2) if old films are not available, it may be estimated relative to the thoracic vertebral interspaces. On the portable radiograph the carina projects over T5, T6, or T7 in 95 per cent of patients (Goodman et al., 1976) (Fig. 2–1). It is rarely higher than the T4-T5 interspace. When the vertebral bodies cannot be accurately counted, the posterior ribs can often be counted and followed medially.

Flexion and extension of the head and neck cause considerable movement of the endotracheal tube tip relative to the carina (Conrardy et al., 1976) (Fig. 2–2). Because the tube is fixed at the nose or mouth, only the distal tip is free to move with head and neck motion. Neck flexion from the neutral position causes approximately a 2-cm descent of the endotracheal tube. Similarly, neck extension from the neutral position causes a 2-cm ascent. This combined excursion of 4 cm is approximately one third the length of the trachea, which measures 12 cm in the average adult. Therefore, a tube that appears to be in good position in the midtrachea

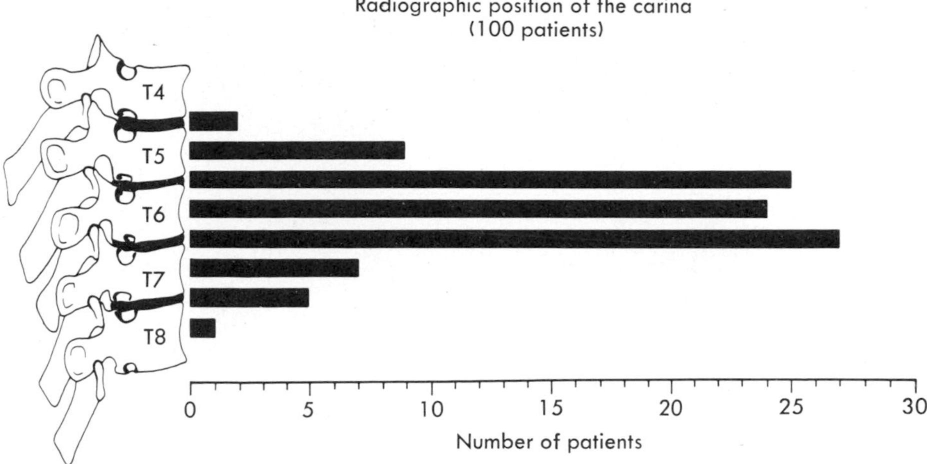

Figure 2–1. The position of the carina relative to the vertebral bodies as seen on the portable chest radiograph (100 patients). (From Goodman: Am. J. Roentgenol. 127:433, 1976.)

when the head and neck are extended may lodge in the right main stem bronchus when the head and neck are flexed.

One can usually determine the posture of the head and neck from the radiograph itself (Goodman et al., 1976). In the neutral position, the inferior border of the mandible is over the lower cervical spine (C5 to C6). In full flexion, the mandible is over the upper thoracic spine; in full extension, the mandible is above C4 (often off the film) (Fig. 2–2A).

Other changes in body position have been shown to slightly alter the endotracheal tube–carina relationship. Lateral rotation of the head from the neutral position causes a 1- to 2-cm ascent of the tube from the carina (Conrardy et al., 1976). When the patient is in Trendelenburg's position or goes from the supine to the sitting position, there is a slight elevation of the carina, causing convergence of the tube tip and the carina (Alberti et al., 1967; Heinonen et al., 1969).

In summary, the following guidelines are suggested for evaluating endotracheal tube position:

1. When the head and neck are in the neutral position, the endotracheal tube tip is ideally in the midtrachea, 5 to 7 cm from the carina.
2. When the head and neck are flexed, the tube has descended maximally, so that it is ideally 3 to 5 cm from the carina.
3. When the head and neck are extended, the tube has ascended maximally, so that it is ideally 7 to 9 cm from the carina.

The ideal endotracheal tube as seen on the radiograph is one half to two thirds the width of the trachea. Wider tubes are associated with an increased incidence of laryngeal injury, and narrower tubes have a significantly increased airway resistance (Pontoppidan et al., 1972). The inflated cuff should fill the tracheal lumen but not bulge the lateral tracheal walls. The cuff should not compress the endotracheal tube wall inward nor deflect the tube bevel toward the lateral tracheal wall.

Potential Complications

In a prospective study of 226 endotracheal intubations, Stauffer et al. (1981) noted 268 complications. The most frequent problems were difficulty in sealing the airway (64 patients), self-extubation (29), right main stem bronchus intubation (21) and aspiration of gastric contents (17). Less frequent complications of radiographic importance included pharyngeal injuries, glottic edema, tooth avulsion, esophageal intubation, and pneumothorax.

Aberrant positioning. Approximately 10 per cent of endotracheal tubes are initially placed in the right main stem bronchus (Stauffer et al., 1981; Zwillich et al., 1974). If radiographed early or if ventilation of the left lung continues via the side hole in the endotracheal tube, the radiograph merely demonstrates the aberrant catheter in the right main stem bronchus (Fig. 2–3). With time, the left lung be-

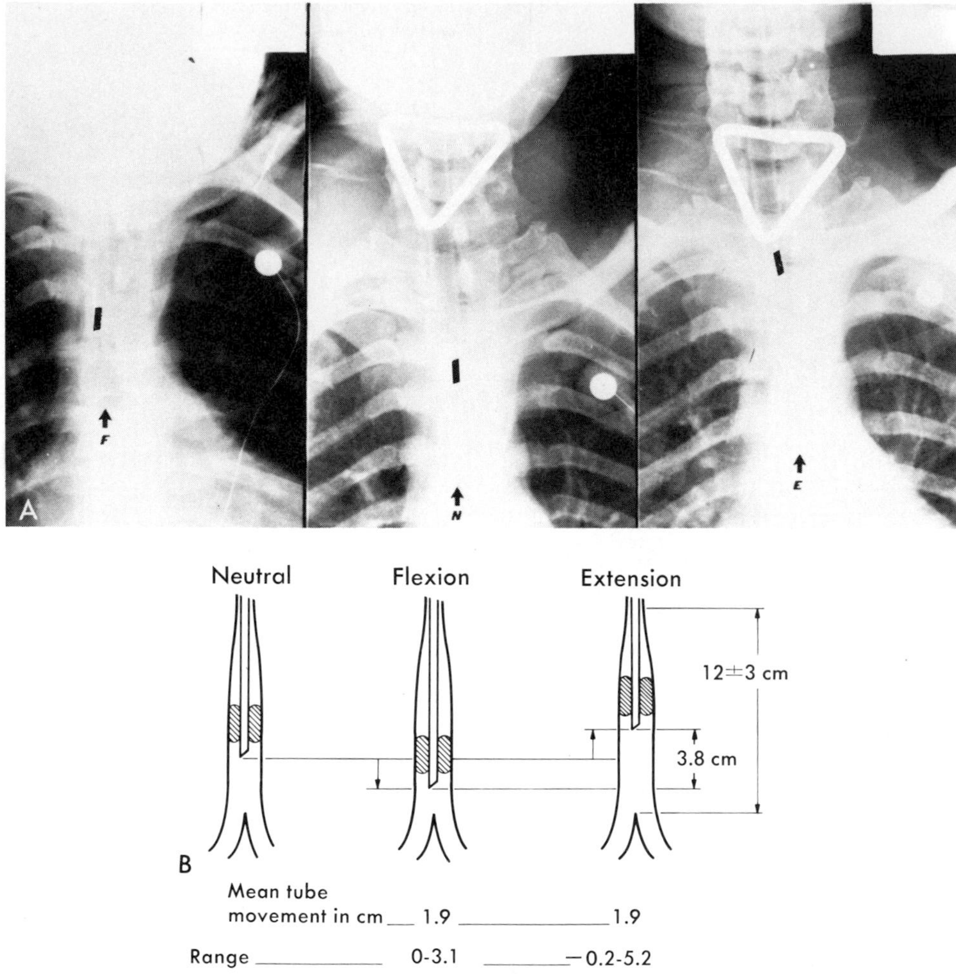

Figure 2–2. *A*, Effects of flexion and extension of the head and neck on endotracheal tube position (↑ = carina). There is an approximately 2-cm descent of the tube when the neck is flexed (*F*) and an approximately 3-cm ascent of the tube when the neck is extended (*E*). In the neutral position (*N*), the mandible is over the lower cervical spine. When the neck is flexed, the mandible is over the upper thoracic spine. When the neck is extended, the mandible is above C4, often off the film. *B*, Mean endotracheal tube movement with flexion and extension of the neck from the neutral position (in 20 patients). The mean tube movement is approximately one third the length of the normal adult trachea. (*B*, From Conrardy et al.: Crit. Care Med. 4:8, 1976. Copyright © 1976, The Williams & Wilkins Co., Baltimore.)

comes atelectatic, the mediastinum shifts to the left, and the right lung becomes hyperlucent (Fig. 2–4). If the endotracheal tube enters the bronchus intermedius, the right upper lobe may also collapse. If the patient is on a ventilator, the right lung is hyperinflated. This may lead to a pneumothorax or tension pneumothorax in as many as 15 per cent of patients (Zwillich et al., 1974). Because the left main stem bronchus branches from the carina at a sharper angle, accidental left main stem bronchus intubation is uncommon.

A tube placed just above the carina may gradually slip downward or may be deflected into the right main stem bronchus when the neck is flexed. Direct carinal irritation will lead to coughing and carinal ulceration. A tube positioned just above the carina will cause the suction catheter to hit the carina at each pass, further abrading the mucosa.

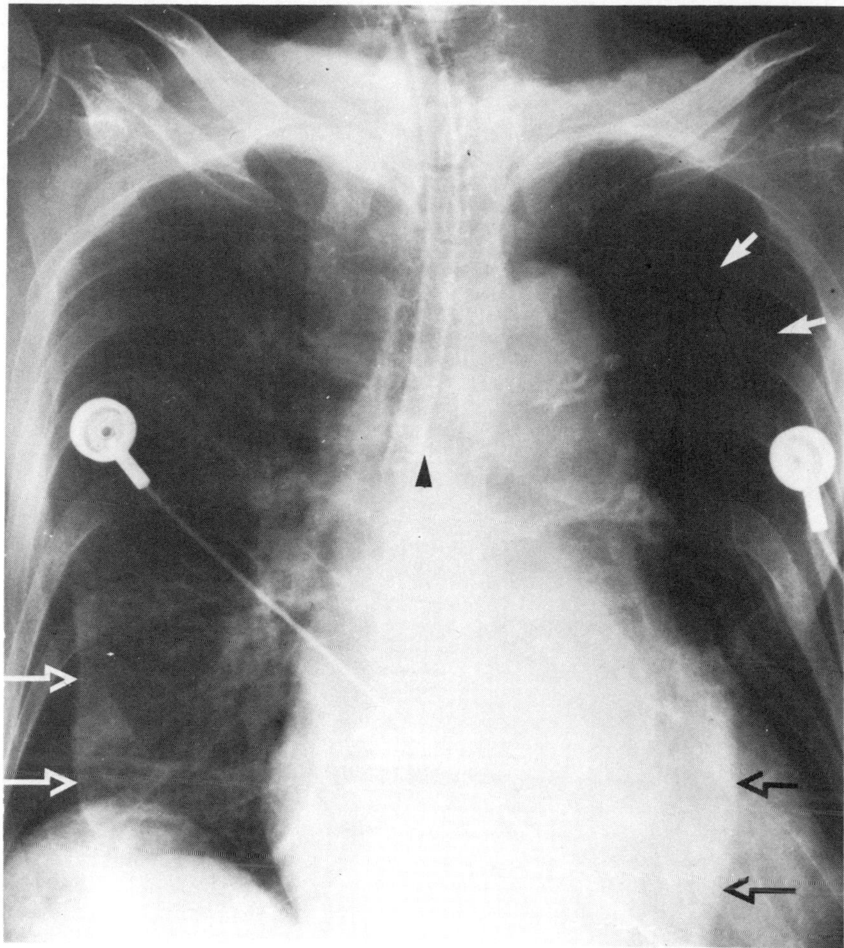

Figure 2–3. Film obtained immediately after intubation demonstrates endotracheal tube in the right main stem bronchus (*arrowhead* = carina). The effects of selective aeration are not yet evident. The density over the heart shadow (*black arrows*) is caused by the breast. A left upper skin fold and the right breast shadow (*white arrows*) mimic a bilateral pneumothorax.

Conversely, several complications may arise when the tube is not placed deeply enough. A tube placed in the pharynx causes ventilatory difficulty and gastric dilatation. Aspiration of gastric content is a frequent sequela (Fig. 2–5). A tube placed just beyond the vocal cords into the cervical trachea may slip into the pharynx when the patient extends his neck or coughs, or when the cuff is inflated. A cuff inflated between or just below the vocal cords frequently causes glottic or subglottic edema or ulceration that may progress to scarring in these areas (Harley, 1971; Zwillich et al., 1974) (Fig. 2–6).

Although superficial injury to the hypopharyngeal or cervical esophageal mucosa is not uncommon at the time of endotracheal intubation, actual perforation is uncommon (Hawkins et al., 1974; Wolff and Kessler, 1973). Perforation is usually into the lateral sinuses or the posterior hypopharyngeal wall (Hirsch et al., 1978). The injury may be apparent immediately or become apparent when delayed complications surface. If the patient develops marked subcutaneous emphysema, pneumomediastinum, or pneumothorax immediately after a difficult intubation, the diagnosis is readily apparent. In other cases the laceration may go unnoticed for days or weeks, until the patient develops signs and symptoms of mediastinitis or a mediastinal or cervical abscess. Radiographic evaluation must include both frontal

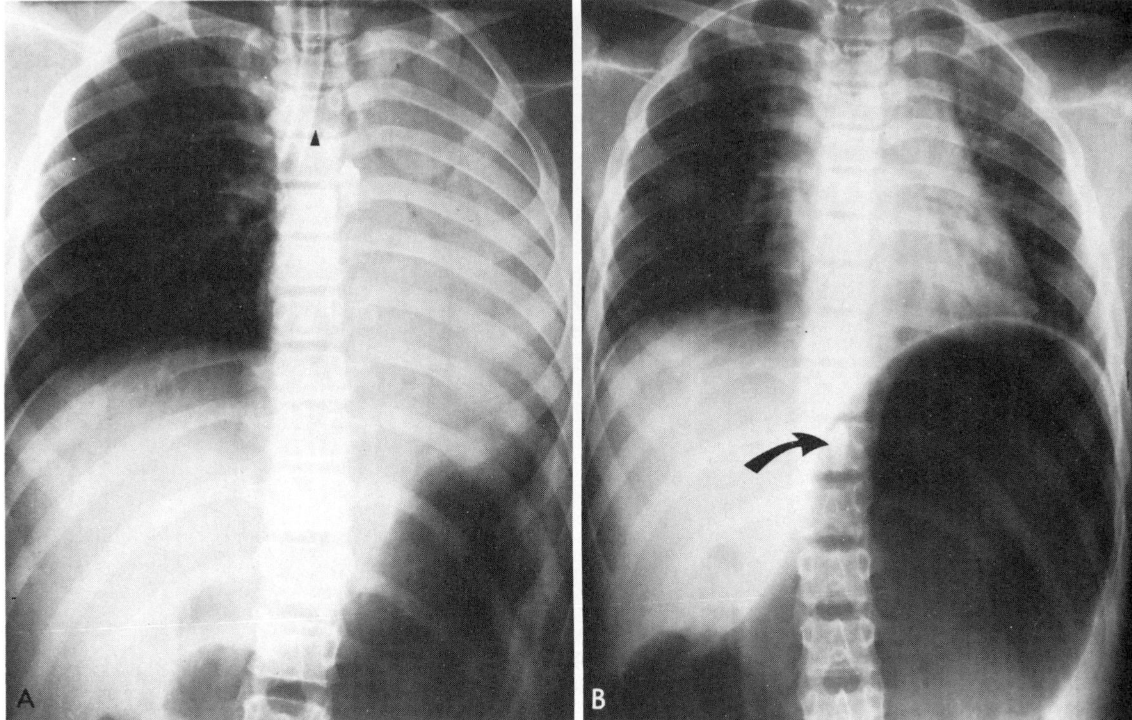

Figure 2–4. Right main stem bronchus intubation. *A*, The endotracheal tube is in the right main stem bronchus (carina = arrowhead). There is complete opacification of the left lung with marked atelectasis. To the left of the spine the radiodensity represents a dislodged tooth in the esophagus. *B*, Twenty-four hours later after the endotracheal tube has been repositioned, there is almost complete re-expansion of the left lung. The mediastinum has returned to midline. Marked gastric distention is noted. The swallowed tooth is now seen near the gastroesophageal junction (*arrow*). (From Goodman, L. R., and Putman, C. E.: Radiological evaluation of patients receiving assisted ventilation. J.A.M.A. 245:858, 1981. Copyright 1981, American Medical Association.)

and lateral chest and neck radiographs in search of air or fluid collections. If erect lateral films cannot be obtained, horizontal beam radiographs with the neck extended are usually adequate to demonstrate air fluid levels within the neck or widening of the prevertebral soft tissue space. Hirsch et al. emphasize that early diagnosis facilitates an early surgical approach and improved outcome. Any patient with suspected hypopharyngeal perforation, regardless of the plain film findings, should have an esophagram.

SECRETIONS AND ATELECTASIS. The clearance of pharyngeal and pulmonary secretions is a serious problem for the intubated patient. Adequate coughing requires an intact, functioning glottis, functioning cilia, adequate respiratory muscles, and a vital capacity at least three times the tidal volume. Despite meticulous suctioning and physical therapy, atelectasis is the most frequent single cause of pulmonary infiltrate in the intubated patient. Except for streaks of discoid atelectasis, differentiation between atelectasis and other alveolar infiltrates is usually impossible on a single radiograph. Rapid changes in the radiographic appearance over hours or days strongly suggest the diagnosis of atelectasis. Films obtained immediately following suctioning or physical therapy often show dramatic improvement in cases of retained secretions (see Chapter 4).

FOREIGN BODIES. The most frequent endotracheal foreign bodies in the intubated patient are mucous plugs or blood clots. These are seldom recognized on the radiograph. Of the exogenous foreign bodies, teeth, fillings, or dentures broken at the time of intubation are the most frequently encountered. Their aspiration may go unnoticed in the patient with a depressed cough reflex. On a well-penetrated radiograph, teeth may be seen in the major bronchi, usually in the gravity-dependent segments (Figs. 2–4, 2–7). Atelectasis may or may not be present.

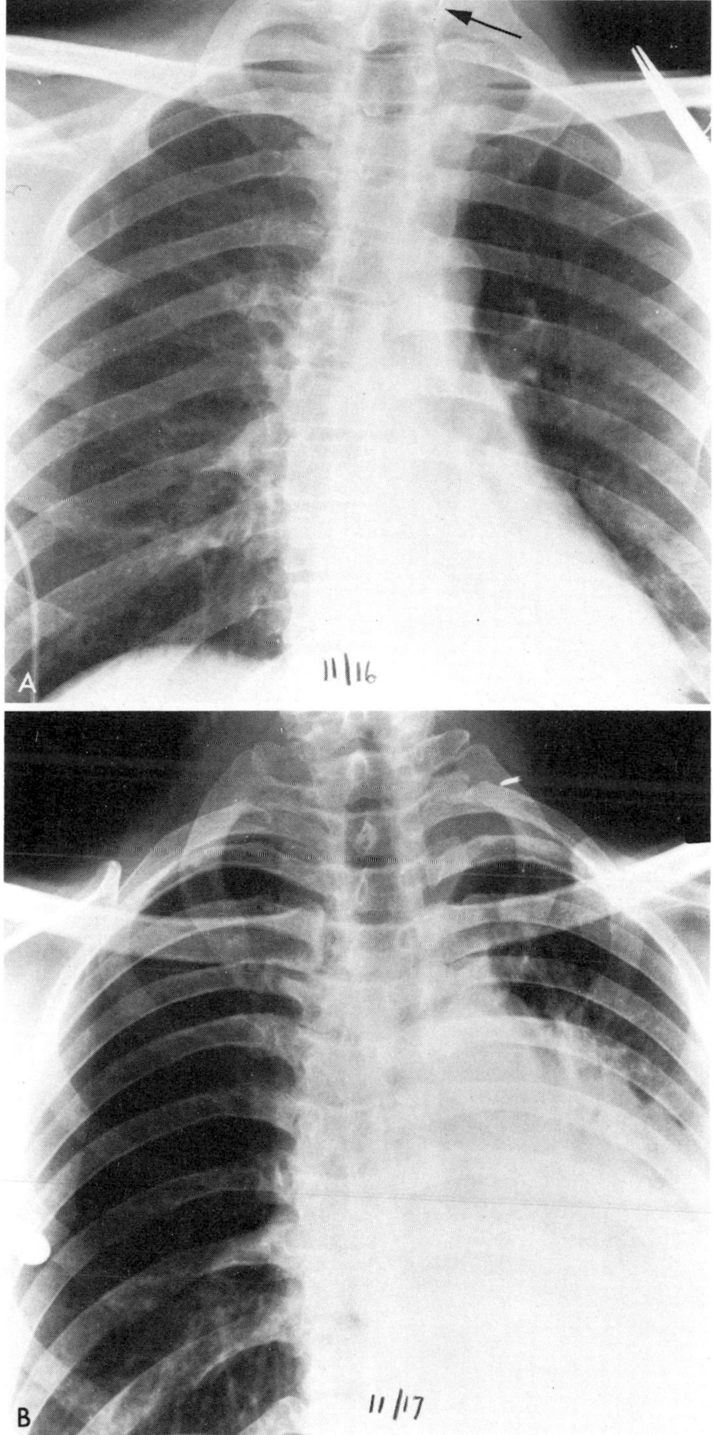

Figure 2–5. Endotracheal tube in the pharynx. *A*, The tip of the endotracheal tube (*arrow*) is above and to the left of the trachea, presumably in the pyriform sinus. There is a left lower lobe infiltrate resulting from aspiration of gastric contents. *B*, The following day, there is more infiltrate and atelectasis on the left side. The tube remains in the pharynx; it is not visible on the radiograph.

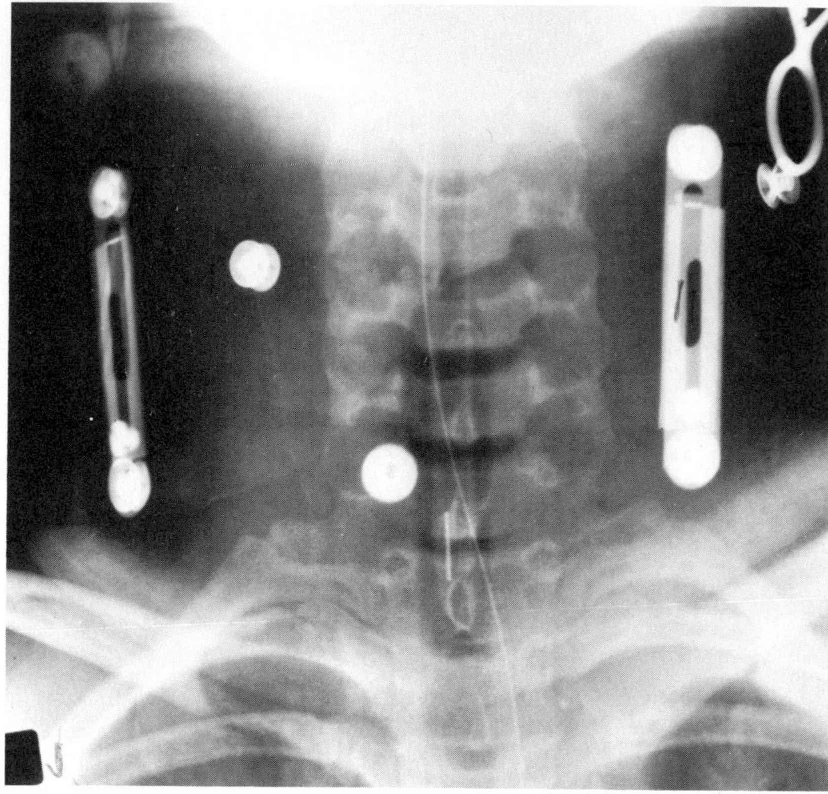

Figure 2–6. Endotracheal tube in the cervical trachea. The tube tip is in the proximal trachea. The inflated cuff is between the vocal cords.

SINUSITIS. Nasal mucosal edema caused by the endotracheal tube may impede sinus drainage and cause sinusitis. Sinusitis may be the cause of unexplained fever or a putrid smell, or it may be the source of aspirated secretions into the lungs. Portable radiographs taken in the upright frontal or Waters position or horizontal beam lateral radiographs will demonstrate air fluid levels in the obstructed sinuses (Arens et al., 1974). Nasal hemorrhage with posterior nasal packing may also cause air fluid levels within the sinuses (Ogawa et al., 1976). Nasal necrosis, an infrequent complication of nasotracheal intubation, is usually diagnosed clinically (Zwillich et al., 1974).

TRACHEOSTOMY AND TRACHEOSTOMY TUBES

Normal Position and Appearance

Tracheostomy, the transtracheal insertion of an artificial airway, is usually performed for long-term ventilatory support or, rarely, to establish an airway below a laryngeal obstruction. The tube tip should be located one half to two thirds the distance between the tracheal stoma and the carina (Fig. 2–8). A tube tip at the level of T3 is usually in satisfactory position. Unlike the endotracheal tube, there is little cephalocaudad movement with flexion and extension of the neck. Ideally, the lumen of the tracheostomy tube should be approximately two thirds the diameter of the trachea: this will minimize airway resistance and ensure that the tube sits straight in the tracheal lumen. As with the endotracheal tube, the cuff should hug, but not distend, the tracheal wall.

Potential Complications

The relatively common surgical procedure of tracheostomy is associated with a surprisingly high morbidity and mortality. The short-term complication rate has been estimated at 30 to

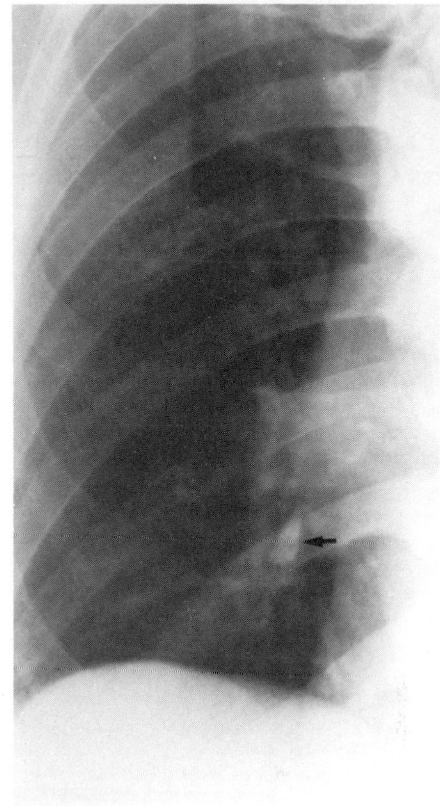

Figure 2–7. Tooth in the right lower lobe bronchus (*arrow*). The tooth was dislodged during intubation.

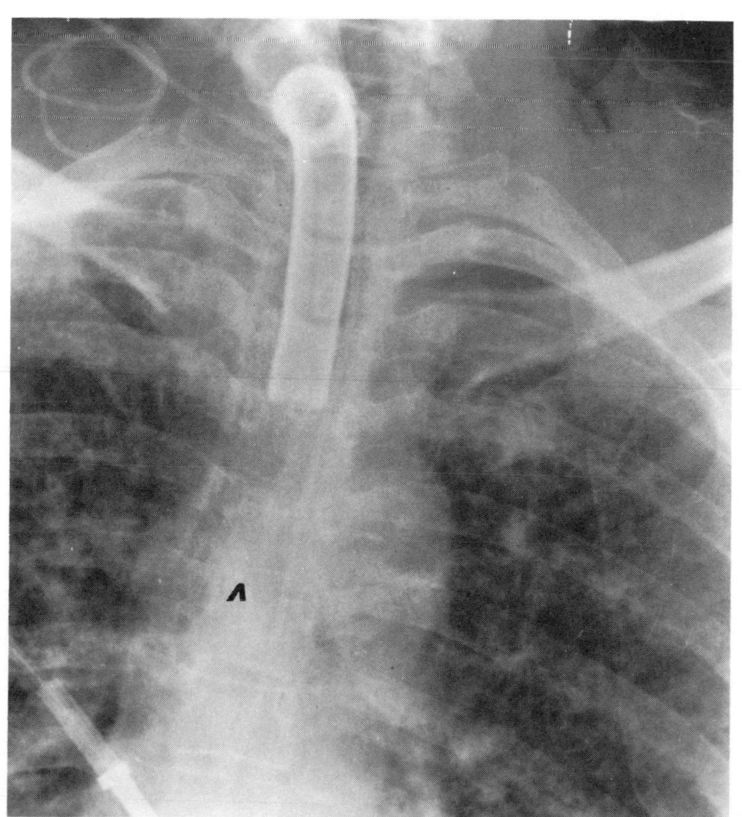

Figure 2–8. Ideally positioned tracheostomy tube. The tracheostomy tube is two thirds the width of the trachea and sits parallel to the long axis of the trachea. The tip is located one half to two thirds the distance between the stoma and the carina.

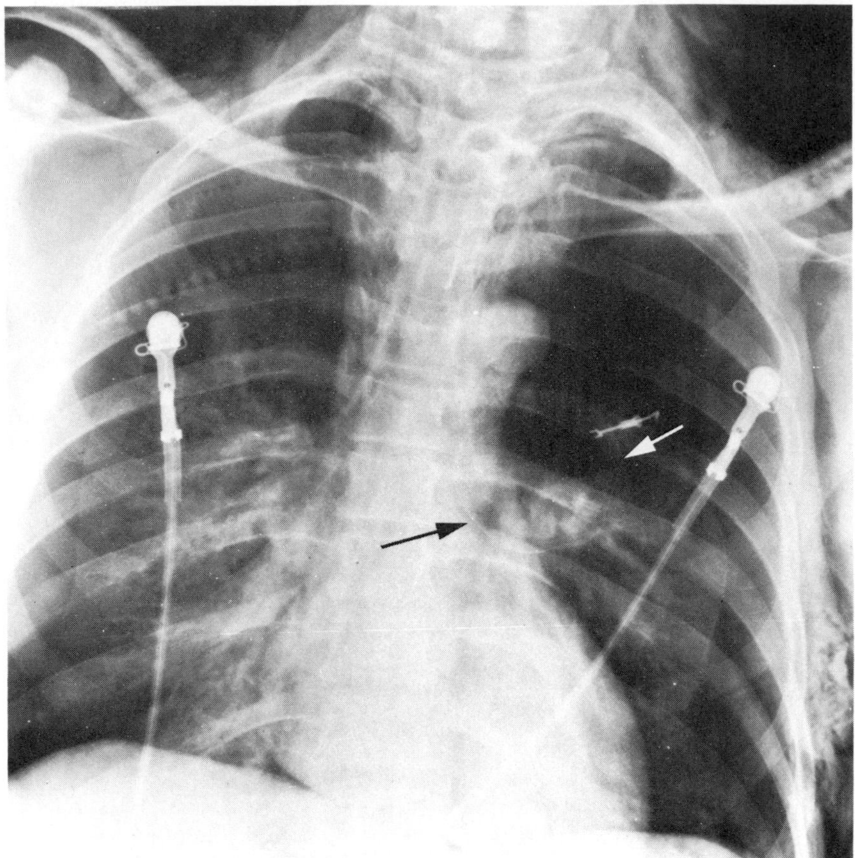

Figure 2–9. Post-tracheostomy pneumothorax. The large bilateral pneumothorax with marked subcutaneous emphysema immediately followed a tracheostomy. The initial tube insertion was paratracheal. The external pressure reservoir of the tracheostomy tube is seen overlying the left hilum (*arrows*).

40 per cent and the long-term complication rate as high as 60 per cent. It is estimated that this procedure causes or contributes to death in 5 to 10 per cent of tracheostomized patients (Mulder and Rubush, 1969; Skaggs and Cogbill, 1969; Stauffer et al., 1981; Stemmer et al., 1976). Many of the complications are preventable, and others may be treated early if recognized on the radiograph. Complications of tracheostomy are best classified as those occurring at the time of surgery, those occurring while the tube is in place, and those occurring following extubation.

COMPLICATIONS AT THE TIME OF INTUBATION. Immediately following the tracheostomy, the radiograph should be closely scrutinized to ensure that the tracheostomy tube is in proper position and that there is no evidence of significant air leaks. Pneumothorax, pneumomediastinum, and subcutaneous emphysema are frequent sequelae of tracheostomy. The leakage of a small amount of air around the tracheostomy stoma is an expected occurrence and is usually of no consequence. However, if the tracheostomy stoma is tightly packed or sutured, air may be trapped in the subcutaneous tissues. Positive pressure therapy or coughing may then cause air to dissect into the mediastinum. Another more serious cause of pneumomediastinum is the inadvertent placement of a tracheostomy tube in the paratracheal soft tissues or through the posterior tracheal membrane (Timmis, 1973) (Fig. 2–9). The pneumomediastinum may progress to a bilateral tension pneumothorax unless the cause is corrected.

Accidental injury to the lung apex at the time of surgery will lead directly to a pneumothorax. This is especially common in patients whose lungs are overinflated because of chronic obstructive pulmonary disease (COPD) or respirator therapy. The cupola of the lung rises into the base of the neck and may be injured when the tracheostomy is performed (Crews and LaPuerta, 1972).

Proper tracheostomy tube position is critical in order to avoid short-term ventilatory difficulties and minimize long-term tracheal injury. A tube placed deeply within the trachea may enter the right main stem bronchus and cause left lung collapse. A tube at the carina will cause carinal irritation and ulceration, and difficulty in suctioning (Fig. 2–10*A*). Conversely, a tube placed not deeply enough may be coughed or pulled out. This potentially fatal complication must be diagnosed at the bedside. Partial extubation, an equally dangerous situation, may escape clinical detection (Stauffer et al., 1981). In this situation, the tracheostomy cuff is partially or totally extruded into the soft tissues of the neck and the tube tip sits at or outside the tracheal stoma (Fig. 2–11). The radiograph demonstrates that the tube tip is above the clavicle, and the cuff is setting in the subcutaneous tissues, often larger than the diameter of the trachea. Subcutaneous emphysema or pneumomediastinum may be present.

Proper alignment of the tracheostomy tube relative to the long axis of the trachea will minimize mucosal damage. This is best ensured by using a tracheostomy tube that is at least two thirds the diameter of the trachea. The tracheostomy stoma serves as a fulcrum for the tube to pivot. If the stoma is eccentric or the tube is narrow relative to the trachea, angulation of the tube is frequent (Fig. 2–10*B*). Acute angulation against the tracheal wall increases airway resistance and decreases the ability to clear secretions. Persistent angulation will erode the tracheal mucosa and may progress to tracheal perforation. Persistent anterior angulation is most often due to a tracheal stoma below the third cartilaginous ring and may be associated with erosion into the innominate artery. Persistent posterior angulation is most often due to an inappropriately short tube or to one where the cuff is partially extruded into the neck. Posterior angulation puts pressure on the posterior tracheal membrane and may cause a tracheoesophageal or tracheomediastinal fistula. Lateral angulation is most often due to a laterally placed tracheostomy stoma (Crews and LaPuerta, 1972; Timmis, 1973). If the clinical situation or anteroposterior (AP) radiograph suggests the possibility of a poorly positioned

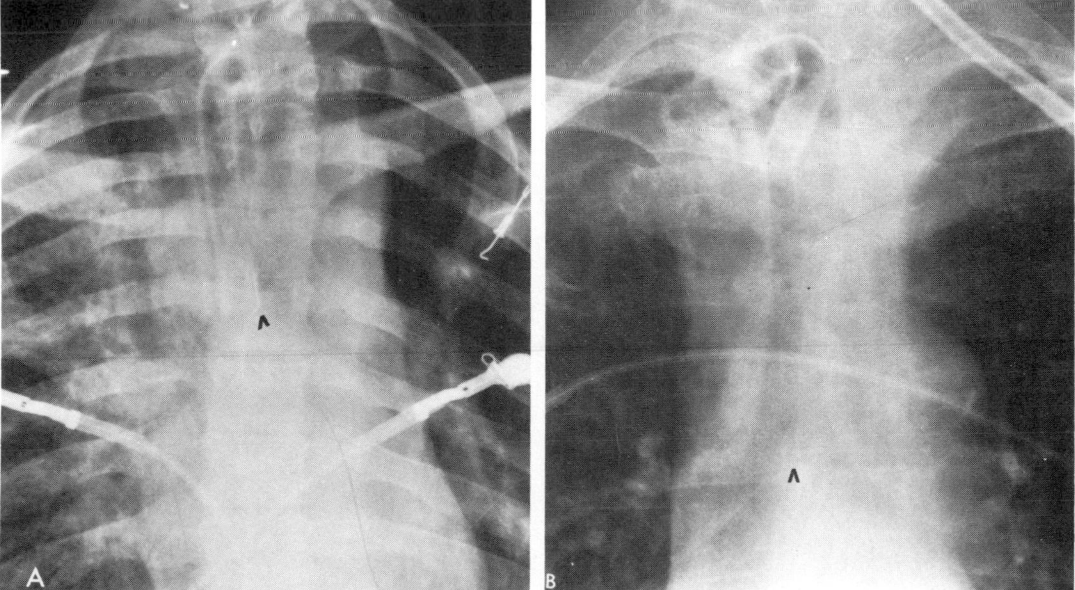

Figure 2–10. *A*, Tracheostomy tube positioned too low. The tip of the tube is at the mouth of the right main stem bronchus. The patient tolerated the tube badly. *B*, Poorly positioned tracheostomy tube. The tube is narrow relative to the width of the trachea. It is not inserted deeply enough, and the tube tip hits the right lateral tracheal wall. There was difficulty in ventilating and suctioning this patient. The tracheostomy stoma had been placed eccentrically to the left.

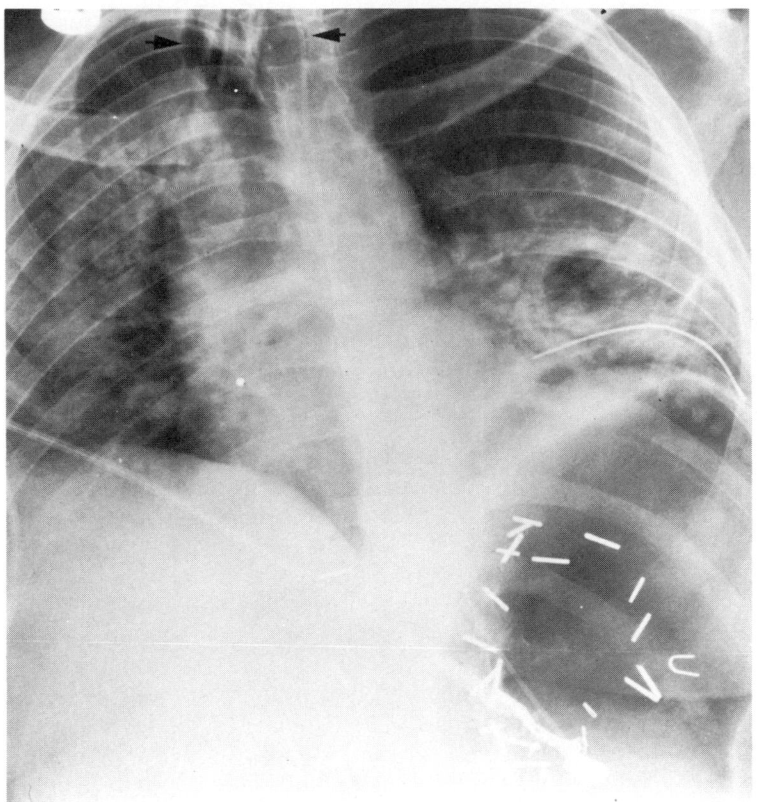

Figure 2–11. Partial extrusion of a tracheostomy tube. The tube is displaced into the cervical trachea with the cuff in the subcutaneous tissue of the neck (*arrows*). The tube tip is above the clavicles, and the cuff is 2½ times the width of the trachea. The cuff and tube were well situated on an earlier film. Also note the marked gastric dilatation. A chest tube, for fluid drainage, is seen above the left diaphragm.

tube, a lateral radiograph is required to check the tube's relation to the trachea in the AP dimension (Fig. 2–12).

Although high-volume, low-pressure (floppy) cuffs have decreased the incidence of tracheal ulceration and scarring, tracheal injury is still a serious complication of tracheostomy (Cooper and Grillo, 1972; Frager and Marshall, 1976). Mucosal ischemia may be minimized by giving careful attention to the radiographic appearance of the cuff relative to the trachea. The oval lucency of the cuff should fill but not acutely dilate the trachea. With prolonged intubation and positive pressure therapy, gradual dilatation of the trachea may be unavoidable. Mild dilatation may not result in permanent damage. However, when the diameter of the cuff is more than one and one half times the diameter of the trachea (measured between the clavicles), severe mucosal ulceration or tracheostenosis occurs in approximately 30 per cent of patients (Khan et al., 1976) (Fig. 2–13).

Airway obstruction due to the inflated cuff is a potentially fatal complication. Most tracheal tubes and cuffs are now constructed as a single unit so that the cuff cannot slide off the end of the tube and obstruct the airway. However, on occasion, the large-volume floppy cuff may "creep" down the sides of the trachea and cover the tube tip (Timmis, 1973). Other cuff-related problems include the eccentric inflation of a cuff deflecting the end hole against the tracheal wall and an overinflated cuff pinching the lumen of the tube shut (Perel et al., 1977). Therefore, on every radiograph the relationship between the cuff and the tube and the cuff and the trachea should be carefully ascertained.

COMPLICATIONS DURING INTUBATION. Numerous complications occur while the tracheostomy tube is in place. In a prospective study of 51 tracheostomies, stomal infection, hemorrhage, or erosion occurred in at least half the patients. Less frequent, but of greater concern to the radiologist, were subcutaneous or mediastinal emphysema, aspiration, mediastinitis, or pneumothorax. Radiographs are usually obtained on a daily basis until the patient's condition stabilizes. Films are then obtained every other day for several days, and then as clinically indicated.

Infection. Colonization of the pharynx and trachea with potential pathogens occurs in the majority of seriously ill patients. In Stauffer's series (1981), cellulitis around the stoma was noted in 36 per cent of patients. In 10 to 20 per cent of patients, tracheal colonization progresses to purulent tracheitis or pneumonia (Mulder and Rubush, 1969; Skaggs and Cogbill, 1969). As noted with endotracheal tubes, atelectasis and retained secretions frequently mimic pneumonia. Differentiation of pulmonary infiltrates is discussed in Chapter 4.

Meteorism. Following the insertion of a nasotracheal or tracheostomy tube, the patient may swallow large amounts of air (Cooper and Malt, 1972; Timmis, 1973). This is most frequent when the inflated cuff puts pressure on the esophagus, or when the patient is receiving positive pressure therapy. Gastric dilatation is often associated with restlessness and elevation of the left hemidiaphragm accompanied by diminished lung function on that side (Figs. 2–4, 2–11). Gastric reflux and aspiration may follow. Marked gastric dilatation seen on the chest radiograph should be noted so that appropriate therapeutic measures may be taken. If gastric dilatation persists, the possibility of a tracheoesophageal fistula or gastric outlet obstruction should be considered.

Tracheal Ulceration or Perforation. Although the incidence and severity of tracheal injury has decreased with increasing awareness of the problem and with the use of the high-volume, low-pressure cuff, inflammation and ulceration of the tracheal mucosa is still a serious problem (Andrews and Pearson, 1971; Cooper and Grillo, 1972; Frager and Marshall, 1976; Stauffer et al., 1981). Several factors combine to assault the tracheal mucosa in the intubated patient:

1. The tube and cuff are prolonged mechanical irritants.
2. The materials used to make or sterilize the tube may irritate the mucosa.
3. Cuff pressures of greater than 25 mm Hg cause mucosal ischemia.

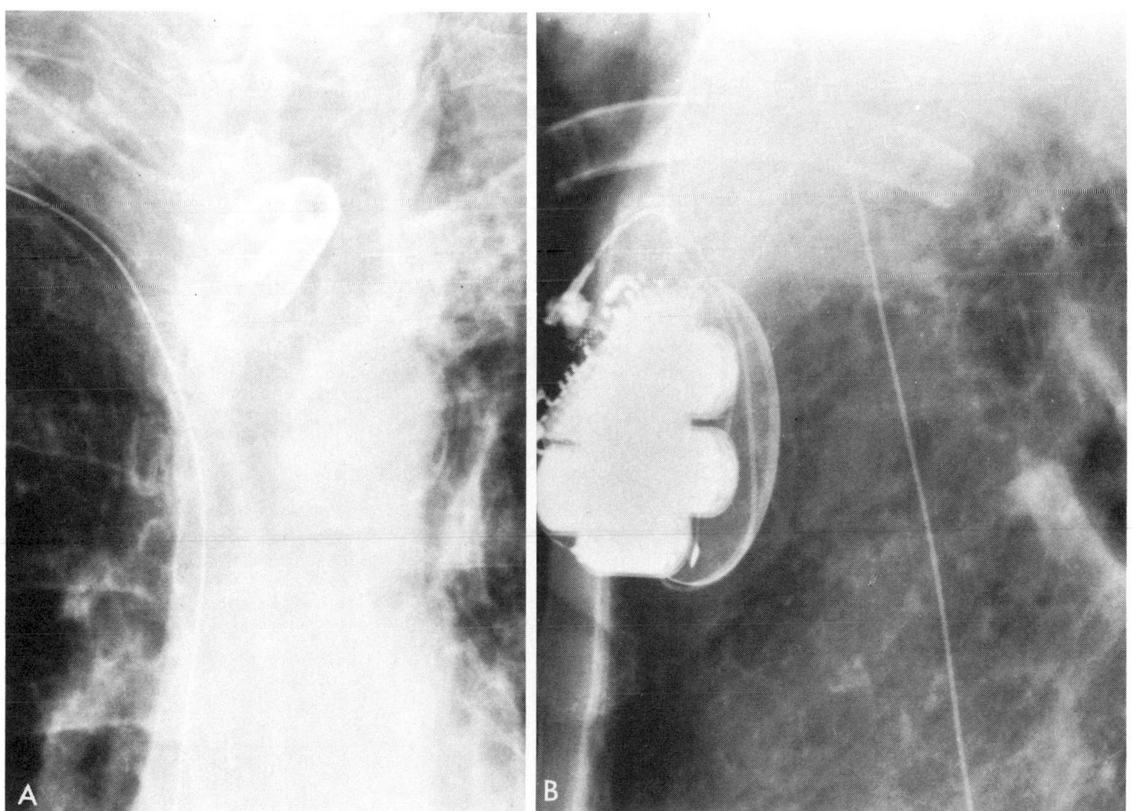

Figure 2–12. Potential posterior tracheal membrane perforation. *A,* In the anteroposterior (AP) projection, the tube appears parallel to the x-ray beam. *B,* Lateral view demonstrates that the tracheostomy tube is too short and a potential danger to the posterior tracheal membrane. (Note post-tracheostomy pneumomediastinum.)

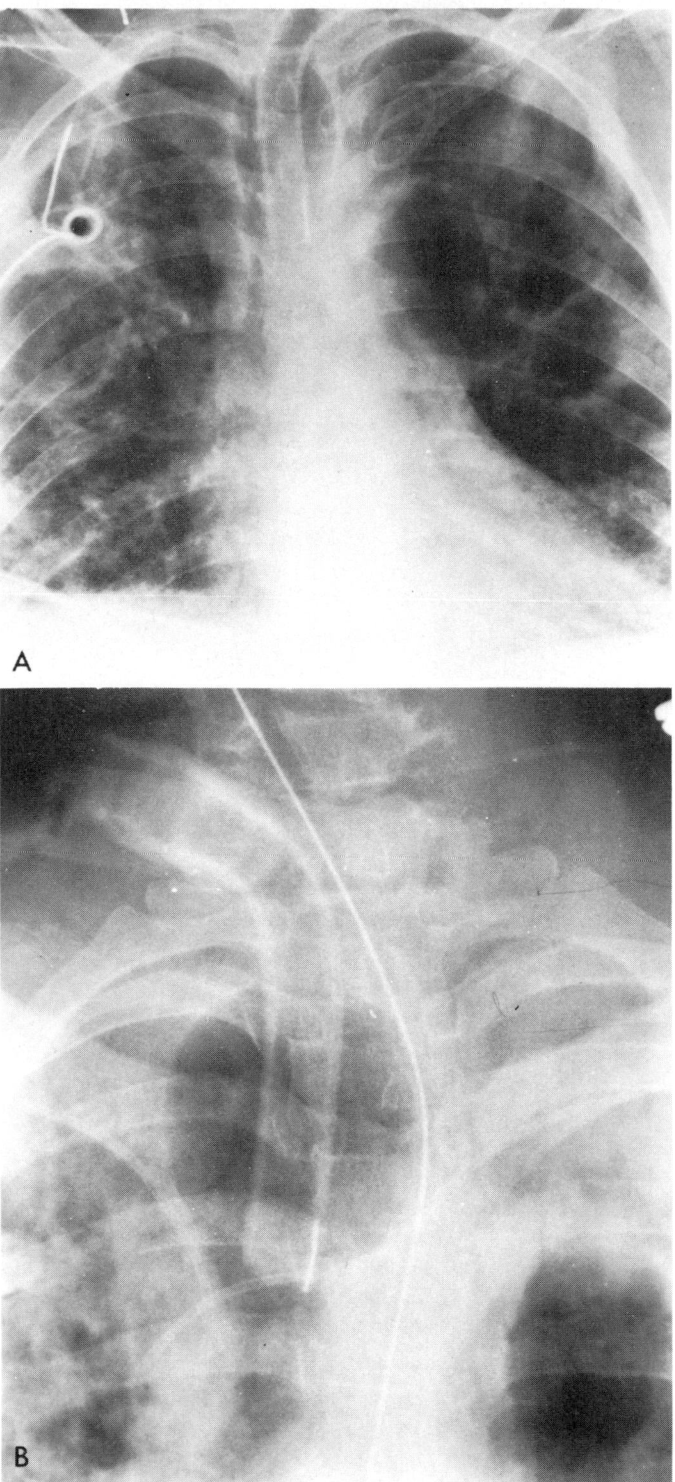

Figure 2–13. *A*, Mild dilatation of the trachea by the cuff. *B*, Same patient six weeks later with severe tracheal dilatation by the cuff. Autopsy showed destruction of the tracheal cartilage in this area.

4. Bacterial colonization of the trachea is frequent and may lead to infection of the damaged mucosa.

5. Secondary factors such as cachexia, hypotension, steroid or broad-spectrum antibiotic administration, and the use of positive pressure ventilators increase the likelihood of tracheal complications (Frager and Marshall, 1976).

In a few patients, ulceration progresses to tracheal perforation. An infrequent but potentially lethal sequela of tracheal erosion is the tracheoinnominate fistula, which is due to erosion of the right anterior lateral tracheal wall at the level of the innominate artery. This complication may be prevented by paying careful attention to the position of the tracheostomy tube tip on each radiograph. Persistent angulation to the right and anteriorly should be scrupulously avoided (Fig. 2–10*B*). This is most often due to a low or eccentric stoma, persistent hyperextension of the neck, or a very asthenic build (Crews and LaPuerta, 1972; Jones et al., 1976; Lane et al., 1975; Timmis, 1973). In two thirds of patients with a tracheoinnominate fistula, massive, usually fatal hemoptysis is the mode of presentation. In the other third, prodromal bleeding of a small-to-moderate amount of arterial blood may precede massive hemoptysis by hours or days. In this latter group, arch aortography may be helpful in confirming the clinical suspicion of a tracheoinnominate artery connection (Conrad et al., 1977).

Erosion through the posterior tracheal membrane leads to tracheoesophageal, tracheopleural, or tracheomediastinal fistula in 0.5 per cent of tracheostomized patients (Harley, 1972). Perforation occurs most often at the level of the tracheostomy cuff, usually at the level of the manubrium sterni. Predisposing conditions include an overdistended cuff, a short tracheostomy tube causing posterior angulation, and the presence of the nasogastric tube in the esophagus (Mulder and Rubush, 1969; Timmis, 1973) (Fig. 2–12). In the majority of patients, perforation occurs during the second to fourth week of intubation. The gradual erosion of the posterior tracheal membrane causes an inflammatory welding between the trachea and the esophagus, resulting in eventual direct tracheoesophageal communication. Therefore, the absence of a pneumomediastinum, mediastinal widening, or a mediastinal abscess does not negate the possibility of a tracheoesophageal fistula. Both the symptoms and the radiographic presentation depend on the relationship of the fistula to the tracheostomy cuff. If the fistula is below the cuff, signs and symptoms are due to the passage of food or refluxed gastric material into the lungs. If the fistula is above the cuff, food or gastric contents will accumulate in the upper trachea. Another characteristic but uncommon sign of a tracheoesophageal fistula is sudden gastrointestinal dilatation with air (Harley, 1972).

The radiographic demonstration of a tracheoesophageal fistula may be difficult. An esophagram using barium or oily Dionosil* is the method of choice. After deflation of the cuff and removal, if possible, careful fluoroscopic monitoring in the extreme oblique or lateral projections is necessary to document a small, anteriorly placed fistula. A videotape or cineradiography may be of great help. Particular attention should be paid to the retromanubrial area, the most frequent level of fistula formation and a difficult site to visualize radiographically. Great care must be taken not to confuse laryngeal aspiration of contrast medium with a tracheoesophageal fistula (Fig. 2–14).

Erosion through the tracheal wall into the mediastinum or pleural space is extremely uncommon. Erosion into the pleural space is associated with a unilateral or bilateral tension pneumothorax. Erosion into the mediastinum may be associated with pneumomediastinum, mediastinitis, or a mediastinal abscess (Harley, 1972; Mulder and Rubush, 1969).

Sequelae of Endotracheal Intubation and Tracheostomy. Injury to the larynx or trachea is almost universal following intubation (Burns et al., 1979; Dane and King, 1975; Stauffer et al., 1981). Fortunately, after extubation, mucosal edema, erythema, and superficial ulcerations usually heal without significant functional impairment. Deep ulcerations of the mucosa may result in permanent laryngeal scarring, tracheal stenosis, and tracheomalacia. Symptoms due to permanent airway compromise usually surface several weeks to many months after extubation. Recognition of the cause of the symptoms is often delayed because they are often attributed to the patient's underlying lung disease (Andrews and Pearson, 1971; Dane and King, 1975; Friman et al., 1976; Pearson et al., 1968).

Laryngeal Injuries. In the vast majority of patients, the laryngeal edema or ulceration caused by endotracheal intubation subsides within a week or two. Permanent glottic damage

*Manufactured by Glaxo Laboratories, Ltd., Middlesex, England. Distributed in the United States by Picker Corp., Falls Church, VA.

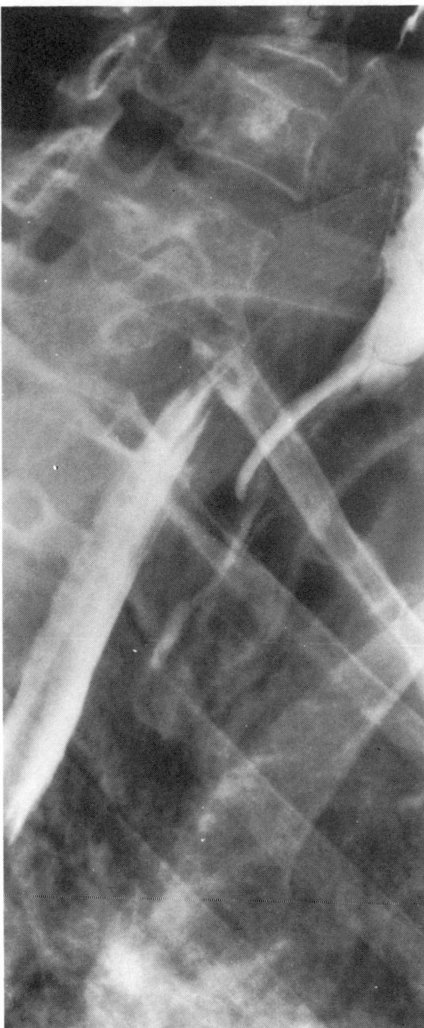

Figure 2–14. This patient was suspected of having a tracheoesophageal fistula because food was repeatedly suctioned from the trachea. No such fistula was demonstrated with a barium swallow, but the patient was noted to aspirate barium around the tube and cuff.

is seen most often after orotracheal intubation and after prolonged intubation (Burns et al., 1979; Dubick and Wright, 1978). The most frequent permanent injuries include scarring of the posterior third of the glottis, fusion of the posterior commissure, arytenoid injury, and subglottic stenosis (Fig. 2–15). Laryngeal injury due to a tracheostomy is uncommon.

Tracheostenosis. Since high-volume, low-pressure cuffs have replaced the high-pressure round balloons, the incidence of symptomatic tracheal injury has fallen considerably from the previously reported levels of 8 to 20 per cent. The vast majority of lesions are at the level of the stoma and the cuff (Fig. 2–16). Lesions at the stoma are usually due to granulation tissue projecting into the lumen or from collapse and fibrosis of the anterior and lateral trachea where the cartilage has been removed or destroyed (Fig. 2–17) (Harley, 1971; James et al., 1970; Stauffer et al., 1981; Weber and Grillo, 1978). Stenosis at the cuff site is usually a circumferential scar 1 to 4 cm long, starting approximately 1.5 cm below the stoma (Harley, 1971; Pearson et al., 1968; Weber and Grillo, 1978). Less frequent areas of stenosis include granulomas of the anterior wall at the site of the tube tip, and subglottic or glottic stenosis from a tracheostomy through the first tracheal ring. Lesions may be multiple or associated with tracheomalacia (Gamsu et al., 1980; Stitik et al., 1978).

Tracheomalacia. When the tracheal cartilage is destroyed, the trachea may not be able to maintain its patency during the respiratory cycle. In the neck, the surgical removal of cartilage or the dissolution of cartilage caused

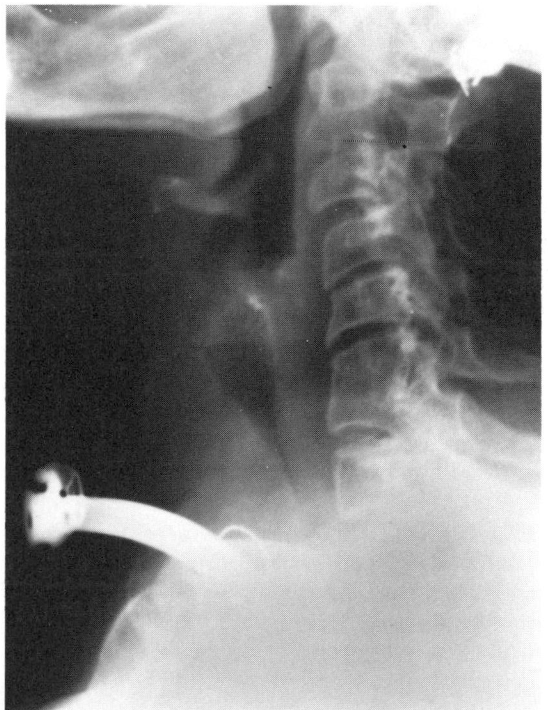

Figure 2–15. Proximal tracheal stenosis. Over the last several years the patient received endotracheal intubation several times for various cardiac problems. Note the severe, almost complete obliteration of the distal cervical trachea. A permanent tracheostomy was required to bypass the obstruction.

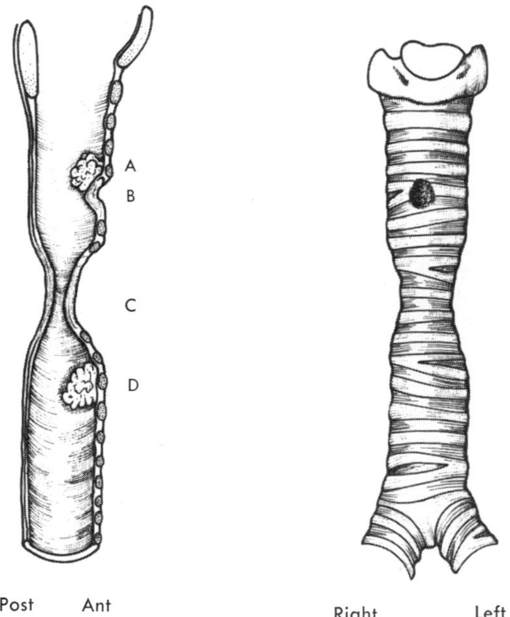

Figure 2–16. Post-tracheostomy lesions. The four common sites of tracheal injury are: *A*, polypoid granuloma above the stoma; *B*, posterior depression of the anterior tracheal wall at the stoma; *C*, circumferential narrowing of the trachea at the cuff site; and *D*, polypoid granuloma along the anterior wall at the tube tip.

by pressure or infection results in softening of the tracheal wall. When the patient inspires, the mobile tissues are sucked inward by the negative intratracheal pressure. Inspiratory stridor results. Within the thorax, dissolution of cartilage is usually at the level of the cuff. The area of malacia is frequently associated with an area of fixed stenosis. Tracheal collapse occurs on expiration, when the intrathoracic pressure exceeds the intratracheal pressure (Gamsu et al., 1980; Geffin et al., 1971; Stitik et al., 1978).

Radiographic Evaluation. The larynx and the cervical and intrathoracic trachea must be studied in each patient. Initial evaluation involves a well-penetrated posteroanterior (PA) and lateral chest radiograph, an AP radiograph of the neck, and a lateral soft tissue radiograph of the neck (James et al., 1970) (Fig. 2–15). If the upper mediastinal trachea cannot be evaluated well on the lateral radiograph, oblique radiographs of the trachea are often helpful. This is the most frequent area of cuff-induced stenosis and must be carefully evaluated. The inner tracheal walls should be parallel and sharply defined in their entire length. In most patients the lumen is slightly narrowed or irregular at the stomal level, but dyspnea is uncommon before there is 50 per cent compromise of the lumen. (If a tracheostomy tube is still present, it must be removed in order to evaluate the trachea properly.)

Conventional tomography in both the AP and lateral projection is required for further evaluation. The entire trachea from cords to carina must be studied, since lesions are often multiple (Fig. 2–17). Fluoroscopy using various respiratory maneuvers is necessary to evaluate cord movement and check for tracheomalacia. In most cases, non-contrast material–enhanced studies adequately define the lesion(s). Positive contrast tracheography is more accurate in defining the extent of the stenosis and identifying tracheomalacic areas (Gamsu et al., 1980; Hemmingsson and Lindgren, 1978; Stitik et al., 1978). Propyliodone (Dionosil), the agent most often used, may cause mucosal edema, which may further compromise the airway. As little contrast material as possible should be used, and one must be prepared to reintubate the patient should respiratory embarrassment develop (James et al., 1970). In view of its potential hazards, tracheography should be reserved for complex cases in which surgery is contemplated or in which the radiographic findings do not correlate with the bronchoscopy or pulmonary function tests (flow-volume loop). If tantalum powder is available, it provides excellent tracheal detail without inciting mucosal edema (Fig. 2–18). The role of CT in evaluating these lesions has not been fully evaluated.

POSITIVE PRESSURE THERAPY DEVICES

The institution of positive pressure therapy may markedly alter the appearance of the chest radiograph. Because a respirator is usually set to deliver a volume of gas larger than the patient has when breathing spontaneously, the radiograph taken at the peak of forced inspiration reflects greater lung inflation. When PEEP is added, the inspiratory lung volume increases further. The increased lung volume may reexpand atelectatic areas and will spread an existing infiltrate over a larger volume (McLoud et al., 1977) (Fig. 2–19). Zimmerman et al. (1979) noted that the addition of PEEP either “cleared” or “diminished” the radiographic appearance of lung disease in over half their patients. Infiltrates disappeared, vessels became sharper and smaller, and areas of

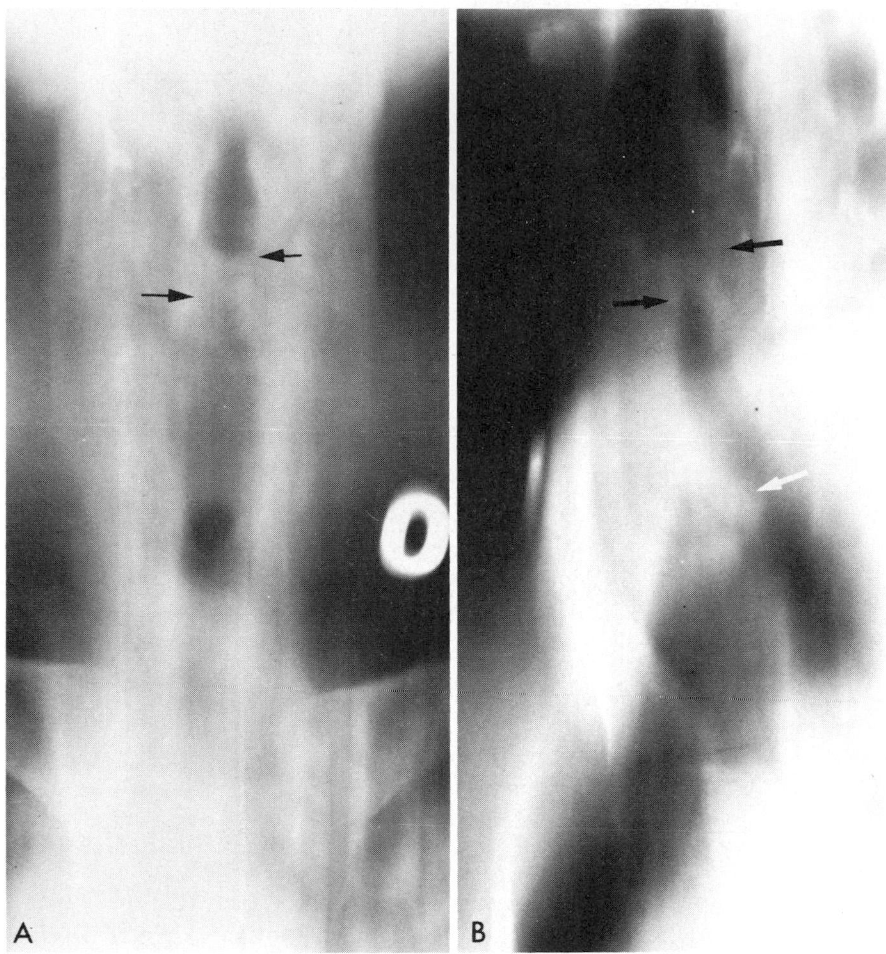

Figure 2–17. Suprastomal stenosis. The patient fractured her cervical spine and injured her upper trachea in an auto accident. A tracheostomy was performed shortly after admission. Several weeks later she could not tolerate extubation. *A*, AP tomogram shows complete occlusion of the trachea (*arrows*) several centimeters above the stoma (*lead marker*). The true and false cords on the right are thickened. *B*, Lateral tomogram confirms the complete obstruction of the upper trachea (*upper arrows*) and also demonstrates the polypoid granuloma at the level of the tracheostomy stoma (*lower arrow*).

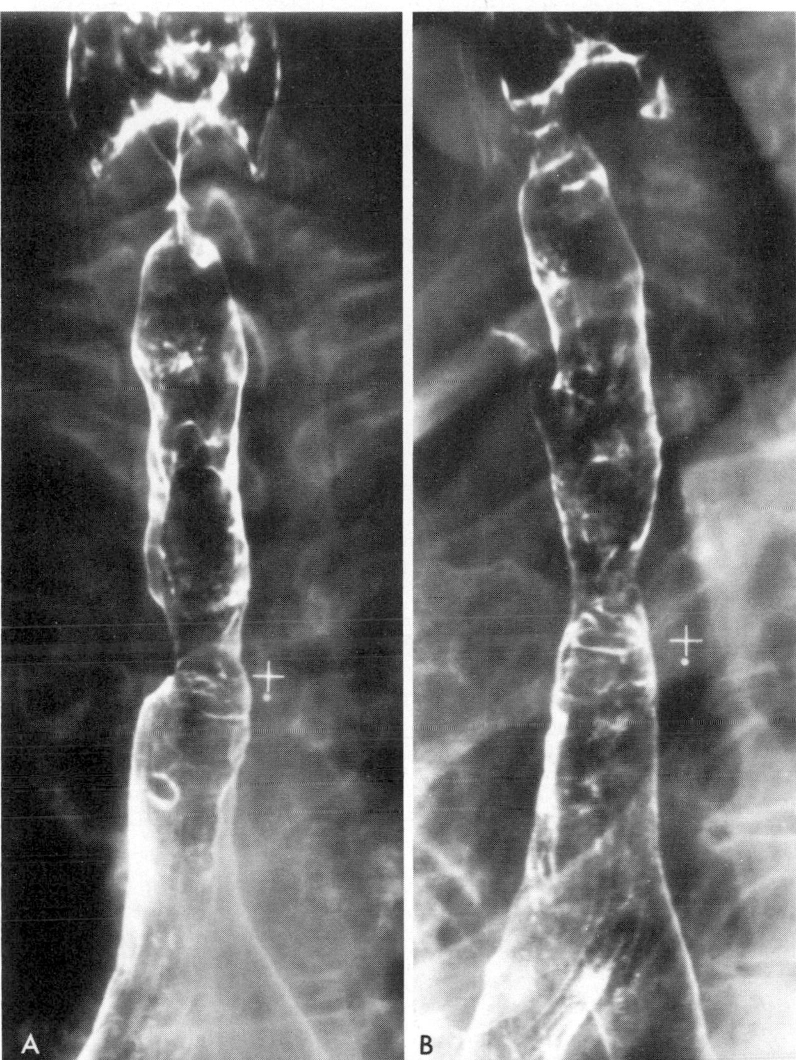

Figure 2–18. Tracheostenosis. *A*, Tantalum tracheogram demonstrates moderate asymmetric tracheostenosis of the midtrachea. Mild narrowing is present at the level of the stoma. The vocal cords and subglottic area appear normal. *B*, Oblique tracheogram confirms the above findings. A small amount of tantalum outlines the residual stomal tract. (Courtesy of Frederick Stitik, M.D., Virginia Beach, VA.)

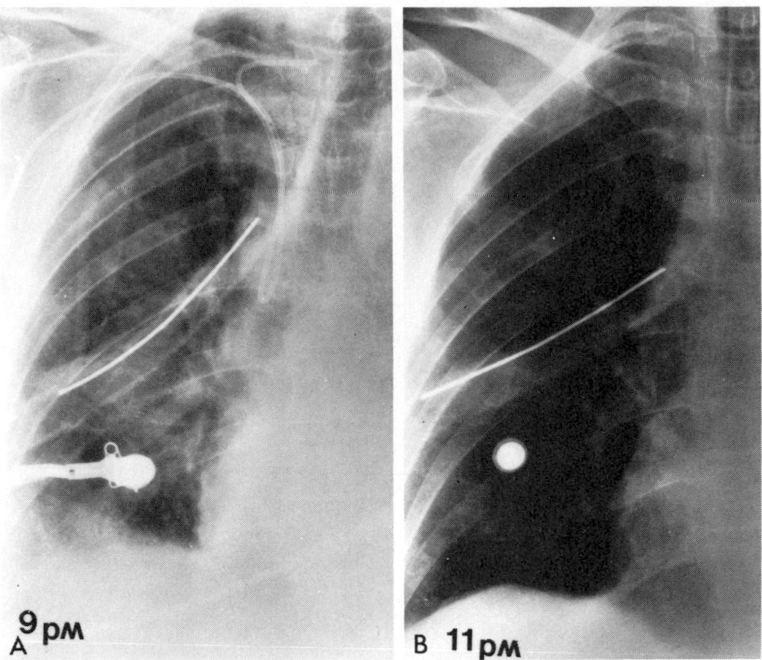

Figure 2–19. Effect of respiratory therapy. *A*, Focal pulmonary infiltrates are noted in the right mid- and right lower lung field. A CVP catheter is coiled in the superior vena cava. A chest tube is noted over the right midlung field. Note that both the opaque and nonopaque wall of the chest tube is visible. *B*, Two hours later the CVP catheter has been removed, an endotracheal tube has been inserted, and positive pressure therapy has been instituted. Note the complete resolution of the pulmonary infiltrates. This probably represents re-expansion of atelectatic areas.

silhouetting disappeared. These radiographic changes, which reversed when PEEP was removed, appeared to be most marked in patients with diffuse edema rather than other types of pulmonary infiltrates (see Fig. 1–4). Therefore, it is imperative that the radiologist know whether the patient was receiving positive pressure therapy at the time the radiograph was taken. On occasion, one must replace the patient on the respirator and re-radiograph to determine whether the apparent worsening is real or reflects a decreased tidal volume.

Potential Complications

Barotrauma. Pulmonary barotrauma, the extra-alveolar escape of air, is seen in 0.5 to 15 per cent of patients receiving positive pressure therapy (Altman and Johnson, 1979; Cullen and Caldera, 1979; Kumar et al., 1973; Rohlfing et al., 1976; Steier et al., 1974; Zwillich et al., 1974). Except for the initial post-tracheostomy period, when air leaks are frequently due to the surgical procedure itself, most air leaks are due to disruption of the pulmonary parenchyma. A small airway or alveolus ruptures, and air dissects along the bronchovascular connective tissue into the mediastinum and then ruptures into the pleural space (Macklin and Macklin, 1944). Approximately two thirds of the pneumothoraces occurring in patients on respirators are tension pneumothoraces (Kumar et al., 1973; Rohlfing et al., 1976; Steier et al., 1974; Zwillich et al., 1974). Only a small percentage of pneumothoraces result from a direct rent in the pleura.

Respirator-induced barotrauma is more frequent in patients on volume respirators than in those on pressure respirators and in patients receiving high tidal volumes. Ventilator pressures less than 25 cm H_2O seldom cause air leaks, whereas pressures above 80 cm H_2O frequently rupture the lung (Nennhaus et al., 1967). In patients with large areas of atelectasis, volume intended to ventilate the entire lung may be delivered to nonatelectatic areas only (Fig. 2–20) (Altman and Johnson, 1979). The role of PEEP in the production of barotrauma remains uncertain. Some studies have reported the incidence of air leaks to be no higher with PEEP than with other positive pressure thera-

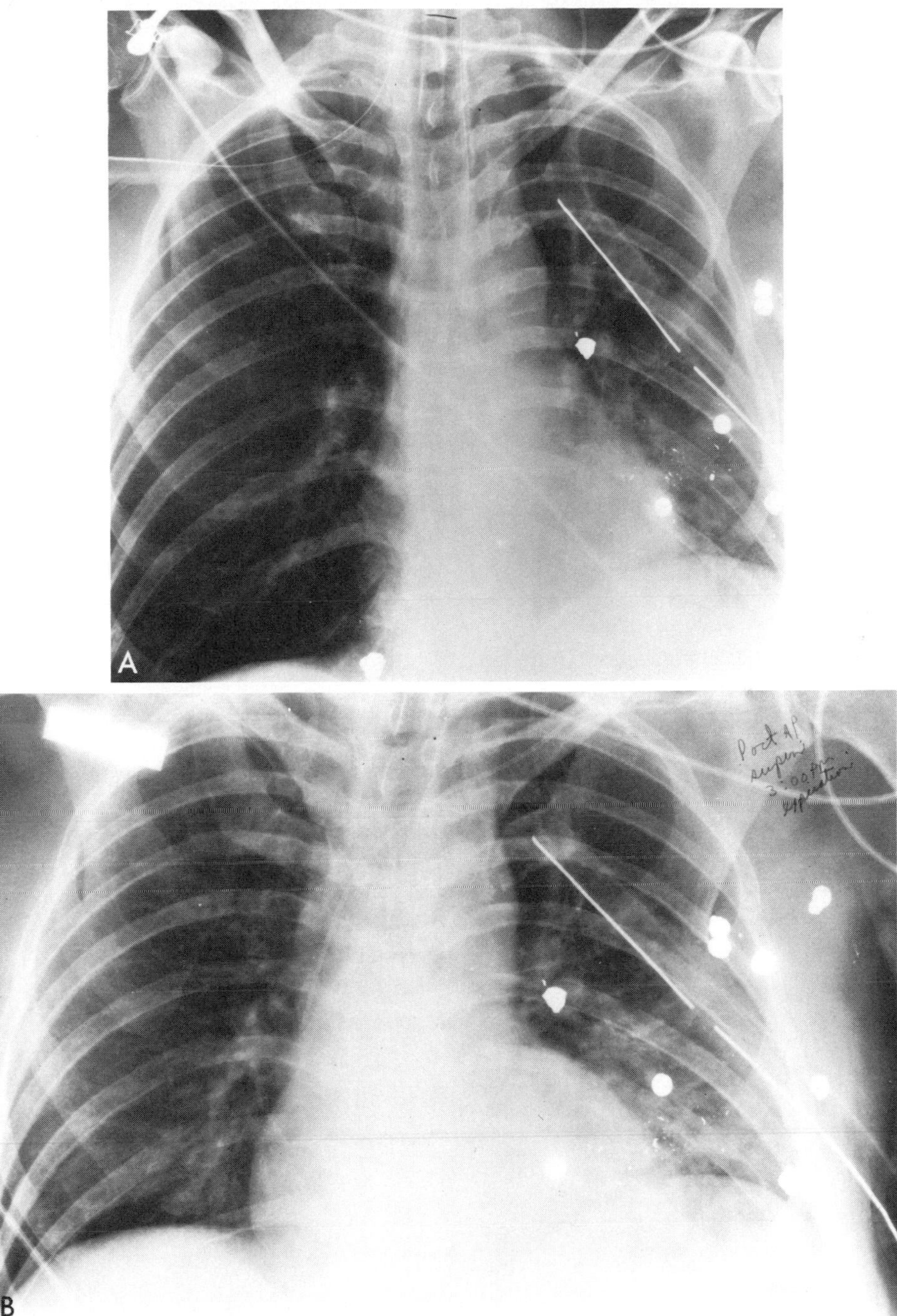

Figure 2–20. Patient with a pneumothorax and lung laceration following a buckshot wound. *A*, Radiograph demonstrates marked hyperinflation of the right lung. The patient was on a volume respirator. *B*, Expiration film shows normal deflation of the right lung. This indicates that hyperinflation is due to uneven ventilation rather than to a "ball-valve" obstruction on the right.

pies, whereas other reports have indicated that PEEP increases the incidence of air leaks (Cullen and Caldera, 1979; Kumar et al., 1973; Steier et al., 1974; Zwillich et al., 1974).

Certain lung diseases predispose the patient to pulmonary barotrauma, and their presence should alert the clinician to a potential pneumothorax. Air leaks occur most often in patients with obstructive lung disease, interstitial fibrosis (decreased compliance), or cavitary lung disease. In a patient on a respirator the day-to-day enlargement of a "hole" in the lung (abscess, bulla, pneumatocele, or interstitial air cyst) indicates that a pneumothorax is imminent. (The radiographic features of barotrauma are discussed in Chapter 4.)

Water retention. Patients receiving positive pressure therapy tend to be in positive water balance. Hypervolemia is reflected clinically in a deteriorating respiratory status (decreased compliance) without apparent cause, a decrease in hematocrit value, a low serum sodium concentration, and gradual weight gain (Davis, 1972; Pontoppidan et al., 1972; Sladen et al., 1968; Manny et al., 1978). Both the clinical and radiographic changes are subtle and may take days or weeks to develop. Serial radiographs reveal the slowly progressive changes of interstitial edema (fuzzy vessels, prominent interstitial markings, perihilar or lower lung field haze) without cardiomegaly or vascular redistribution. Day-to-day radiographic changes may be imperceptible, yet changes over several days may be obvious. Therefore, one must use the films of the previous week as well as those of the previous day for comparison. The edema usually occurs in gravity-dependent areas and may change with changes in the patient's positioning. If the patient is radiographed after lying on his side for several hours, the radiograph will show increased edema on the dependent side (Leeming, 1968; Zimmerman et al., 1982) (see Figs. 4–17,4–18).

The cause of the inappropriate water retention remains controversial. It does, however, appear to be related to the positive pressure therapy itself, since patients receiving negative pressure (iron lung) therapy tend to be in negative water balance. Suggested causes of fluid retention include inappropriate antidiuretic hormone (ADH) secretion, hypoalbuminemia, increased airway pressure, decreased intrathoracic venous pressure, reduction of lymphatic fluid return, subclinical congestive heart failure, reduction of pulmonary blood flow, and insensible water gain due to nebulized fluid.

"Respirator lung." Patients receiving respirator therapy on a long-term basis may develop nonspecific interstitial infiltrates and alveolar hyaline membranes. This was initially attributed to the respirator therapy itself. It is now recognized that these changes are those of oxygen toxicity or the adult respiratory distress syndrome (ARDS) and are not related to the ventilator alone (Pontoppidan et al., 1972). (ARDS is discussed in Chapter 5.)

PLEURAL DRAINAGE TUBES

In the bedridden patient, intrapleural air collects beneath the sternum and intrapleural fluid collects posteriorly. The ideal position for the thoracostomy tube is therefore anterosuperior for a pneumothorax (Fig. 2–20) and posteroinferior for a hydrothorax (Fig. 2–21). In reality, tubes in less than ideal position often function well in the adhesionless chest. Anteroposterior and lateral radiographs are usually obtained to document proper tube position.

If only an AP radiograph is obtained, a tube inserted into the subcutaneous tissues of the chest or into the oblique fissure will appear to be in satisfactory position. Webb and Godwin have shown that the non-opaque wall of an intrathoracic chest tube is usually seen because of air in the tube and adjacent lung or pleural space (Figs. 2–19, 2–20). When positioned in the subcutaneous tissue, the non-opaque wall is "silhouetted" by chest wall, which is similar in density to the plastic tube. When the tube is in the major fissure, the tip of the tube is further from the cassette than the rest of the tube. It will appear magnified (Milne, 1980). In addition, one should check the radiograph to ensure that the side hole of the tube (the break in the opaque strip) projects within the thorax (Fig. 2–21).

After removal of the tube, residual pleural lines often delineate the former tube position. They represent areas of pleural thickening around the tube track (Fig. 2–22*A*). They are rarely significant but may be confusing. A review of previous films will demonstrate the position occupied by the tube. On occasion, the radiodense pleural stripe are seen parallel to the lateral rib cage and may closely simulate a pneumothorax. The thickened pleura may actually form a space that, when partially filled

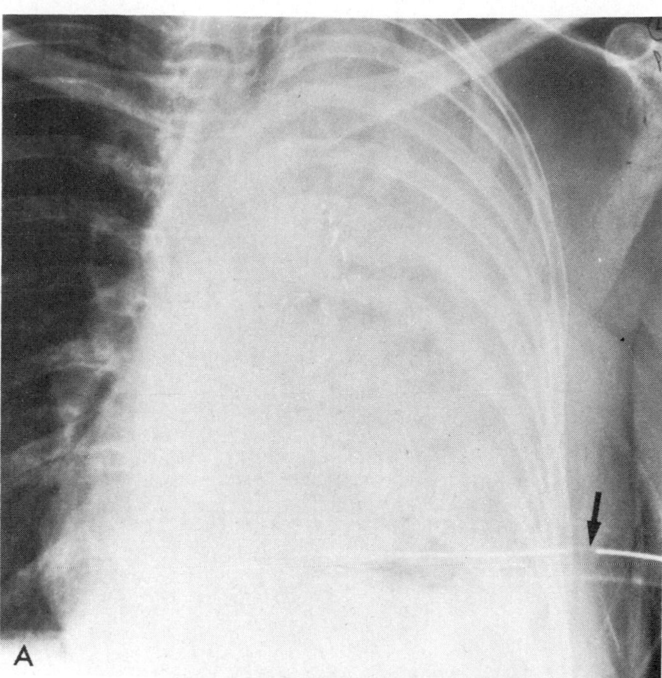

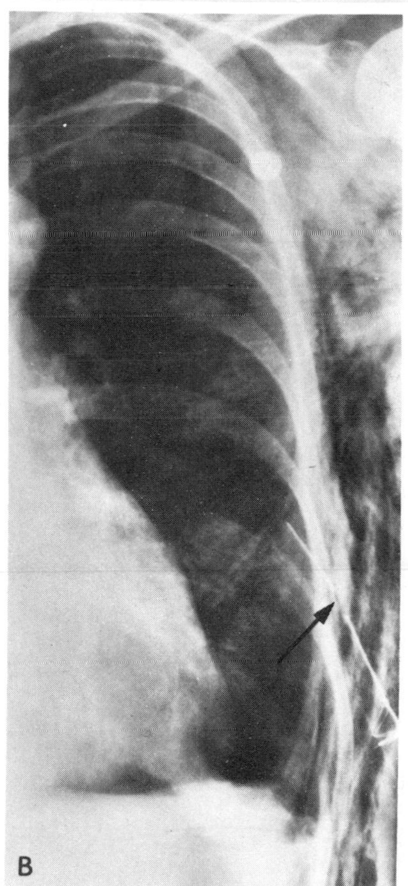

Figure 2–21. Malfunctioning pleural drainage tube. *A*, The tube is properly placed at the lung base to drain the patient's effusion. However, the side hole is seen lateral to the ribs (*arrow*) and air in the chest wall. The tube was replaced, and drainage improved. *B*, Another patient, showing marked subcutaneous emphysema. Note that side hole of catheter is in the subcutaneous tissue (*arrow*).

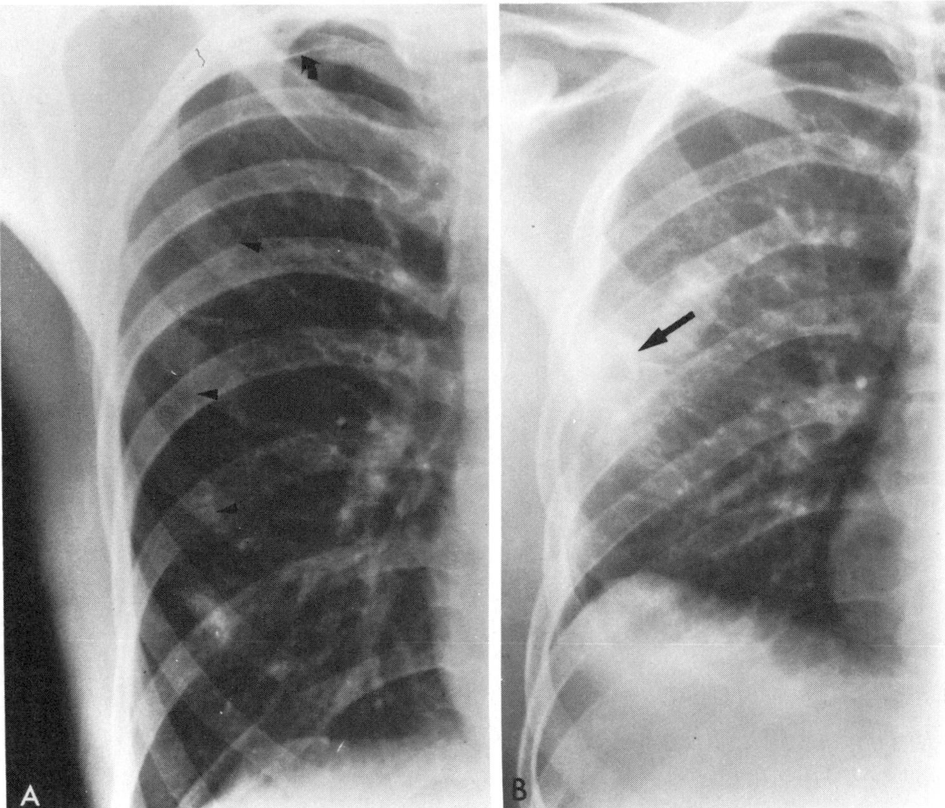

Figure 2–22. *A,* Tube track following the removal of a chest tube. A line of pleural thickening is seen along the path of the tube (*arrows*), simulating a pneumothorax. The density over the anterior fifth rib is the site of insertion of the tube. A small pneumothorax remains (*upper arrow*). *B,* Infected tube track (different patient). Fever and leukocytosis developed two days after removal of the chest tube. Note the diffuse pleural thickening plus the focal right midlung density with a central lucency (*arrow*). Purulent drainage was positive for *Staphylococcus aureus.*

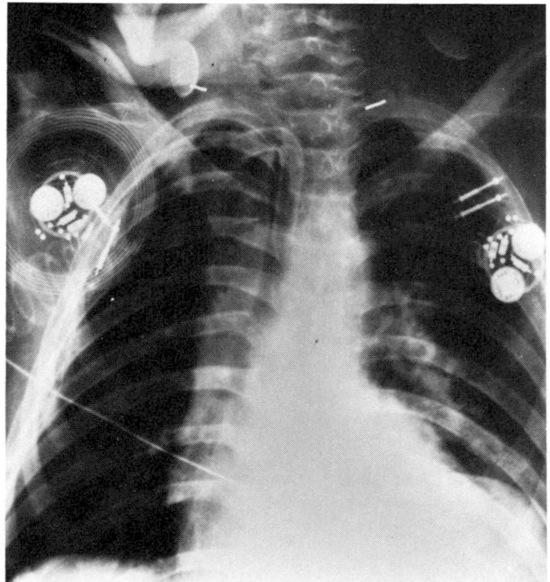

Figure 2–23. Diaphragmatic pacers. The platinum phrenic nerve electrodes are seen over the transverse processes of T-1. A very fine wire leads from each electrode to each receiver. (Case of Dr. Carl Ravin, Durham, NC.)

with fluid, may mimic an abscess. If completely filled, it may be seen as a dense linear band "within the lung." These fluid collections usually decrease in size or disappear completely within days or weeks. An enlarging tube track in a patient with an unexplained fever should raise the possibility of an empyema (Fig. 2–22*B*).

DIAPHRAGM PACING

Diaphragmatic pacing is of value in chronic ventilatory insufficiency, when the phrenic nerves, lung, and diaphragm are functional (for example, quadriplegia, central alveolar hypoventilation, COPD). A radiofrequency receiver is implanted into the subcutaneous tissue of the anterior chest wall and connected to a platinum electrode placed on the phrenic nerve behind the clavicle (Fig. 2–23). An external radiofrequency transmitter sends signals through the intact skin to the receiver, which sends an electrical signal to the phrenic nerve (Glenn, 1978). Complications of radiographic interest include infection around the implanted receiver and breakage of the electrode.

REFERENCES

Alberti, J., Hanafee, W., Wilson, G., et al.: Unsuspected pulmonary collapse during neuroradiologic procedures. Radiology 89:316, 1967.

Altman, A. R., and Johnson, T. H.: Roentgenographic findings in PEEP therapy. Indicators of pulmonary complications. J.A.M.A. 242:727, 1979.

Andrews, M. J., and Pearson, F. G.: Incidence and pathogenesis of tracheal injury following cuffed tube tracheostomy with assisted ventilation; analysis of a two-year prospective study. Ann. Surg. 173:249, 1971.

Arens, J. F., LeJeune, F. E., Jr., and Webre, D. R.: Maxillary sinusitis; a complication of nasotracheal intubation. Anesthesiology 40:415, 1974.

Burns, H. P., Dayal, V. S., Scott, A., et al.: Laryngotracheal trauma: observations on its pathogenesis and its prevention following prolonged orotracheal intubation in the adult. Laryngoscope 89:1316, 1979.

Conrad, M. R., Cameron, J., and White, R. I., Jr.: The role of angiography in the diagnosis of tracheal–innominate artery fistula. Am. J. Roentgenol. 128:35, 1977.

Conrardy, P. A., Goodman, L. R., Laing, R., et al.: Alteration of endotracheal tube position. Crit. Care Med. 4:8, 1976.

Cooper, J. D., and Grillo, H. C.: Analysis of problems related to cuffs on intratracheal tubes. Chest 62 (Aug. Suppl.):21S, 1972.

Cooper, J. D., and Malt, R. A.: Meteorism produced by nasotracheal intubation and ventilatory assistance. N. Engl. J. Med. 287:652, 1972.

Crews, E. R., and LaPuerta, L.: A Manual for Respiratory Failure. Springfield, IL, 1972, Charles C Thomas.

Cullen, D. J., and Caldera, D. L.: The incidence of ventilator-induced pulmonary barotrauma in critically ill patients. Anesthesiology 50:185, 1979.

Dane, T. E. D., and King, E. G.: A prospective study of complications after tracheostomy for assisted ventilation. Chest 67:398, 1975.

Davis, T. J.: The influence of intrathoracic pressure on fluid and electrolyte balance. Chest 62 (Nov. Suppl.):118S, 1972.

Dubick, M. N., and Wright, B. D.: Comparison of laryngeal pathology following long-term oral and nasal endotracheal intubations. Anesth. Analg. Cleve. 57:663, 1978.

Frager, M. E., and Marshall, R. D.: Tracheal dilatation. Anesthesia 31:470, 1976.

Friman, L., Hedensteirna, G., and Scheldt, B.: Stenosis following tracheostomy. Anesthesia 31:479, 1976.

Gamsu, G., Borson, D. B., Webb, W. R., and Cunningham, J. H.: Structure and function in tracheal stenosis. Am. Rev. Respir. Dis. 121:519, 1980.

Geffin, B., Grillo, H. C., Cooper, J. D., et al.: Stenosis following tracheostomy for respiratory care. J.A.M.A. 216:1984, 1971.

Glenn, W. W. L.: Diaphragm pacing: present status. PACE 1:357, 1978.

Goodman, L. R., Conrardy, P. A., Laing, F., et al.: Radiographic evaluation of endotracheal tube position. Am. J. Roentgenol. 127:433, 1976.

Harley, H. R. S.: Laryngotracheal obstruction complicating tracheostomy or endotracheal intubation with assisted respiration: critical review. Thorax 26:493, 1971.

Harley, H. R. S.: Ulcerative tracheo-eosophageal fistula during treatment by tracheostomy and intermittent positive pressure ventilation. Thorax 27:338, 1972.

Hawkins, D. B., Seltzer, D. C., Barnett, T. E., et al.: Endotracheal tube perforation of the hypopharynx. West. J. Med. 120:282, 1974.

Heinonen, J., Takki, S., and Tammisto, T.: Effect of the Trendelenburg tilt and other procedures on the position of endotracheal tubes. Lancet 1:850, 1969.

Hemmingsson, A., and Lindgren, P. G.: Roentgenologic examination of tracheal stenosis. Acta Radiol. [Diagn.] (Stockh.) 19:753, 1978.

Hirsch, M., Abramowitz, H. B., Shapiro, S., and Barki, Y.: Hypopharyngeal injury as a result of attempted endotracheal intubation. Radiology 128:37, 1978.

James, A. E., Jr., Macmillan, A. S., Jr., Eaton, S. B., et al.: Radiological considerations of granuloma and stenosis at the site of tracheostomy. Radiology 96:513, 1970.

Jones, J. W., Reynolds, M., Hewitt, R. L., et al.: Tracheoinnominate artery erosion; successful surgical management of a devastating complication. Ann. Surg. 184:194, 1976.

Khan, F., Reddy, N., and Khan, A.: Cuff/trachea ratio as an indicator of tracheal damage. Chest 70:431(abstr.), 1976.

Kumar, A., Pontoppidan, H., Falke, K. J., et al.: Pulmonary barotrauma during mechanical ventilation. Crit. Care Med. 1:181, 1973.

Lane, E. E., Temes, G. D., and Anderson, W. H.: Tracheal-innominate artery fistula due to tracheostomy. Chest 68:678, 1975.

Leeming, B. W. A.: Radiological aspects of the pulmonary complications resulting from intermittent positive pressure ventilation (I.P.P.V.). Australas. Radiol. 12:361, 1968.

Macklin, M. T., and Macklin, C. C.: Malignant interstitial emphysema of the lungs and mediastinum. Medicine 23:281, 1944.

Manny, J., Patten, M. T., Liebman, P. R., and Hechtman,

H. B.: The association of lung distention, PEEP and biventricular failure. Ann. Surg. 187(2):151, 1978.
McLoud, T. C., Barash, P. G., and Ravin, C. E.: PEEP: radiographic features and associated complications. Am. J. Roentgenol. 129:209, 1977.
Milne, E. N. C.: Chest radiology in the surgical patient. Surg. Clin. North Am. 60(6):1503, 1980.
Muhm, J. R., and Crowe, J. K.: The evaluation of tracheal abnormalities by tomography. Radiol. Clin. North Am. 14(1):95, 1976.
Mulder, D. S., and Rubush, J. L.: Complications of tracheostomy; relationship to long-term ventilatory assistance. J. Trauma 9:389, 1969.
Nennhaus, H. P., Javid, H., and Julian, O. C.: Alveolar and pleural rupture; hazards of positve pressure respiration. Arch. Surg. 94:136, 1967.
Ogawa, T. K., Bergeron, R. T., Whitaker, C. W., et al.: Air-fluid levels in the sphenoid sinus in epistaxis and nasal packing. Radiology 118:351, 1976.
Pearson, F. G., Goldberg, M., and de Silva, A. J.: Tracheal stenosis complicating tracheostomy with cuffed tubes. Arch. Surg. 97:380, 1968.
Perel, A., Katzenelson, R., Klein, E., and Cotev, S.: Collapse of endotracheal tubes due to overinflation of high-compliance cuffs. Anesth. Analg. (Cleve.) 56(5):731, 1977.
Pontoppidan, H., Geffin, B., and Lowenstein, E.: Acute respiratory failure in the adult. N. Engl. J. Med. 287:690, 1972.
Rohlfing, B. M., Webb, W. R., and Schlobohm, R. M.: Ventilator-related extra-alveolar air in adults. Radiology 121:25, 1976.
Skaggs, J. A., and Cogbill C. L.: Tracheostomy; management, mortality, complications. Am. Surg. 35:393, 1969.
Sladen, A., Laver, M. B., and Pontoppidan, H.: Pulmonary complications and water retention in prolonged mechanical ventilation. N. Engl. J. Med. 279:448, 1968.
Stauffer, J. L., Olson, D. E., and Petty, T. L.: Complications and consequences of endotracheal intubation and tracheotomy; a prospective study of 150 critically ill adult patients. Am. J. Med. 70:65, 1981.
Steier, M., Ching, N., Roberts, E. B. R., et al.: Pneumothorax complicating continuous ventilatory support. J. Thorac. Cardiovasc. Surg. 67:17, 1974.
Stemmer, E. A., Oliver, C., Carey, J. P., et al.: Fatal complications of tracheotomy. Am. J. Surg. 131:288, 1976.
Stitik, F. P., Bartelt, D., James, A. E., Jr., and Proctor, D. F.: Tantalum tracheography in upper airway obstruction: 100 experiences in adults. Am. J. Roentgenol. 130:35, 1978.
Timmis, H. H.: Tracheostomy; an overview of implications, management and morbidity. Adv. Surg. 7:199, 1973.
Tisi, G. M., Twigg, H. L., and Moser, K. M.: Collapse of left lung induced by artificial airway. Lancet 1:791, 1968.
Webb, W. R., and Godwin, J. D.: The obscured outer edge: a sign of improperly placed pleural drainage tubes. AJR 134:1062, 1980.
Weber, A. L., and Grillo, H. C.: Tracheal stenosis: an analysis of 151 cases. Radiol. Clin. North Am. 26:291, 1978.
Wolff, A. P., and Kessler, S.: Iatrogenic injury to the hypopharynx and cervical esophagus; an autopsy study. Ann. Otol. Rhinol. Laryngol. 82:778, 1973.
Zimmerman, J. E., Goodman, L. R., and Shahvari, M. B. G.: Effect of mechanical ventilation and positive end-expiratory pressure (PEEP) on chest radiographs. AJR133:811, 1979.
Zimmerman, J. E., Goodman, L. R., St. Andre, A. C., and Wyman A. C.: Radiographic detection of mobilizable lung water: the gravitational shift test. AJR 138:59, 1982.
Zwillich, C. W., Pierson, D. J., Creagh, C. E., et al.: Complications of assisted ventilation; a prospective study of 354 consecutive episodes. Am. J. Med. 57:161, 1974.

Chapter 3

CARDIOVASCULAR MONITORING AND ASSIST DEVICES

by Carl E. Ravin

CENTRAL VENOUS PRESSURE CATHETERS

A critical factor in the management of seriously ill patients is maintenance of an optimal blood volume; that is, one that will produce adequate circulation to critical organs without overloading cardiac pumping capability. Monitoring central venous pressure (CVP) via an intravenous (IV) catheter is one method by which this important relationship between intravascular blood volume and cardiac pumping capacity can be assessed (Wilson et al., 1962). The physiologic principles involved are discussed in Chapter 1.

In addition to monitoring CVP, these catheters also serve as a secure route for IV administration of fluids. They ensure a more consistent venous flow than peripheral veins, which may vasoconstrict, particularly during periods of cardiovascular collapse, when access to the circulatory system is most needed.

The catheter employed for such monitoring is generally a 16-gauge polyethylene tube 24 to 36 inches in length. It is inserted either percutaneously through a 14-gauge needle or via a cutdown into a peripheral vein (usually in the upper extremity) and advanced into the central venous system. Use of subclavian venipuncture for access to the central venous system is discussed later.

Ideal Position

Correct positioning of the CVP catheter is of utmost importance. It must be located within the true central venous system, beyond all the valves that interfere with direct transmission of right atrial pressure to the catheter (Wilson et al., 1962). The most proximal of these valves are found in the subclavian vein and in the internal jugular vein approximately 2.5 cm from their junction to form the brachiocephalic vein (Goss, 1976). The location of the last valve in the subclavian vein is closely approximated by the anterior first rib (Ravin et al., 1976); thus, in order for a catheter to monitor CVP accurately, it must lie medial to the anterior portion of the first rib (demonstrated on the chest radiograph). The optimal location is at the junction of the brachiocephalic veins to form the superior vena cava or within the superior vena cava itself (Langston, 1971; Wilson et al., 1962) (Figs. 1–6, 3–6).

Potential Complications

Aberrant positioning. Prospective studies have shown that as many as one third of CVP catheters are incorrectly placed at the time of initial insertion (Langston, 1971). The most common aberrant locations include the internal jugular vein (Fig. 3–1); the right atrium or ventricle; or various extrathoracic locations, including the upper extremities (Fig. 3–2) or the hepatic veins (Fig. 3–3).

Positions within the right atrium are undesirable because of an increased incidence of cardiac perforation by the catheter. Continued infusion of fluid through the catheter into the pericardial space following perforation can rapidly produce fatal cardiac tamponade (Brandt et

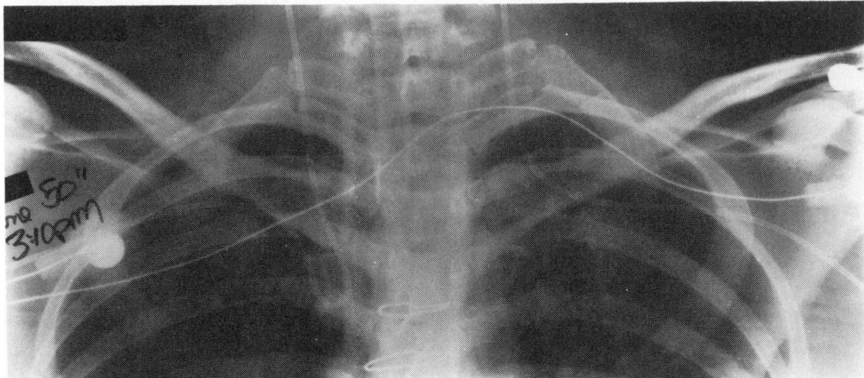

Figure 3–1. Bilateral central venous pressure (CVP) catheters inadvertently positioned in the internal jugular veins. True CVP cannot be monitored with this catheter position. (From Ravin, C. E., Putman, C. E., and McLoud, T. C.: Am. J. Roentgenol. 126:423, 1976.)

al., 1970; Friedman and Jurgeleit, 1968; Bone et al., 1973). Positioning distal to the tricuspid valve more often causes cardiac arrhythmias because of irritation of the endocardium, but it can also cause perforation (Kline and Hofman, 1968).

An important problem of all aberrant catheter positioning is that true CVP is not monitored; rather, some other pressure bearing no constant relationship to CVP is assessed. Such pressures can vary widely from the true CVP (Langston, 1971). Attempts to regulate the patient's intravascular blood volume on the basis of these erroneous measurements can lead to serious errors in patient management (Fig. 1–4).

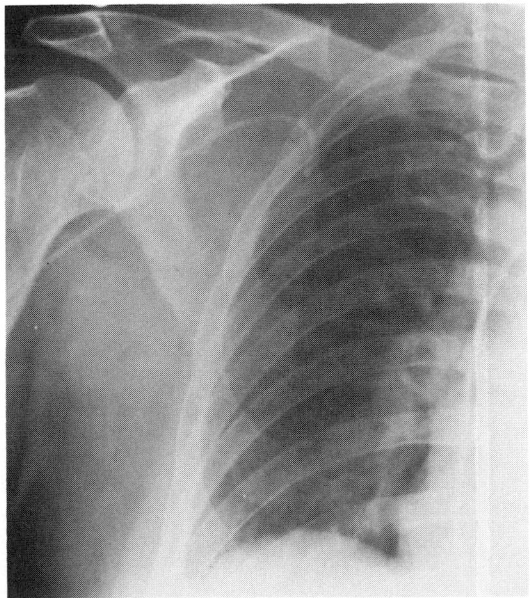

Figure 3–2. CVP catheter inserted into the basilic vein of the right upper extremity and terminating in an extrathoracic vein.

Additional complications of aberrant positioning are theoretically possible from infusion of potentially toxic substances (some antibiotics and hypertonic hyperalimentation solutions) directly into the liver or heart rather than into the central venous system, where rapid dilution can take place (Daly et al., 1975). Finally, the unusual torque resulting from aberrant catheter positioning can result in perforation or erosion of the catheter through the venous wall, with subsequent significant bleeding (Langston, 1971).

Therefore, if the CVP catheter is in a less than optimal position, attempts should be made to reposition it. Fluoroscopy is helpful in making such adjustments, but unfortunately is not generally available in intensive care units (ICUs). After any attempt at repositioning, the position of the catheter should be confirmed by appropriate radiographs.

It is important to realize that catheters frequently change position after initial placement because of patient motion, manipulation of the catheter by physicians or nursing personnel, or straightening or bending of the catheter itself within the vascular system. Position changes resulting from patient motion or alterations of the catheter course are more likely to occur if the catheter crosses a joint (especially the elbow) (Brandt et al., 1970) or follows a circuitous route to the central venous system. (To avoid these problems, some physicians have advo-

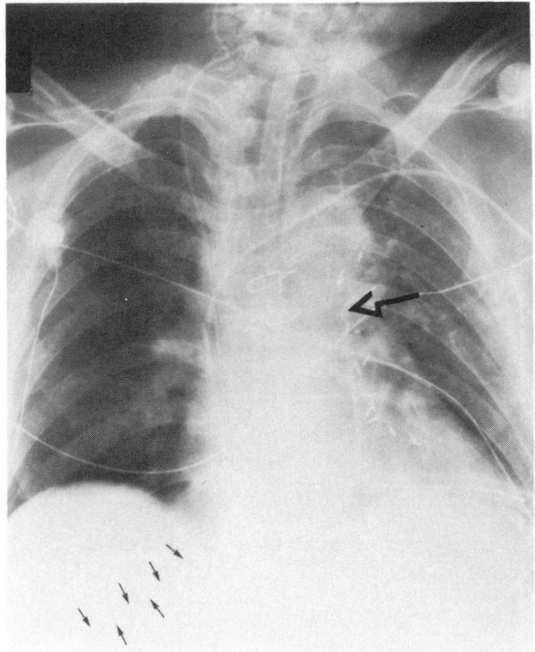

Figure 3–3. CVP catheter extending from the right internal jugular vein through the superior vena cava, the right atrium, and the proximal inferior vena cava to terminate in a hepatic vein. The photograph has been retouched to enhance demonstration, but the catheter was easily visualized on the original radiograph. The Swan-Ganz catheter, inserted via the left subclavian vein, has its tip in the main pulmonary artery (*open arrow*). (From Ravin, C. E., Putman, C. E., and McLoud, T. C.: Am. J. Roentgenol. 126:423, 1976.)

cated the subclavian approach discussed below.) It is, therefore, important to check the position of the catheter on each film obtained. One should not assume that because the catheter was correctly positioned on the initial examination it will remain so; periodic radiographic confirmation of the catheter position is recommended.

CATHETER EMBOLIZATION. Another potentially serious complication is that of catheter breakage and embolization. This can result from laceration of the catheter by the needle used to insert it, fracture at a point of stress, or detachment of the catheter from its hub (Al-Abrak and Samuel, 1974; Blair et al., 1970). Following such an event the catheter fragment may lodge in the vena cava, in the right side of the heart, or in the pulmonary artery (Figs. 9–29, 9–30) and result in thrombosis, infection, or perforation (Blair et al., 1970). To facilitate detection of broken fragments, it is strongly recommended that only radiopaque catheters be employed in ICUs. Frequently it is possible to retrieve such radiopaque catheter fragments under fluoroscopic control (see Chapter 9), although on occasion thoracotomy is required (Blair et al., 1970).

SUBCLAVIAN CATHETERS

Subclavian catheters have proved to be extremely useful in providing rapid access to the central venous system (Fontenelle et al., 1971), particularly in those patients in whom there is peripheral vascular collapse. Because of its large size and consistent anatomic location, the subclavian vein is readily available for venipuncture even when peripheral vessels are not. Its size and rapid blood flow allow a catheter to be left in place for prolonged periods without significant risk of thrombosis—a great advantage in situations requiring hyperalimentation (Dudrick et al., 1969). Moreover, because the catheters employed in this technique are shorter (6 to 8 inches) than the previously discussed CVP catheters and because no moving joints are traversed, changes in catheter position after initial placement are far less frequent. On the other hand, differences in the method of insertion of the subclavian catheters predispose patients to several unique complications.

Ideal Position

The ideal position for the subclavian catheter is identical to that of the CVP catheter discussed previously.

Potential Complications

ANATOMIC AND TECHNICAL CONSIDERATIONS. An understanding of the potential complications related to the use of the subclavian catheter is facilitated by knowledge of the regional anatomy. The subclavian vein enters the thorax over the anterior portion of the first rib, and lies between the rib and the overlying clavicle. It is separated from its companion artery by the intervening scalenus anticus muscle. The pleura covering the apex of the lung lies approximately ½ cm deep to the subclavian vein. In addition, the phrenic nerve as well as the nerves of the brachial plexus, particularly its inferior trunk, lie in close proximity to both the vein and the artery.

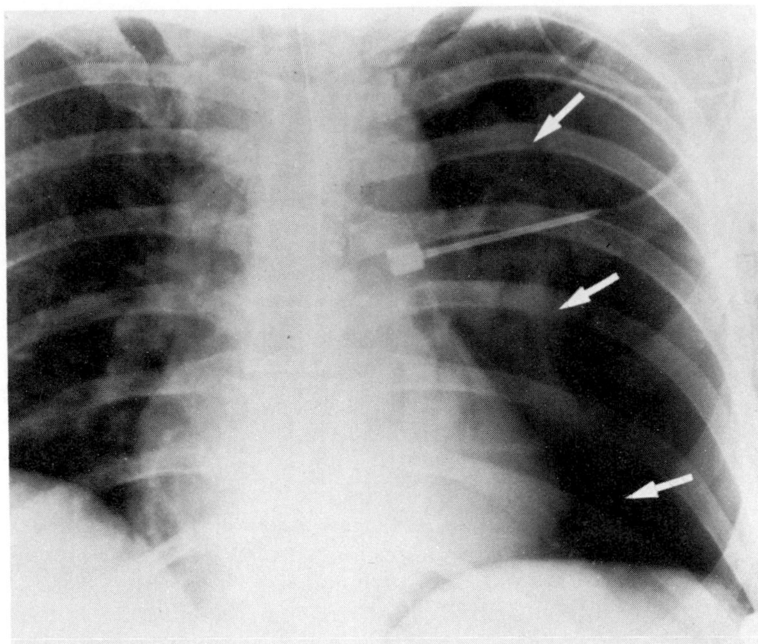

Figure 3–4. Anteroposterior (AP) portable chest film demonstrating a large left pneumothorax accompanied by complete collapse of the left lung (*arrows*). This pneumothorax was not detected clinically, although the patient had been examined on several occasions before the film was obtained. Successful placement of the subclavian line had required several attempts and it is thought that the pneumothorax resulted from one of the early unsuccessful attempts. (From Ravin, C. E, Putman, C. E., and McLoud, T. C.: Am. J. Roentgenol. 126:423, 1976.)

The standard subclavian approach is to insert a needle under the inferior border of the clavicle at its midpoint and direct it toward the suprasternal notch. Its course will carry it into the subclavian vein just beneath the sternoclavicular joint (Davidson et al., 1963). Prospective studies indicate that the number of complications encountered in the placement of subclavian lines relates to the experience of the physician doing the venipuncture (Bernard and Stahl, 1971), and, as expected, complications are a function of the time available for insertion of the catheter—they are more frequent in emergency settings.

PNEUMOTHORAX. The complication most frequently discovered by radiologists is pneumothorax (Fig. 3–4). This is often difficult to detect clinically; therefore, it is strongly recommended that a chest film (upright, with the patient in expiration, if possible) be obtained whenever placement of a subclavian catheter has been attempted. Should initial placement fail, it is imperative that a film be obtained before placement is attempted on the opposite side, since failure to recognize the pre-existing pneumothorax may result in creation of bilateral pneumothoraces when contralateral placement is attempted (Fig. 3–5) (Maggs and Schwaber, 1977).

ECTOPIC INFUSION. Another potential complication is ectopic infusion of fluid into the mediastinum (Adar and Mozes, 1970) (Fig. 3–6) or pleural space (Aulenbacher, 1970 (Fig. 3–7). Although this can also occur with CVP catheters, in my experience it has more frequently been associated with the use of subclavian catheters. This probably reflects the greater chance of perivascular catheter placement with the subclavian approach. Infusion of fluid into mediastinal or pleural spaces produces a radiographic appearance suggestive of significant intrathoracic bleeding. In most cases, however, the rapid accumulation of such fluid after insertion of a subclavian catheter should suggest the diagnosis of ectopic infusion. This can be confirmed by thoracentesis, if the fluid is accumulating in the pleural space, or by injection of water-soluble contrast medium through the catheter itself, particularly if fluid is accumulating in the mediastinum. Confirmation of ectopic infusion by these methods avoids the more involved angiographic procedures required to exclude major arterial or venous bleeding. In general, mediastinal bleeding resulting from catheter injury tends to tamponade itself, and only rarely is surgical repair of the laceration required.

MISCELLANEOUS COMPLICATIONS. A multitude of other complications have been infrequently associated with subclavian venipuncture. Of these, the most common is inadvertent puncture of the subclavian artery (Bernard and

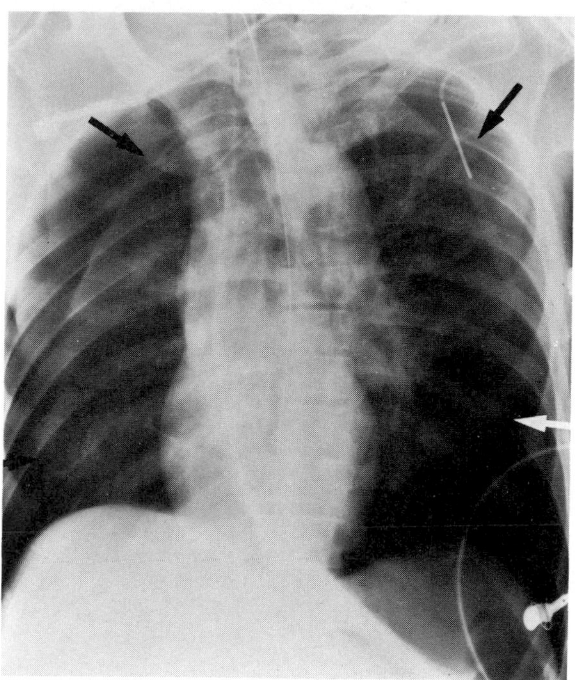

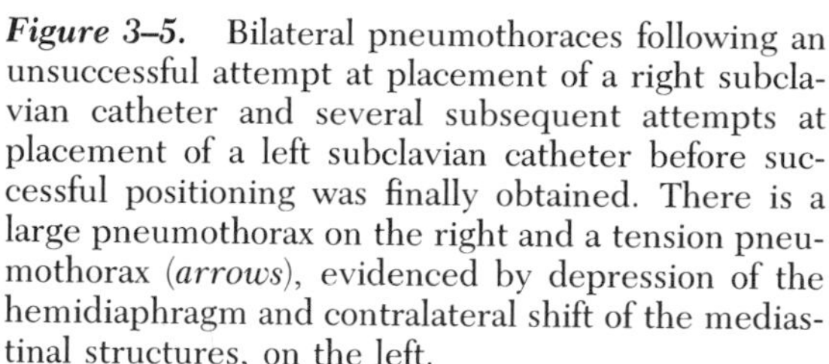

Figure 3–5. Bilateral pneumothoraces following an unsuccessful attempt at placement of a right subclavian catheter and several subsequent attempts at placement of a left subclavian catheter before successful positioning was finally obtained. There is a large pneumothorax on the right and a tension pneumothorax (*arrows*), evidenced by depression of the hemidiaphragm and contralateral shift of the mediastinal structures, on the left.

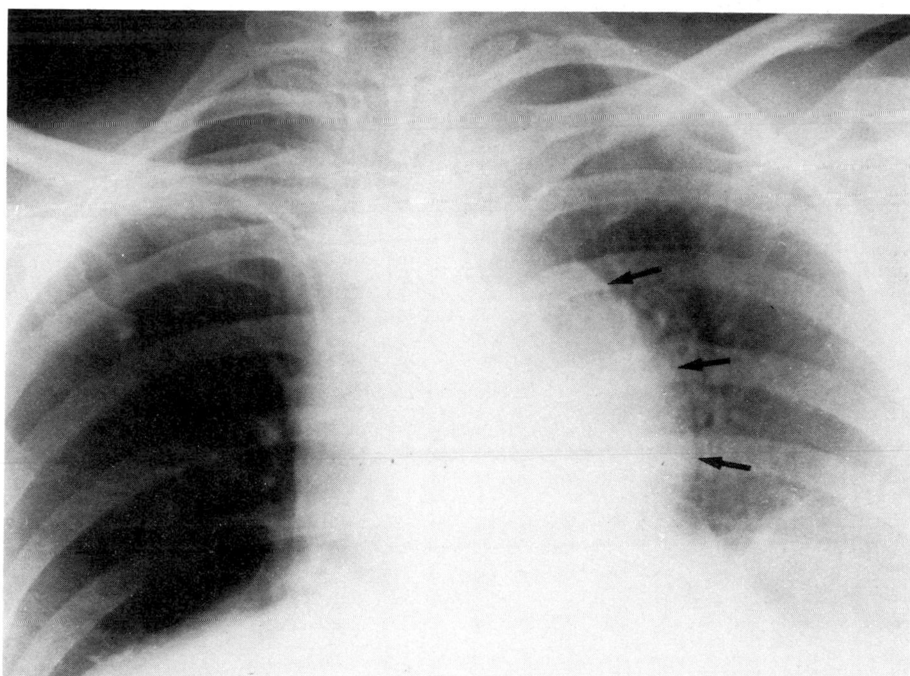

Figure 3–6. Hemorrhage after an unsuccessful left subclavian catheter insertion. The right subclavian catheter is in normal position in the superior vena cava. The right lung is normal. On the supine film, fluid is seen over the entire left lung. There is marked widening of the mediastinal shadow on the left (*arrows*). These findings were not present on a previous radiograph. Since no fluid was ever infused through the left catheter, these changes are presumably due to bleeding. The mass regressed with time.

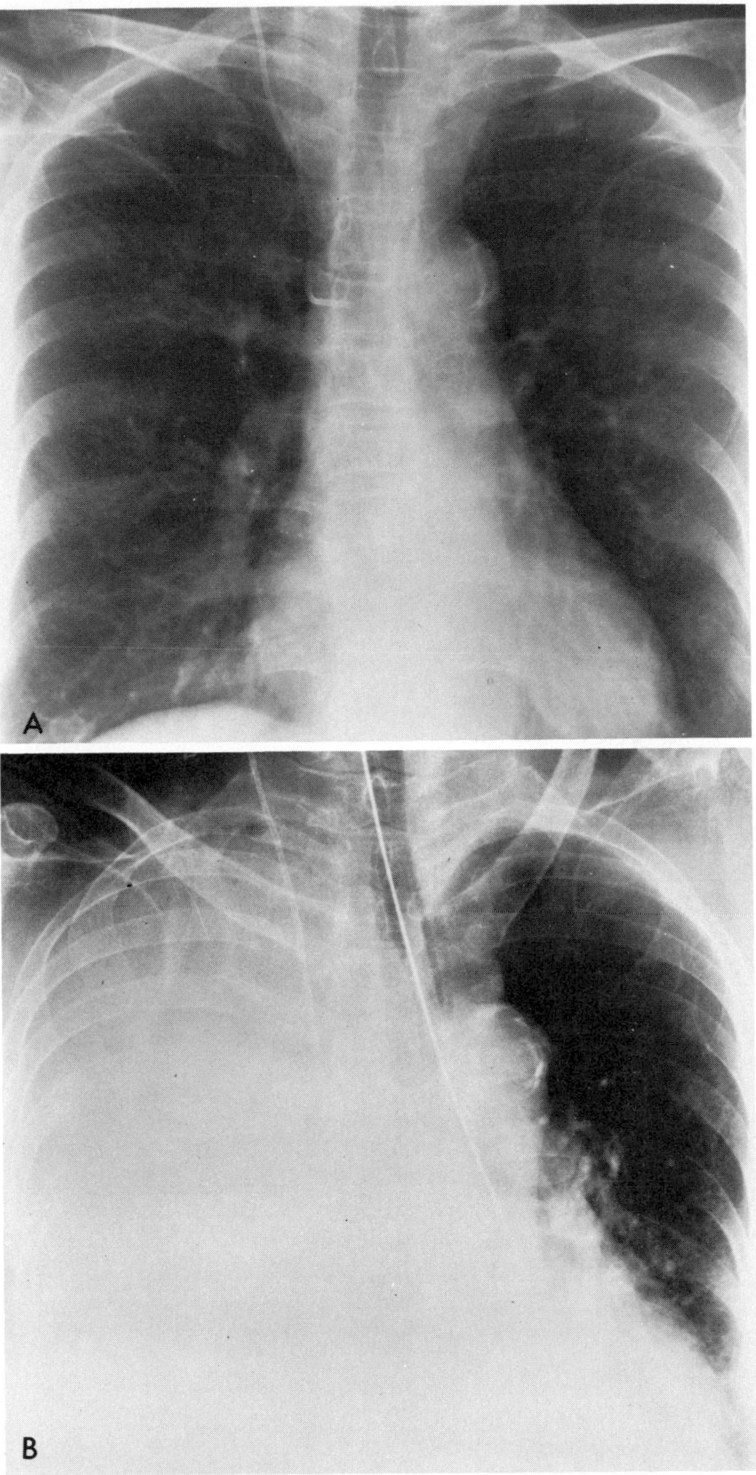

Figure 3–7. A, PA radiograph demonstrating a CVP catheter inserted via the right internal jugular vein. The distal tip makes an unusual curve medially. *B*, Following intravenous administration of several liters of fluid through the catheter, complete opacification of the right hemithorax was noted. Diagnostic thoracentesis demonstrated the pleural fluid to be identical to that being infused through the catheter.

Stahl, 1971). In the vast majority of instances, the resultant bleeding is of no clinical significance and is readily controlled by direct pressure. Infrequently, more significant bleeding with hematoma formation may occur, and on rare occasions surgical intervention is required to repair a lacerated subclavian artery (Lefrak and Noon, 1972). In addition to bleeding, infrequent fatal air embolism (Flanagan et al., 1969) and injury to the phrenic nerve (Drachler et al., 1976) or to branches of the brachial plexus have been reported. Clot frequently forms in the veins with prolonged catheterization (Fig. 3–8). However, symptomatic venous obstruction or pulmonary embolism is uncommon. With experience and careful attention to technique, the incidence of complications resulting from the use of the subclavian technique can be markedly reduced (Merk and Rush, 1975).

SWAN-GANZ CATHETERS

As noted previously, one of the most important factors in the management of critically ill patients is maintenance of optimal blood volume. Monitoring of the CVP to determine the optimal volume has several significant limitations (see Chapter 1). More accuracy has been obtained by monitoring pulmonary capillary wedge (PCW) pressures through use of the flow-directed Swan-Ganz catheter (DeLaurentis et al., 1973; Fisher et al., 1975; Humphrey et al., 1976). The basic catheter consists of a central channel for pressure monitoring and a second, smaller channel connected to an inflatable balloon at the catheter tip (Swan and Ganz, 1975) (see Chapter 1). Recent modifications of the catheter also allow determinations of cardiac output and CVP (Forrester et al., 1972). The catheter can be inserted at the bedside and "floated" to the pulmonary artery without need for fluoroscopic monitoring. It is distinguished radiographically from standard IV catheters by the presence of a radiopaque stripe down its center.

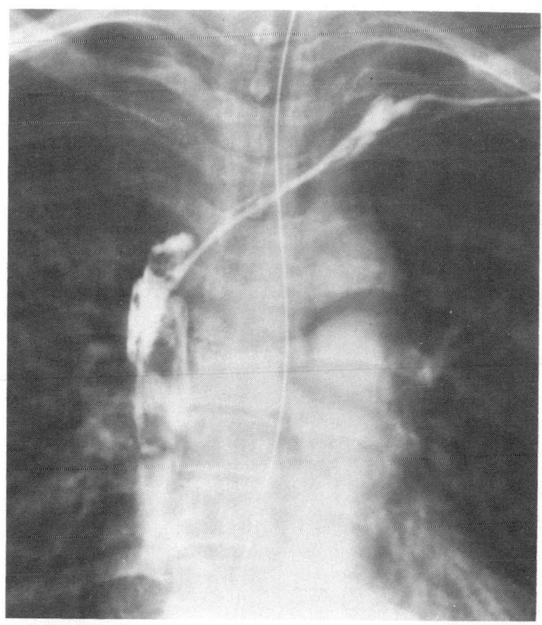

Figure 3–8. Superior vena cava thrombosis after prolonged catheterization. Venogram through the offending catheter demonstrates a large clot in the SVC and innominate vein.

Ideal Position

Ideally, the catheter is positioned so that it lies within the right or left main pulmonary artery (Swan and Ganz, 1975) (Figs. 1–6, 3–3). Inflating the balloon causes the catheter to "float" downstream into a wedge position, and deflating the balloon allows the catheter to "recoil" into the central pulmonary artery. Excessive intravenous or intracardiac slack enhances the likelihood of distal migration of the catheter, which increases the incidence of complications.

Potential Complications

PULMONARY INFARCTION. The most common significant complication associated with use of the Swan-Ganz catheter is pulmonary infarction distal to the catheter tip (Foote et al., 1974; Sise et al., 1981) (Figs. 3–9 and 3–10). Infarction occurs as a result of occlusion of the pulmonary artery by the catheter itself or as a result of clot formation in or about the catheter (McLoud and Putman, 1975; Ravin et al., 1976; Yorra et al., 1974) (Fig. 3–8).

Another potential cause of in situ thrombosis is inadvertent failure to deflate the catheter balloon (Foote et al., 1974) (Fig. 3–11). The balloon is seen as a 1-cm rounded radiolucency located at the tip of the catheter. Because of its size, a persistently inflated balloon can potentially obstruct a major pulmonary artery and lead to significant pulmonary infarction. The radiographic patterns of pulmonary infarction

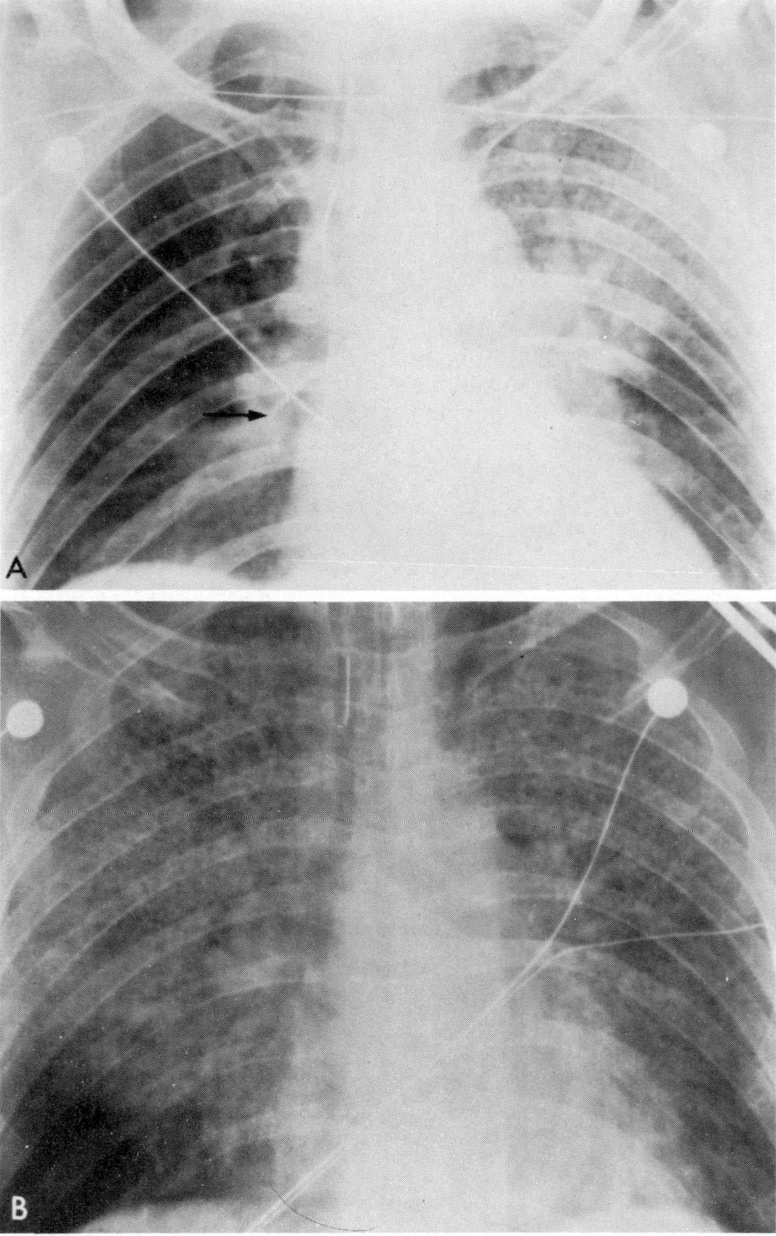

Figure 3–9. *A*, AP radiograph demonstrating a Swan-Ganz catheter in the right lower lobe pulmonary artery, where it had been positioned for several days (*arrow*). There is some air space consolidation in the left upper lobe on this film, consistent with pulmonary edema. *B*, Radiograph obtained the next day, demonstrating diffuse pulmonary edema sparing the portion of the right lower lobe supplied by the pulmonary artery in which the Swan-Ganz catheter had been positioned. It is likely that a pulmonary embolus from the catheter blocked blood flow to this portion of the lung and prevented the development of pulmonary edema in this area. The remaining portions of the lung, which had unobstructed perfusion, became edematous when the patient developed congestive heart failure.

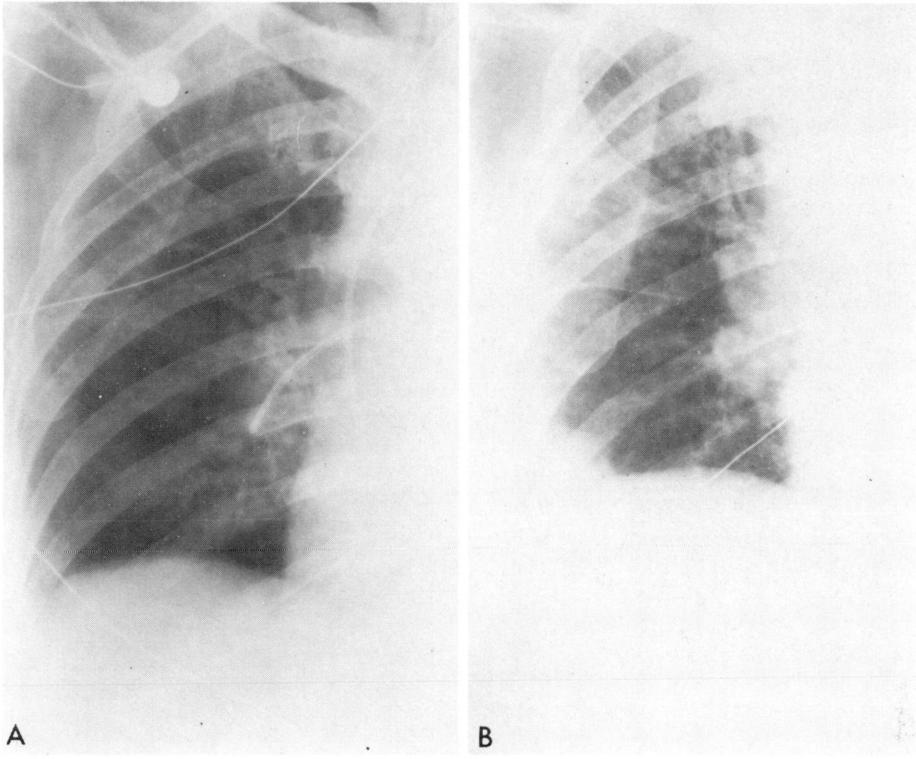

Figure 3–10. *A*, Swan-Ganz catheter positioned in a basilar segmental artery of the right lower lobe. *B*, Follow-up examination two days later, demonstrating a pleural-based density in the right costophrenic angle with a convex upper border consistent with pulmonary infarction. (From Ravin, C. E., Putman, C. E., and McLoud, T. C.: Am. J. Roentgenol. 126:423, 1976.)

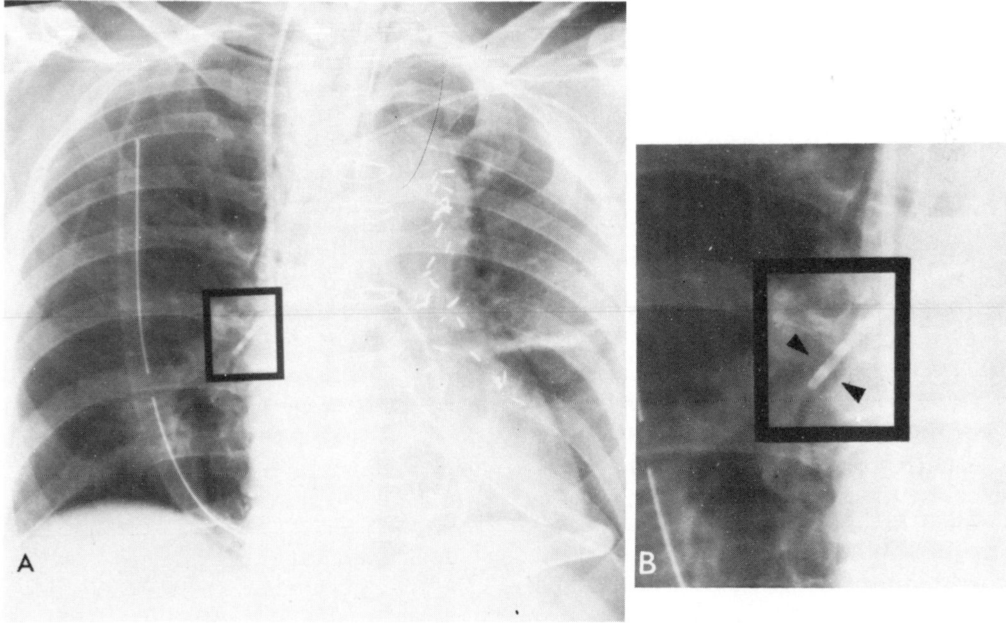

Figure 3–11. *A*, AP portable radiograph demonstrating a Swan-Ganz catheter making several loops in the right ventricle. The area outlined in the box, *B*, shows that the balloon (*arrows*) at the tip of the catheter remains partially inflated, creating the potential for massive thrombosis. (From Ravin, C. E., Putman, C. E., and McLoud, T. C.: Am. J. Roentgenol. 126:423, 1976.)

are similar to those seen with infarction from other causes (McLoud and Putman, 1975). Most consist of patchy airspace infiltrates involving the area of the lung supplied by the pulmonary artery in which the catheter lies. On occasion, Hampton's hump configuration is identified. Often, however, no definite radiographic manifestation of infarction is noted, although evidence of it can be found at autopsy.

If recognized or suspected, pulmonary infarction is treated by removal of the Swan-Ganz catheter. Systemic heparinization is not required, since the source of the emboli and obstruction has been removed.

Arrhythmias. Passage of Swan-Ganz catheters through the right side of the heart has been infrequently associated with both atrial (Geha et al., 1973) and ventricular (Cairns and Holder, 1975) arrhythmias, as well as with complete heart block (Abernathy, 1974). In addition, insertion of an excessive length of catheter can lead to coiling or redundancy in the right side of the heart (Figs. 3–11, 3–12), resulting in irritation of the conducting bundle and production of premature ventricular contractions.

Miscellaneous complications. Rare instances of pulmonary arterial rupture (Chun and Ellestad, 1971; Lapin and Murray, 1972), pulmonary artery to bronchial tree fistula (Rubin and Puckett, 1974), intracardiac knotting of the catheter (Lipp et al., 1971), and balloon rupture (Swan et al., 1970) have been reported with use of the Swan-Ganz catheter. Most of these complications can be avoided, however, if the recommendations for use and positioning of the catheter are strictly followed.

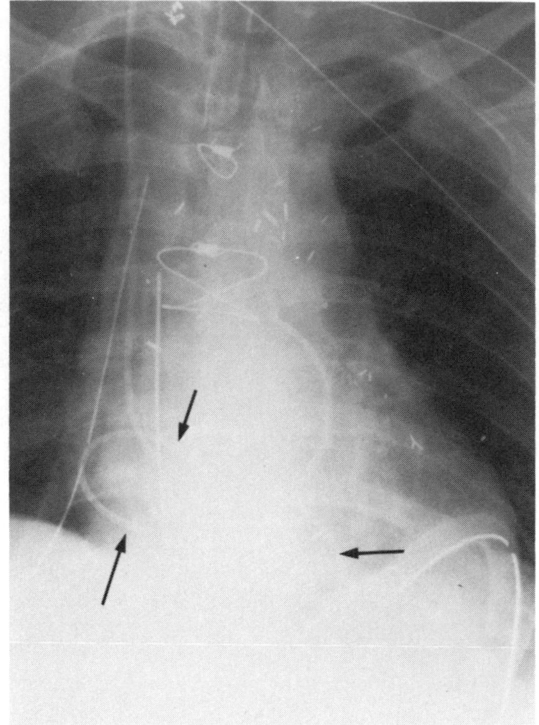

Figure 3–12. Inadvertent insertion of an excessive length of Swan-Ganz catheter resulted in coiling of loops in the right atrium and right ventricle (*arrows*). This condition frequently produces arrhythmias that are refractory to drug therapy; these are readily corrected, however, by straightening the catheter. The tip of the catheter is in the right main pulmonary artery.

INTRA-AORTIC COUNTERPULSATION BALLOON

The intra-aortic counterpulsation balloon (IACB) is being employed with increasing frequency in order to improve cardiac function in the setting of cardiogenic shock or high-risk cardiac surgery (Cleveland et al., 1975; Weber and Janicki, 1974). The device consists of a fusiform inflatable balloon approximately 26 cm in length surrounding the distal end of a centrally placed catheter. The balloon is inflated with approximately 40 ml of gas during diastole and is forcibly deflated during systole. Inflation-deflation timing is linked to the electrocardiogram (ECG). Inflation during diastole increases diastolic pressure in the proximal aorta, thereby increasing perfusion of the coronary arteries and increasing oxygen delivery to the myocardium. The pattern of balloon deflation is such that it starts the column of aortic blood moving distally, thereby decreasing the afterload against which the left ventricle must eject its stroke volume, and diminishing left ventricular work and oxygen requirements. The overall effect of balloon pumping, therefore, is increased oxygen delivery to the myocardium and decreased left ventricular work, resulting in overall improvement in cardiac function (Dunkman et al., 1972).

Radiographically, the device appears as a catheter surrounded at its distal end during diastole by an oblong, gas-filled balloon (Hyson et al., 1977) (Fig. 3–13). During systole, the balloon is deflated and is not visualized radiographically.

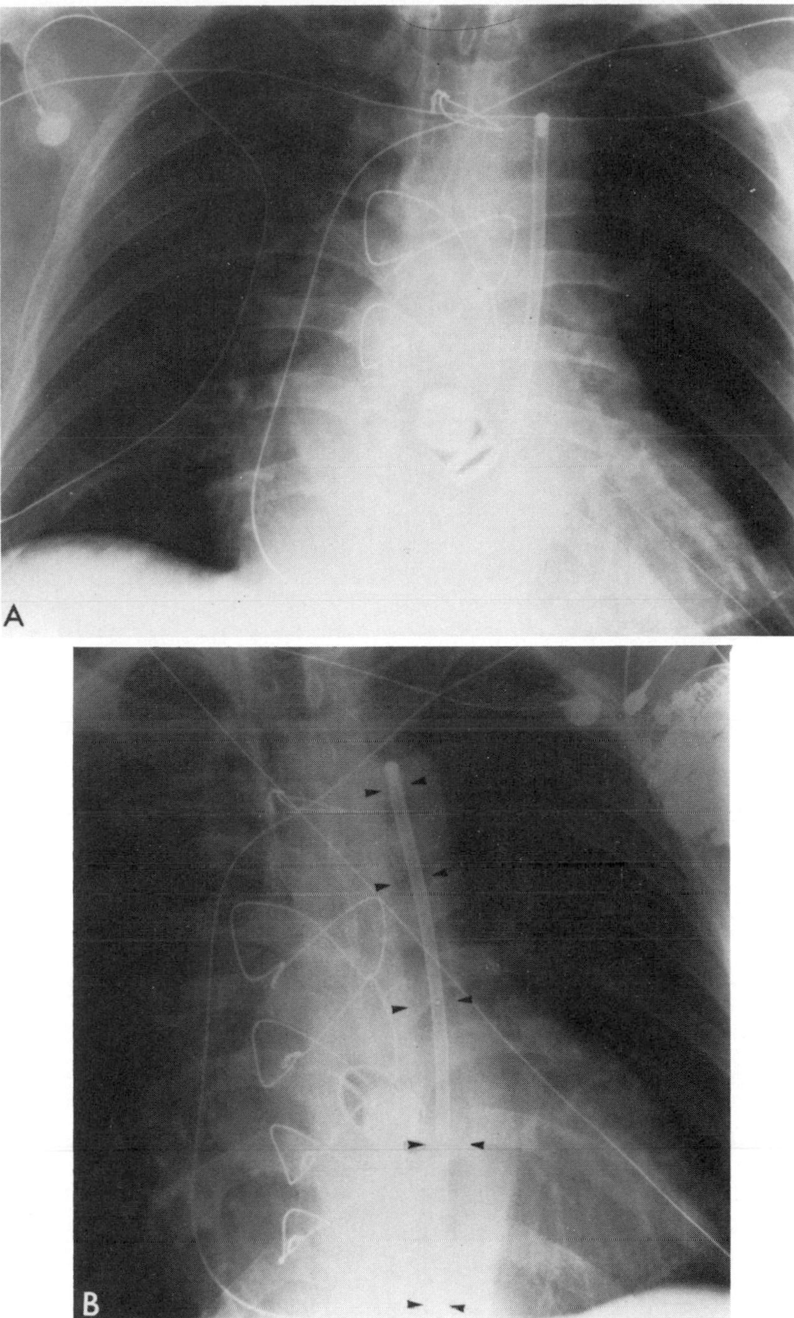

Figure 3–13. IACB correctly positioned with its tip at the level of the aortic arch. *A*, During systole the balloon is deflated and is not visualized radiographically. *B*, During diastole, the balloon is inflated and is seen as a radiolucent filling defect within the aortic lumen. A ball valve mitral prosthesis is visible in systole in *A* and diastole in *B*. (From Hyson et al.: Am. J. Roentgenol. 128:915, 1977.)

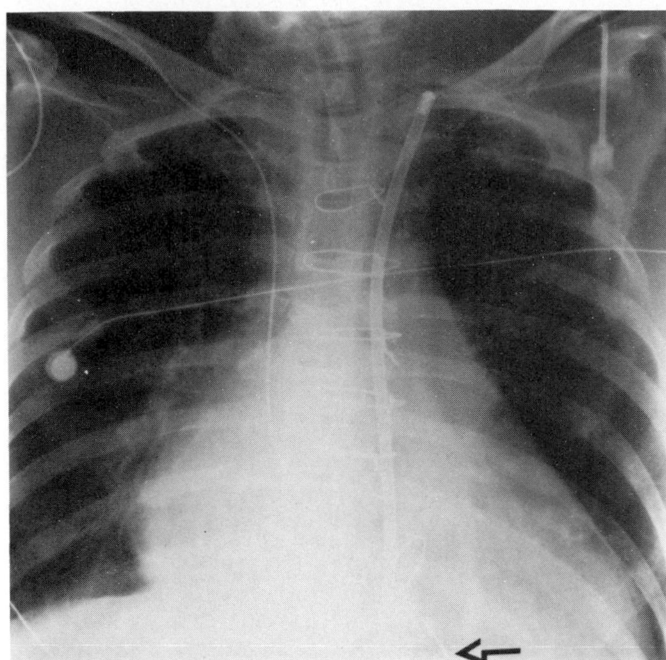

Figure 3–14. IACB has been advanced too far and its tip lies in the left subclavian artery. The transvenous pacer wire is in the right ventricle, not at the apex, however (*arrow*). (From Ravin, C. E., Putman, C. E., and McLoud, T. C.: Am. J. Roentgenol. 126:423, 1976.)

Ideal Position

The IACB is inserted through a Dacron graft placed end-to-side to the common femoral artery and then advanced retrograde to the thoracic aorta (Kantrowitz et al., 1968). Ideally, the tip of the catheter should be placed just distal to the left subclavian artery (Fig. 3–13). This allows maximal augmentation of diastolic pressures in the proximal aorta, and decreases the risk of embolization of the cerebral vessels. In clinical practice, the tip of the device is placed so that it projects at the level of the aortic knob on the frontal radiograph (Hyson et al., 1977). At present, this is achieved by having the surgeon estimate the length of catheter needed to reach from the site of insertion in the femoral artery to the level of the aortic knob. In most cases, this has been satisfactory, although attempts are currently being made to use fluoroscopic monitoring to ensure ideal positioning.

Potential Complications

ABERRANT POSITIONING. If the catheter is advanced too far, it either may enter and obstruct the left subclavian artery (O'Rourke and Shepherd, 1963) (Fig. 3–14) or may be positioned in the aortic arch, increasing the risk of cerebral embolus. More commonly, the aorta proves to be more tortuous than anticipated and the balloon does not reach the level of the aortic knob, but is positioned more distally (Fig. 3–15). This results in less effective counterpulsation, and, if too distal, the balloon may obstruct the major abdominal vessels when inflated. Thus, following placement of the IACB, a film is strongly recommended to determine accurately its position and any need for adjustment.

AORTIC DISSECTION. Another potential complication of the IACB is dissection into or through the aortic wall at the time of insertion. Several cases have been described in which such dissection occurred but was of no clinical consequence (Dunkman et al., 1972), although in other instances dissection has been followed by death (Pace et al., 1976). A history of difficulty in inserting the device or complaints of pain by the patient during the procedure should alert the radiologist to this potential complication. In addition, loss of definition of the descending thoracic aorta on the chest radiograph following placement of the IACB may occasionally be an early clue to intramural positioning (Hyson et al., 1977) (Fig. 3–16). Aortography is generally required to confirm this ectopic location. The angiographer should be aware that

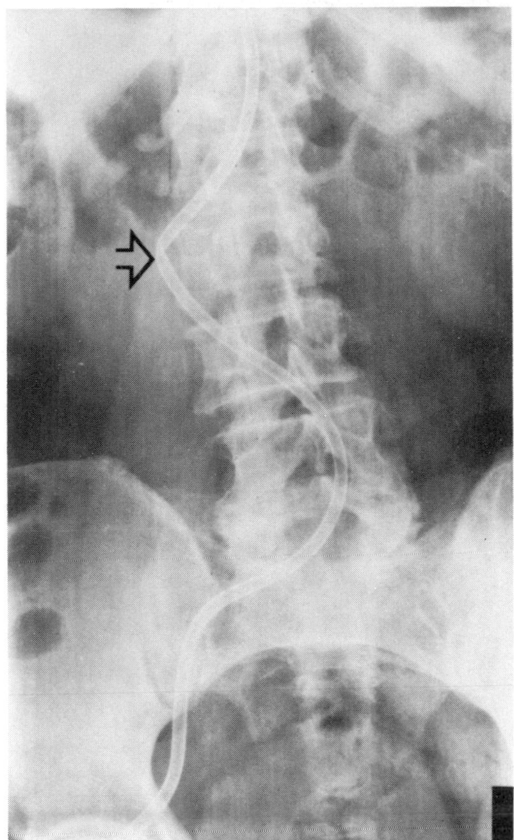

Figure 3–15. AP radiograph of the abdomen demonstrating the markedly circuitous course of the IACB owing to tortuosity of the abdominal aorta. There is also a kink (*arrow*) in the balloon catheter. (From Hyson et al.: Am. J. Roentgenol. 128:915, 1977.)

patients undergoing balloon pumping are fully heparinized, and that performance of arteriography is therefore more complicated and the risk of postprocedure bleeding increased.

MISCELLANEOUS COMPLICATIONS. Other risks associated with use of the IACB include reduction of platelets, red blood cell destruction, emboli, balloon rupture with gas embolus, and vascular insufficiency of the catheterized limb (Weber and Janicki, 1974). Most of these complications are not recognized radiographically, although confirmation of vascular insufficiency may require arteriography.

TRANSVENOUS PACEMAKERS

Since its introduction in the late 1950's, transvenous endocardial pacing has become the method of choice for maintaining cardiac rhythm in patients with heart block or other bradyarrhythmias (Chung, 1976). The pacemaker electrode catheter is inserted into the external jugular vein or the cephalic vein and directed under fluoroscopic control to the apex of the right ventricle.

Ideal Position

Ideally, the catheter is positioned in the apex of the right ventricle and is wedged beneath the trabeculae carneae area to ensure stability as well as intimate contact with the endocardium (Fig. 3–20). Sharp angulation in the course of the catheter from the pulse-generator unit to the distal tip should be avoided, since such areas are under increased mechanical stress and may fracture (McHenry and Grayson, 1970). Gentle curves of the catheter through the veins and heart are also desirable to help avoid catheter recoil. Radiographs in both frontal and lateral projections are required to assess positioning completely. On the frontal view the catheter should project at the apex of the right ventricle, and on the lateral view the tip of the catheter should lie anteriorly 3 to 4 mm beneath the epicardial fat stripe (Ormond et al., 1971).

Potential Complications

ABERRANT POSITIONING. The most common abnormality recognized radiographically is malpositioning. Common aberrant locations include the coronary sinus, the right atrium, the pulmonary outflow tract, and the pulmonary artery (Figs. 3–14, 3–17). Of these, the most difficult to assess radiographically is placement in the coronary sinus. In this location the catheter often appears to be ideally positioned on the frontal projection, but is directed posteriorly rather than anteriorly on the lateral projection. If only a frontal view can be obtained, however, a clue to ectopic placement in the coronary sinus is an upward deflection of the catheter tip as it follows the sinus around the posterior atrioventricular groove (Hall and Rosenbaum, 1971).

On occasion, pacemakers are intentionally placed in the coronary sinus in order to achieve atrial rather than ventricular pacing. This is done primarily in investigation of various bradyarrhythmias and tachyarrhythmias (Hewitt et al., 1981). However, for the most part, such

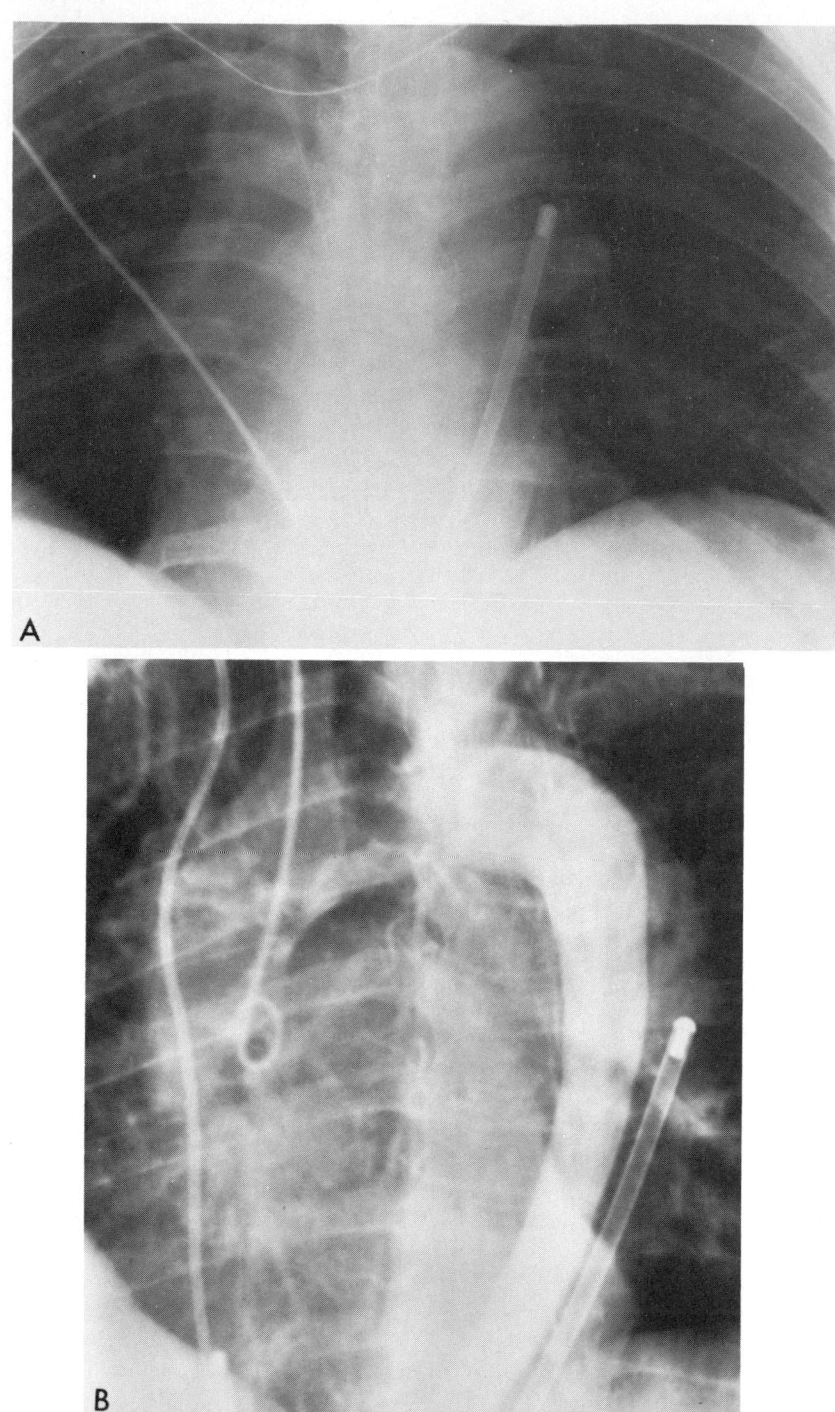

Figure 3–16. *A*, Following treatment of an IACB, the border of the descending aorta is indistinct. The patient complained of pain at the time of insertion. *B*, Aortogram demonstrating the extraluminal position of the IACB. (From Hyson et al.: Am. J. Roentgenol. 128:915, 1977.)

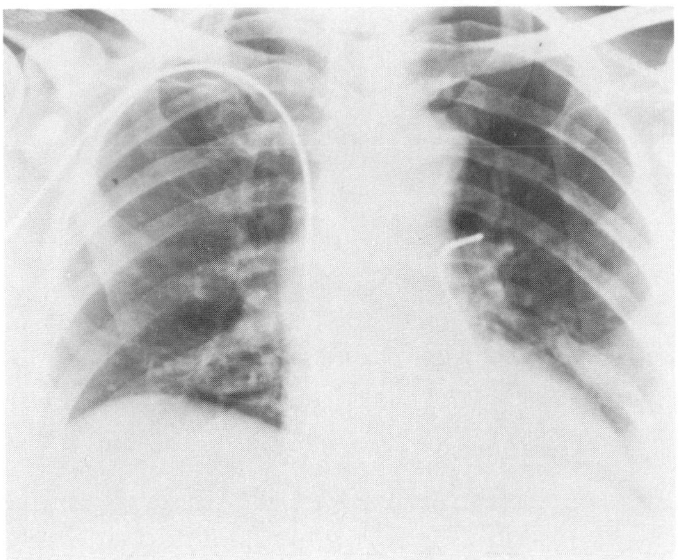

Figure 3–17. Transvenous pacer wire inadvertently advanced to the left pulmonary artery.

investigations are not carried out in the ICU, and thus positioning in the coronary sinus (Fig. 3–18) should be viewed with suspicion in this setting.

MYOCARDIAL PERFORATION. Another potential complication is perforation of the myocardium by the catheter itself. This may be difficult to recognize unless the catheter clearly projects outside the myocardium (Fig. 3–19) or anterior to the epicardial fat stripe (Ormond et al., 1971). Although hemopericardium accompanied by cardiac tamponade can occur, most such perforations are not of great clinical significance, since withdrawal of the catheter will correct the

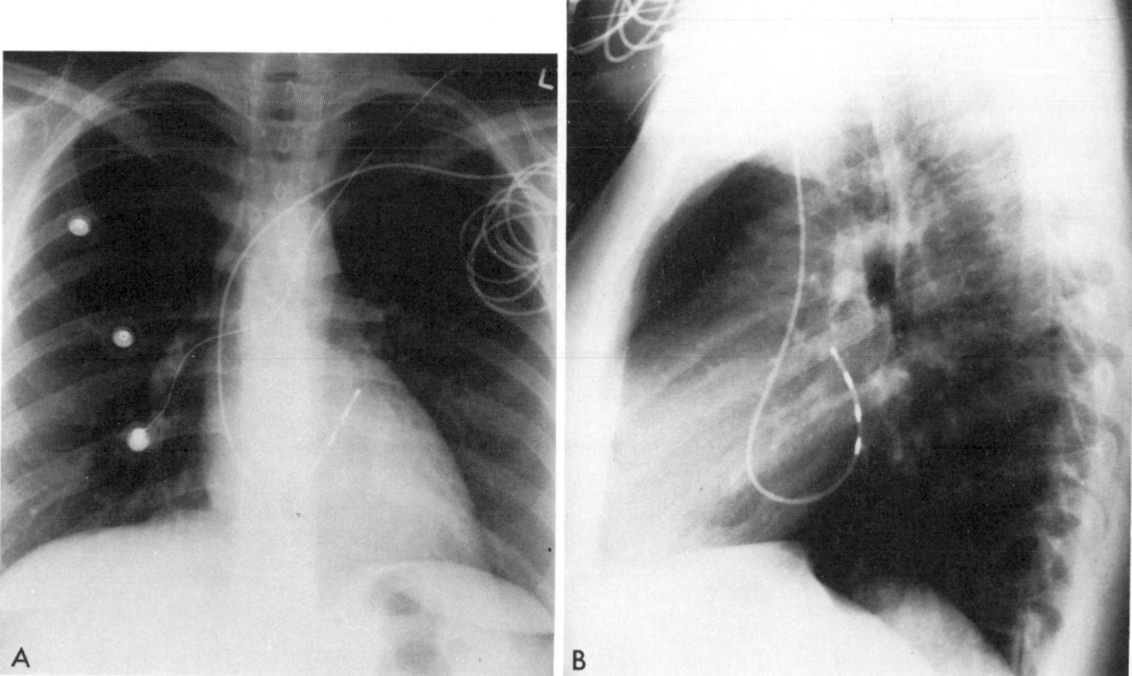

Figure 3–18. *A*, Note upward direction of the catheter tip, which is positioned in the coronary sinus. The sinus runs in the posterior atrioventricular groove. *B*, The lateral view confirms positioning in the coronary sinus as evidenced by the posterior location of the catheter.

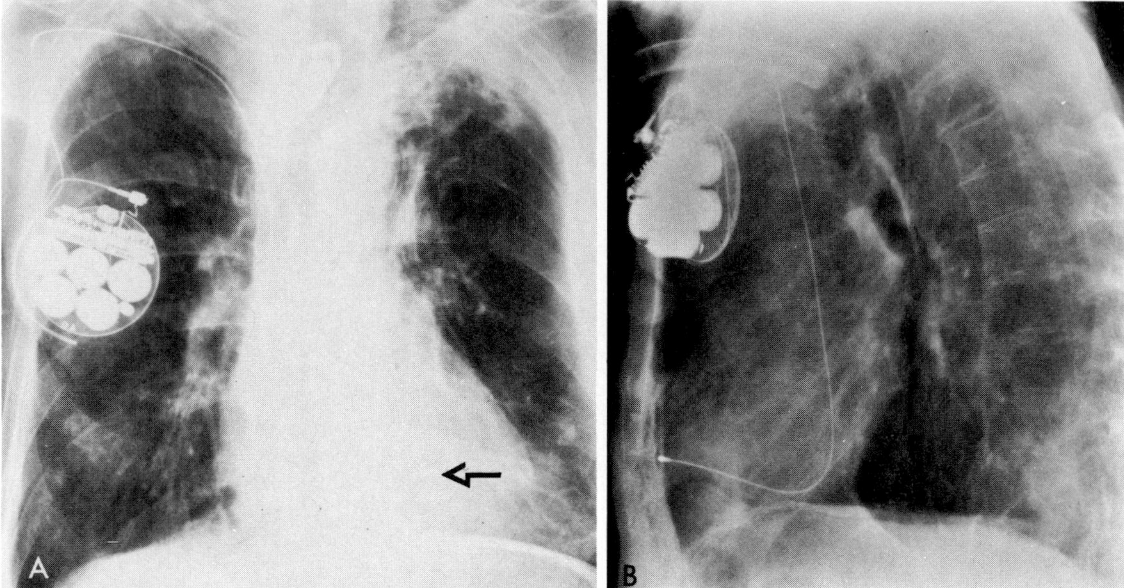

Figure 3–19. *A*, PA chest radiograph of a patient with a transvenous pacemaker who developed a pneumomediastinum following tracheostomy. The tip of the pacing electrode is barely visible projecting over the right ventricle *(arrow)*. *B*, Lateral view showing the pacemaker tip extending beyond the myocardium into the pericardial space. This had not been clinically suspected before the patient developed a pneumomediastinum. (*Note*: tracheostomy tube is poorly positioned in the trachea.)

position and not cause significant bleeding (McHenry and Hopkins, 1968; Sorkin et al., 1976).

Mechanical problems. In the clinical setting of inadequate pacing, the radiologist must also be alert to the possibility of fracture of the electrode wires or detachment of the pacemaker wires from the pulse unit. Although detachments can be readily recognized, electrode fracture (Fig. 3–20) may be more difficult to define because the insulating sheath can hold the broken ends close enough together to escape detection (Hall and Rosenbaum, 1971). Fluoroscopy, if available, is sometimes useful to better evaluate pacemaker electrodes for fracture.

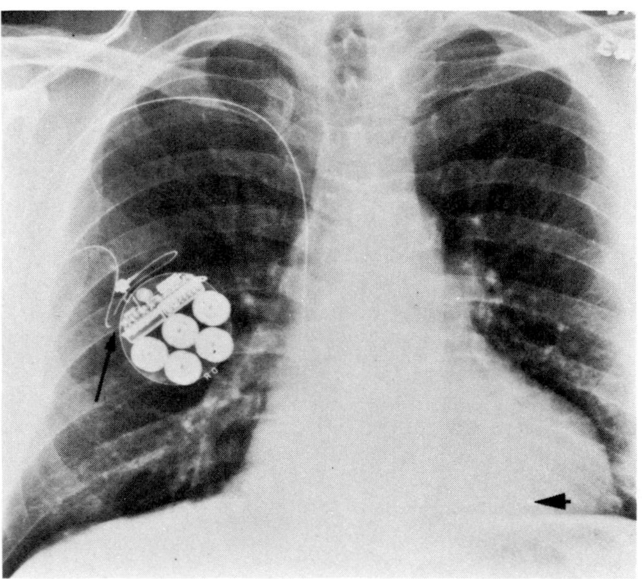

Figure 3–20. PA chest radiograph in a patient who had symptoms of congestive failure and was not pacing satisfactorily. The pacer wire is fractured *(arrow)* just distal to the pacer unit. The electrode tip projects over the apex of the right ventricle *(arrowhead)*.

Inadequate pacing may also result from failure of the pulse-generator due to battery failure. Although initial reports enthusiastically outlined radiographic criteria by which battery failure could be determined (Lillehei et al., 1965), in actual practice such techniques are difficult to apply (Sorkin et al., 1976). The major drawback has been difficulty in obtaining perfectly aligned views of the batteries. Any angulation of the battery with reference to the x-ray beam distorts the image and produces a picture similar to that described in battery failure (that is, irregularity or obliteration of the radiolucent rings and central core of the battery). Thus, it is usually easier, particularly in the ICU setting, to measure the electronic output of the pacer directly in order to determine battery failure.

SUMMARY

Although development of various cardiovascular monitoring and assist devices during the past 10 to 15 years has contributed significantly to improved management of seriously ill patients, the devices are not without potential complications of their own. Many of these complications are difficult, if not impossible, to detect clinically but are readily apparent on standard radiographs. Knowledge of the purpose of a device, its ideal position, and the potential complications facilitates better interpretation of radiographs obtained in the ICU and leads to early detection of the complications.

REFERENCES

Abernathy, W. S.: Complete heart block caused by the Swan-Ganz catheter. Chest 65:349, 1974.

Adar, R., and Mozes, M.: Hydromediastinum. J.A.M.A. 214:372, 1970.

Al-Abrak, M. H., and Samuel, J. R.: An unusual cause of breaking of a central venous catheter. Anaesthesia 29:585, 1974.

Aulenbacher, C. E.: Hydrothorax from subclavian vein catheterization. J.A.M.A. 214:372, 1970.

Bernard, R. W., and Stahl, W. M.: Subclavian vein catheterizations; a prospective study. 1. Noninfectious complications. Ann. Surg. 173:184, 1971.

Blair, E., Hunziker, R., and Flanagan, M. E.: Catheter embolism. Surgery 67:457, 1970.

Bone, D. K., Maddrey, W. C., Eagan, J., and Cameron, J. L.: Cardiac tamponade, a fatal complication of central venous catheterization. Surgery 106:868, 1973.

Brandt, R. L., Foley, W. J., Fink, G. H., et al.: Mechanism of perforation of the heart with production of hydropericardium by a venous catheter and its prevention. Am. J. Surg. 119:311, 1970.

Cairns, J. A., and Holder, D.: Ventricular fibrillation due to passage of a Swan-Ganz catheter. Am. J. Cardiol. 35:509, 1975.

Chun, G. M. H., and Ellestad, M. H.: Perforation of the pulmonary artery by a Swan-Ganz catheter. N. Engl. J. Med. 284:1041, 1971.

Chung, E. K.: Artificial cardiac pacing. Postgrad. Med. 59:83, 1976.

Cleveland, J. C., LeFemine, A. A., Madoff, I., et al.: The role of intraaortic balloon counterpulsation in patients undergoing cardiac operations. Ann. Thorac. Surg. 20:652, 1975.

Daly, J. M., Ziegler, B., and Dudrick, S. J.: Central venous catheterization. Am. J. Nurs. 75(5):820, 1975.

Davidson, J. T., Ben-Hur, N., and Nathen, H.: Subclavian venipuncture. Lancet 2:1139, 1963.

DeLaurentis, D. A., Hayes, M., Matsumoto, T., et al.: Does central venous pressure accurately reflect hemodynamic and fluid volume patterns in the critical surgical patient? Am. J. Surg. 126:415, 1973.

Drachler, D. H., Koepke, G. H., and Weg, J. G.: Phrenic nerve injury from subclavian vein catheterization. J.A.M.A. 236:2880, 1976.

Dudrick, S. J., Wilmore, D. W., Vars, H. M., et al.: Can intravenous feeding as the sole means of nutrition support growth in the child and restore weight loss in an adult? An affirmative answer. Ann. Surg. 169:974, 1969.

Dunkman, W. B., Leinbach, R. C., Buckley, M. J., et al.: Clinical and hemodynamic results of intra-aortic balloon pumping and surgery for cardiogenic shock. Circulation 46:465, 1972.

Fisher, M. L., DeFelice, C. E., and Parisi, A. F.: Assessing left ventricular filling pressure with flow-directed (Swan-Ganz) catheters. Chest 68:542, 1975.

Flanagan, J. P., Gradisar, I. A., Gross, R. J., et al.: Air embolus—a lethal complication of subclavian venipuncture. N. Engl. J. Med. 281:488, 1969.

Fontenelle, L. T., Dooley, B. N., and Cuello, L.: Subclavian venipuncture and its complications. Ann. Thorac. Surg. 11:331, 1971.

Foote, G. A., Schabel, S. I., and Hodges, M.: Pulmonary complications of the flow-directed balloon-tipped catheter. N. Engl. J. Med. 290:927, 1974.

Forrester, J. S., Ganz, W., Diamond, G., et al.: Thermodilution cardiac output determination with a single flow-directed catheter. Am. Heart J. 83:306, 1972.

Friedman, B. A., and Jurgeleit, H. C.: Perforation of atrium by polyethylene CV catheter. J.A.M.A. 203:1141, 1968.

Geha, D. E., Davis, N. J., and Lappas, D. G.: Persistent atrial arrhythmias associated with placement of a Swan-Ganz catheter. Anesthesiology 39:651, 1973.

Goss, C. M.: Gray's Anatomy (ed. 29). Philadelphia, 1976, Lea & Febiger, pp. 697 and 704.

Hall, W. M., and Rosenbaum, H. B.: The radiology of cardiac pacemakers. Radiol. Clin. North Am. 9:343, 1971.

Hewitt, M. J., Chen, J. T. T., Ravin, C. E., and Gallagher, J. J.: Coronary sinus atrial pacing: radiographic considerations. AJR 136:323, 1981.

Humphrey, C. B., Oury, J. H., Virgilio, R. W., et al.: An analysis of direct and indirect measurements of left atrial filling pressure. J. Thorac. Cardiovasc. Surg. 71:643, 1976.

Hyson, E. A., Ravin, C. E., Kelley, M. J., et al.: The intra-aortic counterpulsation balloon; radiographic considerations. Am. J. Roentgenol. 128:915, 1977.

Kantrowitz, A., Phillips, S. J., Butner, A. N., et al.:

Technique of femoral artery cannulation for phase-shift balloon pumping. J. Thorac. Cardiovasc. Surg. 56:219, 1968.

Kline, I. K., and Hofman, W. I.: Cardiac tamponade from CVP catheter perforation. J.A.M.A. 206:1794, 1968.

Langston, C. S.: The aberrant central venous catheter and its complications. Radiology 100:55, 1971.

Lapin, E. S., and Murray, J. A.: Hemoptysis with flow-directed cardiac catheterization. J.A.M.A. 220:1246, 1972.

Lefrak, E. A., and Noon, G. P.: Management of arterial injury secondary to attempted subclavian vein catheterization. Ann. Thorac. Surg. 14:294, 1972.

Lillehei, C. W., Cruz, A. B., Johnsrude, I., et al.: New method of assessing state of charge of implanted cardiac pacemaker batteries. Am. J. Cardiol. 16:717, 1965.

Lipp, H., O'Donoghue, K., and Resnekov, L.: Intracardiac knotting of a flow-directed balloon catheter. N. Engl. J. Med. 284:220, 1971.

Maggs, P. R., and Schwaber, J. R.: Fatal bilateral pneumothoraces complicating subclavian vein catheterization. Chest 71:552, 1977.

McHenry, M. M., and Grayson, C. E.: Roentgenographic diagnosis of pacemaker failure. Am. J. Roentgenol. 109:94, 1970.

McHenry, M. M., and Hopkins, D. M.: Cardiac tamponade as a result of infusion; complication of transvenous pacing. J.A.M.A. 203:1071, 1968.

McLoud, T. C., and Putman, C. E.: Radiology of the Swan-Ganz catheter and associated pulmonary complications. Radiology 116:19, 1975.

Merk, E. A., and Rush, B. F.: Emergency subclavian vein catheterization and intravenous hyperalimentation. Am. J. Surg. 129:266, 1975.

Ormond, R. S., Rubenfire, M., Anbe, D. T., et al.: Radiographic demonstration of myocardial penetration by permanent endocardial pacemakers. Radiology 98:35, 1971.

O'Rourke, M. F., and Shepherd, K. M.: Protection of the aortic arch and subclavian artery during intra-aortic balloon pumping. J. Thorac. Cardiovasc. Surg. 65:543, 1963.

Pace, P., Tilney, N., Couch, N., et al.: Peripheral arterial complications of intra-aortic balloon counterpulsation (abstr.). Circulation 54:11, 1976.

Ravin, C. E., Putman, C. E., and McLoud, T. C.: Hazards of the ICU. Am. J. Roentgenol. 126:423, 1976.

Rubin, S. A., and Puckett, R. P.: Pulmonary artery–bronchial fistula. A new complication of Swan-Ganz catheterization. Chest 75:515, 1979.

Sise, M. J., Hollingsworth, P., Brimm, J. E., et al.: Complications of the flow-directed pulmonary-artery catheter: a prospective analysis in 219 patients. Crit. Care Med. 9:315, 1981.

Sorkin, R. P., Schuurmann, B. J., and Simon, A. B.: Radiographic aspects of permanent cardiac pacemakers. Radiology 119:281, 1976.

Swan, H. J. C., and Ganz, W.: Use of a balloon flotation catheter in critically ill patients. Surg. Clin. North Am. 55:501, 1975.

Swan, H. J. C., Ganz, W., Forrester, J., et al.: Catheterization of the heart in man with use of a flow-directed balloon-tipped catheter. N. Engl. J. Med. 283:447, 1970.

Weber, K. T., and Janicki, J. S.: Intraaortic balloon counterpulsation. Ann. Thorac. Surg. 17:602, 1974.

Wilson, J. N., Grow, J. B., Demong, C. V., et al.: Central venous pressure in optimal blood volume maintenance. Arch. Surg. 85:563, 1962.

Yorra, F. H., Oblath, R., and Jaffe, H.: Massive thrombosis associated with use of the Swan-Ganz catheter. Chest 65:682, 1974.

Chapter 4

CARDIOPULMONARY DISORDERS IN THE CRITICALLY ILL

by Lawrence R. Goodman

Although cardiopulmonary problems encountered in the intensive care unit (ICU) are not unique to this setting, several factors make the radiographic evaluation of these complications difficult and at times impossible. Portable radiographs do not provide the detail and reproducibility achieved by stationary equipment. The lung or cardiac abnormalities visualized are frequently the result of more than one disease process. An acute cardiac or respiratory disorder is frequently superimposed on chronic obstructive pulmonary disease (COPD) In the presence of COPD, the clinical and radiographic findings of pneumonia, edema, congestive heart failure, and so on are often atypical and difficult to evaluate (Hublitz and Shapiro, 1969; Rosenow and Harrison, 1970; Tillotson and Lerner, 1968; Ziskind et al., 1970). The lung or heart may be one of several failing organ systems, and the changes on the chest radiograph may be the reflection of extrathoracic disease (for example, renal failure, coagulopathy, or sepsis). In addition, various support and monitoring devices may alter the appearance of the heart and lungs on the radiograph.

This chapter reviews the major cardiopulmonary disorders encountered in the ICU. Many of the radiographic changes are nonspecific and require careful attention to the time of onset, speed of progression, and location of the abnormality. Serial radiographs must be viewed for day-to-day changes as well as more general trends. An ongoing dialogue between the radiologist and the referring physician is vital for proper interpretation.

Although portable radiographs add to the difficulty of diagnosis, modern mobile units and the recent addition of phototimed cassettes make it possible to obtain adequate films for most patients. An upright, inspiratory radiograph is the ideal, but a motion-free supine film is preferable to a struggling, semislouched expiratory film. In patients undergoing cardiac surgery, a preoperative supine film is often of great help in interpreting the postoperative films (Harris, 1980). The liberal use of lateral, lateral decubitus, and oblique positions and the use of horizontal beam radiographs is often more rewarding than repeating the anteroposterior (AP) film "one more time." Radiographs obtained after various therapeutic or diagnostic maneuvers (for example, diuresis, bronchoscopy, thoracentesis) often aid greatly in establishing the diagnosis.

PULMONARY INSUFFICIENCY

Acute respiratory failure is defined as "the sudden inability of the respiratory apparatus to maintain adequate arterial oxygenation and adequate carbon dioxide elimination" (Petty, 1971). Although seldom seen as completely separate disorders, carbon dioxide retention is most frequently due to inadequate ventilation (the mechanics of breathing), and hypoxia is usually secondary to impaired gas exchange (Table 4–1).

Acute pulmonary insufficiency is responsible for approximately one half of ICU admissions. Although ICU therapy has resulted in a dra-

TABLE 4–1.

Pathologic States Primarily Producing Hypercapnia*

- A. Central nervous system
  1. Pharmacologic depression of the respiratory center (by barbiturates, morphine, tranquilizers, tromethamine [THAM], alcohol, and so on)
  2. Cerebrovascular accident
  3. Meningitis and encephalitis
  4. Severe intracranial hypertension (head trauma, intracranial tumor, and so on)
- B. Diseases of nerves and muscles
  1. Guillain-Barré
  2. Muscular dystrophy
  3. Myasthenia gravis
  4. Insecticide poisoning
  5. Curare toxicity
  6. Tetanus
  7. Chronic progressive polyneuropathy
  8. Diphtheric polyneuritis
  9. Poliomyelitis
- C. Diseases of the chest wall
  1. Flail chest
  2. Kyphoscoliosis
- D. Metabolic diseases
  1. Severe hypothyroidism
  2. Starvation
  3. Severe obesity
  4. Severe electrolyte disturbance
- E. Pulmonary causes
  1. Chronic obstructive disease of the lung
     - a. Pulmonary emphysema
     - b. Chronic bronchitis
  2. Acute obstructive disease of the lung
     - a. Severe asthmatic attack
     - b. Acute bronchiolitis
     - c. Mechanical obstruction of the airways by water (drowning), blood (hemoptysis), pus, or other material
     - d. Pulmonary edema
  3. Massive disease of the lung parenchyma
  4. Restrictive disease of the pleura
  5. Severe pain or diaphragmatic embarrassment after abdominal surgery
- F. Mechanical obstruction of the large airways
  1. Upper respiratory tract obstruction
  2. Obstruction of the trachea or large bronchi

Pathologic States Primarily Producing Hypoxia*

1. Pulmonary emphysema and chronic bronchitis
2. Extensive pneumonic consolidation, extensive pulmonary tumors, and extensive granulomatous processes
3. Pulmonary atelectasis
4. Aspiration pneumonia
5. Diffuse parenchymatous diseases, such as diffuse interstitial fibrosis, alveolar proteinosis, sarcoidosis, and lymphangitic spread of carcinoma
6. Pulmonary infarction
7. Status asthmaticus
8. Adult respiratory distress syndrome

*Adapted from Crews, E., and LaPuerta, L.: A Manual of Respiratory Failure. Springfield, IL, 1972, Charles C Thomas.

matic decrease in the morbidity and mortality from pulmonary insufficiency, mortality is still 10 to 20 per cent. In patients with pulmonary insufficiency and COPD, mortality as high as 30 to 40 per cent has been reported (Nunn et al., 1979; Pontoppidan et al., 1972; Rogers et al., 1972).

A potentially life-threatening respiratory disorder may be present in the face of a normal radiograph. The "sick patient–normal radiograph syndrome" is frequently an aid in diagnosing the underlying problem. In patients with central nervous system (CNS) disease, neuromuscular disorders, most drug overdoses, and metabolic derangement, the initial and subsequent radiographs are normal unless a secondary complication such as aspiration pneumonia or atelectasis develops. In other disorders such as pulmonary embolus, sepsis, viral pneumonia, smoke inhalation (Fig. 4–1), and adult respiratory distress syndrome (ARDS), the speed at which the radiograph turns "positive" may help confirm or refute the initial impression (Eaton et al., 1973; Fraser and Paré, 1979). Patients with severe COPD frequently have potentially fatal pulmonary insufficiency with little or no radiographic evidence of an acute process superimposed upon their emphysema.

ATELECTASIS

The most frequent radiographically demonstrable infiltrate in the ICU patient is atelectasis. Numerous factors, such as depressed consciousness, debility, pain, tracheal intubation, and respirator therapy, decrease the ability to cough and alter mucociliary clearance of secretions (Donnenfeld, 1971; Gamsu et al., 1976; Mulder and Rubush, 1969; Sackner et al., 1975). Mucosal edema or secretions in the smaller airways obstruct airflow, and diminished lung surfactant potentiates alveolar collapse. Atelectasis is especially common in the postoperative period, especially after thoracotomy or upper abdominal surgery (Pierce, 1977). Most infiltrates appearing within the first 48 hours after surgery are due to atelectasis if aspiration can be ruled out clinically or endoscopically.

The radiographic appearance of atelectasis varies from a slight decrease in lung volume without visible infiltrate (microatelectasis) to complete opacification and collapse of a segment, lobe, or lung (Figs. 4–2*A*, 4–3*A*). Atelectasis appearing as linear densities parallel or oblique to the diaphragm presents few diagnostic problems. Larger areas of atelectasis are often patchy and ill defined and may be single or multiple. Differentiation between atelectasis and pneumonia on a single radiograph often is not possible. The correct diagnosis is made by observing rapid changes in size, shape, or location of infiltrates on serial radiographs. The diagnosis of atelectasis can be made with certainty if films are taken before and after physical therapy, suctioning, or bronchoscopy (Fig. 4–2*B*, 4–3*B*). A dramatic improvement indicates that pooled secretions are the primary problem. Other parenchymal disorders, although benefited by these maneuvers, do not show rapid radiographic improvement (Bryant et al., 1973).

The presence or absence of an air bronchogram in a collapsed lobe or segment may help to predict the value of bronchoscopy and physical therapy. Marini et al. (1979) found frequent improvement after bronchoscopy when air bronchograms were absent, and rare improvement when they were present. These authors reasoned that when air bronchograms are absent, mucus amenable to removal is present in the large airways, and that when air bronchograms are present, the major airways are clear.

Left lower lobe infiltrates or areas of atelectasis are of particular importance in the ICU because they occur frequently after upper abdominal or cardiac surgery and are easily overlooked behind the magnified cardiac silhouette. On well-penetrated radiographs, air bronchograms in the retrocardiac area, the loss of pulmonary markings, or the loss of the lateral border of the descending aorta are reliable indicators of a pulmonary infiltrate. Left lower lobe volume loss is documented by crowded retrocardiac vessels or air bronchograms and by the elevation of the diaphragm. A shift of the mediastinum to the left, depression of the left hilus, or visualization of a triangular-shaped density behind the heart indicates marked volume loss (Fig. 4–4). The left upper lobe may appear hyperlucent.

The silhouette sign applied to the diaphragm, however, is not always reliable on the portable radiograph. The diaphragm may be silhouetted by an enlarged heart on a supine or semierect radiograph. An x-ray beam not perfectly tangent to the dome of the diaphragm (for example, lordotic film) will also cause a pseudosilhouette sign. Great variation among patients in the carinal angle makes depression of the left main stem bronchus of limited value in detecting left

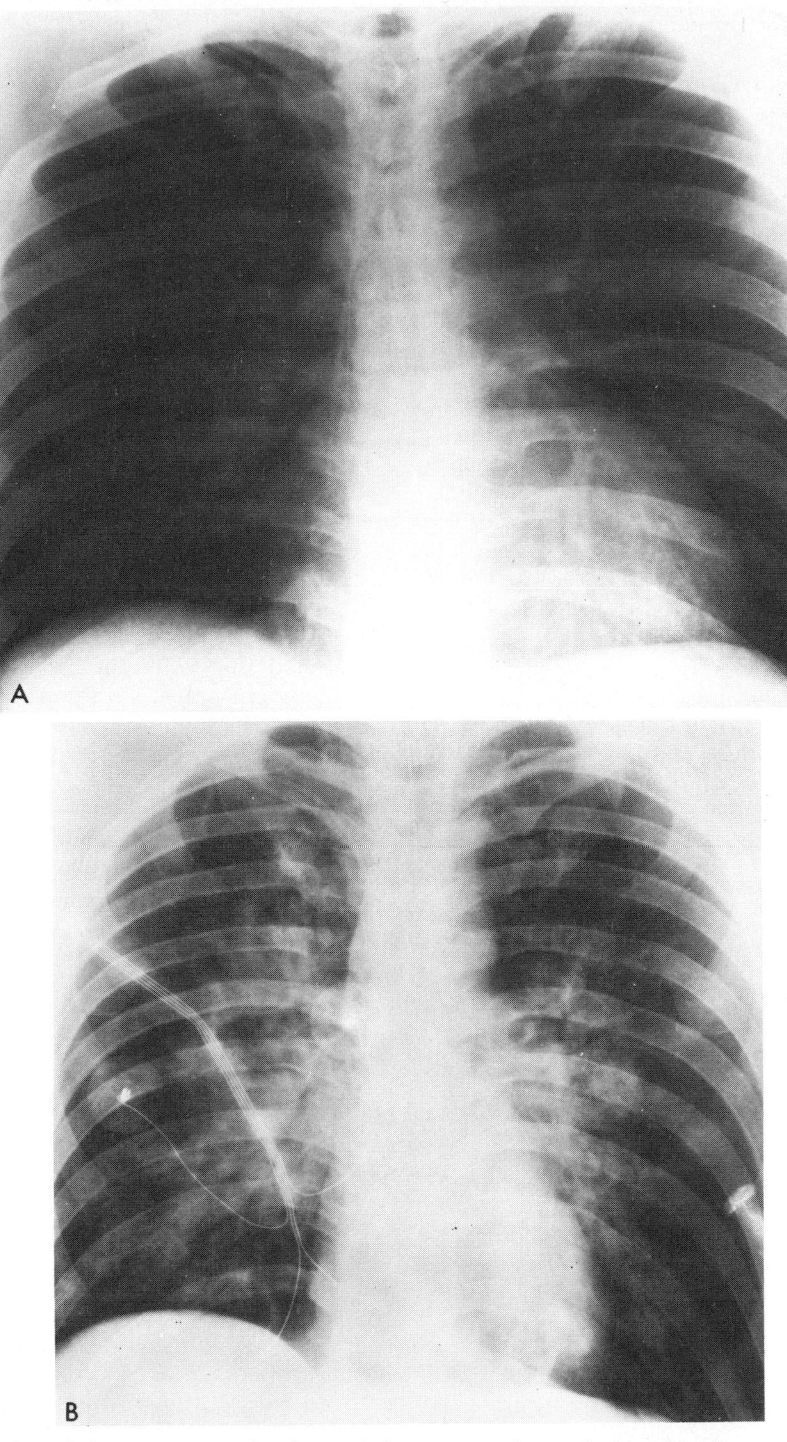

Figure 4–1. Smoke inhalation. *A*, Initial radiograph (approximately two hours after the patient inhaled large amounts of burning electrical insulation fumes) is normal. *B*, Approximately eight hours later, there is severe bilateral alveolar edema. The patient died of pulmonary insufficiency within 36 hours of admission.

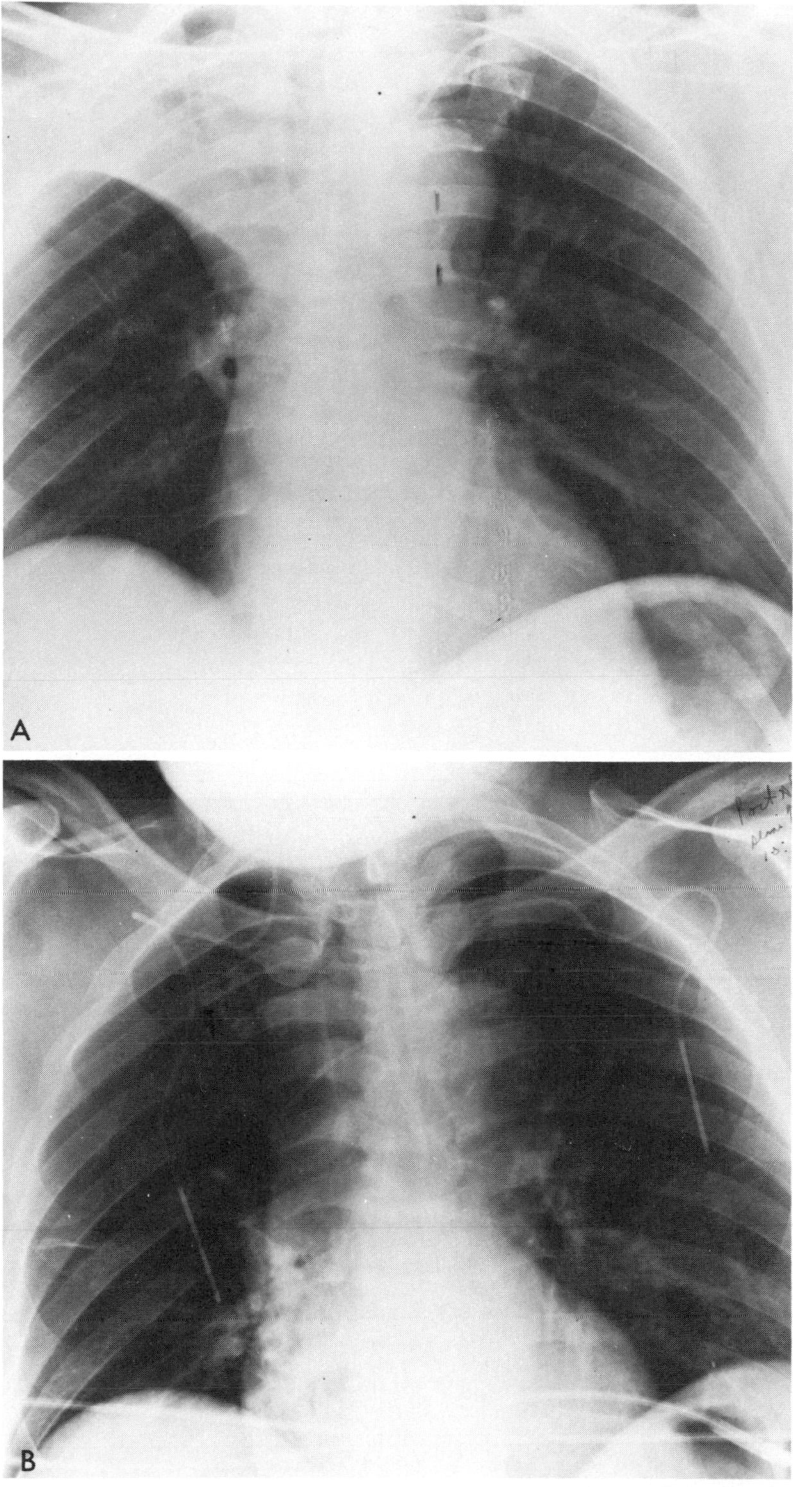

Figure 4–2. Atelectasis. *A*, There is total opacification and partial collapse of the right upper lobe. No air bronchogram is seen. A radiograph two days earlier had been normal. *B*, Following physical therapy and suctioning, there is complete clearing of the right upper lobe. Note that the subclavian catheter is in the right jugular vein. The left CVP catheter is in the superior vena cava.

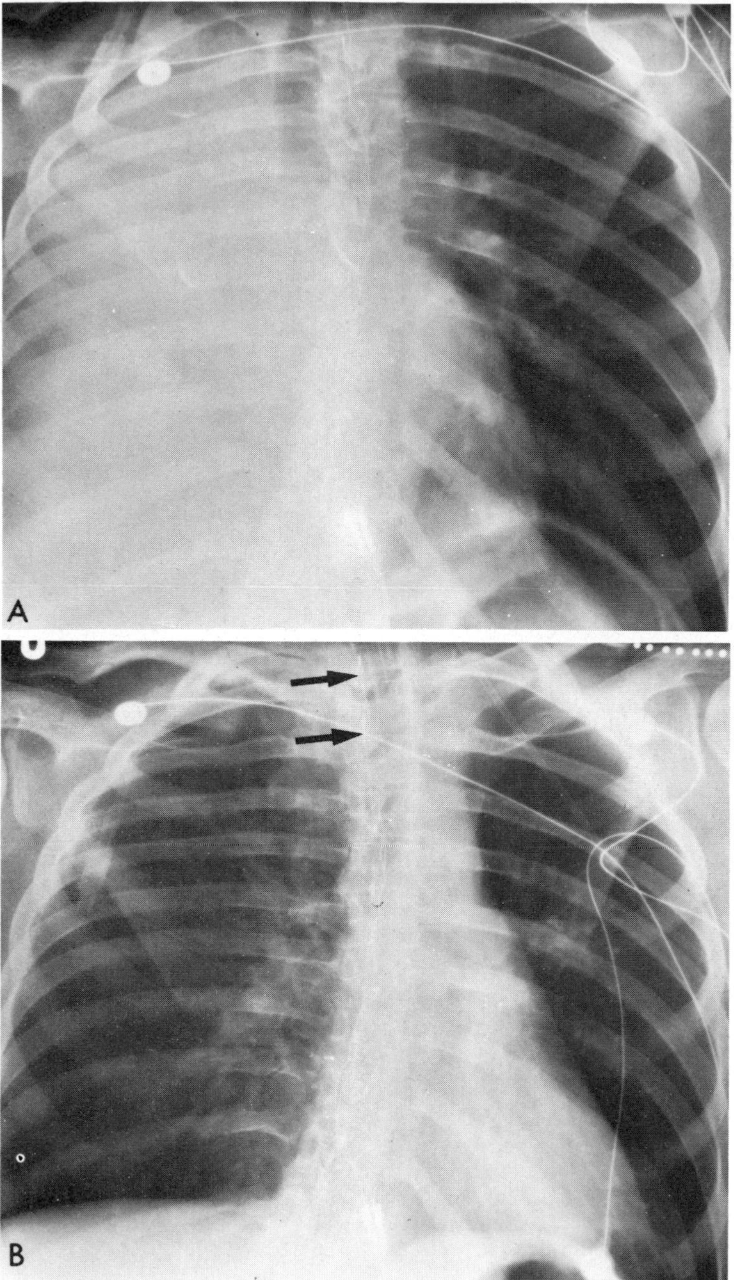

Figure 4–3. Right lung atelectasis. This young quadriplegic entered the hospital with increasing shortness of breath and a low-grade fever. *A*, The AP radiograph reveals total opacification of the right hemithorax with no visible air bronchograms. The mediastinum is shifted to the right and the left lung is hyperinflated. *B*, Fiberoptic bronchoscopy revealed tenacious secretions in all the large airways. This radiograph, obtained 14 hours after bronchoscopy and suctioning, reveals almost total re-expansion of the right lung. There is no evidence of pneumonia. Incidentally noted is flattening of the upper margins of the third, fourth, and fifth posterior ribs on the right owing to pressure from the scapula, a common finding in long-standing quadriplegia. The electrodes noted over the first and second thoracic vertebrae are those of the dorsal column stimulator, used for intractable pain (*arrows*).

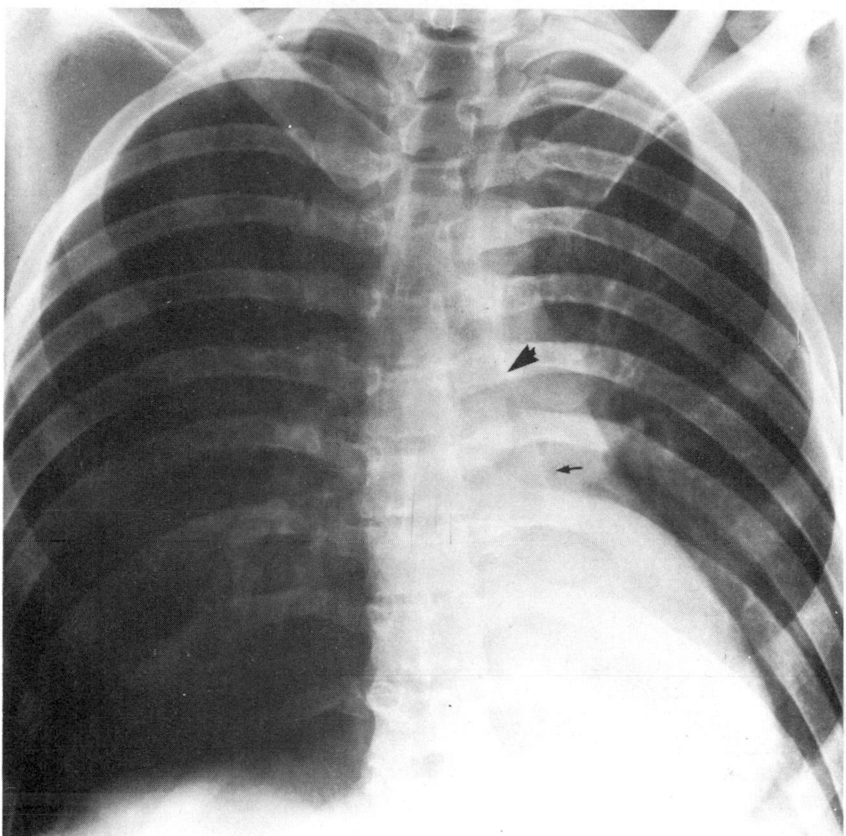

Figure 4–4. Left lower lobe collapse. The mediastinum is shifted to the right. The left diaphragm is elevated and obscured. The descending aorta cannot be visualized. There is a homogeneous density in the retrocardiac area, and the left main stem (*upper arrow*) and left lower bronchus (*lower arrow*) are depressed and moved medially.

lower lobe collapse unless the changes are gross or earlier portable radiographs are available to document a change. In questionable cases, an overpenetrated AP radiograph or a film with the patient turned 15° to 30° to the right will demonstrate the retrocardiac area more clearly. A right lateral decubitus radiograph will suspend the left lung in inspiratory apnea, facilitating retrocardiac evaluation (Lerner, 1978).

In the postoperative patient, hypoxemia and diminished compliance are frequently present in the face of a normal chest radiograph. Changes in the breathing patterns during general anesthesia lead to diminished surfactant and peripheral lung collapse (microatelectasis). This may be accompanied by ventilation-perfusion mismatch and shunting (Pierce, 1977). In most cases, these changes are reversible with assisted ventilation. In addition to microatelectasis, the normal radiograph and hypoxemia may suggest a pulmonary embolus or early ARDS.

PNEUMONIA

Lung infections occur in approximately 10 to 20 per cent of ICU patients. Although pneumonia may be the cause of hospitalization, most patients develop pneumonia while in the hospital for other illnesses (Feingold, 1970; Stevens et al., 1974). The majority of infections contracted outside the hospital are due to viruses, mycoplasma, or gram-positive cocci, whereas at least half of hospital-acquired pneumonias are due to mixed anaerobic organisms or to aerobic gram-negative bacteria. In nosocomial infections, *Staphylococcus* is the most frequent gram-positive organism, and aerobic rods (*Hemophilus influenzae, Escherichia coli, Klebsiella,* and *Pseudomonas* spp.) are the most frequent gram-negative organisms (Sanford and Pierce, 1979).

Hospital-acquired infection often follows an atypical clinical course, has atypical radiographic features, and is frequently antibiotic-

TABLE 4–2. Factors That Compromise Host Defense Mechanisms*

A. Basic diseases
  1. Hodgkin's disease
  2. Other lymphomas and leukemias
  3. Multiple myeloma
  4. Carcinomas and sarcomas
  5. Inherited and acquired primary immunodeficiency diseases
B. Superimposed conditions
  1. Altered physical barriers
    a. Indwelling intravenous and urethral catheters
    b. Gastrointestinal mucosal toxicity
    c. Nebulizers with intermittent positive pressure breathing apparatus
    d. Local mechanical disruption of tissues, membranes, and blood vessels by tumor growth and necrosis
  2. Altered indigenous microbial flora
    a. Broad-spectrum antibiotic therapy
  3. Leukopenia
    a. Immunosuppressives
    b. Cytotoxic chemotherapy
    c. Irradiationm
  4. Altered leukocyte response
    a. Decreased migration
    b. Diminished phagocytosis
    c. Decreased bactericidal capacity
  5. Impaired T- and/or B-cell–mediated immunity
    a. Corticosteroid therapy
    b. Cytotoxic chemotherapy
    c. Irradiation
    d. Antilymphocyte globulin

*From Bode, F. R., Paré, J. A. P., and Fraser, R. G.: Pulmonary Diseases in the Compromised Host. Medicine 53:255, 1974. Copyright© 1974, The Williams & Wilkins Co., Baltimore.

resistant (Heineman, 1974). Since hospital-acquired infections occur in patients with other serious illnesses, mortality is extremely high. Patients with pneumonias developed in the ICU have a mortality of approximately 50 per cent. In one study, mortality from gram-positive cocci, gram-negative rods, and *P. aeruginosa* pneumonia was 5, 30, and 70 per cent, respectively (Stevens et al., 1974). Others have reported death rates from *P. aeruginosa* pneumonia as high as 90 per cent (Flick and Cluff, 1976; Rose et al., 1973).

Numerous factors contribute to the high incidence and grave prognosis of pneumonia in the ICU. Almost every ICU patient can be considered a "compromised host" with decreased resistance to infection (see Table 4–2). The patient's primary disease (for example, malignancy, diabetes, or COPD) may leave him more susceptible to infection. Prolonged hospitalization and debility are associated with gradual alteration of the normal pharyngeal flora to flora rich in gram-negative organisms (Sanford and Pierce, 1979). Previous antibiotic therapy or steroid administration may accelerate the colonization of the pharynx. Finally, normal physical barriers to infection may be bypassed by various tubes and catheters. Most patients with intratracheal tubes develop tracheal colonization within several days of intubation (Shapiro, 1975). Respirators, suctioning apparatus, nebulizers, portable x-ray equipment, and hospital personnel are potential sources of infection. Thus, aspiration of infected nasal, oral, or tracheal secretions is a prime source of endogenous pneumonia.

The complex spectrum of pulmonary and systemic disease seen in the ICU makes the correct diagnosis of pneumonia a difficult one. Pathogens are frequently cultured from the sputum and infiltrates seen on the radiograph when, in fact, pneumonia is not present. In a study of 60 patients believed by their primary physician to have pneumonia, Bryant and associates (1973) found the diagnosis to be in error in approximately two thirds of the cases. Misdiagnosis was based on transient fevers or on abnormalities found on physical or chest radiographic examination. In 58 to 60 patients, a potentially pathogenic organism was recovered from the sputum. Diseases most frequently misdiagnosed as pneumonia are atelectasis, atypical patterns of congestive heart failure, and pulmonary embolus (Sanford and Pierce, 1979).

The incidence of pneumonia tends to parallel that of atelectasis. Many patients with persistent volume loss will develop an infection four to ten days after the onset of atelectasis. Therefore, any persistently atelectatic area or any area that appears worse after initial improvement should be suspected of being infected. Similarly, if aspiration pneumonitis fails to clear after several days, secondary infection is likely.

In the immunologically normal patient, a combination of fever, leukocytosis, sputum rich in leukocytes and bacteria, and a stable or progressive infiltrate seen on the chest radiograph is required for the diagnosis of pneumonia (Shapiro, 1975). In patients with compromised immunity due to a primary disorder or immune-depressing medication, the usual clinical, laboratory, and radiographic signs of pulmonary infection may be absent. When pneumonia is present, the radiograph may demonstrate pulmonary infiltrates in the absence of clinical signs and symptoms. In neutropenic patients, conversely, pulmonary infection may be present in the absence of radiographically demonstrable pulmonary disease (Zornoza et al., 1976). Differentiation between infectious and noninfectious pulmonary disease in this group is also difficult. In a review of lung disease in immunocompromised patients, Greenman and associates (1975) found "no significant correlation with fever, white cell count, nature of immunosuppression or duration, character or extent of x-ray findings. Roentgenographic presentation and course influenced the pre-biopsy differential diagnosis, but in only 44 per cent of the patients was [the primary clinical diagnosis confirmed by biopsy]. . . ."

The radiograph is a helpful adjunct for following the progress of pneumonia. The infiltrate should stabilize within a few days of appropriate antibiotic therapy and should gradually clear within the following few days to weeks. Progression of the infiltrate or volume loss should raise a question as to the effectiveness of the antibiotics, the possibility of a superinfection, the presence of retained secretions, or the presence of an associated pulmonary process. Other complications of pneumonia, such as abscess, empyema, broncho-pleural fistula, and so on, should be sought (Goodman et al., 1980).

The radiographic patterns of pneumonia are, in general, nonspecific and require bacteriologic confirmation. It is beyond the scope of this book to review the radiographic patterns of the numerous common and opportunistic types of pneumonia found in the ICU. Several recent reviews are available on this subject (Castellino and Blank, 1979; Goodman et al., 1980; Williams et al., 1976). *P. aeruginosa* pneumonia, however, because of its prevalence and virulence in the ICU, is discussed in more detail.

Pseudomonas aeruginosa Infection

The ubiquitous organism *P. aeruginosa* is often cultured from both hospital personnel and patients. In patients with the predisposing causes discussed previously, *P. aeruginosa* tracheal colonization often progresses to pulmonary infection. *P. aeruginosa* bacteremia with secondary pulmonary involvement is also a frequent occurrence in the ICU, with the urinary tract the most frequent site of infection.

The onset of symptoms is usually abrupt and includes fever, chills, and copious sputum production. Primary nonbacteremic *P. aeruginosa* pneumonia usually appears as a diffuse, nodular, bilateral lower lobe infiltrate that rapidly progresses to involve most of the lung (Joffe, 1969; Renner et al., 1972; Tillotson and Lerner, 1968) (Fig. 4–5). A bilateral symmetric pattern simulating pulmonary edema is not uncommon. Small, central lucencies, representing uninvolved lung or focal air trapping, frequently simulate the presence of multiple microabscesses. The nodules rapidly coalesce into large confluent areas, and at this stage one or more true abscesses may appear (Rose et al., 1973). Empyemas are not uncommon (Fig. 4–6). Unilateral infiltrates, interstitial infiltrates, or focal masses are unusual. Pneumonia due to *P. aeruginosa* septicemia also initially appears with discrete nodules, but rapidly progresses to a picture indistinguishable from the primary pneumonic form.

Lung Biopsy Techniques

If sputum staining and transtracheal aspiration fail to diagnose the cause of the infection, fluoroscopically guided percutaneous thin-needle aspiration or transcricoid bronchial brushing are often helpful. Percutaneous aspiration of *focal* pulmonary infiltrates yields one or more infectious agents in approximately 75 per cent of patients (Fig. 4–7). Unfortunately, a

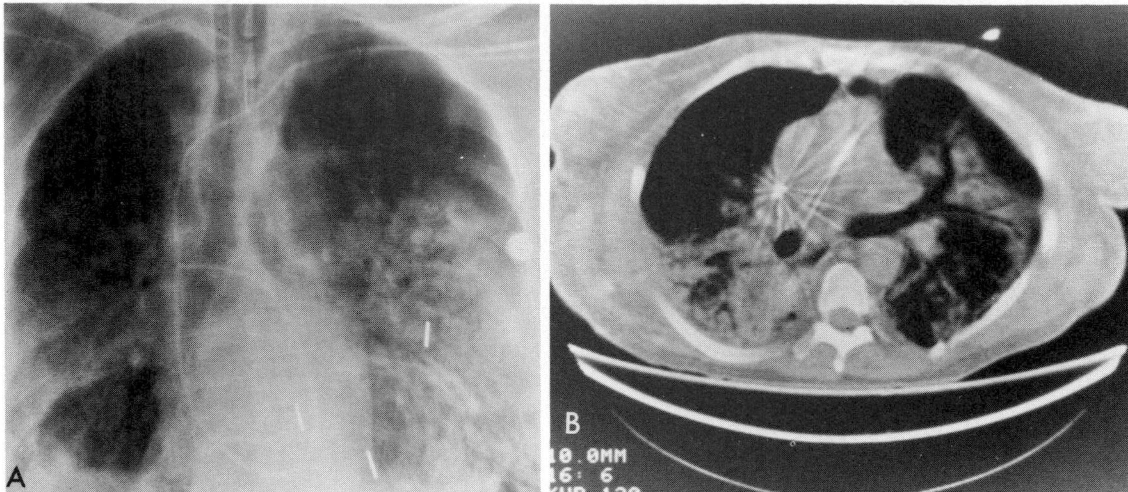

Figure 4–5. *Pseudomonas* pneumonia. *A*, Diffuse bilateral symmetric infiltrates are noted in the lower two thirds of both lungs. The heart does not appear enlarged. The wedge pressure was normal. Cultures repeatedly grew *Pseudomonas*. *B*, After some initial improvement the patient's condition worsened. Clinically and radiographically a right-sided empyema could not be excluded. CT scan shows diffuse parenchymal infiltrates. Little or no pleural effusion is noted. No empyema is present.

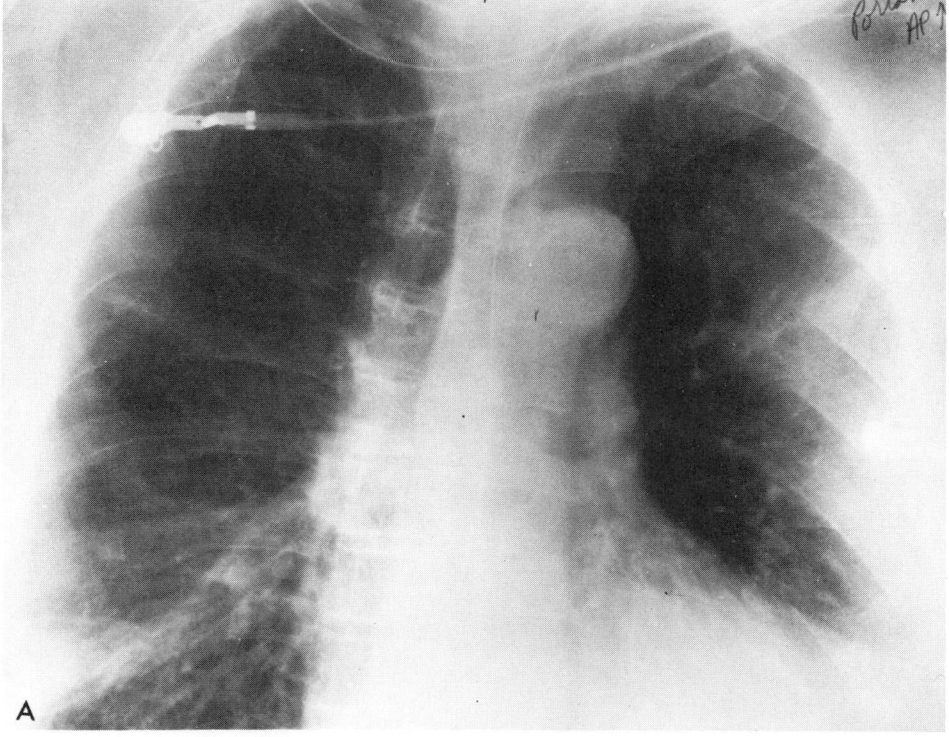

Figure 4–6. *See legend on opposite page*

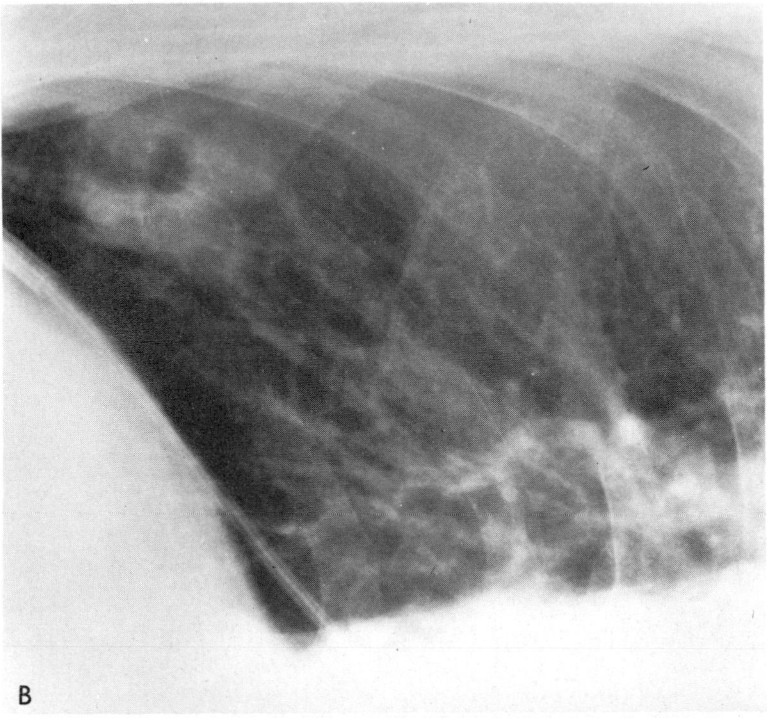

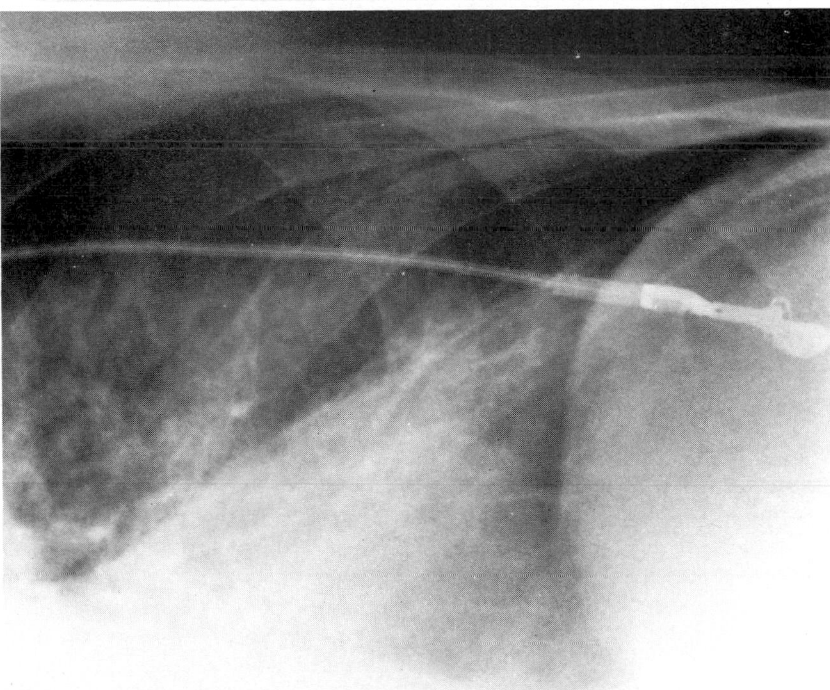

Figure 4–6. *P. aeruginosa* abscess. *A*, AP radiograph demonstrates a focal infiltrate at the right costophrenic angle and diffuses haziness at the left costophrenic angle, suggesting a left effusion. *B*, Left lateral decubitus film. For technical reasons, the left side was not visualized well. However, the right side shows an air fluid level in the lateral infiltrate, indicating an abscess. *C*, Right lateral decubitus film. The left costophrenic angle is seen to be clear, indicating that the density on the AP film is due to a pleural effusion.

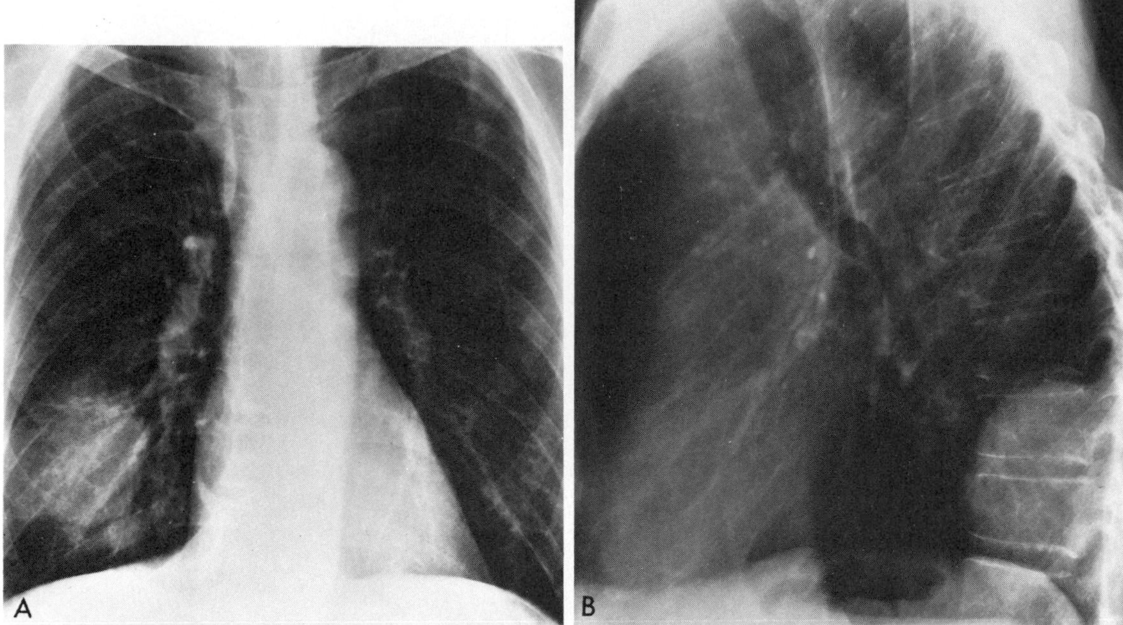

Figure 4–7. Percutaneous needle biopsy in an asymptomatic patient with a diagnosis of glioblastoma, one month following craniotomy. *A*, Chest radiograph shows a mass in the right lower lobe. *B*, In a lateral projection the mass is located posteriorly. Aspiration needle biopsy yielded a pure culture of streptococcus. Complete resolution followed penicillin therapy.

negative aspiration does not exclude a pulmonary infection. In experienced hands the pneumothorax rate is approximately 25 per cent, with one in three pneumothoraces requiring chest tube drainage. If the prothrombin time is over 60 per cent of control value, bleeding is rarely a serious complication (Castellino and Blank, 1979; Matthay and Moritz, 1981; Sagel et al., 1978).

Transcricoid bronchial brushing is performed through an angiogram catheter inserted over a guidewire via the cricothyroid membrane. The brush is passed, under fluoroscopic control, into the area in question. The bronchus is brushed and aspirated, and a selective lobar bronchogram is performed as the catheter is withdrawn. This is especially valuable when an endobronchial lesion, an abscess, or bronchiectasis is suspected (Fig. 4–8).

Open lung biopsy is the procedure of choice in patients with diffuse lung infiltrates, when a noninfectious etiology is considered, or in patients with focal disease in whom the more conservative procedures have failed to establish a diagnosis. Open lung biopsy is also safest when the patient has a bleeding disorder, has severe bullous disease, or is on a respirator.

ASPIRATION SYNDROMES

Another frequent cause of pulmonary infiltrates is that of "aspiration pneumonitis." This term combines three distinct clinical entities that have very different clinical and radiographic presentations and vary widely in prognosis (Bartlett and Gorbach, 1975). Pulmonary disease may be produced by the aspiration of toxic fluids, bland fluids or particles, or secretions contaminated with a heavy inocula of organisms from the upper airways. Each type behaves differently; the only common denominator is the breakdown of the normal protective mechanism of the pharynx and larynx. Predisposing factors include general anesthesia, depressed consciousness, neuromuscular disorder, esophageal disease, or the presence of a nasogastric or intratracheal tube (Mendelson, 1946; Tinstman et al., 1973).

Aspiration of Toxic Fluids

The aspiration of low pH gastric contents (pH less than 2.5), hydrocarbons, alcohol, mineral oil, or water-soluble contrast agents causes a marked inflammatory reaction in the lungs. The initial radiographic and clinical changes are due to a chemical pneumonitis that may resolve or become secondarily infected. Mortality rates are in the 20 to 30 per cent range (LeFrock, 1979; Tinstman et al., 1973).

When a large quantity of gastric juice is aspirated, fever, tachypnea, and rales usually present within one to two hours. In one third of patients, cyanosis, bronchospasm, shock, or apnea may follow (Bynum and Pierce, 1976; LeFrock, 1979). In general, infiltrates are present on the radiograph within the first six hours and often progress for the next 24 hours. The initial radiograph usually shows poorly defined nodular or patchy densities that often become confluent (Fig. 2–5). These are most often perihilar or basilar in location, often bilateral. After massive aspiration, a bilateral, rapidly progressing edema pattern may be evident. Differentiation from congestive heart failure may be difficult (Fig. 4–9*A*, *B*). In aspiration pneumonitis, however, the heart and vessels do not enlarge (Landay et al., 1978).

Most patients will stabilize and start to show progressive clearing within a few days. After clearing has started, any worsening suggests a secondary infection, or retained secretions or

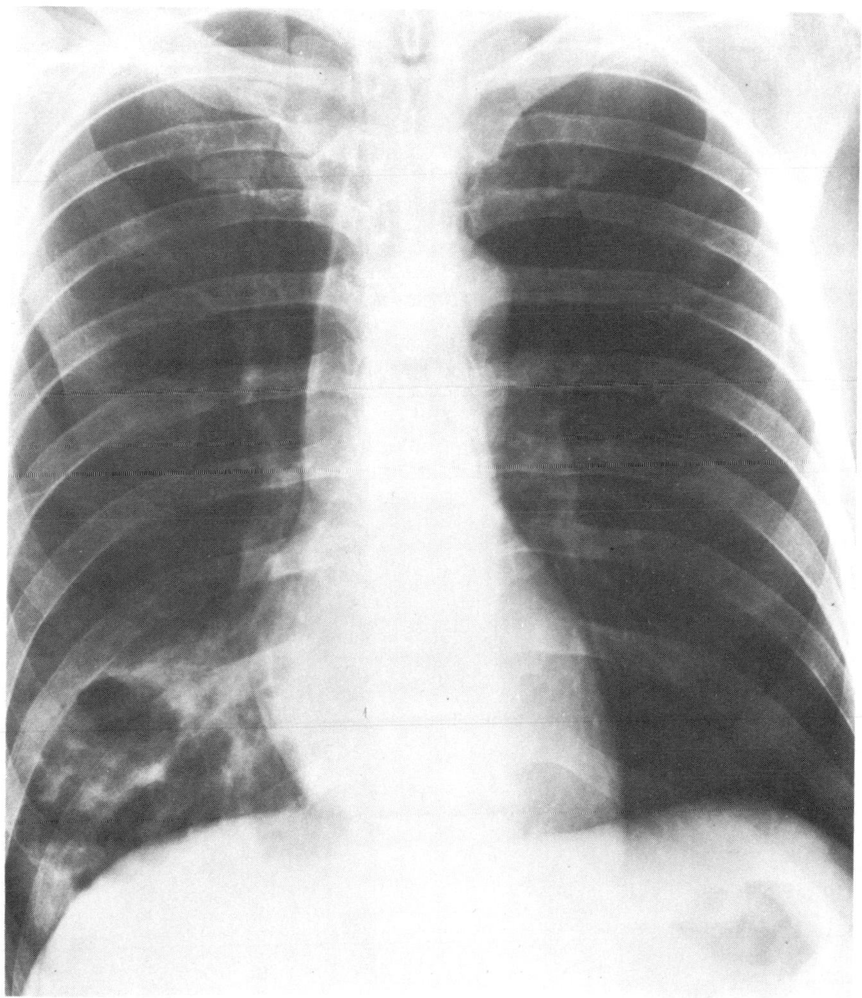

Figure 4–8. Bronchial brushing for infection. A middle-aged man with several weeks' history of fever and cough, in whom there was no response to antibiotic therapy. There is a cavitary lesion in the right lower lobe. The presence of the cavity indicates a communication with the bronchus and therefore the strong likelihood that a successful diagnosis could be made via the bronchus. Bronchial brushing was positive for tuberculosis. A bronchogram demonstrated patent bronchi and multiple cavities (*not shown*).

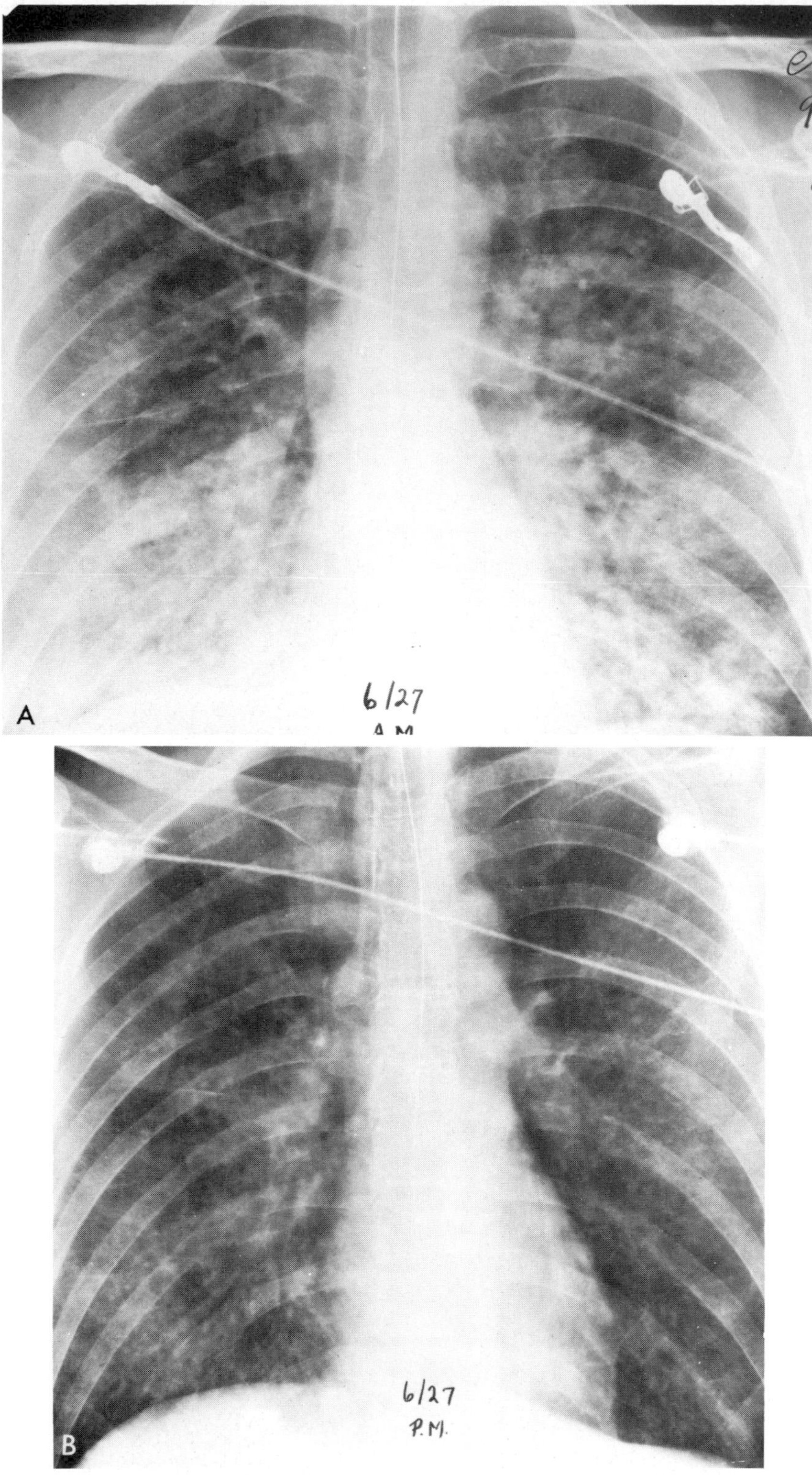

Figure 4–9 *See legend on opposite page*

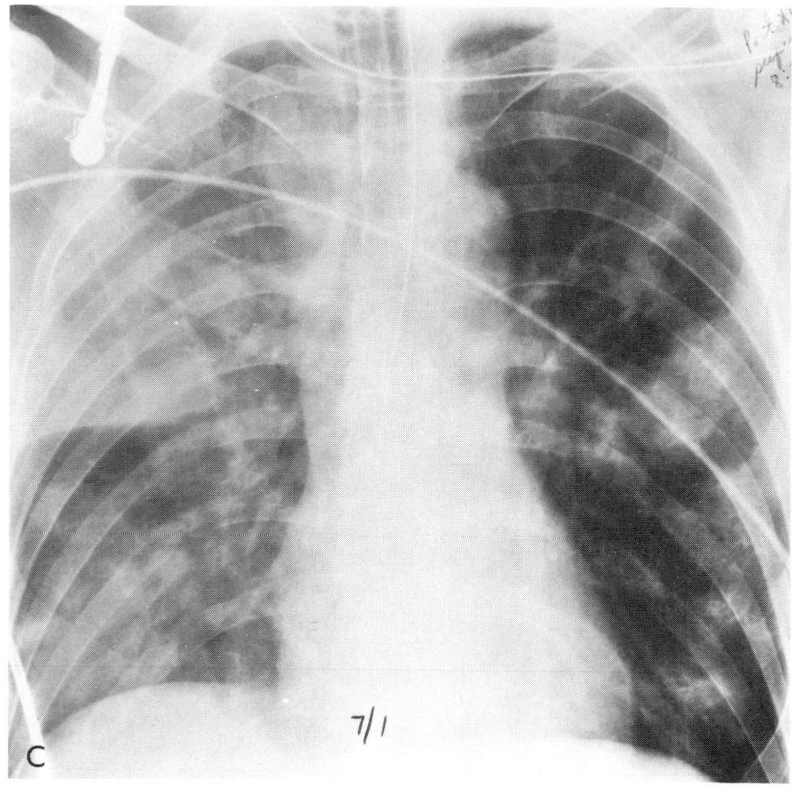

Figure 4–9. Aspiration pneumonia. *A*, Diffuse, fluffy, bilateral alveolar infiltrates are demonstrated several hours after gastric acid aspiration. The rapid onset and the radiographic distribution suggest pulmonary edema, but the cardiac silhouette is small. *B*, Eighteen hours later, there is considerable clearing of the fluffy, bilateral pulmonary infiltrates. (Part of the improvement is undoubtedly due to a deeper inspiration.) *C*, Four days later, diffuse pulmonary infiltrates are noted, as well as lobar consolidation of the right upper lobe. *Klebsiella* organisms were cultured from the sputum.

food particles (Fig. 4–9*C*). Other complications include cavitation, empyema, pneumothorax, or ARDS.

Repeated small aspirations of gastric contents, frequently at night, are more difficult to diagnose. Recurrent bouts of lower lobe atelectasis, pneumonitis, or cavitation without apparent cause should lead one to consider this possibility. Sputum may fail to yield the causative organism or may repeatedly grow "mixed" or "normal" organisms (LeFrock, 1979).

Aspiration of Bland Fluids or Solids

Fluids such as blood, water, barium, and neutralized gastric acid do not cause chemical pneumonitis. Transient respiratory distress is due either to the volume of fluid aspirated (asphyxiation) or to a reflex lung reaction to a foreign substance (Bartlett and Gorbach, 1975). The radiograph is often normal unless large volumes of fluid are aspirated. If infiltrates are present, they rapidly disappear following coughing, suctioning, or positive pressure therapy (Fig. 4–10).

The aspiration of food particles or blood clots usually excites a bout of coughing due to direct bronchial irritation. A large inoculum may cause wheezing, dyspnea, or cyanosis. The initial radiograph may be normal or may demonstrate areas of atelectasis or focal overinflation. Fluoroscopy or expiratory films accentuate areas of inspiratory or expiratory obstruction. Blood clots usually lyse or are coughed up, whereas food particles may remain in the bronchi despite the cessation of acute symptoms. If there is clinical or radiographic evidence of persistent airway obstruction, early bronchoscopic removal of the offending foreign body will prevent delayed complications such as pneumonia, bronchiectasis, lung abscess, or empyema.

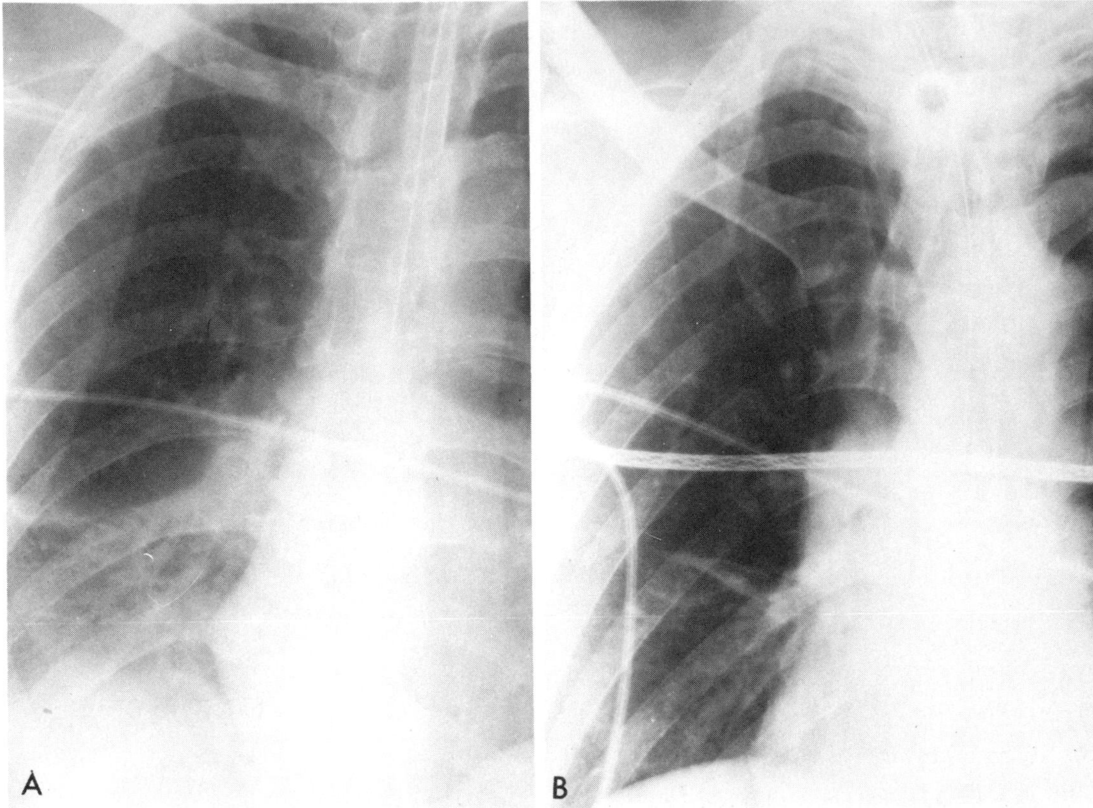

Figure 4–10. Aspiration of blood. *A*, There is consolidation and volume loss in the right lower lobe. The patient was aspirating blood from multiple facial fractures. *B*, A tracheostomy was performed to protect the trachea and to facilitate suctioning. Film taken 18 hours later shows almost complete clearing of the right lower lobe infiltrate and atelectasis.

Aspiration of Infected Secretions

As previously mentioned, the upper airways of the hospitalized patient are frequently colonized by various saprophytic and pathogenic organisms (Sanford and Pierce, 1979). These most frequently are enteric gram-negative organisms (*Klebsiella* organisms or *Escherichia coli*), *Pseudomonas aeruginosa*, or *Staphylococcus* organisms. When they are aspirated into the lung, an indolent or fulminant pneumonia may ensue. Although the radiographic appearance of the infiltrates is nonspecific, occurrence in gravity-dependent segments (posterior segment of the upper lobes, superior and posterior basal segments of the lower lobes) may give a clue to the cause (Fig. 4–11). Cavitation and empyema are frequent sequelae, and healing is often slow (Bartlett and Gorbach, 1975). Cultures from these pneumonias or abscesses usually yield mixed aerobic and anaerobic flora. Gram's stain is often of major importance in the differentiation of colonization from true infection.

PULMONARY EDEMA

Congestive Heart Failure

When left ventricular failure is the obvious clinical diagnosis, the radiograph does little more than confirm the diagnosis, check for secondary complications, and offer visual means of following the patient's progress. On the other hand, before the development of alveolar edema, the radiograph may indicate interstitial edema before clinical signs and symptoms are present. The upright portable radiograph provides a method of evaluating the pulmonary venous pressure and may obviate the need for intravascular pressure monitoring. Portable radiographic technique, however, must be modified to maximize our ability to detect increased pulmonary venous pressure and interstitial pulmonary edema. This section considers the physiologic-radiologic correlates of left ventricular failure, as well as the techniques for maximizing radiographic information.

Congestive heart failure (CHF) occurs when the left ventricle fails to eject a normal volume of blood during systole. Decreased ejection results in increased ventricular end-diastolic volume, increased pressure, and slight cardiac enlargement. Initially, this stretches the myocardium, causing increased strength of contraction (Frank-Starling curve; see Fig. 1–7). Eventually, stretching becomes counterproductive, contractions decrease in force, and the ventricle dilates further. Although left ventricular enlargement is the hallmark of left ventricular failure, it may be absent in acute myocardial infarction, acute arrhythmias, or rapid volume overload (Chait et al., 1972; Shapiro and Hublitz, 1974). Mild-to-moderate cardiac enlargement may escape detection on portable radiographs unless serial films are available for comparison (Harrison et al., 1971). Conversely, cardiac enlargement may be present without left ventricular failure.

Because of the variability of heart size, radiographic signs of increased pulmonary venous pressure, not cardiomegaly, are the primary diagnostic criteria. Using portable, semierect AP radiographs exposed at 40 inches, McHugh and associates (1972) found the following correlations between the radiographs and the pulmonary capillary wedge (PCW) pressures:

1. The radiograph is normal when the PCW is less than 12 mm Hg.

2. When the PCW is 12 to 18 mm Hg (mild CHF), there is redistribution of flow to the upper lobes (West et al., 1965) (Fig. 4–12*A*).

3. As the PCW increases from 18 to 22 mm Hg, the peripheral vessels dilate. The radiograph shows interstitial edema, which is most reliably demonstrated by blurring of the margins of the medium-size vessels, peribronchial cuffing, and a perihilar or basilar haze (Fig. 4–13).

4. Further elevation of the PCW is associated with periacinar rosette formation, the result of fluid in the alveoli (Fig. 4–12*B*). This may progress to diffuse alveolar edema.

5. Cardiomegaly, pleural effusion, and Kerley lines are inconsistent findings on the port-

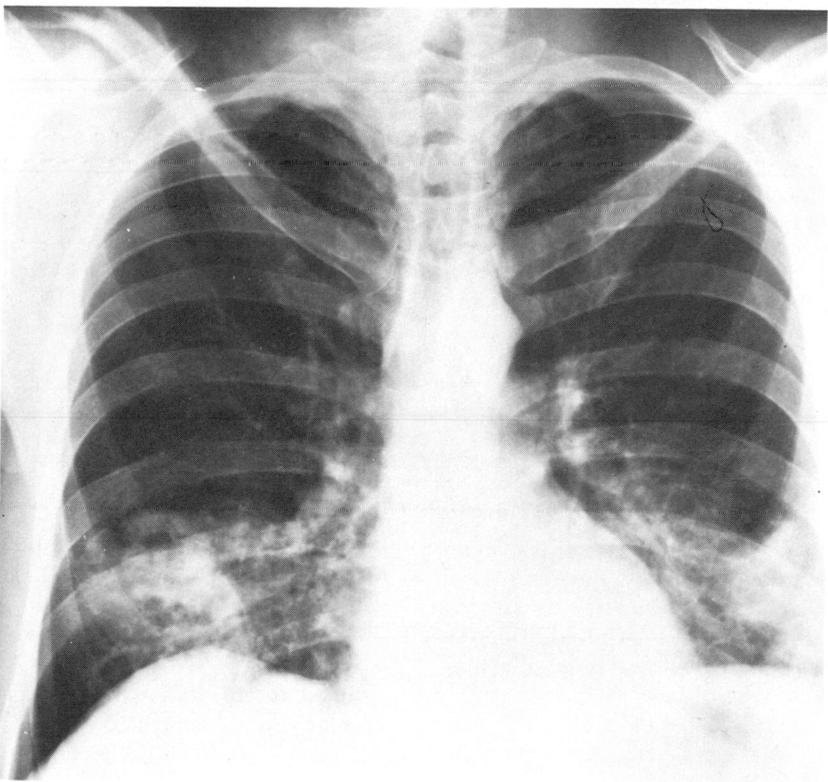

Figure 4–11. Aspiration of infected secretions. Bilateral lower lobe infiltrates and cavities are due to aspiration of infected secretions from the trachea. Cultures repeatedly grew mixed flora.

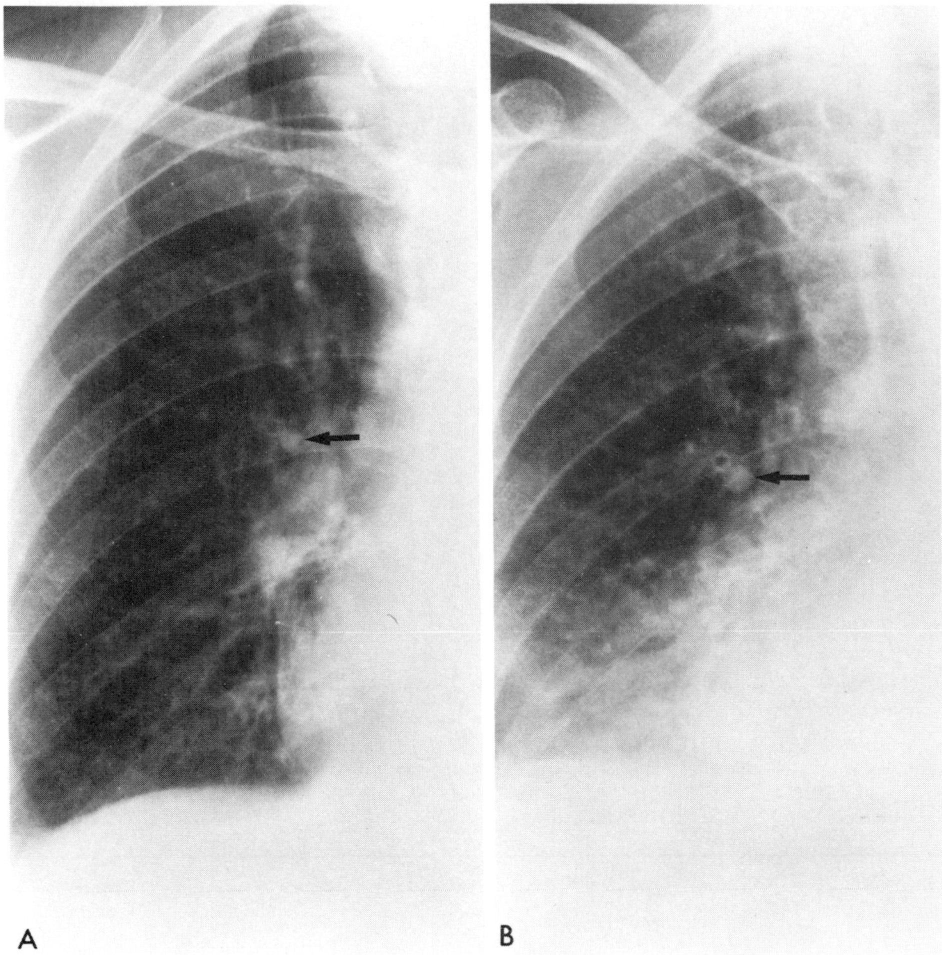

Figure 4–12. Congestive heart failure (CHF). *A*, There is redistribution of the pulmonary circulation. The upper lobe vessels are larger than the lower lobe vessels. The artery seen on end (*arrow*) is slightly larger than the corresponding bronchus on end. *B*, Two days later, with the patient in severe pulmonary edema, the perivascular edema obscures all the vessels. The vessel on end (*arrow*) is now considerably larger than the corresponding bronchus on end. The bronchus on end is thickened by peribronchial edema. Lower lobe alveolar edema is also visualized.

able radiograph (Harrison et al., 1971; McHugh et al., 1972).

6. In 10 per cent of cases the chest radiograph–PCW correlation is poor. The radiograph may lag several hours behind the PCW early in the patient's course ("preclinical failure") or immediately following treatment ("post-therapeutic lag"). When the vascular integrity is compromised (for example, in hypoxia or uremia), interstitial or alveolar edema may occur at lower PCWs.

In the ICU, atypical patterns of CHF may be as frequent as the "classic" patterns. Numerous factors, such as gravity, pulmonary parenchymal disease, and the integrity of the pulmonary vascular bed, influence the distribution of the edema fluid. The largest group of patients developing atypical pulmonary edema are those with COPD. The diagnosis of COPD *and* CHF may be elusive both clinically and radiographically (Liebman et al., 1978; Rosenow and Harrison, 1970; Unger et al., 1975). Hublitz and Shapiro (1969) have called attention to two basic atypical radiographic patterns of heart failure in patients with emphysema. One pattern consists of overt pulmonary edema, but in a bizarre distribution corresponding to the areas of relatively normal blood flow (Fig. 4–14). In the other pattern, fluid is confined to the interstitium of the lung and gives a hazy, reticular, or miliary nodular pattern, a reflection of disordered fluid drainage (Figs. 4–15, 4–16). The picture is further confused by the frequent absence of visible cardiomegaly in COPD. Careful comparison with earlier radiographs is often of great help in detecting subtle interstitial changes, the distribution of the patient's bullous disease, and subtle changes in heart size. Each bout of heart failure tends to have the same atypical radiographic appearance.

Other disorders that disturb the pulmonary vascular bed also cause atypical pulmonary edema patterns. Disorders such as congenital pulmonary vascular disease, the Swyer-James syndrome, pulmonary arterial compression, or pulmonary embolus will cause unusual edema patterns. In the bedridden adult with pulmonary edema who has a definite segmental or lobar sparing, the possibility of a recent pulmonary embolus to that area should be seriously considered (Fig. 3–9) (Hyers et al., 1981).

It is often difficult to distinguish cardiogenic pulmonary edema, atypical edema, or overhydration from bilateral infiltrates of other causes (pneumonia, ARDS, and so forth). Since the distribution of cardiogenic edema is dependent on hydrostatic pressure, gravity may be used as a diagnostic aid. If the patient is placed in the decubitus position for two hours, and then sat up and re–x-rayed, edema will increase on the dependent side and diminish on the contralateral side (Fig. 4–17). Other infiltrates will not shift (Fig. 4–18). Zimmerman et al. (1982) have shown that a positive shift test has a predictive value of 0.85 and a negative test a predictive value of 0.78.

Just as increased left-sided pressures are reflected in the pulmonary veins, increased right-sided pressures are reflected in the azygos vein or superior vena cava. However, dilatation of the superior vena cava is difficult to recognize on the AP radiograph, and dilatation of the azygos vein as seen on the supine film is extremely insensitive to pressure changes (Preger et al., 1969). Despite these limitations, severe dilatation of either vein or dilatation demonstrated on serial erect radiographs accurately reflect systemic venous hypertension. In addition to right-sided heart failure, a markedly dilated azygos vein or superior vena cava may

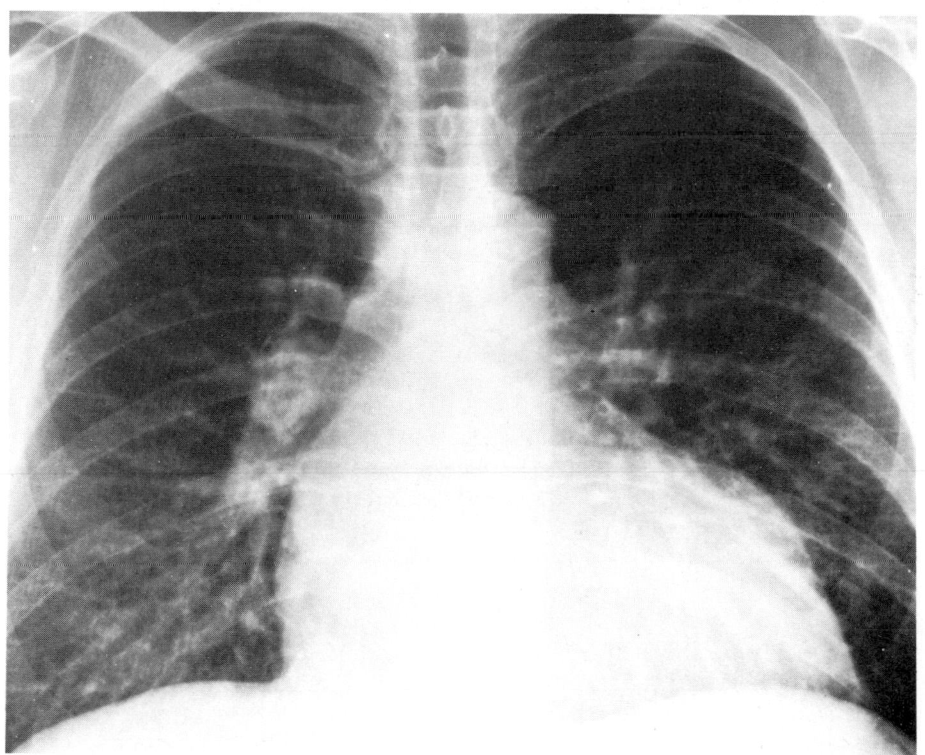

Figure 4–13. CHF. The cardiac contour is enlarged. There is a bulge along the left ventricular contour, indicating a left ventricular aneurysm. The upper lobe pulmonary vessels are prominent. The hila and lower lobe vessels are fuzzy because of perivascular edema. The interstitial markings in the mid- and lower lung fields are accentuated and the minor fissure is slightly thickened. The azygos vein also appears slightly prominent.

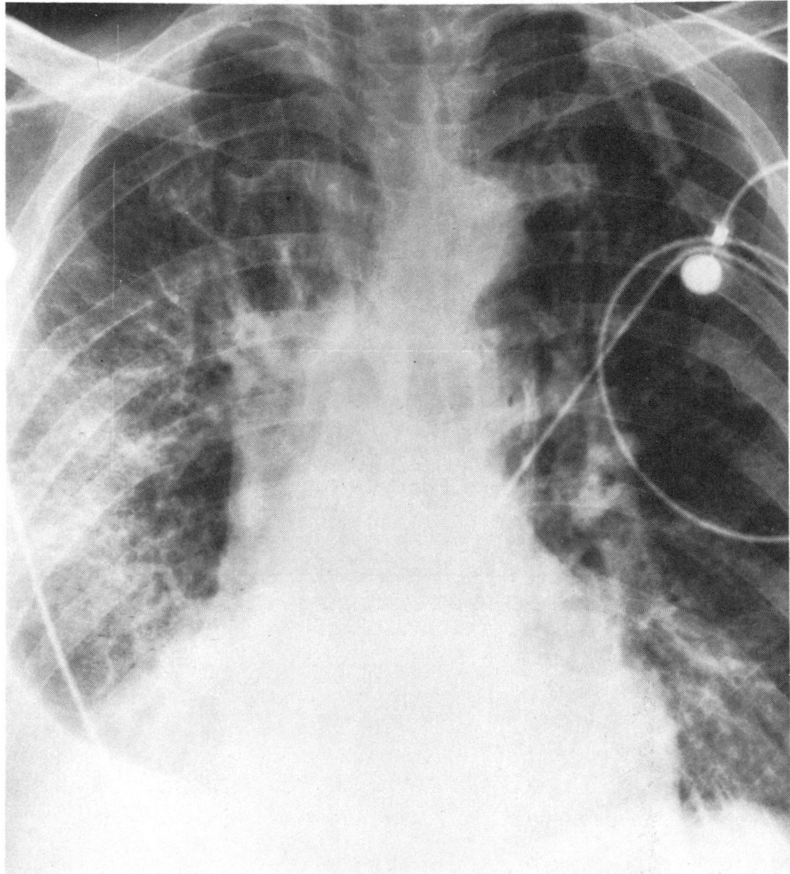

Figure 4–14. Atypical CHF. There is alveolar edema involving the entire right lung and the left lower lobe. A right-sided effusion is also visualized. The heart is at the upper limits of normal. The distribution of the edema represents fluid forming in those areas of the lung that have relatively normal perfusion in this patient with chronic obstructive pulmonary disease (COPD).

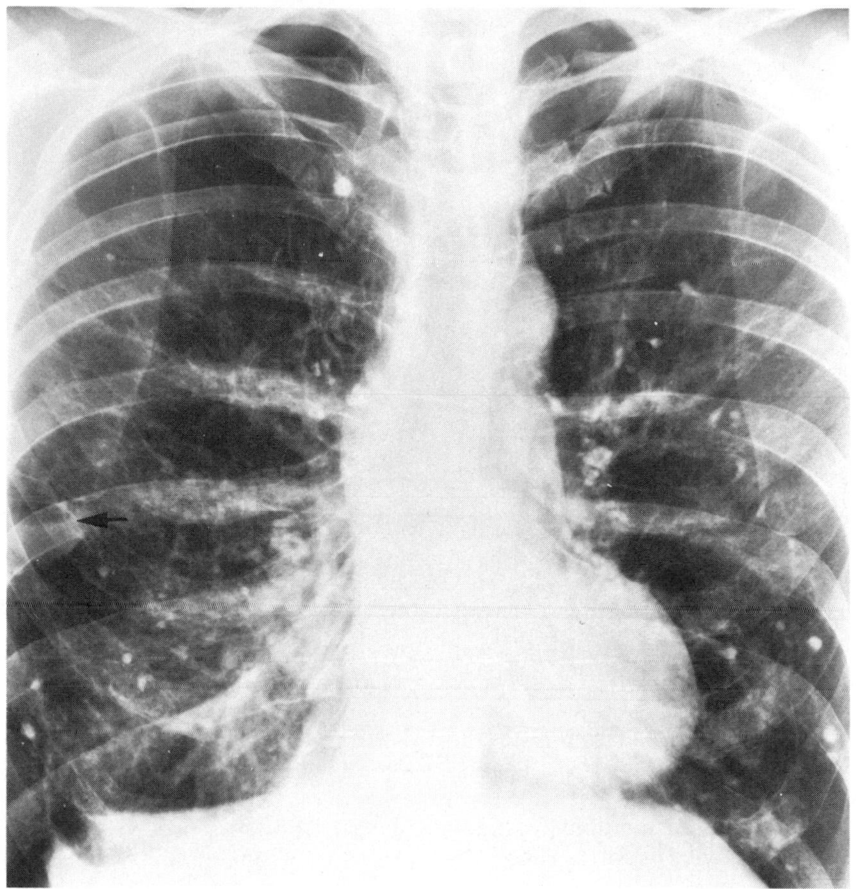

Figure 4–15. Atypical CHF. The interstitial markings on the right are more prominent than those on the left. On earlier films they were equal. In addition, there is now an air fluid level in the bulla in the right midlung (*arrow*). Clinically, the patient appeared to have CHF, not pneumonia. Following appropriate treatment, the interstitial pattern on the right returned to baseline. Clearing of the fluid from the bulla took several weeks. Multiple granulomas, presumably histoplasmosis, are also seen.

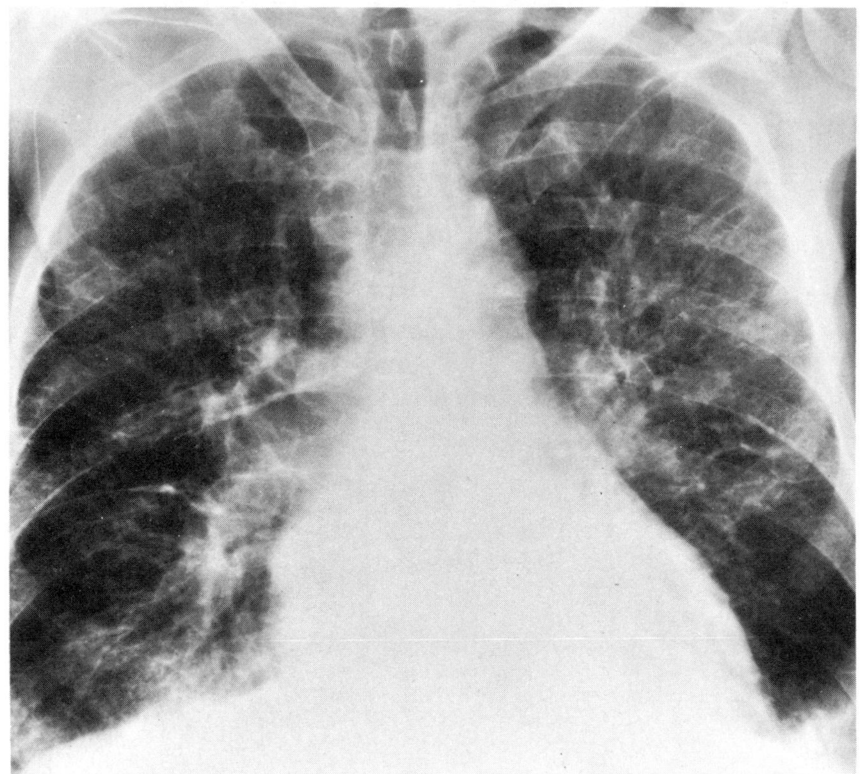

Figure 4–16. Atypical CHF. On the right side there is predominantly interstitial thickening and thickening of the minor fissure. On the left side there is evidence of intra-alveolar edema. The left base remains hyperlucent in this patient with COPD.

be seen in cardiac tamponade or tricuspid valve disease.

Chait and associates (1972) have emphasized the value of upright portable radiographs in the diagnosis of mild subclinical interstitial edema. In their study, two thirds of patients with radiographic but no clinical evidence of CHF eventually developed overt failure. These authors strongly recommend the use of an upright posteroanterior (PA) portable radiograph at a 6-foot target film distance. The patient sits at the bedside, and the film is supported in a commercial or homemade film holder (Lame and Redick, 1970). Portable equipment must be capable of taking radiographs at 0.05 second or less. This technique is applicable to most patients with cardiac disease and to other ICU patients, even though they may be tethered with multiple tubes.

Anteroposterior radiographs exposed with a 40- to 48-inch target film distance cannot be properly evaluated for CHF. Short target film distances cause magnification and geometric unsharpness, which simulate peribronchial edema. The heart is also magnified. With the patient in the supine position, the most valuable sign of increased pulmonary venous pressure, pulmonary vascular redistribution, is lost. Thus, the AP supine film can mimic the major radiographic changes of CHF. Every effort must be made to obtain an erect or semierect radiograph. If this is not possible, the supine film may be of some value when serial changes are sought from day to day. This may be used to some advantage in patients undergoing cardiac surgery or in those who are expected to develop postoperative cardiac problems. In this group, an AP supine film should be obtained preoperatively for a standard of comparison (Harris, 1980).

Noncardiac Pulmonary Edema

Pulmonary edema, the transudation of fluid from the capillaries into the interstitium or alveoli, may be due to numerous causes other than increased pressure in the pulmonary veins. Any disorder that increases pulmonary capillary

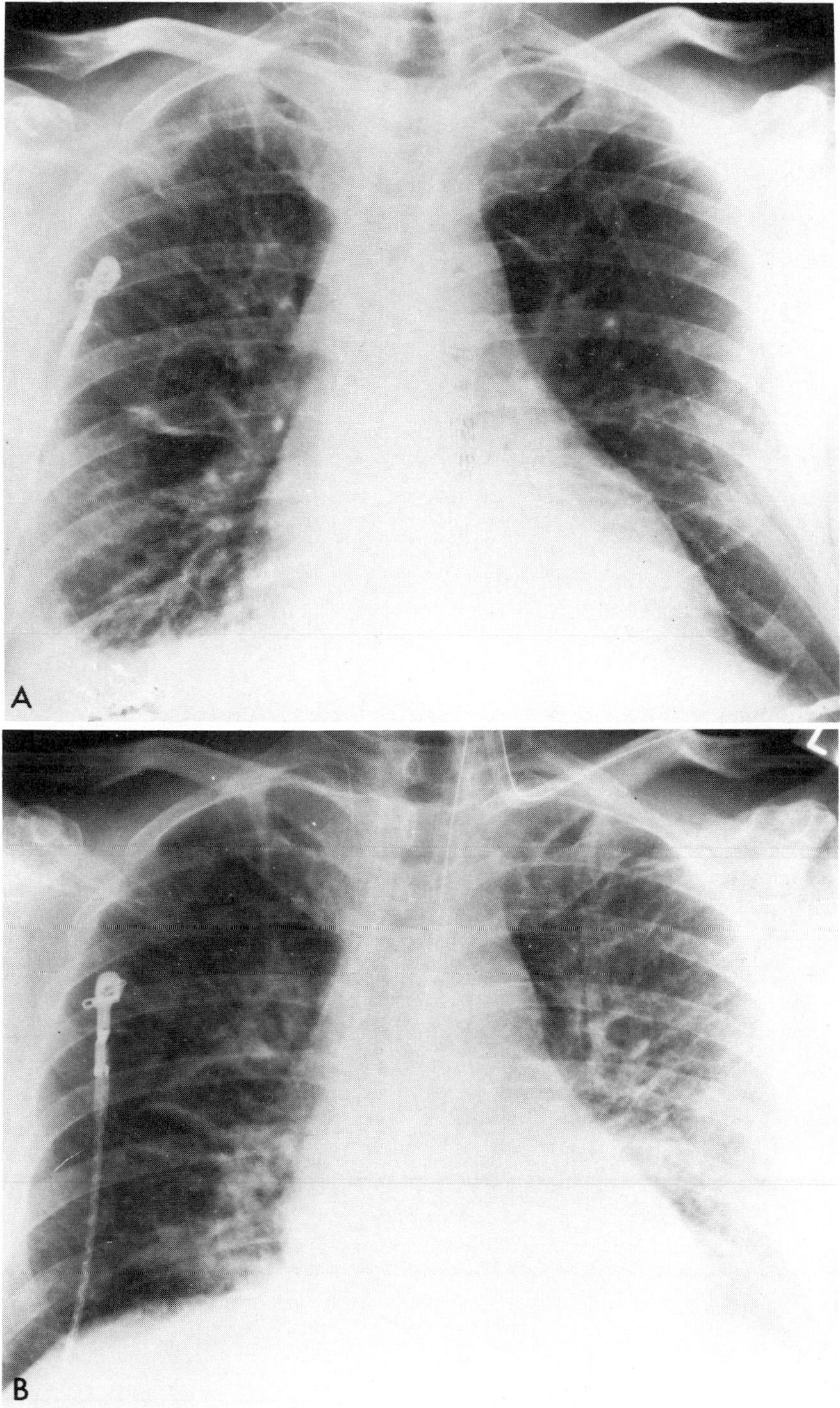

Figure 4–17. Heart failure: positive shift test. *A*, Erect AP radiograph of patient with prominent vessels and interstitial markings plus a small effusion on the right. He is believed to have unilateral pulmonary edema. *B*, After two hours on the patient's left side, a repeat erect AP radiograph shows clearing on the right and shift of edema to the left. He was subsequently proved to be in heart failure due to excess fluid administration. (From Zimmerman et al.: Am. J. Roentgenol., 138:59, 1982.)

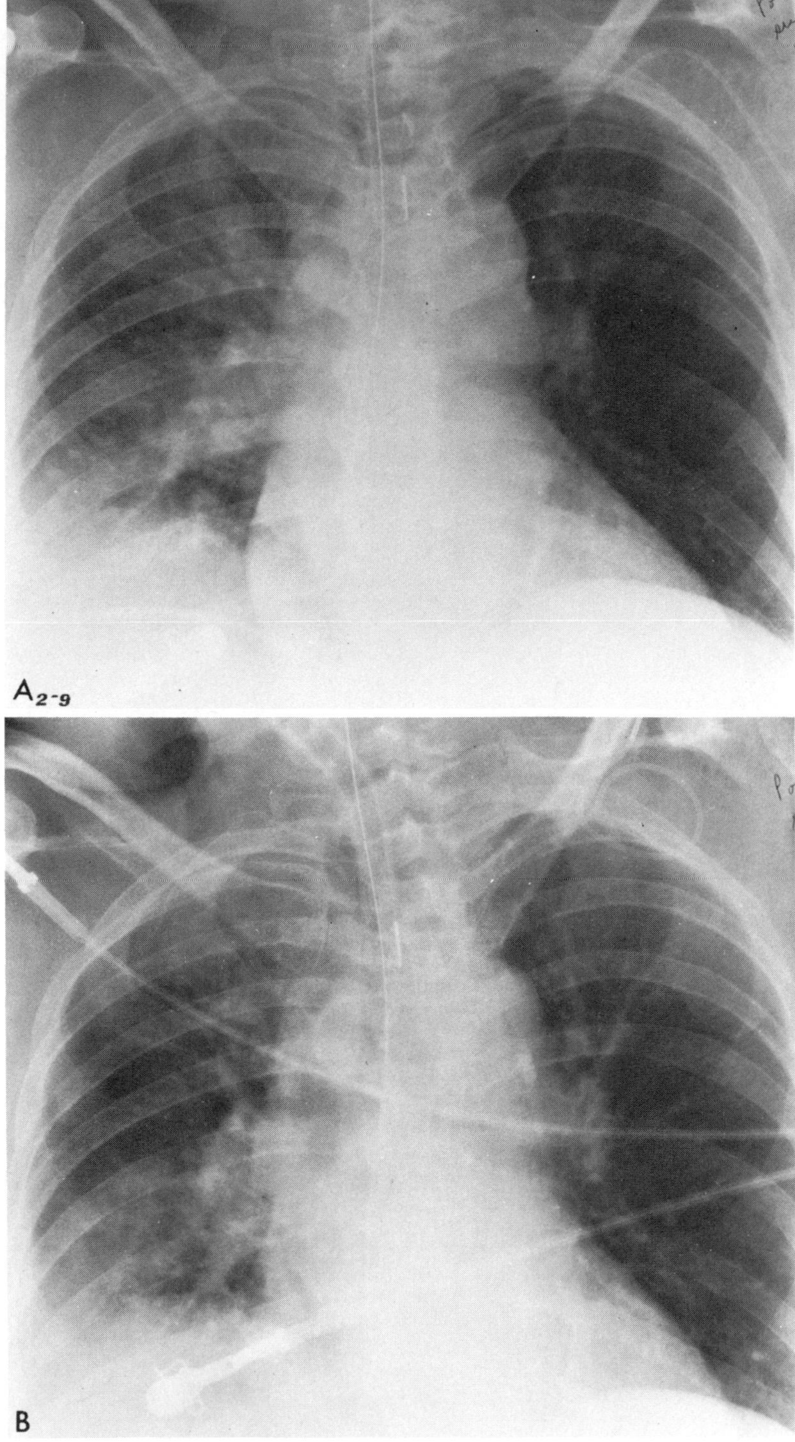

Figure 4–18. Pneumonia: negative shift test. *A*, There is a diffuse infiltrate involving the right side; this is most prominent at the right base. Clinically, it was suspected that the patient may have had an atypical pulmonary edema pattern. *B*, AP radiograph taken after the patient had lain on the left side for several hours indicates no change in the distribution of the pulmonary infiltrate. The patient was eventually shown to have a bacterial pneumonia.

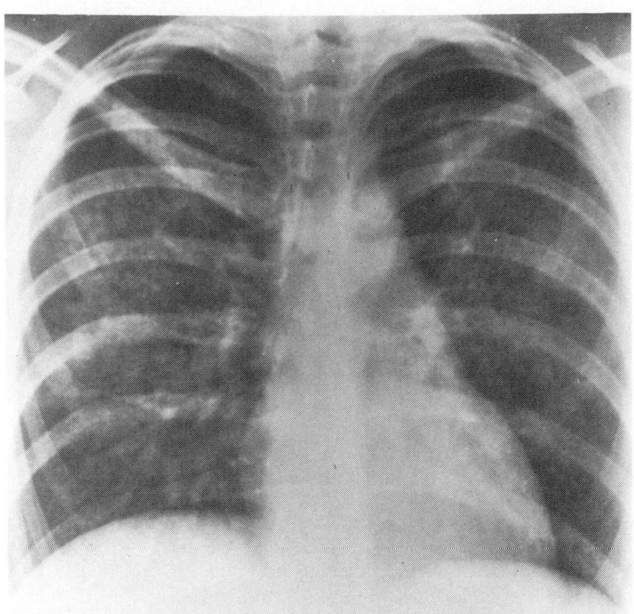

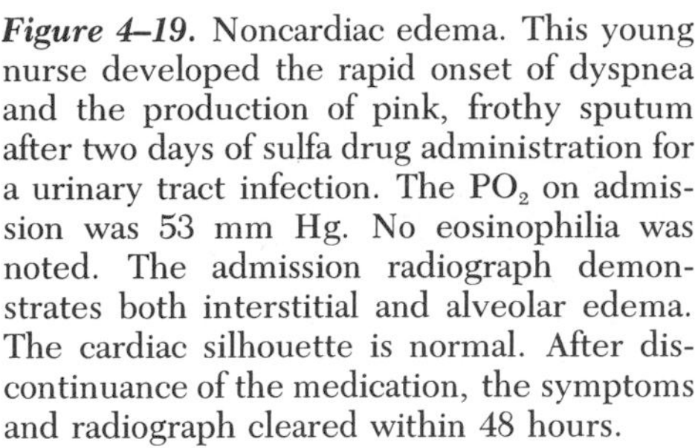

Figure 4–19. Noncardiac edema. This young nurse developed the rapid onset of dyspnea and the production of pink, frothy sputum after two days of sulfa drug administration for a urinary tract infection. The PO_2 on admission was 53 mm Hg. No eosinophilia was noted. The admission radiograph demonstrates both interstitial and alveolar edema. The cardiac silhouette is normal. After discontinuance of the medication, the symptoms and radiograph cleared within 48 hours.

permeability, that decreases the plasma oncotic pressure, or that decreases lymphatic or venous drainage will cause fluid to accumulate in the lung. The radiographic signs of interstitial or alveolar edema are identical to those of CHF, whereas the signs of increased pulmonary venous pressure (vascular redistribution) or cardiomegaly are normally absent (Figs. 4–1, 4–19). Frequent causes of noncardiac edema in the ICU include uremia, sepsis, drug reactions, and ARDS. Table 4–3 summarizes the major causes of edema.

PULMONARY EMBOLISM

Pulmonary embolism is common and difficult to diagnose in the bedridden ICU patient. Predisposing factors include a history of previous embolism, venous or cardiac disease, COPD, obesity, malignancy, dehydration, and "the pill." Pulmonary emboli account for 5 per cent of postoperative deaths and are especially frequent after hip, gynecologic, and prostate surgery (Hartsuck and Greenfield, 1973). Only one third of patients with clinically suspected emboli have positive angiograms, and in patients with emboli documented at autopsy, only 50 per cent were suspected during life (Smith et al., 1964). Adding further to the difficulty of management of the ICU patient is the frequent occurrence of bleeding from anticoagulation (Cheely et al., 1981).

The chest radiograph may be normal or may demonstrate nonspecific changes such as an elevated hemidiaphragm, atelectasis, or patchy infiltrates. The infiltrates tend to be peripheral (Fig. 4–20A). Those that appear and disappear rapidly are due to edema or hemorrhage, and those that persist are likely to be infarcts. Pleural effusions occur in about half the patients, most often associated with infarction. Typically the effusions are small to moderate in size, are unilateral, and are associated with the recent onset of chest pain. After several days the effusions regress (Bynum and Wilson, 1978). Large pulmonary emboli may cause hypoperfusion, unilateral edema, a large pulmonary artery with an abrupt cut-off, or generally enlarged pulmonary arteries (Fig. 4–21). These abnormalities occur infrequently and are seldom recognized on portable radiographs obtained in the ICU (Viamonte et al., 1980). The chest radiograph also serves to exclude other pulmonary disorders that may mimic pulmonary embolism, and is essential for proper interpretation of abnormal perfusion scans.

The radioisotope perfusion scan is the most

TABLE 4–3. Causes of Pulmonary Edema Based on Mechanism*

A. Increased capillary hydrostatic pressure
   1. Left ventricular failure
   2. Mitral valve obstruction
   3. Pulmonary venous obstruction
   4. Hypertransfusion
B. Increased capillary permeability
   1. Toxic inhalants: Carbonyl chloride (phosgene), metallic oxides, paraquat, oxides of nitrogen (silo-filler's disease), ozone, high oxygen atmosphere, smoke inhalation, aspiration of fluids, drowning and near-drowning
   2. Circulating toxins: Alloxan, monocrotaline, alpha-naphthylthiourea, snake venom, pulmonary fat emboli, iodized oil (lymphangiography), histamine, serotonin and kinins
   3. Immunologic reactions: Rheumatic edema, Goodpasture's syndrome, systemic lupus, transfusion reactions
   4. Drug idiosyncracy: Nitrofurantoin (Furadantin), sulfonamides, hydralazine, hexamethonium, methotrexate, busulfan
   5. Infections: Bacterial, viral
   6. Radiation injury
   7. Uremia
   8. Adult respiratory distress syndromes: Wet lung, shock lung, stiff lung, diffuse capillary leak syndrome — after surgery, trauma, burns, hemorrhage, shock, cardiopulmonary bypass
   9. Disseminated intravascular coagulation: Heat stroke, malaria, eclampsia, endotoxemia
C. Decreased plasma osmotic pressure — hypoalbuminemia: Renal, hepatic, protein-losing enteropathy, nutritional disorders
D. Lymphatic insufficiency
E. Unknown or speculative
   1. High altitude
   2. Neurogenic
   3. Narcotic overdose (heroin, methadone)
   4. Cardioversion
   5. Pulmonary embolism

*From CRC Critical Reviews in Clinical Radiology and Nuclear Medicine, J. H. Shapiro and U. F. Hublitz, Vol. 5, p. 389, 1974. © CRC Press, Inc., 1974. Used by permission of CRC Press, Inc.

sensitive, albeit nonspecific, diagnostic tool for examination for pulmonary embolism. In the normally perfused lung, the radionuclide image is homogeneous. In the presence of emboli, the lung scan demonstrates discrete areas of decreased perfusion corresponding to the distribution of the obstructed arteries (Fig. 4–20*B*). These focal areas of hypoperfusion typically have a lobar or segmental distribution. Perfusion defects that result from emboli are frequently multiple and occur most often in the lower lobe. If the chest radiograph is normal and the lung scan demonstrates lobar or segmental perfusion defects, 75 to 90 per cent of patients will have angiographically demonstrable pulmonary emboli (Jackson et al., 1975; Poulose et al., 1970). If patchy, nonsegmental defects are demonstrated on the lung scan, only 25 per cent of patients will have demonstrable emboli. A negative scan essentially eliminates the diagnosis of pulmonary embolism (Novelline et al., 1978).

In the ICU, where COPD, atelectasis, and pneumonia are so common, the meaning of segmental and smaller defects is even less certain. Ventilation scanning, if possible, may demonstrate matched defects, making pulmonary emboli less likely. Other noninvasive tests, such as blood gas analysis, analyses of fibrin degradation products, impedance plethysmography, Doppler evaluation, and isotope venography, although helpful, are not specific for pulmonary emboli (Cheely et al., 1981; Viamonte et al., 1980).

Since ventilation and perfusion scans are safer and easier than angiography, these studies should be done first whenever possible. A negative scan essentially rules out an embolus, and a lobar ventilation-perfusion mismatch strongly suggests emboli (Fig. 4–22). In others, the diagnosis remains uncertain. In patients with severe COPD or diffuse severe pulmonary consolidation, angiography without scanning is usually indicated (Cavaluzzi et al., 1979; Neuhaus et al., 1978). Similarly, patients with suspected massive emboli requiring thrombectomy should receive angiographic examination without delay. Angiography is also required whenever there is a contraindication to anticoagulation or interruption of the inferior vena cava is contemplated.

Pulmonary angiography remains the most de-

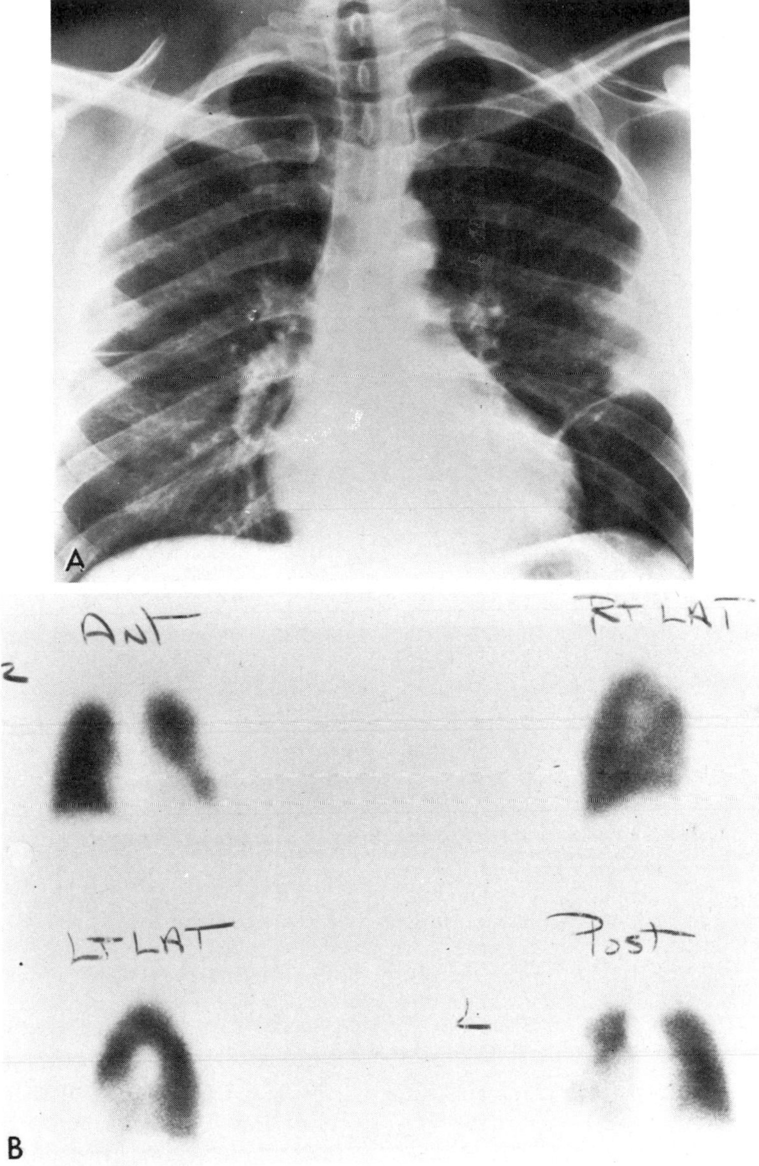

Figure 4–20. Pulmonary embolism and infarction in a 37-year-old man with long leg cast for fractures. Chest pain and minimal dyspnea developed 36 hours earlier. *A*, The PA radiograph shows a peripheral left alveolar density abutting the pleura. A streak of atelectasis is noted lateral to the left heart border. *B*, A perfusion scan shows a segmental perfusion defect in the area of the infiltrate. Because of the strong history and the above findings, a pulmonary angiogram was not performed.

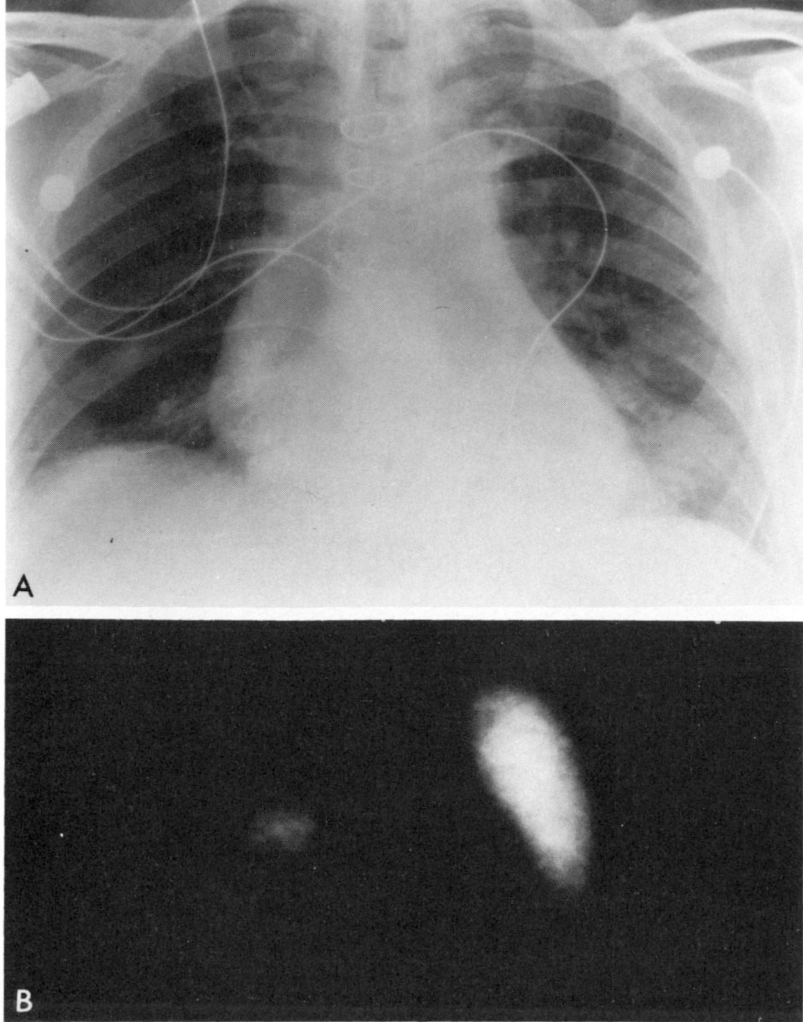

Figure 4–21. Pulmonary emboli with unilateral edema. This 49-year-old coronary artery bypass patient developed severe dyspnea and tachycardia approximately ten days after cardiac surgery. *A*, The AP radiograph reveals a diffuse left-sided infiltrate (new) and a normal right lung. *B*, The AP perfusion scan shows a normal left lung. Minimal perfusion is noted at the right base. No perfusion is noted elsewhere on the right. Follow-up scans nine days later demonstrated partial return of perfusion (*not shown*).

finitive diagnostic tool available. Clinically significant emboli too peripheral to visualize by high-quality, selective angiography are rare (Novelline et al., 1978).

Pulmonary angiography can be performed by a cutdown of the brachial vein or by faster percutaneous puncture of the femoral vein. If the femoral route is used, the iliac veins and inferior vena cava must be well visualized to verify the absence of clots before the catheter is advanced. The reliability of bedside segmental angiography via the Swan-Ganz catheter and intravenous digital angiography has yet to be demonstrated (Dougherty et al., 1980).

Pulmonary arterial pressure should be monitored before high-pressure injections of contrast medium are given. In the presence of markedly elevated pressure (greater than 50 mm Hg), the pressure used for injection and the volume of contrast medium should be reduced and selective studies performed. The catheter may also be withdrawn into the right atrium for injection. Injections into the right ventricle induce cardiac arrhythmias and should be avoided. Precautions and complications of angiography are discussed in Chapters 9 and 10.

Main pulmonary artery or right atrium injec-

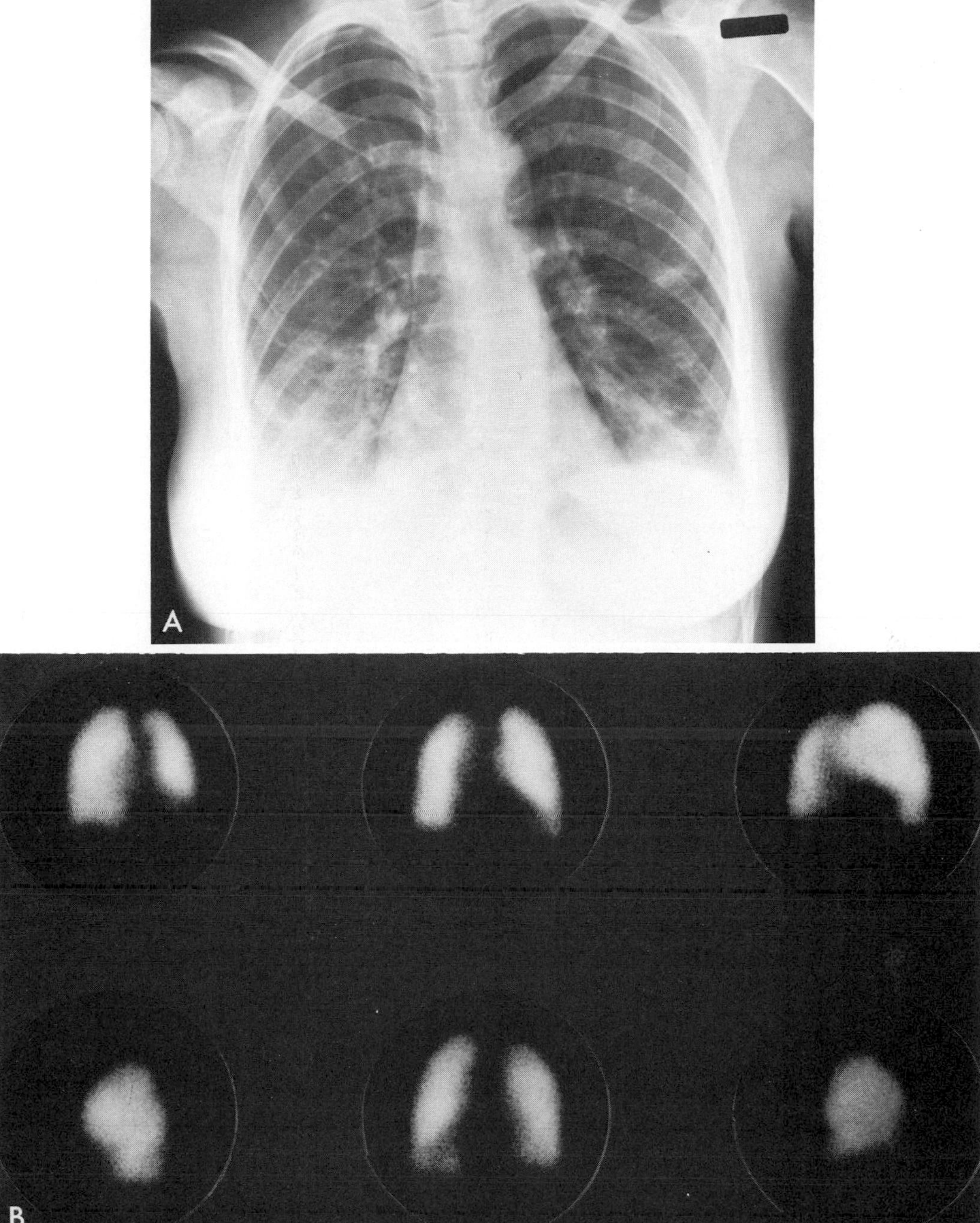

Figure 4–22. Suspected pulmonary embolism. *A*, AP radiograph shows some minimal patchy infiltrates at the lung bases and a suggestion of a right effusion. The heart was normal in size and the pulmonary vessels unremarkable. *B*, Perfusion scan on the same day shows normal perfusion, virtually excluding a pulmonary embolism.

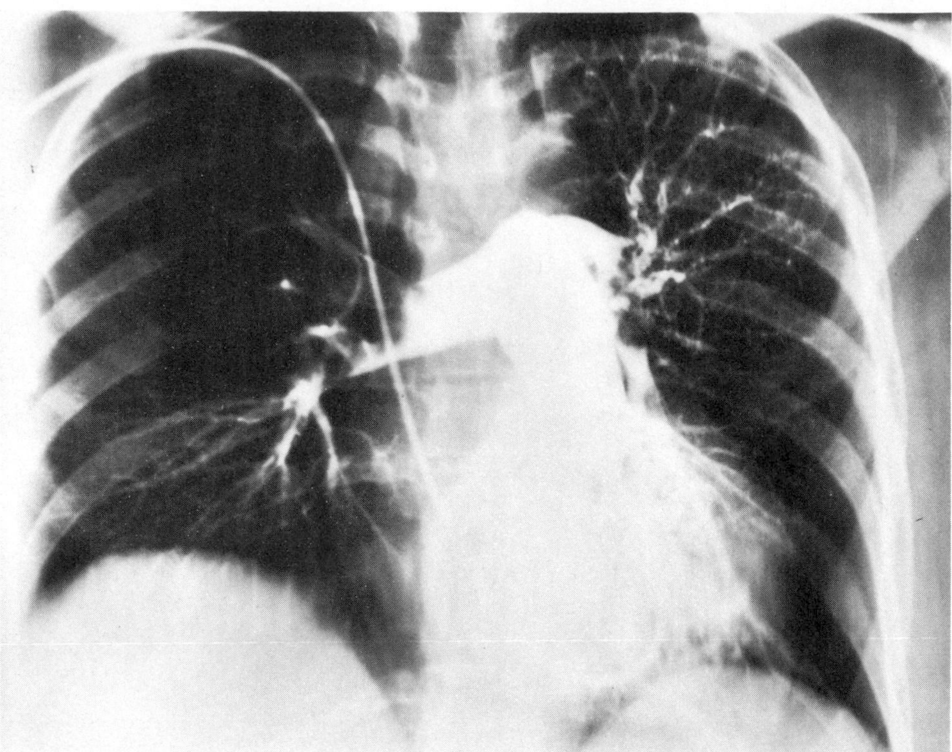

Figure 4–23. Main pulmonary artery injection revealing multiple bilateral intraluminal clots and abrupt cut-off of the right upper and middle lobe pulmonary arteries. The patient's chest radiograph was normal (*not shown*).

tions are usually adequate to demonstrate large emboli on angiographic examination. If no embolus is seen, selective oblique studies must be performed. The lung scan, the mainstream pulmonary angiogram, or the patient's symptoms dictate the side to be selectively injected. The oblique projection diminishes superimposition of arteries, and geometric magnification improves the visualization of defects in the small vessels.

The only definitive angiographic sign of pulmonary embolism is demonstration of the embolus itself. When obstruction is complete, there is a crescentic cut-off of the affected artery (Fig. 4–23). Emboli that do not cause complete obstruction produce a well-marginated lucency within the opacified artery. Secondary signs of pulmonary embolism include pruned or rapidly tapering arteries, peripheral arterial tortuosity, regional diminution of arterial or venous flow rate, and regional hypovascularity. Although these signs may be present in patients with pulmonary embolism, they may also be noted in many other pulmonary diseases. They are helpful, however, because they often serve to direct attention to a particular lobe or segment that can then be examined more selectively.

ABNORMAL AIR COLLECTIONS

Extra-alveolar air collections (EAA) are a frequent and potentially lethal problem in the ICU. They may occur spontaneously, follow trauma, or be due to diagnostic or therapeutic maneuvers. The incidence of iatrogenic air leaks has increased greatly with the more aggressive management of the critically ill patient. Steier and associates (1973) have documented a sevenfold increase in the incidence of iatrogenic pneumothorax over a six-year period without a corresponding increase in spontaneous or post-traumatic EAA. Positive pressure therapy, closed-chest cardiac massage, and subclavian vein catheterization are the three most frequently implicated procedures. The overall incidence of pulmonary barotrauma in patients receiving mechanical ventilation has been estimated at 5 to 15 per cent (Rohlfing et al., 1976). When a pneumothorax develops in these patients, approximately two thirds are under tension. The presence of bullae or blebs, asthma, emphysema, pulmonary infarction, interstitial fibrosis, aspiration pneumonia, necrotizing pneumonia, or pulmonary metastasis in the spontaneously breathing patient predisposes him to air leaks. The application of positive pressure to any of the above conditions will further increase the frequency of EAA. The early recognition of EAA allows for modification of therapy so as to avoid or prepare for the possibility of a tension pneumothorax (Zimmerman et al., 1975).

In any patient suspected of having EAA, or following any procedure known to cause air leaks, a portable erect radiograph should be obtained. Supine or semierect films are not adequate to rule out a small or moderate pneumothorax. If upright films cannot be obtained, lateral decubitus films with the side in question elevated are adequate substitutes. A supine oblique radiograph may at times be helpful in demonstrating air anterolateral to the lung. A horizontal beam lateral radiograph may demonstrate air beneath the sternum or mediastinal air outlining the ascending aorta. Retrosternal lucency per se may be difficult to interpret because a pneumothorax, pneumomediastinum, or large retrosternal space due to hyperinflation may have a similar radiographic appearance (Cimmino, 1967). The pleural line or anterior inferior tip of the lung must be seen to confirm the diagnosis.

The pathogenesis of pneumothorax is frequently oversimplified, with the lung collapse being likened to that of an over-inflated balloon that has ruptured. This certainly happens in spontaneous pneumothorax associated with a rupture of apical blebs, with needle puncture of the lung, or when infected lung parenchyma is weakened by abscess formation. However, the visceral pleura is extremely resilient and ruptures with difficulty. A second mechanism of equal importance is the rupture of alveoli with dissection of gas along the vessel sheaths into the mediastinum. (Zimmerman et al., 1975.)

Since the mediastinal tissue planes are continuous with those of the neck and the retroperitoneum, air may dissect along these planes. Rupture of the mediastinal parietal pleura will lead to a pneumothorax, and rupture of the parietal peritoneum will lead to a pneumoperitoneum (Macklin and Macklin, 1944). Because interstitial air dissection is the most frequent cause of pneumothorax in the patient receiving respiratory therapy, the discussion in this section is structured to follow the course of air along the interstitial tissues into the mediastinum and then into the subcutaneous tissues, the pleural space, and the pericardium.

Interstitial Emphysema

Following rupture of the alveoli, air dissecting along the interstitial tissues may cause little in the way of clinical symptoms or may cause marked respiratory and circulatory embarrassment. Although interstitial air dissection presumably precedes most cases of pneumomediastinum, the radiographic documentation of interstitial air is difficult in the adult (Leeming, 1968). It appears radiographically as an irregular radiolucent mottling in the medial half to two thirds of the lower lung field. It may be streaky or cleftlike, or may show multiple small bubbles of air (Fig. 4–24). Unlike air bronchograms, interstitial air is irregular in distribution and does not taper progressively (Westcott and Cole, 1974). A pathognomonic but rare sign of interstitial emphysema is visualization of a radiolucent "halo" of air around a pulmonary vessel seen on end (Fig. 4–24).

A more frequent sign of interstitial emphysema is the round or oval subpleural air cyst, which is a collection of air in the loose connective tissue beneath the pleura (Fig. 4–25). Such air cysts develop rapidly, change rapidly, are thin-walled, and may appear in an area previously free of disease. They are seen most often along the diaphragmatic or visceral pleural surfaces (Rohlfing et al., 1976; Westcott and Cole, 1974). Air loculated in the infrahilar region may be trapped in the inferior pulmonary ligament. If these cysts appear only in a diseased area, differentiation from a thin-walled abscess or pneumatocele may be impossible. Edema or pulmonary infiltrate around a pre-existing bullae may give a similar appearance. Bullae, which are usually stable in size as the parenchymal diseases comes and goes, may also be identified elsewhere in the lung or on old films. In any event, air cysts, abscesses, pneumatoceles, and bullae should be followed carefully for signs of enlargement. Enlargement indicates a potential rupture and should lead to a reassessment of the need for positive pressure respiration or for preparation for the eventuality of a pneumothorax (Zimmerman et al., 1975) (Fig. 4–25).

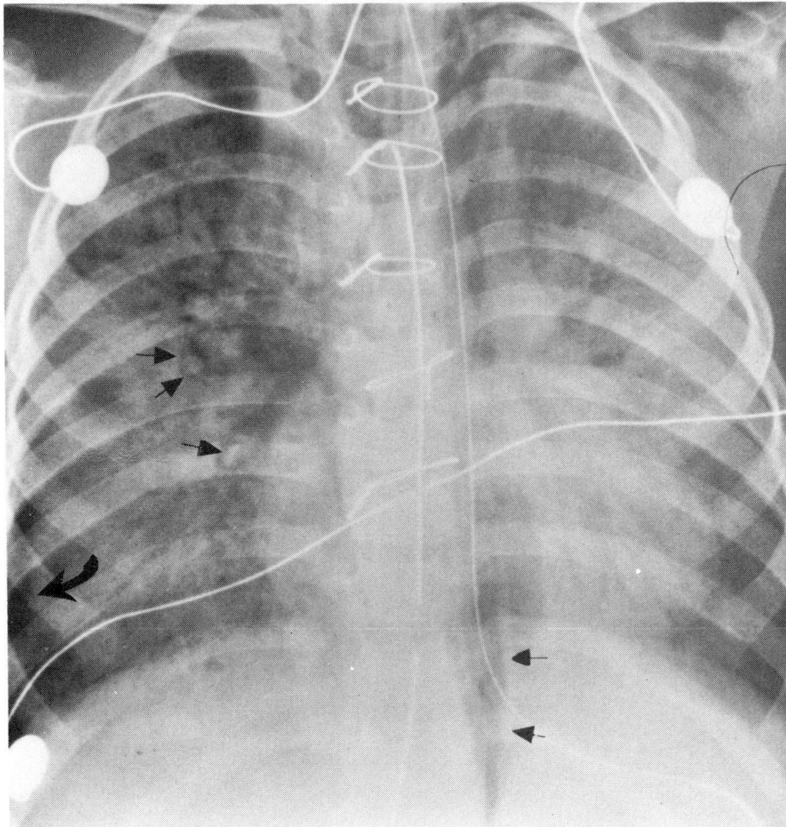

Figure 4–24. Interstitial emphysema and pulmonary edema in a young child. Diffuse alveolar edema is noted bilaterally with multiple streaky and bubbly lucencies throughout the right lung. Unlike air bronchograms, the lucencies do not taper and branch symmetrically. Two vessels on end surrounded by a halo of air are seen on the right (*arrows*). A small pneumothorax is seen laterally on this supine film (*curved arrow*). Air is seen entering the retroperitoneum on the left (*arrows*). This pattern of interstitial emphysema is seldom seen in adults. (Courtesy of B. Rohlfing, M.D., San Francisco, CA.)

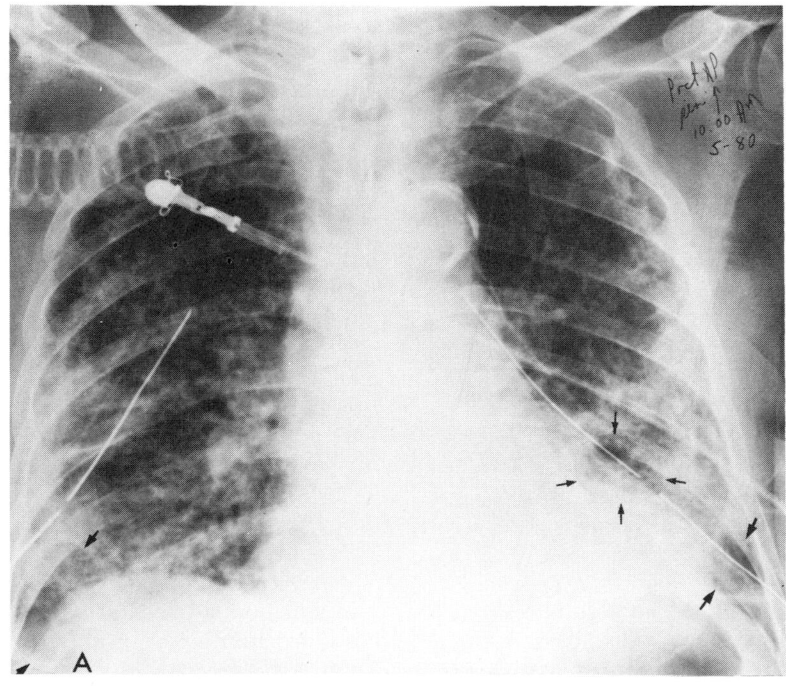

Figure 4–25 *See legend on opposite page*

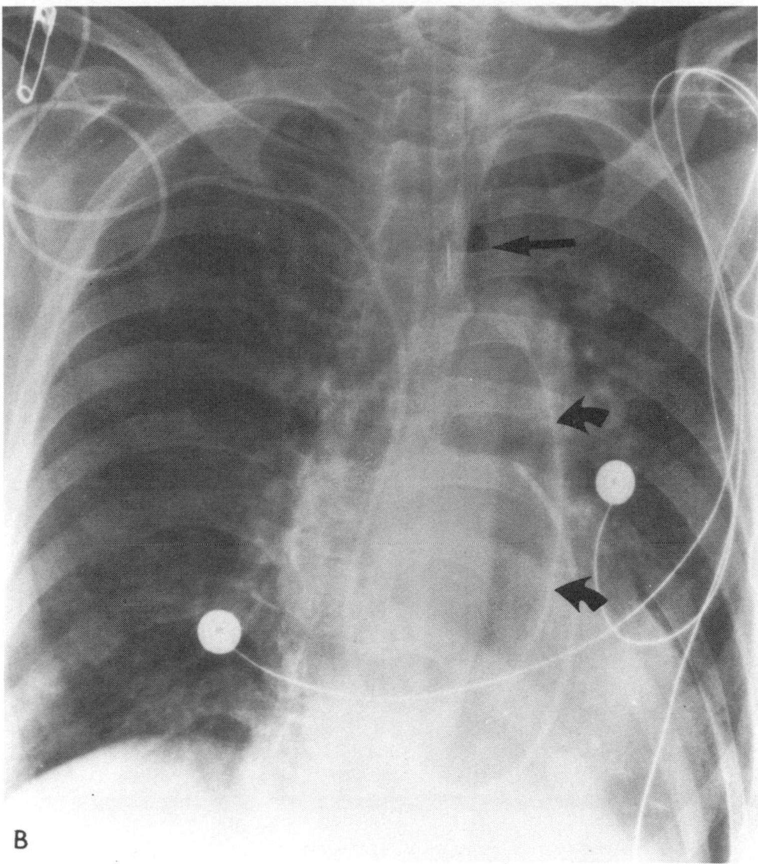

Figure 4–25. Interstitial air cysts (2 patients). *A*, Air has dissected in the interstitial tissues and has collected subpleurally (*arrows*). These collections develop rapidly and differentiation from pneumatocele may be difficult. Chest tubes are draining bilateral pneumothoraces. *B*, A film 18 hours earlier showed a left lower infiltrate. Now, in addition to the infiltrate, there is a large collection of air in the retrocardiac area (*curved arrows*). This presumably represents an interstitial air cyst. It is too high to be air in the inferior pulmonary ligament. An area suspect for a pneumomediastinum (*upper arrow*) is also seen. On the following day a radiograph (*not shown*) revealed a tension pneumothorax. The focal air collection was no longer present.

Pneumomediastinum

Air may reach the mediastinum from the lung, the neck, or the abdomen or from rupture of the esophagus or trachea. In the patient with obstructive airway disease or who is receiving respirator therapy, pneumomediastinum is usually the first radiographic sign of interstitial air dissection and may be the precursor to a pneumothorax. Air in the neck or retroperitoneum due to surgery, trauma, or infection may dissect along the tissue plains into the mediastinum. Tracheal or esophageal rupture may also cause mediastinal emphysema.

Large collections of mediastinal air cause a wide lucent band around the heart and mediastinum, delineated by the reflected visceral and parietal pleura. This usually presents little diagnostic difficulty, although differentiation from a medial pneumothorax in a supine patient may be difficult (Fig. 4–26). When the pneumomediastinum is small, more subtle signs must be sought.

1. A thin, very sharp lucent line around the heart or an "unusually clear" heart border may be the first indicator of a pneumomediastinum. The pleural reflection must be seen delineating this lucency laterally (Fig. 4–26). If not, care must be taken to distinguish this lucency from the "kinetic halo" often seen separating the heart, aorta, and diaphragm from a pulmonary infiltrate or pulmonary edema (Fig. 4–27). This

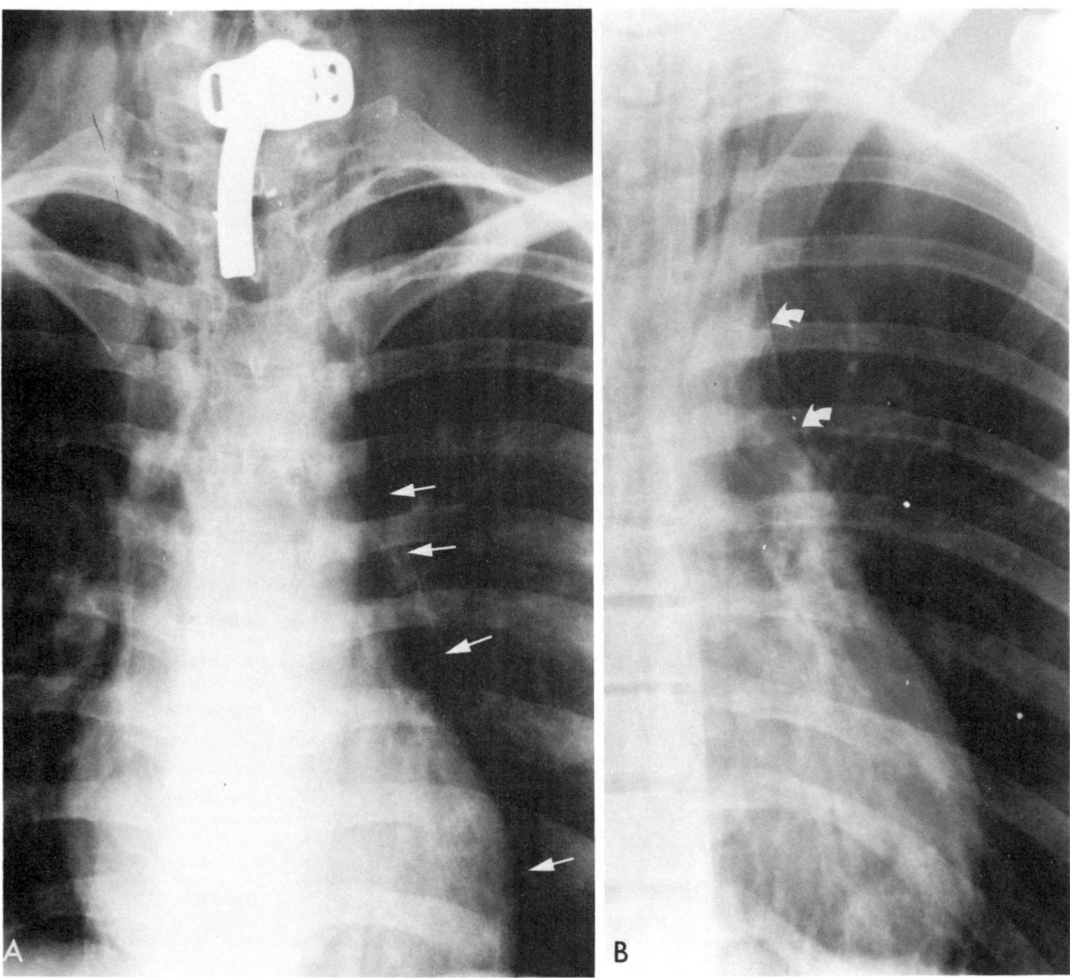

Figure 4–26. Pneumomediastinum (2 patients). *A*, A large lucency is seen adjacent to the left border of the heart, delineated by the pleura (*arrows*). Subcutaneous air is seen in the neck. *B*, The reflected mediastinal pleura is outlined by arrows. No other abnormalities were identified. (Courtesy of C. Ochs, M.D., Birmingham, Ala.)

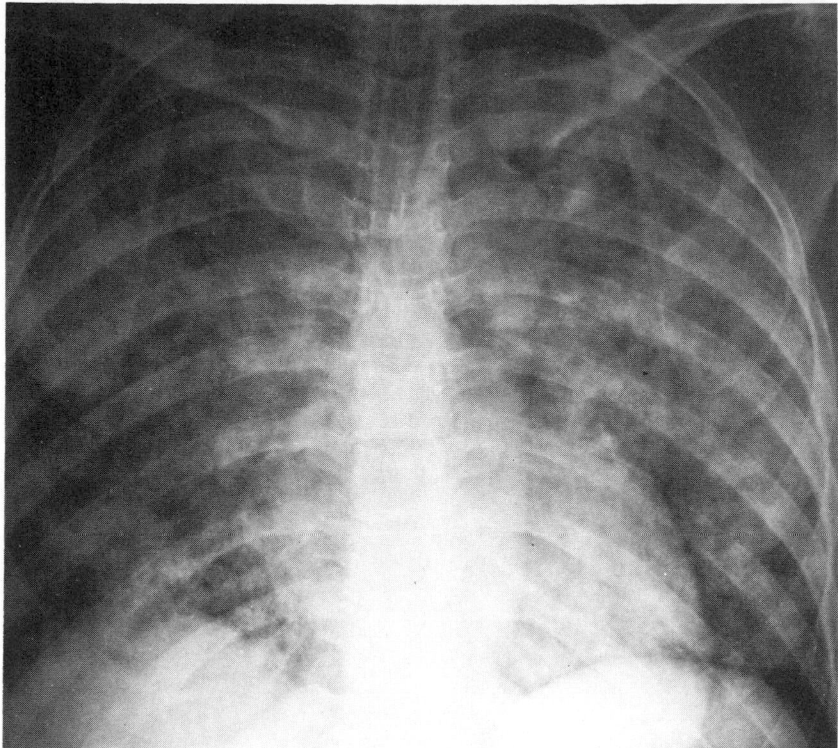

Figure 4–27. "Kinetic halo." A radiolucency is seen around the heart border, the transverse and descending aorta, and both hemidiaphragms. The pleural reflection is not seen in any of these locations.

halo is only moderately lucent and does not have a pencil-sharp lateral border. It is postulated that it is caused by increased reabsorption of edema fluid due to the milking action that the beating heart, aorta, and diaphragm have on the adjacent lung tissue (Steckel, 1974). The Mach effect may also contribute to the apparent lucency.

2. On the frontal film, a thin crescent of air may outline the aortic knob or a thin black stripe may delineate the descending aorta (Figs. 2–12*A*, 4–25*B*, 4–28). On a lateral radiograph a sharp lucent line may outline the ascending aorta, the great vessels, and possibly the thymus and prevertebral soft tissues.

3. Rarely, in adults, air dissects between the parietal pleura and the diaphragm. A lucent stripe is then seen between the lung base and the diaphragm. The undersurface of the heart may be outlined and the diaphragm seen as a continuous structure across the midline (Levin, 1973). If the individual muscle slips of the diaphragm can be distinguished, this indicates that air has dissected between the parietal pleura and diaphragm (extrapleural) or between the parietal peritoneum and diaphragm (extraperitoneal) (Christensen and Landay, 1980).

4. Air in the soft tissues of the neck or retroperitoneum offers indirect confirmation of a pneumomediastinum.

Subcutaneous Air

Air collecting in the subcutaneous tissues of the neck and shoulder may be due to local trauma (tracheostomy, transtracheal aspiration) or may be secondary to a pneumomediastinum. Subcutaneous emphysema after tracheostomy is usually self-limited but may on occasion dissect downward into the mediastinum. This is most likely to occur in the ventilated patient whose tracheostomy stoma has been sutured or packed tightly. Subcutaneous emphysema due to pulmonary barotrauma may be the first clinical or radiographic sign of extra-alveolar air (Figs. 4–26*A*, 4–29).

The radiograph reveals sharply etched linear lucencies that parallel the tissue planes or multiple lucent bubbles in the soft tissues. Individual muscles or muscle slips are often visible. Air must be differentiated from fat lucencies that are seen outlining the muscle planes on ideally exposed radiographs. Extensive air in

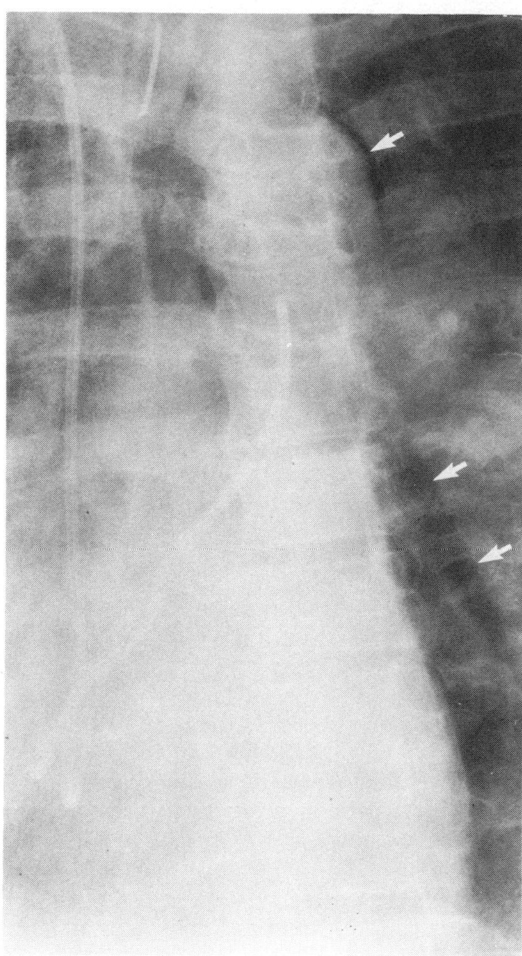

Figure 4–28. Pneumomediastinum. A small crescent of air is seen outlining the aorta. The aortic pleural reflection is faintly seen (*upper arrow*). The lower arrows delineate the left lower lobe bronchus on this badly rotated film. Several redundant loops of the Swan-Ganz catheter are seen in the right ventricle.

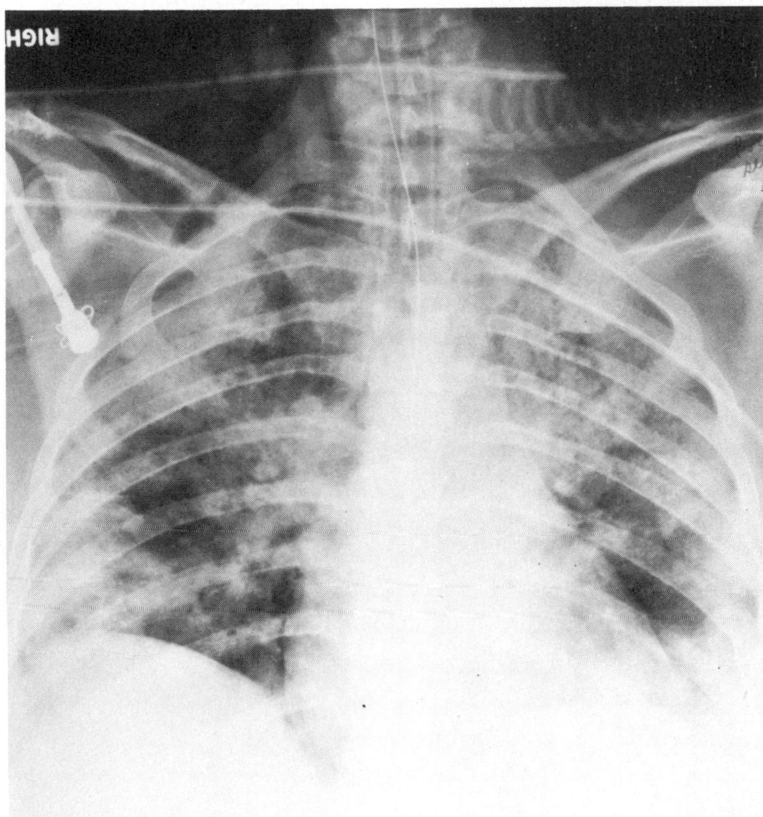

Figure 4–29. Subcutaneous emphysema. Air accumulated in the right side of the neck of this patient, who was being ventilated for *Pneumocystis carinii* pneumonia. No definite pneumomediastinum, interstitial air, or pneumothorax developed. Numerous pleural adhesions were encountered when a prophylactic tube was inserted into the right hemithorax.

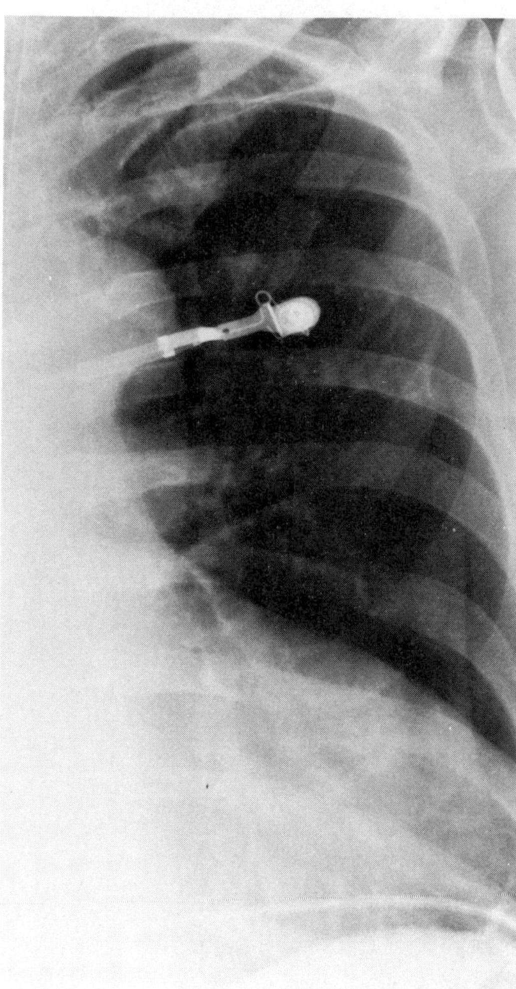

Figure 4–30. Skin fold. The redundant fold of skin closely mimics a pneumothorax. The pulmonary vessels are difficult to see beyond the skin fold without a bright light. Note that the skin fold appears as a broad white band bordered by a thin lucent line laterally.

the soft tissues of the chest may mimic or obscure pulmonary parenchymal disease.

A small amount of subcutaneous air may be seen alongside a thoracostomy drainage tube and is of no clinical significance. However, a progressive increase in subcutaneous air indicates the presence of a bronchopleural fistula or a chest tube that is malfunctioning (Fig. 2–21). Subcutaneous air in the soft tissues around the rib cage of patients with blunt thoracic trauma may be the only indication that the integrity of the pleura has been breached. Even in the absence of a visible pneumothorax, a prophylactic thoracostomy tube should be considered before the patient is placed on a respirator (Fig. 4–29).

Pneumothorax

Every effort should be made to obtain an upright expiratory radiograph when a pneumothorax is being considered. In addition to the absence of pulmonary markings in the lung apex, the radiodense pleural stripe must be visualized. In patients with COPD or who are hyperinflated by the ventilator, apical pulmonary markings are often sparse, simulating a pneumothorax. In such instances, the absence of apical vessels is usually bilateral and the pleural stripe is not seen. In obese patients or in those with poor skin tone, air trapped in skin folds frequently mimics a pneumothorax (Figs. 2–3, 4–30). This usually appears as a radiodense band with a radiolucent line on the outer margin. The band often extends beyond the confines of the thorax. Lung markings are usually visible lateral to the lucency.

If the patient is radiographed in the supine position, air will rise anteriorly. If the air collects medially, between the lung and the heart, it will mimic a pneumomediastinum or pneumopericardium (Cimmino, 1967) (Fig. 4–31). Air collecting between the lung base and the diaphragm will show as a radiolucent band or an unusually deep costophrenic angle laterally or medially (Gordon, 1980; Kurlander and Helman, 1966) (Fig. 4–32). Air collecting in the lateral anterior costophrenic sulcus may appear as a focal "subdiaphragmatic" lucency over the lateral aspect of the liver or spleen (Rhea et al., 1979) (Fig. 4–33). Air may also collect in the minor fissure. If any of these signs are present, horizontal beam radiographs should be obtained to ascertain the size of the pneumothorax (Figs. 4–32*B*, 4–33, 4–34). The absence of all the above signs does *not* exclude a pneumothorax on a supine film.

A tension pneumothorax should be diagnosed clinically. Treatment should not await radiographic confirmation. If it is diagnosed by the radiograph, immediate therapy must be instituted. The usual combination of a totally collapsed lung and a mediastinal shift to the contralateral side is readily diagnosed. Great care should be exercised in interpreting mediastinal shifts on AP radiographs because slight degrees of rotation or scoliosis can appear as large mediastinal shifts. In these cases, the demonstration of a flat or inverted diaphragm allows the diagnosis of tension pneumothorax in spite of rotation (Figs. 3–5, 4–35). In the ICU, a tension pneumothorax is not infrequently present without complete collapse of the lung. The severely diseased lung may be too rigid to collapse completely, or pleural adhesions may fix areas of lung to the chest wall. Again, the depressed diaphragm is a helpful aid in diagnosis.

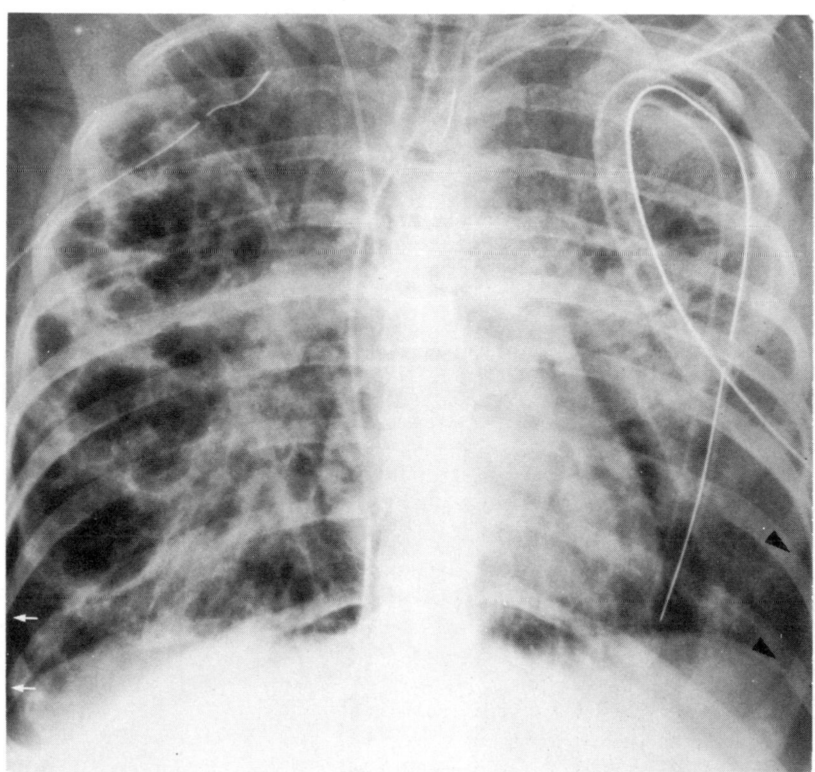

Figure 4–31. Pneumothorax. On the supine radiograph on the left side, the intrapleural air is seen adjacent to the heart, simulating a pneumomediastinum or pneumopericardium. The air in the left costophrenic angle confirms the pneumothorax (*arrowheads*). Without this air, an upright or decubitus film would be necessary to distinguish the pneumothorax from a pneumomediastinum or pneumopericardium. On the right side, air is seen along the right lateral lung margin (*white arrows*). A central venous pressure (CVP) catheter is seen entering the inferior vena cava. The left thoracostomy tube is poorly positioned to relieve a pneumothorax.

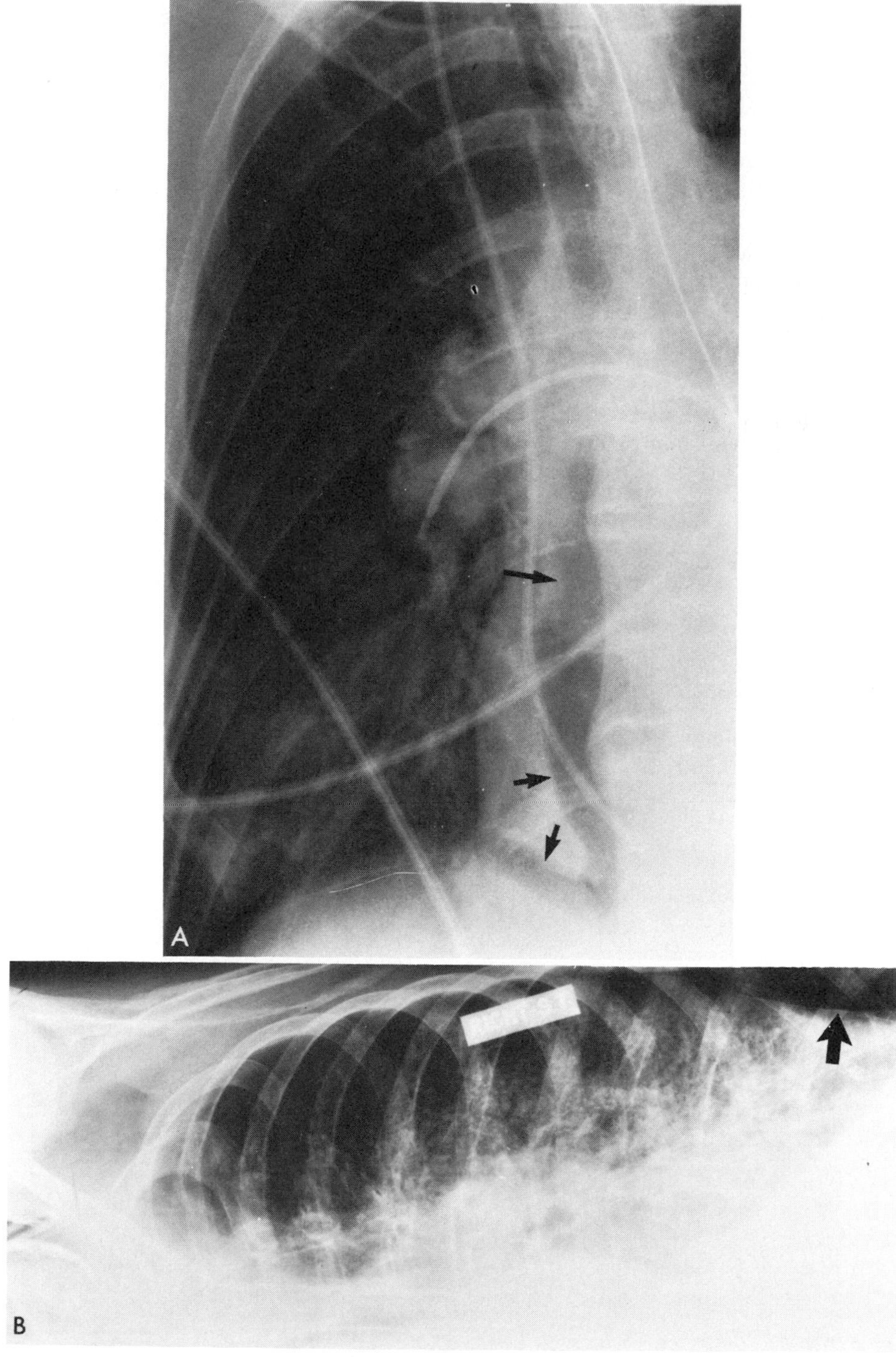

Figure 4–32. Pneumothorax. *A*, Supine radiograph shows a radiolucent band to the right of the spine (*horizontal arrows*), continuous with a thin radiolucency between the lung base and the hemidiaphragm (*vertical arrows*). *B*, Decubitus film demonstrates a small collection of air between the lung and the ribs in the costophrenic angle (*arrows*).

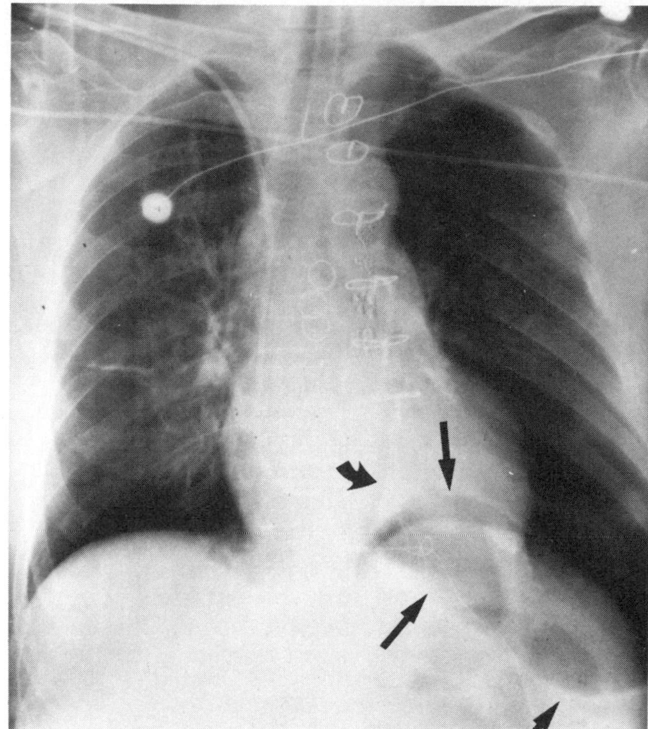

Figure 4–33. Pneumothorax. On the supine film a large collection of air is seen over the left upper quadrant (*straight arrows*). The lucency is due to air collecting along the anterior chest wall in the anterior costophrenic angle. A small amount of air is also seen in the medial pleural space (*curved arrow*).

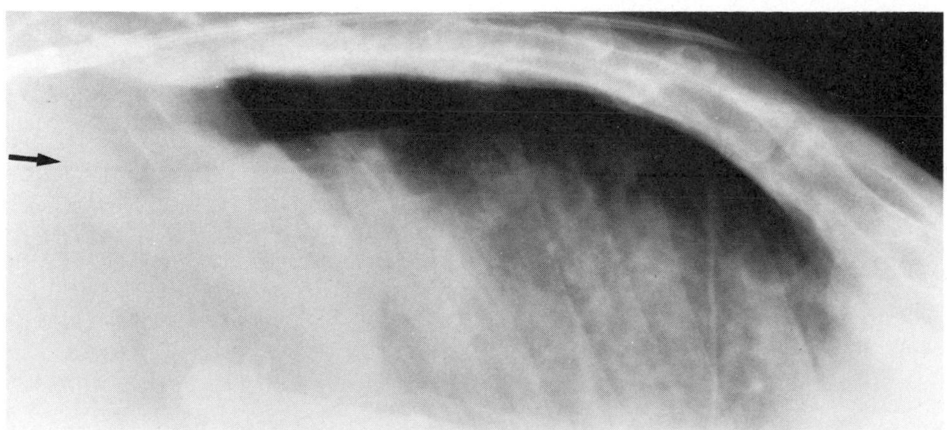

Figure 4–34. Pneumothorax. Horizontal beam lateral (across the bed) radiograph demonstrates air beneath the sternum and the anteroinferior angle of the lung (*arrow*).

Pneumopericardium

Pneumopericardium in adults is almost always due to surgery, trauma, or infection and rarely, if ever, results from a pneumomediastinum (Cimmino, 1967). In the adult, the radiolucent rim around the heart is usually outlined by a thickened pericardium and usually presents little diagnostic difficulty. On the upright radiograph, the air extends to or includes the proximal pulmonary artery and aorta but does not extend above this level (Fig. 4–36). On the supine radiograph, a pneumopericardium, a pneumothorax, and a pneumomediastinum may have a similar appearance. In the absence of a visibly thickened pericardium, a lucency around the heart is most likely due to air between the visceral and parietal pleura (pneumothorax) or to air between the parietal pericardium and the parietal pleura (pneumomediastinum). In doubtful cases, a lateral decubitus or horizontal beam lateral radiograph will aid in the differentiation of pleural, mediastinal, and pericardial air.

Abscess vs. Empyema

The cause of an air fluid level on an upright chest radiograph can usually be ascertained by the clinical history and a review of serial films. On occasion, however, differentiation between a lung abscess and an air fluid level due to a loculated empyema may be difficult. As a general rule, empyemas have a long air fluid level that is not very dense, a reflecton of the long, flat configuration of most intrapleural collections. Most empyema collections are posterior and appear on the AP radiograph as an air fluid level that traverses most of the chest and reaches the lateral chest wall. Lateral radiographs demonstrate a narrow AP diameter to the collection as well as the tapering pleural margins (Fig. 4–37). The air fluid level again reaches the chest wall (Friedman and Hellekant, 1976; Schachter et al., 1976). Lateral loculations are broad in their AP diameter and narrow in their lateral dimension. Demonstration of an air fluid level crossing a fissure on an upright or lateral decubitus film is diagnostic of an extrapulmonary collection. Conversely, abscesses tend to be round, have air fluid levels that do not reach the end of the surrounding infiltrate (Fig. 4–6*B*), and do not cross fissures on the horizontal beam radiograph.

When the diagnosis is uncertain, computerized tomography (CT) is often of great help. Abscesses are characterized by an irregular shape; multiple side-pockets; a ragged, thick wall; and an irregular interface with the normal lung. Empyemas tend to be regular, smooth, and without side-pockets and have a sharp interface with the lung (Fig. 6–3*B*, *C*). Empyemas may change shape with changing position, whereas an abscess tends to remain unaltered (Baber et al., 1980). CT is also of value in determining the presence or absence of fluid when there is dense parenchymal consolidation (Fig. 4–5).

ABNORMAL FLUID COLLECTIONS

Pleural Effusions

The spectrum of diseases causing pleural effusions in the ICU patient is similar to that in other hospitalized patients. Two additional problems, however, are worthy of comment. Following abdominal surgery, approximately 50 per cent of patients develop small pleural effusions in the first several postoperative days (Light and George, 1976). In 20 per cent of patients the effusion is bilateral. An effusion is more likely to occur after upper abdominal surgery, on the side of the surgery, in patients with postoperative atelectasis or with ascites. The effusions are usually small to moderate in size, are exudates, and are of little apparent clinical significance. They usually resolve within a week or two. Unless there is strong clinical reason to suspect a pulmonary embolus, subphrenic abscess, empyema, or the like, no further work-up is usually required. These effusions contrast with those due to subphrenic abscess. The latter generally appear during or after the *second* postoperative week, and are often associated with fever and upper abdominal symptoms.

Another unusual cause of pleural effusions in the ICU relates to intravenous (IV) infusion catheters. Catheters may perforate the mediastinal veins and enter the pleural space. Fluid or blood then rapidly accumulates on that side. This is discussed more fully in Chapter 3.

Pleural effusions may be difficult to detect on radiographs taken with the patient sitting in bed. Even in the absence of an effusion, the costophrenic angles are often shallow and the diaphragm may appear flattened or elevated. Differentiation between fluid and posterior basal atelectasis may be difficult (Savoca et al.,

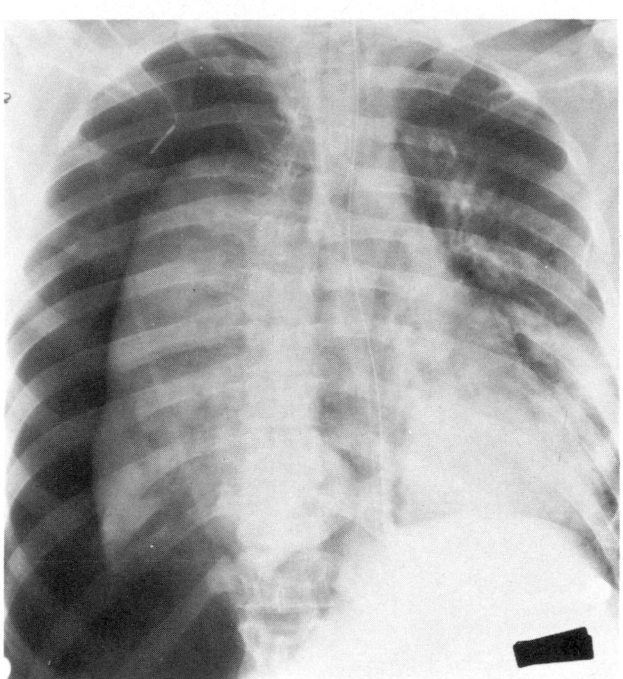

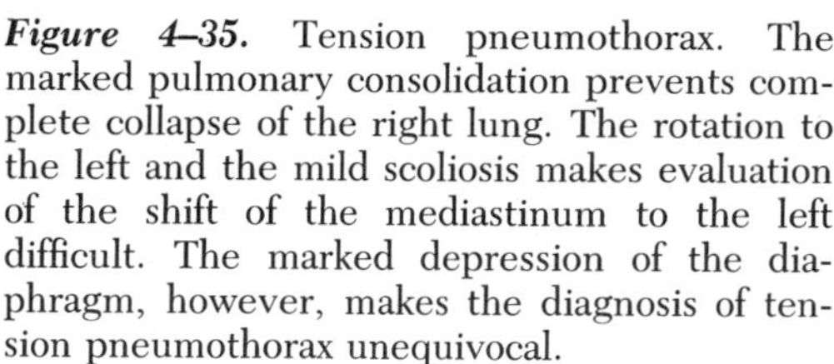

Figure 4–35. Tension pneumothorax. The marked pulmonary consolidation prevents complete collapse of the right lung. The rotation to the left and the mild scoliosis makes evaluation of the shift of the mediastinum to the left difficult. The marked depression of the diaphragm, however, makes the diagnosis of tension pneumothorax unequivocal.

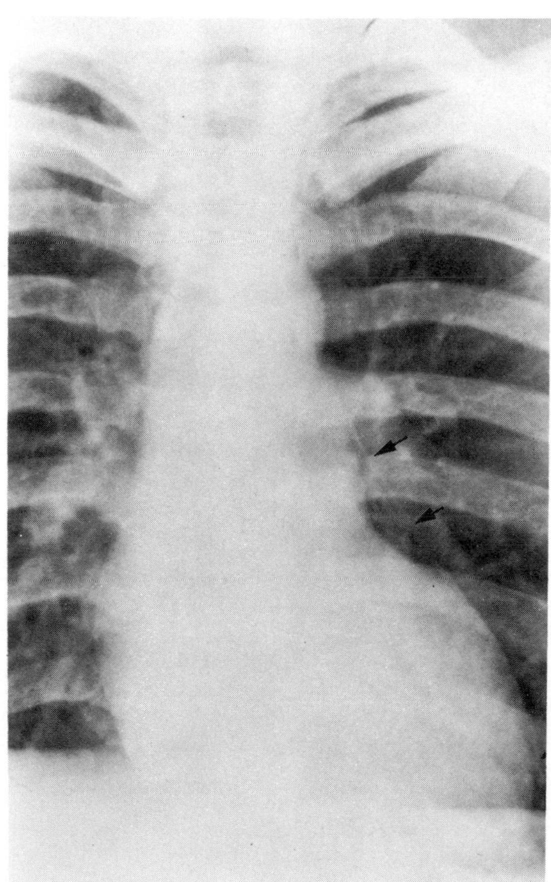

Figure 4–36. Pneumopericardium. There is a lucency along the left border of the heart that does not extend beyond the pulmonary artery. The combined density of the pericardium and the visceral and parietal pleura are seen (*arrows*). In this unusual case following a battlefield blast injury, air was demonstrated within the pericardium, but pneumomediastinum, pneumothorax, and subcutaneous emphysema never developed. (Courtesy of C. Ochs, M.D., Birmingham, MA.)

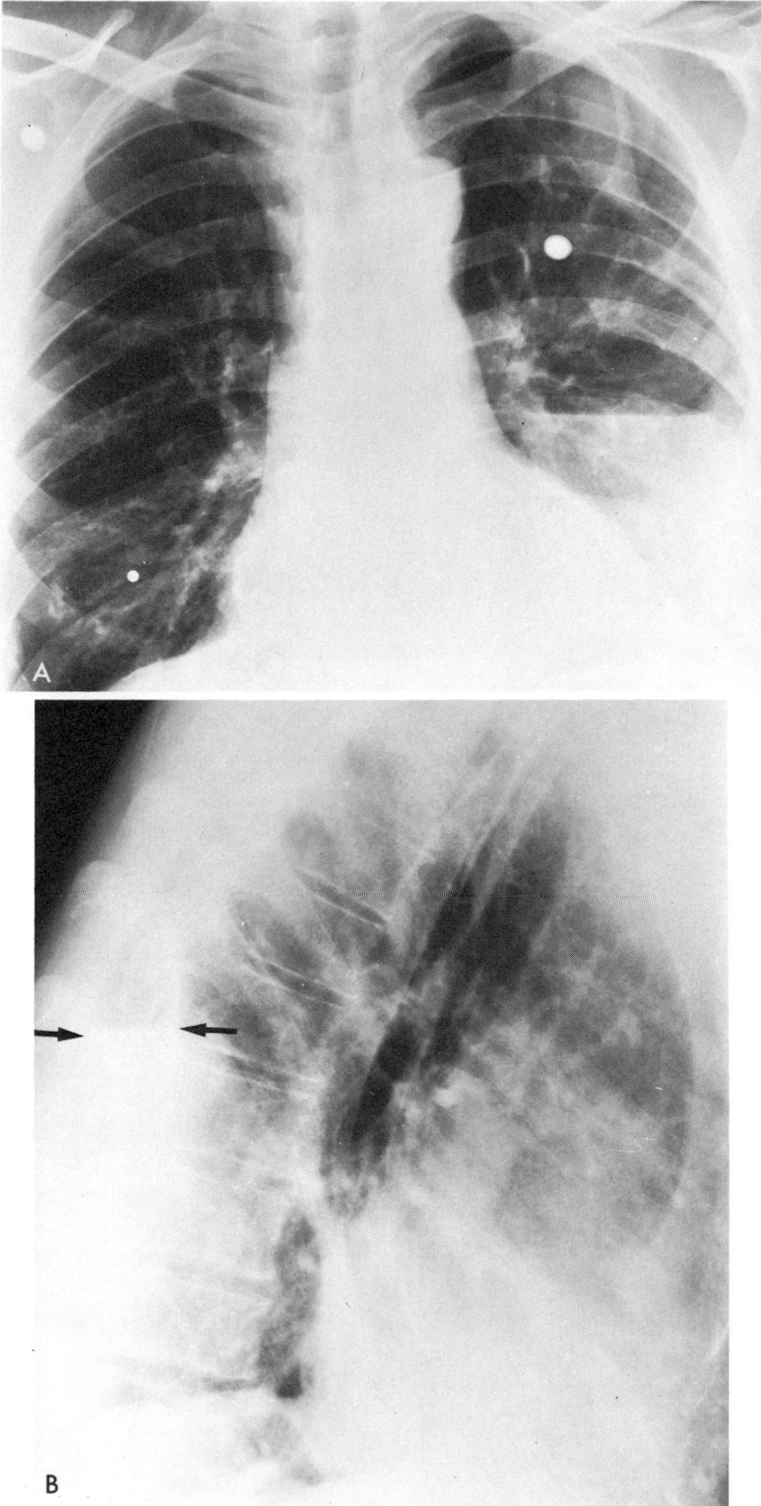

Figure 4–37. Bronchopleural fistula. *A*, AP upright film demonstrates an air fluid level across the entire hemithorax. In this case, it does not quite reach the lateral chest wall. A fluid collection is also noted over the left scapula. *B*, Lateral radiograph demonstrates a sharp air fluid level running the entire length of the lesion (*arrows*). The lesion is long and flat, and the margins taper because of its intrapleural location.

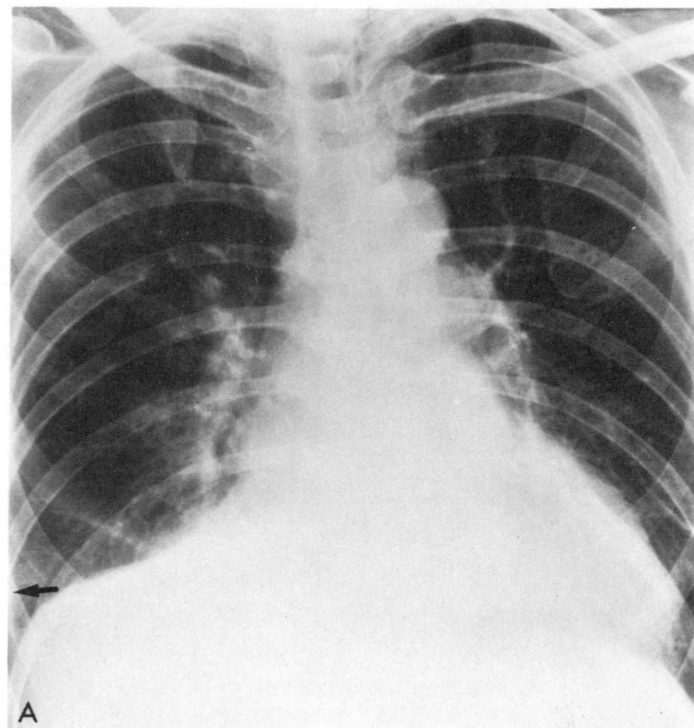

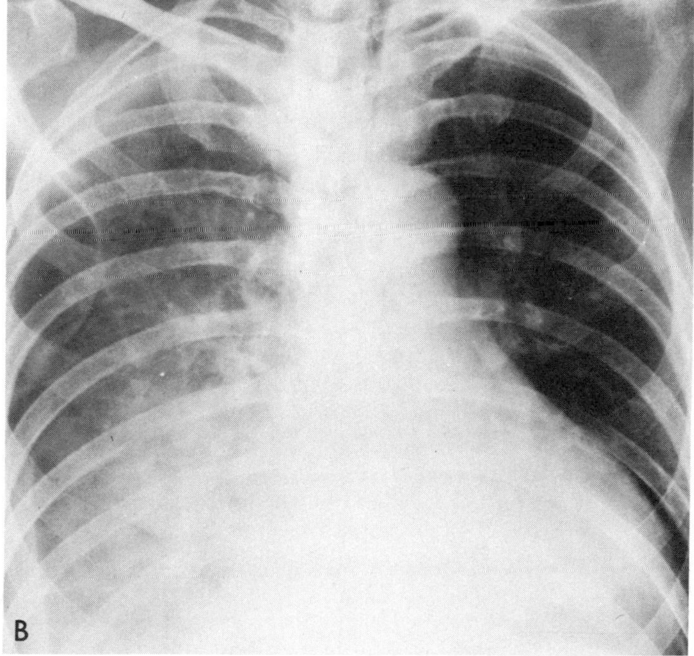

Figure 4–38. Pleural effusion. *A*, AP upright radiograph demonstrates a density adjacent to the right border of the heart, representing either a right middle lobe collapse or medial fluid. In addition the right hemidiaphragm is elevated, and there is minimal thickening of the lateral pleural space (*arrow*). *B*, Supine film taken several hours later demonstrates the fluid layering out over the entire right hemithorax along the lateral lung and into the apex. In addition there is an infiltrate at the right base medially, as demonstrated by the increased density and the air bronchogram.

1978). With slight angulation of the x-ray tube cephalad, the right hemidiaphragm, which is normally higher anteriorly, spuriously appears elevated in comparison with the left one. On the left side the anterior part of the diaphragm may be projected higher than the stomach bubble, falsely suggesting a left subpulmonic effusion. Slight thickening of the lateral or medial pleural stripe or a small meniscus is often the first clue to a small-to-moderate effusion (Figs. 4–14, 4–38). Fluid tracking up in the major fissure may cause the diaphragm to fade gradually into the lung. On occasion, the superior margin of the major fissure is visualized as an arcuate line approximately parallel to the fifth or sixth posterior rib (Fig. 4–39). Fluid in the

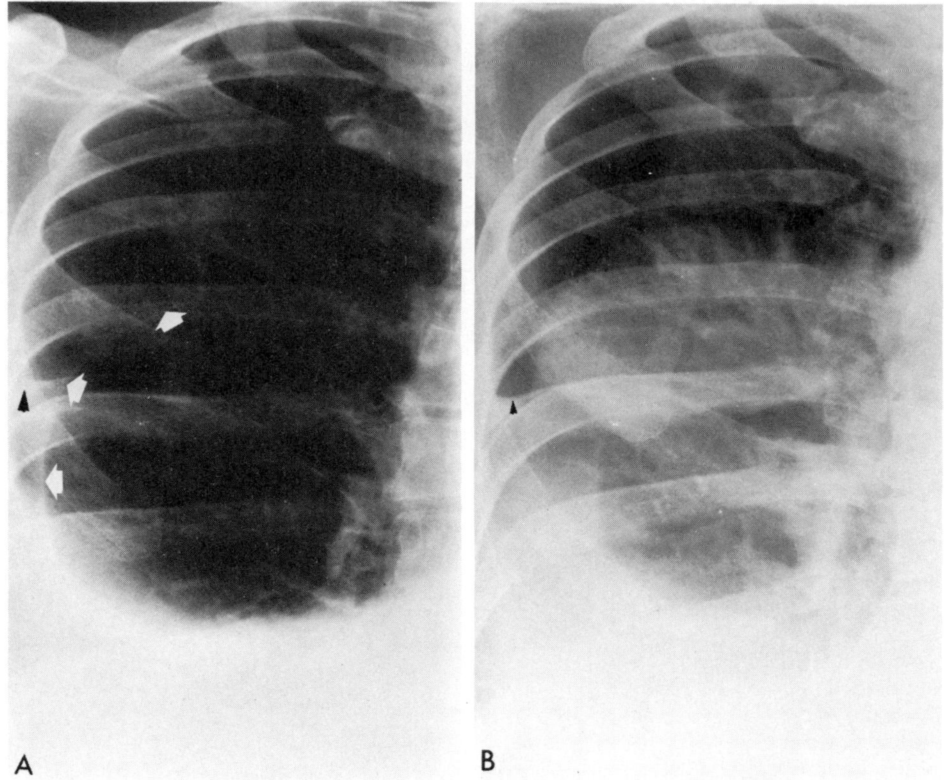

Figure 4–39. Pleural effusion. *A*, Upright portable radiograph demonstrates a large meniscus laterally. The right hemidiaphragm is not seen. There is thickening of both the major (*white arrows*) and minor (*black arrow*) fissures. *B*, Supine radiograph demonstrates fluid trapped in both the major and minor fissures (*arrow*). The fluid delineates the upper extent of the major fissure. Note that the pulmonary vessels can be seen through the effusion.

minor fissure will thicken the fissure. Larger effusions will cause a homogeneous density over the lung bases or the entire hemithorax (Figs. 3–6, 4–38), through which the pulmonary vessels may be seen.

Dandy (1978) has recently emphasized the unusual distribution of fluid that occurs when the major fissure is incomplete. In many patients the medial aspect of the major fissure never forms. Therefore, fluid entering the fissure causes a homogeneous density over the lateral lung while sparing the perihilar area. This may mimic a lateral infiltrate, or the sharply defined medial lucency may be mistaken for a focal air collection (bulla, pneumatocele) (Fig. 4–40).

On the supine radiograph, effusion may thicken the lateral or apical pleural space, thicken the fissures, or cause an overall increased density to the entire hemithorax. On overpenetrated supine radiographs, widening of the left paraspinous line is often visible in the presence of a free effusion (Trackler and Brinker, 1966). Several bedside maneuvers are available to confirm or deny the presence of an effusion. Decubitus films, with the patient lying on a wooden board to prevent sagging, can usually be obtained. Whenever possible, bilateral decubitus films are taken to rule out an unsuspected effusion on the opposite side. If the patient's condition or obesity precludes a decubitus film with the suspected side down, a film with the suspected side up may help differentiate pleural fluid from pleural thickening or lateral lower lobe infiltrate (Fig. 4–6). If decubitus films cannot be obtained, a supine and erect film may demonstrate a generalized increased density on the supine film that disappears when the patient sits erect (Figs. 4–38, 4–39). A supine oblique radiograph may also

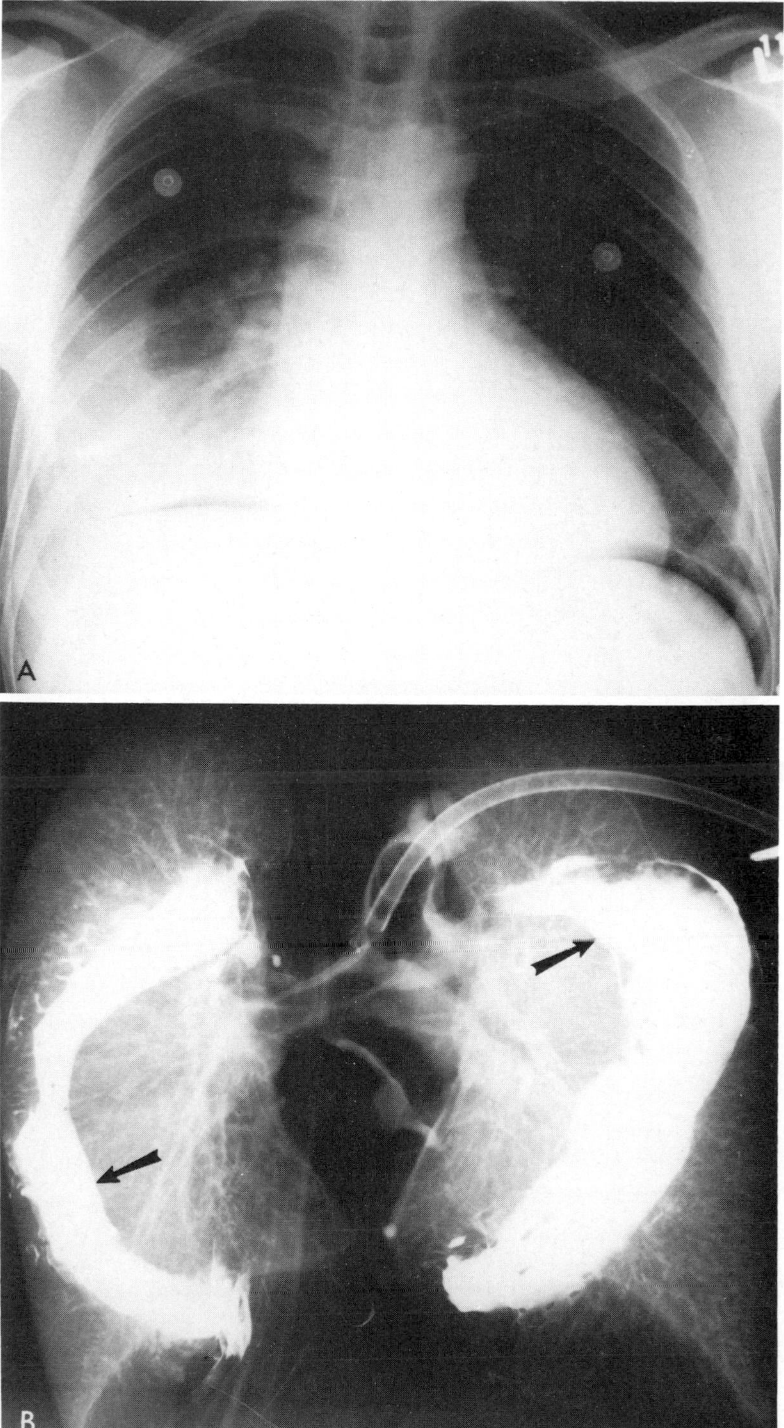

Figure 4–40. Incomplete fissure sign. *A*, Pneumoperitoneum and right hydrothorax after peritoneal dialysis. Fluid fills the lateral half of the major fissure, leaving a lucency medially. This should not be confused with a bulla or other type of abnormal air collection. (Courtesy of Dr. W. E. Dandy, Jr., Baltimore, MD.) *B*, Specimen radiograph of a different patient with barium applied to the major fissures. The clear perihilar areas are due to an incomplete fissure centrally. (From Dandy, W. E., Jr.: Radiology 128:21, 1978.)

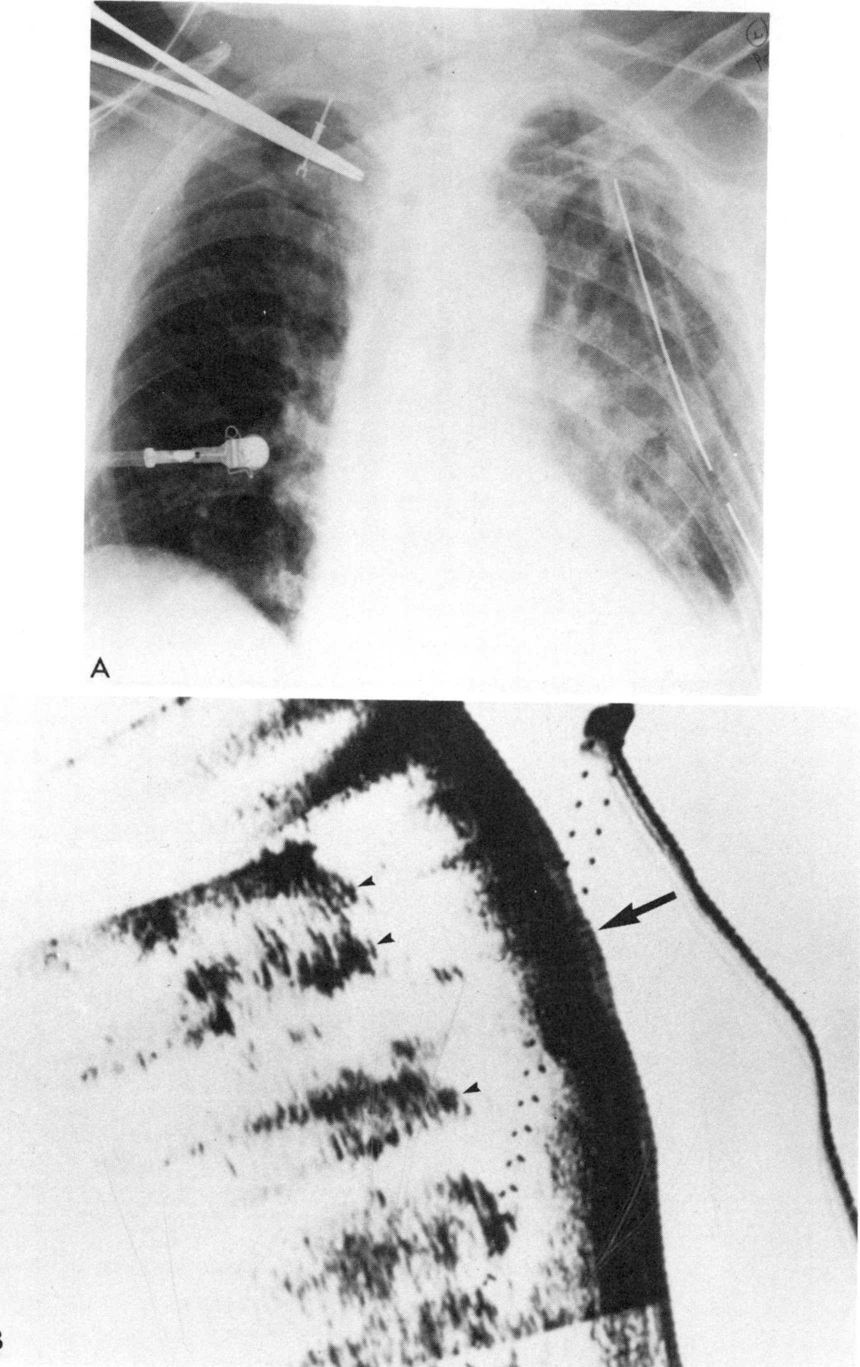

Figure 4–41. Empyema. Several days after initial chest tube insertion, the patient's fever returned. Serial chest radiographs demonstrated an enlarged retrocardiac density. *A*, Portable radiograph shows the chest tube in the left pleural space and a density in the left lower lung field. *B*, Ultrasound demonstrates that the posterior chest wall (*arrow*) is separated from the visceral wall of the empyema sac (*arrowheads*) by fluid. Debris within the empyema produces a few scattered internal echoes. After a chest tube had been inserted under ultrasonic guidance, the empyema drained and the fever diminished.

demonstrate fluid between the lung and the lateral chest wall.

The totally immobilized patient and the individual with small effusions, massive effusions, and loculated collections may present diagnostic difficulties. Ultrasonography can readily detect free effusions and can locate loculated collections. Ultrasonically guided thoracentesis will greatly increase the chances of a successful tap of a local pleural pocket (Fig. 4–41). However, attempts to predict the likelihood of a successful tap based on the echogenicity of the focal collection have not been reliable (some echo-free collections will not yield fluid, whereas many complex collections do) (Laing and Filly, 1978).

Computerized tomography will also graphically demonstrate the extent of the fluid, its loculations, and its relationship to other intrathoracic structures (Figs. 4–5, 4–42, 6–3). CT has repeatedly demonstrated that portable radiographs grossly underestimate the amount of effusion. Collections high in protein or blood may give CT numbers in the soft tissue rather than fluid range (that is, > 20 H.U.), and it may be difficult to distinguish phlegmonous pleura from a focal fluid collection.

Pericardial Effusions

Pericardial effusions are discussed in Chapter 11.

Mediastinal Fluid

Acute widening of the mediastinum is most often due to hemorrhage, false passage of tubes or catheters, or infection. Interpretation of mediastinal widening on portable films is extremely hazardous. If possible, serial 6-foot PA radiographs should be obtained. If AP radiographs must be used, serial films using the same target film distance, the same patient position, and the same degree of inspiration are mandatory for proper evaluation. Mediastinal widening is discussed in Chapter 3 (catheter trauma), Chapter 6 (sternotomy), and Chapters 7 and 9 (aortic disease).

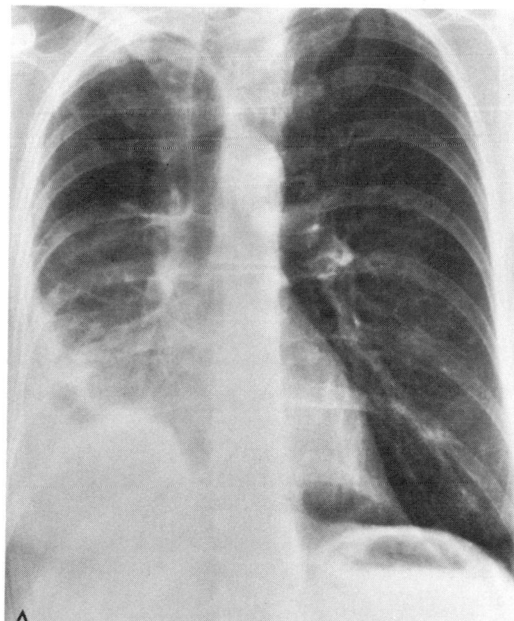

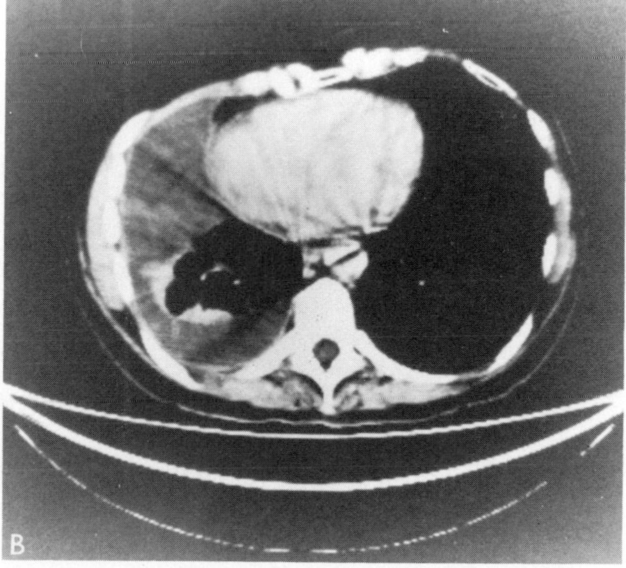

Figure 4–42. Loculated effusion. This patient with ovarian carcinoma developed an unexplained fever. A pneumonia was suspected clinically. *A*, Chest radiograph shows a definite right-sided effusion. A parenchymal process could not be excluded. Decubitus film did not clear the right lower lobe. *B*, CT demonstrates a loculated effusion at the base. Except for some minimal peripheral atelectasis, no parenchymal abnormality was demonstrated. The effusion was tapped and proved to be a sterile transudate. The fever eventually diminished without additional therapy.

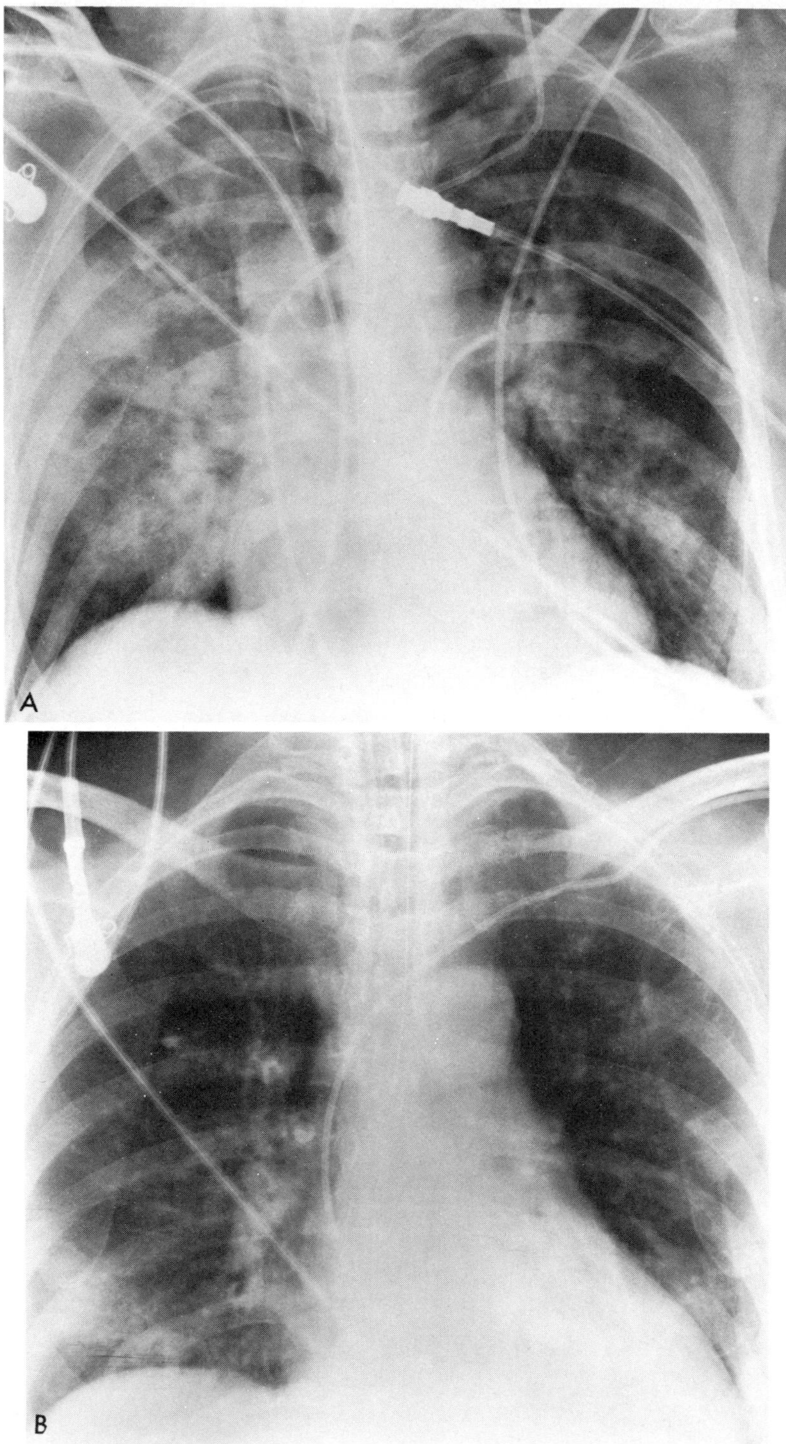

Figure 4–43. Pulmonary hemorrhage. *A*, Diffuse bilateral pulmonary infiltrates developed over 24 hours in this patient with renal failure. During this same period, the hematocrit dropped several points and the patient was found to be thrombocytopenic. *B*, Three days later, the majority of the infiltrates cleared. A small residual infiltrate is seen at both bases.

PULMONARY HEMORRHAGE

Tracheobronchial Bleeding

Small amounts of blood-streaked sputum in the intubated patient or frequently suctioned patient are usually due to direct tracheal injury and do not require radiographic evaluation. As discussed in Chapter 2, short bouts of arterial bleeding in the intubated patient may be a precursor to a tracheoinnominate artery fistula requiring rapid diagnostic work-up.

Parenchymal Bleeding

Pulmonary parenchymal bleeding may be due to a focal pulmonary process, diffuse lung disease, or a coagulation disorder. When such bleeding is due to a local lung process (for example, aspergilloma, bronchiectasis), the combination of radiography and bronchoscopy is usually adequate for localization (Cudkowitz, 1974). In patients with diffuse lung disease, it may be extremely difficult to determine the source of bleeding by conventional methods. In patients with bleeding from inflammatory lung disease (for example, sarcoidosis, tuberculosis, cystic fibrosis, and so on), bronchial angiography often demonstrates areas of hypervascularity and bronchopulmonary anastomosis. Although this technique does not positively define the site of bleeding unless extravasation is seen (which is rare), it does define the area most likely to be bleeding (Ishihara et al., 1974). The bronchial angiogram serves to define the area requiring resection or serves as a guide to catheter embolization of the suspected vessel. Remy et al. (1977) performed bronchial artery embolization in 49 bleeding patients. Bleeding stopped in 41, but six rebled within 7 months. Since the basic lesion is not cured, surgery may be required if rebleeding occurs.

In patients with coagulation disorders, Goodpasture's syndrome, or vasculitis, or in patients receiving anticoagulant therapy, pulmonary parenchymal hemorrhage may occur without preexisting lung disease. The usual presentation is the triad of anemia, hemoptysis, and pulmonary infiltrates. The radiographic pattern varies from mild interstitial thickening to nodulation to consolidation. Most often there is a rapid progression, and when the disorder is bilateral a pulmonary edema pattern may be seen. Shadowing tends to spare the apices and periphery (Bowley et al., 1979b; Palmer et al., 1978) (Fig. 4–43). Within a few days, the infiltrates stabilize and gradually regress as a reticular interstitial pattern replaces the alveolar infiltrate. The interstitial thickening gradually subsides and returns to normal over the following one or two weeks. Repeated bouts of hemorrhage will cause hemosiderin-induced interstitial fibrosis (Robboy et al., 1973).

On occasion, severe pulmonary hemorrhage may occur with little or no hemoptysis. Therefore, the absence of hemoptysis does not exclude the diagnosis. When the clinical or radiographic presentation suggests hemorrhage, further investigation is required. The demonstration of hemosiderin-laden macrophages in bronchial lavage samples supports the diagnosis (Finley et al., 1975). Extravasation of blood into the parenchyma may also be inferred from studies using radionuclide-tagged red blood cells (Benoit et al., 1964). Bowley et al. (1979a) showed that, after pulmonary hemorrhage, carbon monoxide uptake in the lung increased owing to binding in the stagnant extravascular blood pool. These authors noted a good correlation between the radiographic changes and the carbon monoxide retention in the lung.

REFERENCES

Baber, C. E., Hedlund, L. W., Oddson, T. A., and Putman, C. E.: Differentiating empyemas and peripheral pulmonary abscesses. Radiology 135:755, 1980.

Bartlett, J. G., and Gorbach, S. L.: The triple threat of aspiration pneumonia. Chest 68:560, 1975.

Benoit, F. L., Rulon, D. B., Theil, G. B., et al.: Goodpasture's syndrome: a clinicopathologic entity. Am. J. Med. 37:424, 1964.

Bode, F. R., Paré, J. A. P., and Fraser, R. G.: Pulmonary diseases in the compromised host. Medicine 53:255, 1974.

Bowley, N. B., Hughes, J. M. B., and Steiner, R. E.: The chest x-ray in pulmonary capillary haemorrhage: correlation with carbon monoxide uptake. Clin. Radiol. 30:413, 1979a.

Bowley, N. B., Steiner, R. E., and Chin, W. S.: The chest x-ray in antiglomerular basement membrane antibody disease (Goodpasture's syndrome). Clin. Radiol. 30:419, 1979b.

Bryant, L. R., Mobin-Uddin, K., Dillon, M. L., et al.: Misdiagnosis of pneumonia in patients needing mechanical respiration. Arch. Surg. 106:286, 1973.

Bynum, L. J., and Pierce, A. K.: Pulmonary aspiration of gastric contents. Am. Rev. Respir. Dis. 114:1129, 1976.

Bynum, L. J., and Wilson, J. E., III: Radiographic features of pleural effusions in pulmonary embolism. Am. Rev. Respir. Dis. 117:829, 1978.

Cameron, J. L., Reynolds, J., and Zuidema, G. D.: Aspiration in patients with tracheostomies. Surg. Gynecol. Obstet. 136:68, 1973.

Castellino, R. A., and Blank, N.: Etiologic diagnosis of focal pulmonary infection in immunocompromised patients by fluoroscopically guided percutaneous needle aspiration. Radiology 132:563, 1979.

Cavaluzzi, J. A., Alderson, P. O., and White, R. I., Jr.: Pulmonary embolism with unilateral lung scan defects and matching infiltrates. J. Can. Assoc. Radiol. 30:162, 1979.

Chait, A., Cohen, H. E., Meltzer, L. E., et al.: The bedside chest x-ray in the evaluation of incipient heart failure. Radiology 105:563, 1972.

Cheely, R., McCartney, W. H., Perry, J. R., et al.: The role of noninvasive tests versus pulmonary angiography in the diagnosis of pulmonary embolism. Am. J. Med. 70:17, 1981.

Christensen, E. E., and Landay, M. J.: Visible muscle of the diaphragm: sign of extraperitoneal air. AJR 135:521, 1980.

Cimmino, C. V.: Some radio-diagnostic notes on pneumomediastinum, pneumothorax, and pneumopericardium. Va. Med. Month. 94:205, 1967.

Crews, E. R., and LaPuerta, L.: A Manual of Respiratory Failure. Springfield, IL, 1972, Charles C Thomas.

Cudkowitz, L.: The localization and management of pulmonary hemorrhage. *In* Oaks, W. W. (ed.): Critical Care Medicine. New York, 1974, Grune & Stratton.

Dandy, W. E., Jr.: The incomplete pulmonary interlobar fissure sign. Radiology 128:21, 1978.

Donnenfeld, F. S.: Atelectasis. Int. Anesthesiol. Clin. 9(4):103, 1971.

Dougherty, J. E., LaSalla, A. F., and Fieldman, A.: Bedside pulmonary angiography utilizing an existing Swan-Ganz catheter. Chest 77:43, 1980.

Eaton, R. J., Senior, E. M., and Pierce, J. A.: Aspects of respiratory care pertinent to the radiologist. Radiol. Clin. North Am. 11:93, 1973.

Feingold, D. S.: Hospital-acquired infections. N. Engl. J. Med. 283:1384, 1970.

Finley, T. N., Aronow, A., Cosentino, A. M., et al.: Occult pulmonary hemorrhage in anticoagulated patients. Am. Rev. Respir. Dis. 112:23, 1975.

Flick, M. R., and Cluff, L. E.: Pseudomonas bacteremia—review of 108 cases. Am. J. Med. 60:501, 1976.

Fraser, R. G., and Paré, J. A. P.: Diagnosis of Diseases of the Chest, 2nd ed. Philadelphia, 1979, W. B. Saunders Co., pp. 1912–1945.

Friedman, P. J., and Hellekant, A. C. G.: Diagnosis of air-fluid levels in the thorax; radiologic recognition of bronchopleural fistula, part 2. Am. Rev. Respir. Dis. 113:159, 1976.

Gamsu, G., Singer, M. M., Vincent, H. H., et al.: Postoperative impairment of mucous transport in the lung. Am. Rev. Respir. Dis. 114:673, 1976.

Goodman, L. R., Goren, R. A., and Teplick, S. K.: The radiographic evaluation of pulmonary infection. Med. Clin. North Am. 64:553, 1980.

Gordon, R.: The deep sulcus sign. Radiology 136:25, 1980.

Greenman, R., Goodall, P., and King, D.: Lung biopsy in immunocompromised hosts. Am. J. Med. 59:488, 1975.

Harris, R. S.: The pre-operative chest film in relation to post-operative management—some effects of different projection, posture and lung inflation. Br. J. Radiol. 53:196, 1980.

Harrison, M. O., Conte, P. J., and Heitzman, E. R.: Radiological detection of clinically occult cardiac failure following myocardial infarction. Br. J. Radiol. 44:265, 1971.

Hartsuck, J. M., and Greenfield, L. J.: Post-operative thromboembolism—a clinical study with ^{125}I-fibrinogen and pulmonary scanning. Arch. Surg. 107:733, 1973.

Heineman, H. S.: Antibiotics and pulmonary disease. *In* Oaks, W. W. (ed.): Critical Care Medicine. New York, 1974, Grune & Stratton.

Hublitz, U. F., and Shapiro, J. H.: Atypical pulmonary patterns of congestive failure in chronic lung disease. Radiology 93:995, 1969.

Hyers, T. M., Fowler, A. A., and Wicks, A. B.: Focal pulmonary edema after massive pulmonary embolism. Am. Rev. Respir. Dis. 123:232, 1981.

Ishihara, T., Inoue, H., Kobayashi, K., et al.: Selective bronchial arteriography and hemoptysis in nonmalignant lung disease. Chest 66:633, 1974.

Jackson, D. C., Tyson, J. W., Johnsrude, I. S., et al.: Pulmonary embolic disease. J. Can. Assoc. Radiol. 26:139, 1975.

Joffe, N.: Roentgenologic aspects of primary *Pseudomonas aeruginosa* pneumonia in mechanically ventilated patients. Am. J. Roentgenol. 107:305, 1969.

Kurlander, G. J., and Helman, C. H.: Subpulmonary pneumothorax. Am. J. Roentgenol. 96:1019, 1966.

Laing, F. C., and Filly, R. A.: Problems in the application of ultrasonography for the evaluation of pleural opacities. Radiology 126:211, 1978.

Lame, E. L., and Redick, T. J.: A bedside cassette holder for 6-foot PA radiographs in comfort. Radiology 95:698, 1970.

Landay, M. J., Christensen, E. E., and Bynum, L. J.: Pulmonary manifestations of acute aspiration of gastric contents. Am. J. Roentgenol. 131:587, 1978.

Leeming, B. W. A.: Radiological aspects of pulmonary complications resulting from intermittent positive pressure ventilation (I.P.P.V.) Australas. Radiol. 12:361, 1968.

LeFrock, J. L., Clark, T. S., Davies, B., and Klainer, A. S.: Aspiration pneumonia: a ten-year review. Am. Surg. 45:305, 1979.

Lerner, M. A.: Inspiration chest radiography by lateral recumbency. Clin. Radiol. 29:155, 1978.

Levin, B.: The continuous diaphragm sign—a newly recognized sign of pneumomediastinum. Clin. Radiol. 24:337, 1973.

Liebman, P. R., Philips, E., Weisel, R., et al.: Diagnostic value of the portable chest x-ray technic in pulmonary edema. Am. J. Surg. 135:604, 1978.

Light, R. W., and George, R. B.: Incidence and significance of pleural effusion after abdominal surgery. Chest 69:621, 1976.

Macklin, M. T., and Macklin, C. C.: Malignant interstitial emphysema of the lungs and mediastinum. Medicine 23:281, 1944.

Marini, J. J., Pierson, D. J., and Hudson, L. D.: Acute lobar atelectasis: a prospective comparison of fiberoptic bronchoscopy and respiratory therapy. Am. Rev. Respir. Dis. 119:971, 1979.

Matthay, R. A., and Moritz, E. D.: Invasive procedures for diagnosing pulmonary infection; a critical review. Clin. Chest Med. 2:3, 1981.

McHugh, T. J., Forrester, J. S., Adler, L., et al.: Pulmonary vascular congestion in acute myocardial infarction; hemodynamic and radiologic correlations. Ann. Intern. Med. 76:29, 1972.

Mendelson, C. L.: The aspiration of stomach contents into the lungs during obstetric anesthesia. Am. J. Obstet. Gynecol. 52:191, 1946.

Mulder, D. S., and Rubush, J. L.: Complications of tracheostomy; relationship to long-term ventilatory assistance. J. Trauma 9:389, 1969.

Neuhaus, A., Bentz, R. R., and Weg, J. G.: Pulmonary embolism in respiratory failure. Chest 73:460, 1978.

Novelline, R. A., Baltarowich, O., Athanasoulis, C. A., et

al.: The clinical course of patients with suspected pulmonary embolism and a negative pulmonary arteriogram. Radiology 126:561, 1978.

Nunn, J. F., Milledge, J. S., and Singaraya, J.: Survival of patients ventilated in an intensive therapy unit. Br. Med. J. 1:1525, 1979.

Palmer, P. E. S., Finley, T. N., Drew, W. L., and Golde, D. W.: Radiographic aspects of occult pulmonary haemorrhage. Clin. Radiol. 20:139, 1978.

Petty, T. L.: Intensive and Rehabilitative Respiratory Care. Philadelphia, 1971, Lea & Febiger.

Pierce, A. K., and Robertson, J.: Pulmonary complications of general surgery. Annu. Rev. Med. 28:211, 1977.

Pontoppidan, H., Geffin, B., and Lowenstein, E.: Acute respiratory failure in the adult, Part 1. N. Engl. J. Med. 287:690, 1972.

Poulose, K. P., Reba, R. C., Gilday, D. L., et al.: Diagnosis of pulmonary embolism. A correlative study of the clinical, scan, and angiographic findings. Br. J. Med. 3:67, 1970.

Preger, L., Hooper, T. I., Steinbach, H. L., et al.: Width of azygos vein related to central venous pressure. Radiology 93:521, 1969.

Remy, J., Arnaud, A., Fardou, H., et al.: Treatment of hemoptysis by embolization of the bronchial arteries. Radiology 122:33, 1977.

Renner, R. R., Coccaro, A. P., Heitzman, E. R., et al.: Pseudomonas pneumonia; a prototype of hospital-based infection. Radiology 105:555, 1972.

Rhea, J. T., VonSonnenberg, E., and McLoud, T. C.: Basilar pneumothorax in the supine adult. Radiology 133:593, 1979.

Robboy, S. J., Minna, J. D., Colman, R. W., et al.: Pulmonary hemorrhage syndrome as a manifestation of disseminated intravascular coagulation; analysis of ten cases. Chest 63:718, 1973.

Rogers, R. M., Weiler, C., and Ruppenthal, B.: The impact of the respiratory intensive care unit on survival of patients with acute respiratory failure. Chest 62:94, 1972.

Rohlfing, B. M., Webb, W. R., and Schlobohm, R. M.: Ventilator-related extra-alveolar air in adults. Radiology 121:25, 1976.

Rose, H. D., Heckman, M. G., and Unger, J. D.: *Pseudomonas aeruginosa* pneumonia in adults. Am. Rev. Respir. Dis. 107:416, 1973.

Rosenow, E. C., III, and Harrison, C. E.: Congestive heart failure masquerading as primary pulmonary disease. Chest 58:28, 1970.

Sackner, M., Hirsch, J., and Epstein, S.: Effect of cuffed endotracheal tubes on tracheal mucous velocity. Chest 68:774, 1975.

Sagel, S. S., Ferguson, T. B., Forrest, J. V., et al.: Percutaneous transthoracic aspiration needle biopsy. Ann. Thorac. Surg. 26:399, 1978.

Sanford, J. P., and Pierce, A. K.: Current infection problems—respiratory. *In* Proceedings of the International Conference on Nosocomial Infections. Baltimore, 1971, Waverly Press.

Sanford, J. P., and Pierce, A. K.: Lower respiratory tract infections. *In* Bennett, J. R., and Brachman, S., (eds.): Hospital Infections. Boston, 1979, Little, Brown & Co.

Savoca, C. J., Gamsu, G., and Rohlfing, B. M.: Chest radiography in intensive care units. West. J. Med. 129:469, 1978.

Schachter, E. N., Kreisman, H., and Putman, C.: Diagnostic problems in suppurative lung disease. Arch. Intern. Med. 136:167, 1976.

Shapiro, B. A.: Clinical Application of Respiratory Care. Chicago, 1975, Year Book Medical Publishers.

Shapiro, J. H., and Hublitz, U. F.: The radiology of pulmonary edema. Crit. Rev. Clin. Radiol., 5:389, 1974.

Smith, G. T., Dammin, G. J., and Dexter, L.: Postmortem angiographic studies of the human lung in pulmonary embolization. J.A.M.A. 188:143, 1964.

Steckel, R. J.: The radiolucent kinetic borderline in acute pulmonary edema and pneumonia. Clin. Radiol. 25:391, 1974.

Steier, M., Ching, N., Bonfils-Roberts, E., et al: Iatrogenic causes of pneumothorax. NY State J. Med. 73:1296, 1973.

Stevens, R. M., Teres, D., Skillman, J. J., et al.: Pneumonia in an intensive care unit. Arch. Intern. Med. 134:106, 1974.

Tillotson, J. R., and Lerner, A. M.: Characteristics of nonbacteremic Pseudomonas pneumonia. Ann. Intern. Med. 68:295, 1968.

Tinstman, T. C., Dines, D. E., and Arms, R. A.: Postoperative aspiration pneumonia. Surg. Clin. North Am. 53:859, 1973.

Trackler, T., and Brinker, R. A.: Widening of the left paravertebral pleural line on supine chest roentgenograms in free pleural effusions. Am. J. Roentgenol 96:1027, 1966.

Unger, K. M. Shibel, E. M., and Moser, K. M.: Detection of left ventricular failure in patients with adult respiratory distress syndrome. Chest 67:8, 1975.

Viamonte, M., Jr., Koolpe, H., Janowitz, W., and Hildner, F.: Pulmonary thromboembolism—update. J.A.M.A. 243:2229, 1980.

West, J. B., Dollery, C. T., and Heard, B. E.: Increased pulmonary vascular resistance in the dependent zone of the isolated dog lung caused by perivascular edema. Circ. Res. 17:191, 1965.

Westcott, J. L., and Cole, S. R.: Interstitial pulmonary emphysema in children and adults; roentgenographic features. Radiology 111:367, 1974.

Williams, D. M., Krick, J. A., and Remmington, J. S.: Pulmonary infection in the compromised host, Parts 1 and 2. Am. Rev. Respir. Dis. 114:359, 593, 1976.

Zimmerman, J. E., Dunbar, B. S., and Klingenmaier, C. H.: Management of subcutaneous emphysema, pneumomediastinum, and pneumothorax during respiratory therapy. Crit. Care Med. 3:69, 1975.

Zimmerman, J. E., Goodman, L. R., Wyman, A., and St. Andre, A.: Radiographic detection of mobilizable lung water: the gravitational shift test. Am. J. Roentgenol., 138:59, 1982.

Ziskind, M. M., Schwarz, M. E., George, R. B., et al.: Incomplete consolidation in pneumococcal lobar pneumonia complicating pulmonary emphysema. Ann. Intern. Med. 72:835, 1970.

Zornoza, J., Goldman, A. M., Wallace, S., et al.: Radiographic features of gram-negative pneumonias in the neutropenic patient. Am. J. Roentgenol. 127:989, 1976.

Chapter 5

ADULT RESPIRATORY DISTRESS SYNDROME

by Charles E. Putman
and Carl E. Ravin

The term "adult respiratory distress syndrome" (ARDS) is used to describe a heterogeneous group of patients with respiratory insufficiency who develop a characteristic clinical, pathophysiologic, and often radiographic pattern hours to days after a severe local or systemic insult. Although many disease processes (see Tables 5–1 and 5–2) may cause this syndrome (Bergofsky, 1970; Moore et al., 1969; Perkoff et al., 1971; Powers et al., 1972), the common final denominator is increased respiratory effort, severe hypoxemia, and diffuse parenchymal opacities. Although seemingly an all-encompassing term, the concept of ARDS is valuable because, in spite of a wide variety of insults, there is a relatively uniform pulmonary response to injury. It is estimated that approximately 5 per cent of patients hospitalized for respiratory failure fulfill the criteria for ARDS (Gomez, 1968).

In addition to the primary disease, many therapeutic maneuvers appear to contribute to the clinical, pathologic, and radiographic picture. The overzealous use of intravenous (IV) fluids, prolonged ventilatory treatment, high oxygen concentrations, and the excessive use of respiratory depressants aggravate pulmonary insufficiency. Therapeutic errors of omission have also been implicated, especially inadequate control of sepsis, poor control of blood filtration, and suboptimal pulmonary management.

It was formerly thought that hypovolemic shock was the main precipitating factor in ARDS. Although this is present in many ARDS victims, it is now generally agreed that shock is not a prerequisite for development of this syndrome (Meyers et al., 1973). In fact, it is difficult to produce experimentally the characteristic lung changes by hemorrhagic shock alone. In the clinical situation, secondary factors

TABLE 5–1. Diseases Associated With ARDS

Amniotic fluid embolism
Arterial emboli
Aspiration
Bowel infarction
Burns and smoke inhalation
Carcinomatosis
Cardiopulmonary bypass
Clostridial sepsis
Disseminated intravascular coagulation
Drug abuse
Eclampsia
Fat embolism
Fractures
Gram-negative sepsis
Heat stroke
High-altitude pulmonary edema
Major surgery
Malaria
Multiple transfusions
Oxygen toxicity
Pancreatitis
Peripheral vascular disease
Pulmonary contusion
Radiation pneumonitis
Ruptured aneurysm
Shock (hypovolemic or endotoxic)
Transfusion reaction
Transplantation
Trauma
Viral pneumonia (influenza)

TABLE 5–2. Synonyms For ARDS

Adult hyaline membrane disease
Adult respiratory insufficiency syndrome
Bronchopulmonary dysplasia
Congestive atelectasis
DaNang lung
Fat embolism
Hemorrhagic lung syndrome
Oxygen toxicity
Post-perfusion lung syndrome
Post-transfusion lung
Post-traumatic atelectasis
Post-traumatic pulmonary insufficiency
Progressive pulmonary consolidation
Progressive respiratory distress
Pulmonary edema
Pulmonary hyaline membrane disease
Pulmonary microembolism
Pump lung
Respirator lung
Shock lung
Solid lung syndrome
Stiff lung syndrome
Transplant lung
Traumatic wet lung
Wet lung
White lung syndrome

that are often present include endotoxins from gram-negative sepsis, massive trauma with ischemic damage to major muscle masses, foreign surfaces such as cardiopulmonary bypass machines, and transfusion reactions, especially those associated with hemolysis (Blaisdell et al., 1970; Byrne and Dixon, 1971; Jeneveihn and Weiss, 1964).

Although the conditions associated with ARDS have common clinical and pathogenic features, each of them requires specific diagnosis and treatment. Through an understanding of the specific insult and the general course of ARDS, a systematic, physiologically oriented therapeutic approach can be applied (Table 5–3).

The radiographic pattern is not specific, but the radiologist plays a major role in the diagnosis or exclusion of this syndrome. The diagnosis is based on a characteristic temporal radiographic pattern in a specific clinical context. This chapter presents a general review of ARDS with special emphasis on its radiographic features.

CLINICAL FEATURES

There is usually a latent period of 24 to 36 hours following the episode of hemorrhage, trauma, or infection; during this time, no signs of clinical respiratory distress are present. Thereafter, tachypnea develops and progresses to severe respiratory distress accompanied by cyanosis and dyspnea, and is refractory to routine oxygen administration. On auscultation, chest sounds are generally normal during the initial latent phase; thereafter, however, fine crepitations and coarse breath sounds can usually be heard. Blood gases demonstrate severe hypoxemia, hypocapnia, and refractory alkalosis (Ayres et al., 1970; Blaisdell and Schlobohm, 1973). As respiratory insufficiency becomes severe, both respiratory and metabolic acidosis may supervene. The onset of hypercapnia and acidosis is an ominous sign. The most reliable diagnostic index in determining the clinical status of the patient is the level of the alveolar-arterial Po_2 gradient (see Chapter 1) (Tomashefski and Mahajan, 1976). The normal patient receiving 100 per cent oxygen has an alveolar-

TABLE 5–3. Sequence of Events Leading to ARDS

Findings	Phase 1 (0–24 hr)	Phase 2 (24–36 hr)	Phase 3 (36–72 hr)	Phase 4 (72 hr–6 wk)
Clinical	Negative	Tachypnea, dyspnea, decreased O_2, decreased CO_2	Respiratory and metabolic acidosis; increased alveolar-arterial P_{O_2} gradient	Progressive respiratory failure or complete recovery with variable signs of pulmonary disease
Pathologic (gross)	Edema +/− petechiae	Increased edema. congestion	Hepatization	Further hepatization or near normal
Microscopic	Microemboli, periarteriolar hemorrhage	Interstitial and intra-alveolar edema	Congestive atelectasis, intra-alveolar hemorrhage, hyaline membranes	Interstitial fibrosis or no specific findings
Chest radiography	Negative	24 hr: perihilar haze, interstitial edema; 36 hr: pulmonary edema	Little change in radiograph after 36 hr	Little change after 36 hr or focal scarring

arterial Po_2 gradient up to 50 mm, but in patients with ARDS this gradient is greatly increased to levels as high as 300 mm Hg. This is primarily due to intrapulmonary arterial venous shunting, although diffusion and ventilation-perfusion disturbances also contribute to abnormal gas exchange. Mechanical disturbances include an increased respiratory rate, a decreased tidal volume and compliance, and an increase in the dead space relative to tidal volume.

PATHOLOGY

Gross changes in the lungs depend on the time elapsed since the original injury. Immediately following the initial insult, they may appear grossly normal. Within four to six hours, scattered petechial hemorrhages may be evident over the pleura of the lungs. The lungs are heavier than normal and on cut section may appear edematous. By 24 to 36 hours, petechial hemorrhages may be confluent and are most evident in the basilar segments of the lungs. The lungs may become reddened and are congested and hemorrhagic. By three to four days, they appear even darker and have the texture of liver (Martin et al., 1968; Orell, 1971).

Microscopically, during the first six hours following the insult the lungs may be normal except for variable numbers of fibrin and platelet microemboli, which fill capillaries and pulmonary arterioles. At eight to 12 hours, vascular congestion and periarteriolar hemorrhage are present. This is followed at 24 to 36 hours by various degrees of congestion and interstitial and intra-alveolar edema. These are the changes that are primarily responsible for the developing signs and symptoms of pulmonary insufficiency. Scattered areas of focal atelectasis and intra-alveolar hemorrhage may peak at 72 hours. The earliest consistent lesions, therefore, seem to be interstitial alveolar edema and thickening of the alveolar walls due to capillary congestion, diapedesis of erythrocytes, and congestive atelectasis. After 72 hours, increased cellularity in the interstitium and intra-alveolar hyaline membranes may become the predominant lesion, whereas hemorrhage and congestion decrease in prominence. In the areas with hyaline membranes, hypertrophy, proliferation, and desquamation of the alveolar lining cells can be defined. If the patient survives for weeks or months after the initial insult, diffuse pulmonary fibrosis becomes the predominant lesion. In a few cases the lungs may return to normal. Pathologic changes are also modified by various therapeutic maneuvers such as the use of positive end-expiratory pressure (PEEP), by overzealous use of IV fluids, and by the use of various drugs such as antibiotics, steroids, and oxygen.

RADIOGRAPHIC FEATURES

Since both clinical and radiographic features of ARDS are not specific (Joffe, 1974; Ostendorf et al., 1975; Putman et al., 1972), it is imperative that radiologists be aware of the complete clinical course of a patient suspected of having ARDS. It is important to interpret films in a serial fashion, because the initial abnormalities may change from hour to hour and then stabilize after 48 to 72 hours. It is this progression of abnormalities that may suggest ARDS radiographically.

The chest radiographic findings correspond closely to the described pathologic abnormalities. Early on, if there is hypoxia and respiratory distress with a positive chest radiograph the patient probably does not have ARDS at this point. Complicating factors such as aspiration pneumonia, fluid overload, or congestive heart failure (CHF) may be responsible for the radiographic abnormality within the first eight to 12 hours. The first definite radiographic abnormality generally appears about 24 hours after the initial insult. This generally consists of a bilateral perihilar haze with ill-defined linear densities extending from the hilum, consistent with interstitial edema (Fig. 5–1). Often, some of these linear densities coalesce and resemble focal areas of pneumonitis (Fig. 5–2). At this time, differentiation of ARDS from pulmonary edema or diffuse pneumonitis is almost impossible. The radiographs should be correlated with physiologic data such as central venous pressure (CVP) or pulmonary capillary wedge (PCW) pressures. Other radiographic signs of CHF such as cardiomegaly, pulmonary vascular redistribution, and pleural effusion are generally absent.

Serial films reveal rapid progression of the disease, from localized confluent infiltrates to a complete alveolar filling pattern within 24 hours after the onset of pulmonary symptoms (Fig. 5–3). Following the development of the pulmonary edema pattern, there may be little alteration in the radiograph for days. However, the radiographic appearance may be dramatically

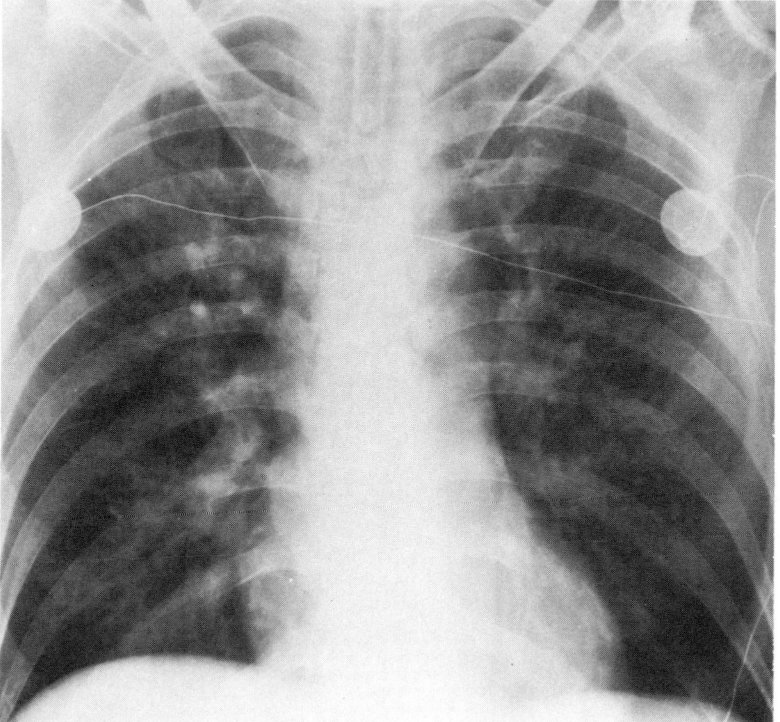

Figure 5–1. Adult respiratory distress syndrome (ARDS), phase 2: a bilateral perihilar haze with linear densities radiating from hila. The endotracheal tube is in good position.

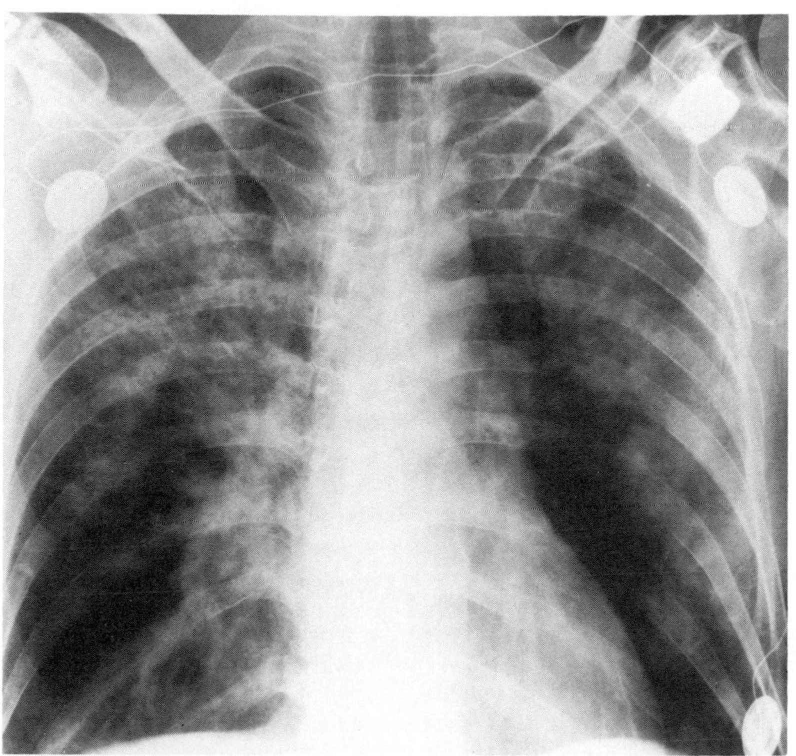

Figure 5–2. ARDS, phase 2 (same patient as in Fig. 5–1): predominant mid- to upper lung airspace process with scattered areas of normal-appearing lung.

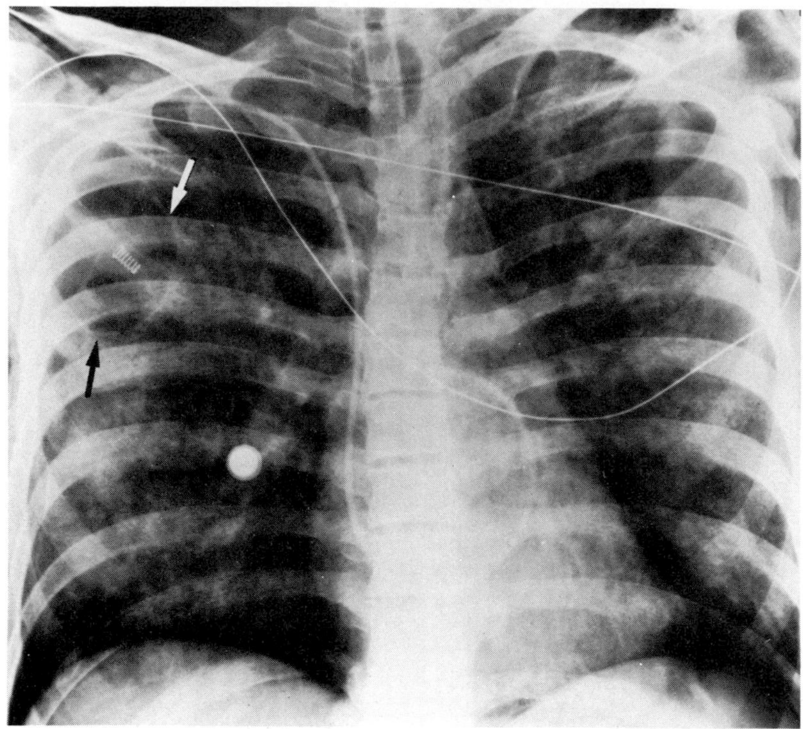

Figure 5–3. ARDS, phase 3 (same patient as in Fig. 5–1): a bilateral patchy airspace process is consistent with pulmonary edema. The heart has not enlarged. A Swan-Ganz catheter is in the main pulmonary artery. The endotracheal tube cuff is overinflated. Its external pressure reservoir is seen over the right lung *(arrows)*. It may simulate a bulla.

altered by treatment. Therapy-related changes may be due to pulmonary oxygen toxicity, barotrauma, and infection (see Chapter 4) (Fig. 5–4). Most notable are improvements in aeration following the use of PEEP (see Chapter 1).

Over a period that may vary from days to weeks, the radiograph may return to a normal baseline or there may be focal areas of scarring consistent with interstitial fibrosis. Patients with underlying chronic obstructive pulmonary disease (COPD) or CHF who also have ARDS will often have radiographic changes more in keeping with the primary disease process.

DIFFERENTIAL DIAGNOSIS

When faced with acute respiratory insufficiency and a radiograph demonstrating a diffuse alveolar or interstitial process, the diagnosis of ARDS is one of exclusion. CHF, pulmonary edema, aspiration pneumonia, oxygen toxicity (Clark and Lambertsen, 1971; Joffe, 1974; Joffe and Simon, 1969), severe infection, lung contusion, pulmonary embolism, and fat emboli frequently mimic ARDS radiographically (Gomez, 1968; Joffe, 1970; Joffe and Simon, 1969). In many instances, the clinical and laboratory data allow for adequate differentiation. Pulmonary embolism and fat embolism, which may be confused with ARDS, are discussed here.

Pulmonary embolism is a frequent diagnostic consideration early in the course of ARDS. In both conditions, the patient has a rapid onset of respiratory insufficiency and a normal or minimally abnormal chest radiograph. The diffuse parenchymal infiltrates that develop in ARDS, however, are rarely seen in pulmonary embolism. The presence of a pleural effusion virtually excludes ARDS, but it is not an uncommon feature with pulmonary embolism. A special problem is the patient with known ARDS who takes a turn for the worse, raising the possibility of a superimposed pulmonary embolism. In such cases, a perfusion lung scan or pulmonary angiogram may be required for confirmation or exclusion of pulmonary embo-

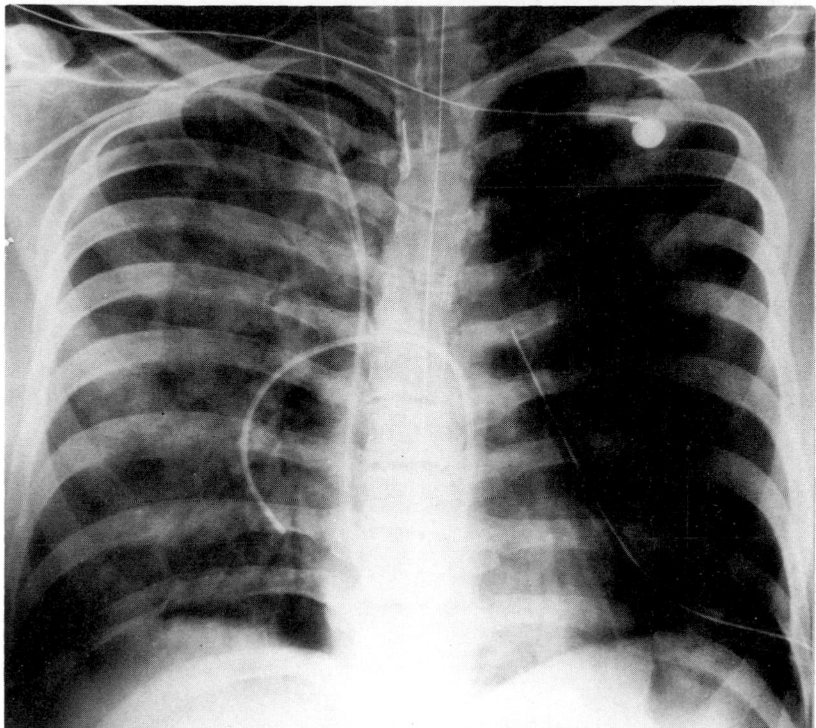

Figure 5–4. ARDS, phase 4 (same patient as in Fig. 5–1): a diffuse airspace process is seen in the right lung and a residual pneumothorax on the left. The endotracheal tube and left chest tube are in satisfactory position. The Swan-Ganz catheter is in the distal right lower lobe pulmonary artery.

lism. In ARDS, the lung scan is normal or diffusely abnormal with multiple subsegmental defects (Fig. 5–5). ARDS alone will not cause segmental defects. When uncertainty persists, pulmonary angiography is required. Pulmonary angiograms in ARDS are free of intraluminal filling defects and cut-off vessels (Newman et al., 1982).

In patients with fat embolism, both clinical and radiographic presentation on occasion may simulate ARDS. Fat embolism syndrome consists of the triad of neurologic dysfunction, respiratory insufficiency, and petechiae following major orthopedic trauma or manipulation. As in ARDS, there is frequently a latent period between the trauma and the clinical syndrome.

Our experience suggests that there are three clinical, pathologic, and radiographic patterns in response to the embolic fat. The more classic pattern is characterized by equivocal chest radiographs, often normal or rarely progressing to an interstitial or alveolar pattern. Histology shows microscopic fat emboli within capillaries, and arterioles with areas of interstitial and alveolar edema. With ventilatory support, most of these patients have an uneventful recovery. The second pattern is characterized by consistently abnormal chest radiographs, progressing from normal to diffuse alveolar consolidation within 24 to 48 hours (Fig. 5–6). Histology demonstrates multiple fat emboli surrounded by fibrin and platelet aggregates, and both interstitial and alveolar hemorrhage, which can progress to hyaline membrane formation and, eventually, to pulmonary fibrosis. This type of response is, therefore, indistinguishable clinically, pathologically, and radiographically from ARDS. The third pattern involves those patients who have massive fat embolism and die within the first 24 hours. These patients usually have evidence of right-to-left shunting; this is due either to sudden rises in right ventricular pressure accompanied by paradoxical embolization, to anatomic shunting through a patent foramen ovale, or to other cardiac defects. This hyperacute form is rarely recognized premortem, and these patients die from sudden changes in right-sided pressure accompanied by terminal arrhythmias. Usually, these radiographs remain normal.

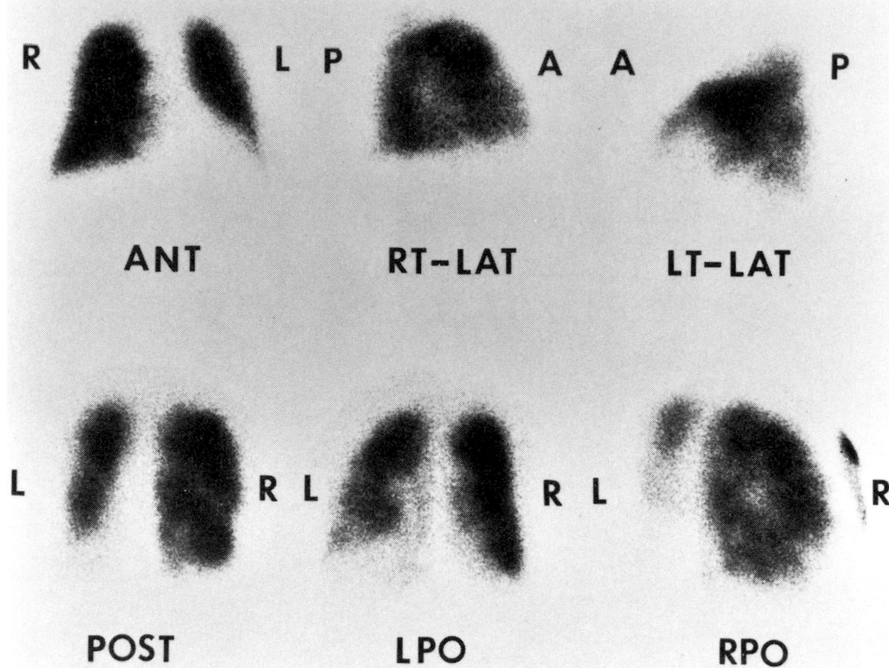

Figure 5–5. Normal perfusion lung scan taken at the same time as that in Figure 5–3 (same patient). This study was done 15 minutes after the diffusely abnormal radiograph was taken. *R*, right; *L*, left; *P*, posterior; *ANT*, anterior; *RT-LAT*, right lateral; *LT-LAT*, left lateral; *POST*, posterior; *LPO*, left posterior oblique; *RPO*, right posterior oblique.

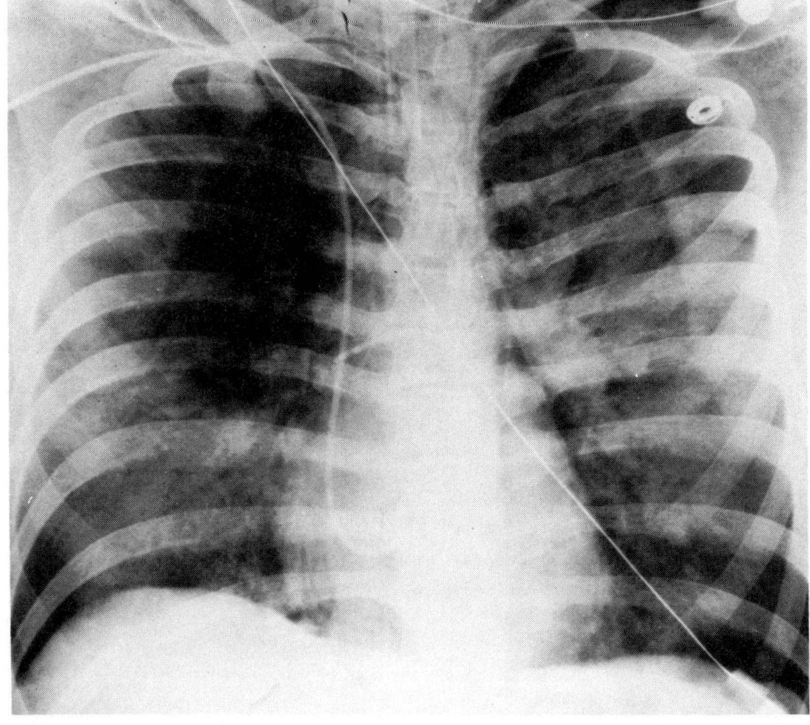

Figure 5–6. Fat embolism. A diffuse airspace process is sparing the right upper lobe. The heart is a normal size. The endotracheal tube and Swan-Ganz catheter are in good position.

TREATMENT

The apparent increased incidence of ARDS primarily reflects our awareness of the syndrome. Current therapy emphasizes early recognition of ARDS, avoidance of known aggravating factors, and vigorous therapy against the precipitating event. If shock has been a contributing factor, it is treated promptly. Pulmonary arterial and pulmonary wedge pressure measurements can be useful guidelines for resuscitation (Petty and Ashbaugh, 1971; Unger et al., 1975).

Ventilatory support to maintain adequate oxygenation is frequently required. Initially, long-term endotracheal intubation is the favored method of airway management, but tracheostomy is performed when ventilatory support is needed for prolonged periods. Volume-regulated ventilators are used to ensure precise volume delivery in the presence of stiff (noncompliant) lungs and to provide optimal levels of PEEP (see Chapter 1). Extracorporeal oxygenation has been used in a few patients with ARDS, but more experience is needed before definite indications for this form of treatment can be made.

Administration of fluids and blood can be carefully monitored by measurement of pulmonary arterial and pulmonary wedge pressure. Overhydration or the overzealous use of hypertonic solutions must be avoided, since these will contribute to the exudation of fluid from the pulmonary capillaries. In a few patients, salt-free albumin can be beneficial in preventing further transfer of water through the alveolar capillary membrane by increasing the serum osmotic pressure. Furthermore, diuretics may aid in eliminating excess water from the lungs and are particularly useful in patients with concomitant left ventricular failure. Despite persistent controversy, corticosteroids are generally used at some time during the course of the syndrome. Steroids are given to prevent an increase in capillary permeability, to prevent leukocytes from adhering to capillary walls, and to prevent the release of lysozymes, which damage capillary endothelium (Clements, 1970; Wilson, 1970). Heparin has been used when consumptive coagulopathy has been documented by appropriate laboratory studies (Blaisdell and Scholobohm, 1973). Prophylactic use of antibiotics plays no role in the treatment of ARDS. Routine cultures and sensitivities of bronchial secretions and serial radiographs are periodically obtained, because bacterial pneumonia is a common secondary problem.

The most important factor in determining a successful outcome in this syndrome is a high degree of suspicion that ARDS may supervene. There are no long-term studies of a large group of survivors of ARDS, but it would appear that lung function returns to normal in most of these individuals despite prolonged mechanical ventilation and high oxygen exposure. Patients with histologic evidence of interstitial fibrosis and abnormal radiographs may also recover, even though pulmonary function may remain abnormal (Fallat et al., 1976; Lamarre et al., 1973). Additional controlled studies are necessary before a more reliable statement can be made about the long-term follow-up of this group of patients.

PATHOGENESIS

Considerable disagreement exists regarding the exact mechanism of the pulmonary damage. It is beyond the scope of this text to delve into each of the proposed theories. Major concepts are presented briefly and referenced.

The precipitating mechanism for ARDS appears to be related to changes in the pulmonary blood vessels or to circulating blood components (Bergofsky, 1970; Murray, 1970; Szidon et al., 1972). Although many researchers agree that pulmonary vessels are the target structures, there is much disagreement on the type of vessels suffering the major damage. Histologic evidence obtained by Veith and associates (1968) indicates injury to the arterioles, whereas Sugg and co-workers (1968) have interpreted their observations to indicate prolonged venoconstriction. Bergofsky found marked reduction in pulmonary capillary blood volume even after total blood volume and pulmonary arterial pressure were fully restored, and implicated direct

TABLE 5–4. Management of ARDS

A. Reversing precipitating event
B. Ventilation and adequate oxygenation
   1. Intubuation
   2. Tracheostomy
   3. PEEP
   4. Extracorporeal oxygenation
C. Proper fluid administration
   1. CVP, Swan-Ganz catheters
   2. Salt-free albumin
   3. Corticosteroids
   4. Diuretics
   5. Heparin
   6. Antibiotics only when indicated by proper cultures and sensitivities

capillary damage as a major determinant in the pathogenesis of ARDS. Microembolism has also been incriminated, since it is easy to demonstrate platelet aggregation, intravascular coagulation, or both, during the initial phase of ARDS (Blaisdell and Schlobohm, 1973; Bo and Hognestad, 1972; Bovier et al., 1970; MacNamara et al., 1972). By means of screen filtration, Swank (1968) demonstrated the presence of platelet microaggregates in experimental traumatic shock. These microaggregates are lodged in the immediate precapillary pulmonary arteriolar region, and may propagate the pathologic processes by damaging vascular endothelium.

Extreme autonomic outflow due to brain hypoperfusion has been suggested as a possible cause of pulmonary arteriolar or venous spasm resulting in ischemic damage and pulmonary edema (Veith et al., 1968). Surfactant deficiency resulting from primary hypoperfusion or injury to surfactant-secreting pneumocytes (alveolar type 2 cells) is another suggested pathogenic mechanism (Greenfield et al., 1968). Deficiency of surfactant leads to diffuse microatelectasis, which in turn decreases compliance and produces venous admixture or shunting through collapsed or edematous alveoli. Tissue hypoxemia and circulating humoral agents, such as histamine and serotonin, have been implicated in the initial insult to the arteriolar capillary pulmonary circulation (Fishman, 1973; Karliner, 1972). Whether the tissue hypoxemia develops because of alteration of capillary tone, precapillary or postcapillary constriction, or alteration of capillary permeability remains unsettled.

REFERENCES

Ayres, S. M., Mueller, H., Giannelli, S., Jr., et al.: Lung in shock; alveolar capillary gas exchange in shock syndrome. Am. J. Cardiol. 26:588, 1970.

Bergofsky, E. H.: The adult acute respiratory insufficiency syndrome following nonthoracic trauma; the lung in shock. Am. J. Cardiol. 26:619, 1970.

Blaisdell, F. W., Lim, R. C., and Stallone, R. J.: The mechanism of pulmonary damage following traumatic shock. Surg. Gynecol. Obstet. 130:15, 1970.

Blaisdell, F. W., and Schlobohm, R. M.: The respiratory distress syndrome; a review. Surgery 74:251, 1973.

Bo, G., and Hognestad, J.: Effects on the pulmonary circulation of suddenly induced intravascular aggregation of blood platelets. Acta Physiol. Scand. 85:523, 1972.

Bovier, C. A., Gaynor, E., Cintron, J. R., et al.: Circulating endothelium as an indication of vascular injury. Thromb. Diath. Haemorrh. (Suppl.) 40:163, 1970.

Byrne, J. P., and Dixon, J. A.: Pulmonary edema following blood transfusion reaction. Arch. Surg. 102:91, 1971.

Clark, J. M., and Lambertsen, C. J.: Pulmonary oxygen toxicity; review. Pharmacol. Rev. 23:37–133, 1971.

Clements, J. A.: Pulmonary surfactant. Am. Rev. Respir. Dis. 101:984, 1970.

Fallat, R. J., Tucker, H. J., and Sgovia, L.: Lung function in long-term survivors from severe respiratory distress. Am. Rev. Respir. Dis. (abstr.) 113:181, 1976.

Fishman, A. P.: Shock lung; a distinctive nonentity. Circulation 47:921, 1973.

Gomez, A. C.: Pulmonary insufficiency in nonthoracic trauma. J. Trauma 8:656, 1968.

Greenfield, L. J., Barkett, G. M., and Coalson, J. J.: The role of surfactant in the pulmonary response to trauma. J. Trauma 8:735, 1968.

Jeneveihn, E. P., Jr., and Weiss, D. I.: Platelet microemboli associated with massive blood transfusion. Am. J. Pathol. 45:313, 1964.

Joffe, N.: Roentgenologic findings in postshock and postoperative pulmonary insufficiency. Radiology 94:369, 1970.

Joffe, N.: The adult respiratory distress syndrome. Am. J. Roentgenol. 122:719, 1974.

Joffe, N., and Simon, M.: Pulmonary oxygen toxicity in the adult. Radiology 92:460, 1969.

Karliner, J. S.: Noncardiogenic forms of pulmonary edema. Circulation 46:212, 1972.

Lamarre, A., Linsao, L., and Reilly, B. J.: Residual pulmonary abnormalities in survivors of idiopathic respiratory distress syndrome. Am. Rev. Respir. Dis. 108:56, 1973.

MacNamara, J. J., Burran, E. L., Larson, E., et al.: Effect of debris in stored blood on pulmonary microvasculature. Ann. Thorac. Surg. 14:133, 1972.

Martin, A. M., Jr., Soloway, H. B., and Simmons, R. L.: Pathologic anatomy of lungs following shock and trauma. J. Trauma 8:687, 1968.

Meyers, J. R., Meyer, J. S., and Baue, A. E.: Does hemorrhagic shock damage the lung? J. Trauma 13:509, 1973.

Moore, F. D., Lyons, J. H., Jr., Pierce, E. C., Jr., et al.: Post-traumatic Pulmonary Insufficiency. Philadelphia, 1969, W. B. Saunders Co.

Murray, J. F.: Shock lung. Calif. Med. 112:44, 1970.

Newman, G. E., Sullivan, D. E., Gottschalk, A., and Putman, C. E.: Scintigraphic perfusion patterns in patients with diffuse lung disease. Radiology 143:227, 1982.

Orell, S. R.: Lung pathology in respiratory distress following shock in the adult. Acta Pathol. Microbiol. Scand. 79:65, 1971.

Ostendorf, P., Birzle, H., Vogel, W., et al.: Pulmonary radiographic abnormalities in shock. Radiology 115:257, 1975.

Perkoff, G., Aach, R., and Kissane, J.: Fat embolism. Am. J. Med. 51:258, 1971.

Petty, T. L., and Ashbaugh, D. G.: Adult respiratory distress syndrome; clinical features, factors influencing prognosis and principles of management. Chest 60:233, 1971.

Powers, S. R., Burdge, R., Leather, R., et al.: Studies of pulmonary insufficiency in nonthoracic trauma. J. Trauma 12:1, 1972.

Putman, C. E., Minagi, H., and Blaisdell, F. W.: Roentgen appearance of disseminated intravascular coagulation (DIC). Radiology 109:13, 1972.

Sugg, W. L., Webb, W. R., Nakae, S. L., et al.: Congestive

atelectasis; an experimental study. Ann. Surg. 168:234, 1968.
Swank, R. L.: Platelet aggregation; its role and cause in surgical shock. J. Trauma 8:872, 1968.
Szidon, J. P., Guiseppe, G., Pietra, G. G., et al.: The alveolar capillary membrane and pulmonary edema. N. Engl. J. Med. 286:1200, 1972.
Tomashefski, J. F., and Mahajan, V.: Managing respiratory distress syndrome in adults. Postgrad. Med. 59:77, 1976.
Unger, K. M., Shiber, E. M., and Moser, K. M.: Detection of left ventricular failure in patients with adult respiratory distress syndrome. Chest 67:8, 1975.
Veith, F. J., Panossian, A., Nehlsen, S. L., et al.: A pattern of pulmonary vascular reactivity and its importance in the pathogenesis of postoperative and post-traumatic pulmonary insufficiency. J. Trauma 8:788, 1968.
Wilson, J. W.: Leukocyte changes in the pulmonary circulation (a mechanism for acute pulmonary injury from various stimuli). Paper presented at the 13th Aspen Emphysema Conference, Aspen, CO, 1970.

Chapter 6

THE POST-THORACOTOMY RADIOGRAPH

by Lawrence R. Goodman

LUNG SURGERY

Following major surgery, it is important to remember that numerous changes in the postoperative chest radiograph merely reflect the procedure performed and are of little clinical significance, whereas other alterations may herald major clinical problems. After recuperation, certain residual radiographic changes are frequently seen and of no importance, while others suggest a delayed complication of surgery. To evaluate the postoperative radiograph properly, one must be familiar with the expected radiographic changes and those that indicate a potential complication. This chapter describes both the expected radiographic changes following pulmonary resection and surgery for acquired heart disease, and the complications of surgery (Goodman, 1980). Other cardiopulmonary complications of surgery such as atelectasis, pneumonia, respiratory insufficiency, and so forth, are covered elsewhere (see Chapters 4 and 5).

Pneumonectomy

After removal of a lung, great care should be taken to expand the remaining lung maximally and to see that the mediastinum has returned to the midline. The immediate postpneumonectomy radiograph should show a fully expanded contralateral lung, an approximately midline trachea, and a vacant hemithorax with little or no fluid. A clamped chest tube may be inserted for use in case of complications (Adkins and Slovin, 1975; Malamed et al., 1977; Pitha and Drapelova, 1970) (Fig. 6–1*A*).

During the first several days, the mediastinum should remain stationary or *gradually* shift *toward* the operated side. A *gradual* shift *away from* the surgical side indicates atelectasis of the remaining lung or the rapid accumulation of fluid on the operative side at a faster rate than that at which the air can be resorbed. This latter problem may require aspiration of air or fluid from the pleural space. A *rapid* mediastinal shift toward the remaining lung usually indicates massive atelectasis or increased tension in the surgical space from a bronchopleural fistula or bleeding (Adkins and Slovin, 1975; Malamed et al., 1977; Pitha and Drapelova, 1970).

The rate of accumulation of fluid in the vacant hemithorax is extremely variable, and standards are difficult to set. Within the first four to seven days the lower half to two thirds of the hemithorax usually fills with fluid (Fig. 6–1*B*, 6–5*A*). Total obliteration of the pleural space usually takes weeks to months (Fig. 6–1*C*). Fluid accumulation may be even more rapid following an extrapleural pneumonectomy or the lysis of multiple adhesions. Under these circumstances, total opacification of the hemithorax may occur over several days. When fluid accumulates more rapidly than air can be resorbed, the mediastinum may shift to the contralateral side and air may be forced through the incision, simulating a bronchopleural fistula. Conversely, total opacification of the thorax may require months to years to occur. Not infrequently, a small cap of air persists at the lung apex without serious consequences.

As the vacant hemithorax fills with fluid, the mediastinum and heart gradually shift *toward* that side. The heart rotates posteriorly and the

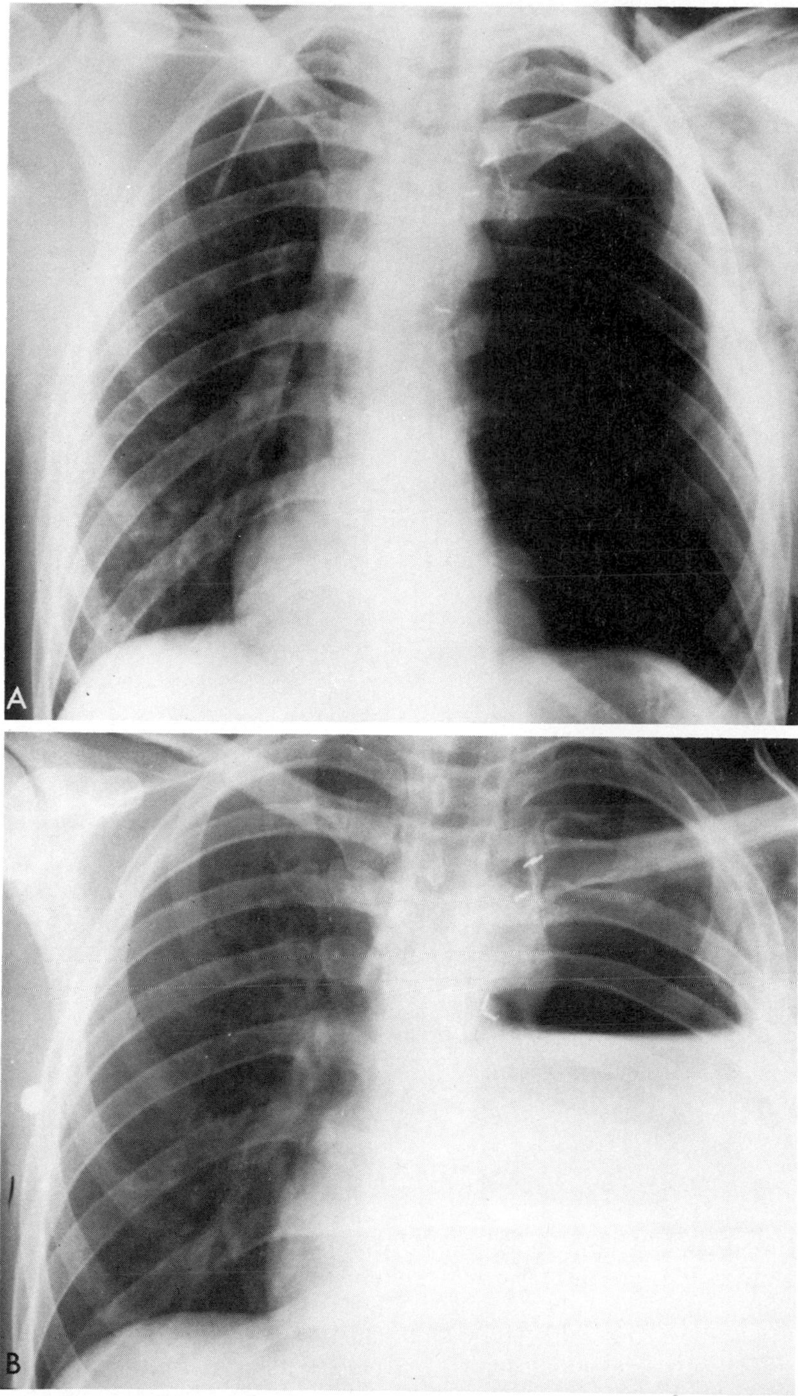

Figure 6–1. After left pneumonectomy for carcinoid tumor. *A*, Postoperative 18 hours. Left pneumothorax, minimal mediastinal shift to the right, and minimal right lower lobe atelectasis. No chest tube. Posterior rib 4 resected, and air in the soft tissues on the left. *B*, Postoperative day 6. Fluid in lower half of left hemithorax; trachea shifted to the midline. Right lower lobe atelectasis cleared; subcutaneous emphysema resolving. *C*, Postoperative day 12. Opaque hemithorax, elevated left hemidiaphragm, and heart and mediastinum shifted further to the left. (From Goodman, L. R.: Am. J. Roentgenol. 134:803, 1980. © 1980, American Roentgen Ray Society.)

Illustration continued on following page

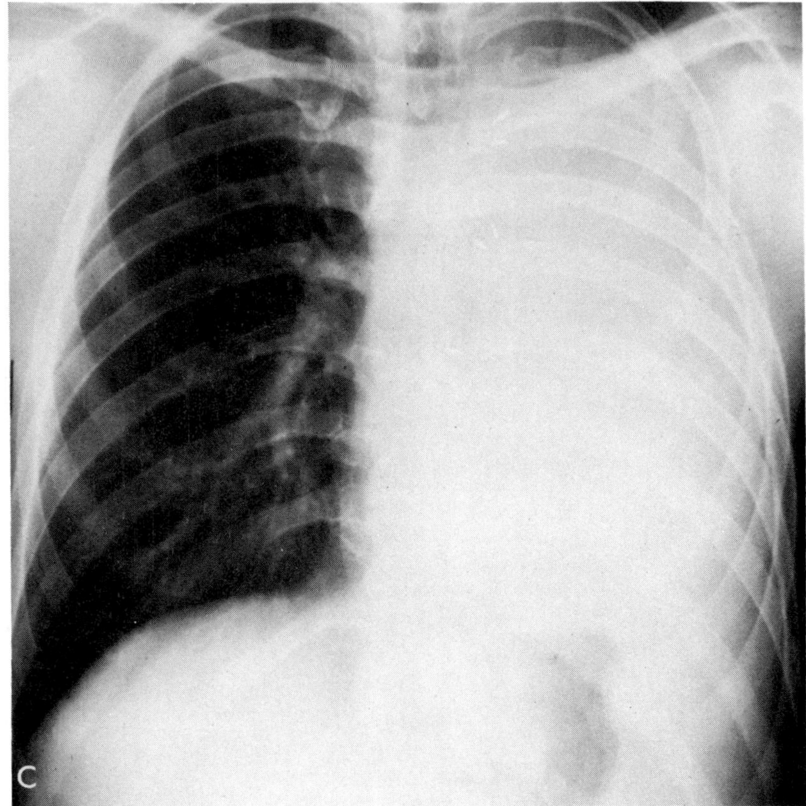

Figure 6–1 *Continued*

remaining lung herniates across the midline, anterior to the heart and aorta. Once the mediastinum has started to shift, any movement *away from* the operated side suggests excess pressure in the operated hemithorax (empyema, bronchopleural fistula) (Barker et al., 1966; Christiansen et al., 1965).

Lobectomy

After the removal of a lobe, the remaining lobes should expand to fill the void. The mediastinum may shift a small amount and the diaphragm may elevate. Marked shifts suggest that fibrosis or atelectasis is preventing hyperinflation of the remaining lobes. Ipsilateral atelectasis, which occurs in as many as one third of patients, must be corrected rapidly before the development of pneumonia or a "pleural peel" that prevents compensatory overexpansion.

If the fissure between the removed lobe and remaining lobes was incomplete, a persistent air leak may develop. This type of air leak usually seals with prolonged chest tube drainage (Adkins and Slovin, 1975; Brooks, 1979; Pitha and Drapelova, 1970). After removal of the chest tube, pleural reaction around the tube track may simulate a pneumothorax, or air and fluid may appear in the tube track and simulate an abscess (see Chapter 2). These radiographic changes are usually of no consequence and disappear within several days. A persistent or increasing density along the tube track suggests a local infection (Fig. 2–22).

Realignment of the remaining lobes after surgery follows a predictable pattern. As a general rule, if one draws a plane through the hilum parallel to the anterior chest wall, lobes and segments ventral to this plane are more mobile than those more dorsal. Thus, after upper or lower lobe resection, the middle lobe or lingula shift into the vacant area. After upper lobectomy, the superior segment of the lower lobe usually elevates, especially on the left. Lingular or middle lobe resection result in minor shifts of both the upper and lower lobes. If the remaining lobes are diseased or if pleural adhesions are present, this normal realignment may not occur and postoperative pleural spaces may remain. Understanding of these shifts ex-

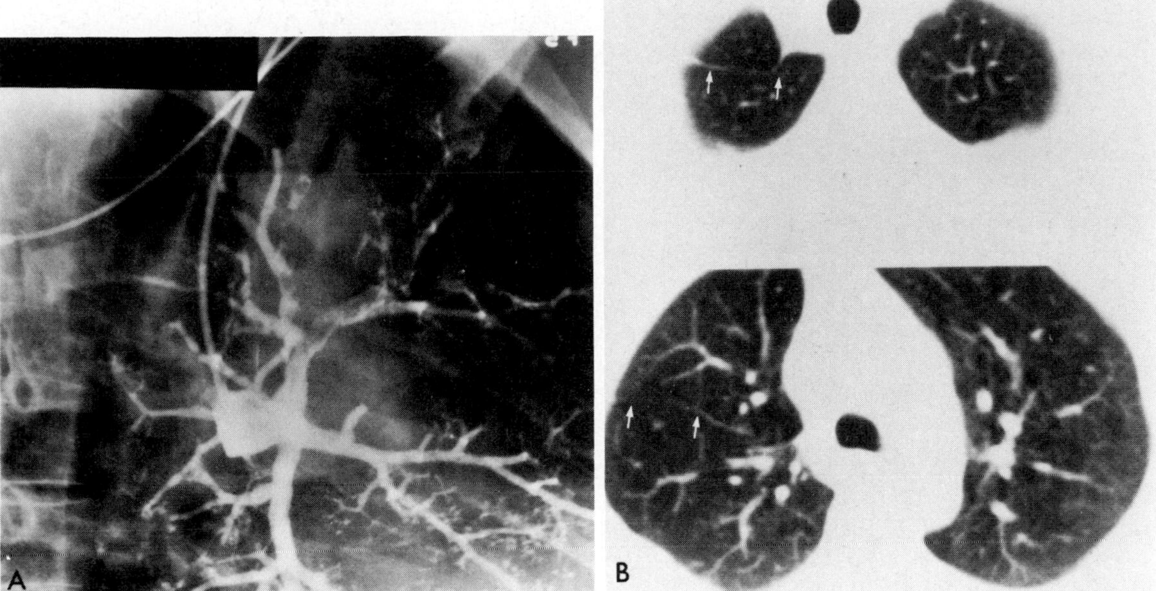

Figure 6–2. Lobar realignment after lobectomy (2 patients). *A*, Oblique radiograph of a left bronchogram after a left lower lobectomy. The apical posterior bronchus supplies the upper third of the lung. The anterior upper lobe bronchus supplies the middle third of the lung, and the lingula bronchus supplies the lower third of the lung. *B*, CT scan of a patient after right upper lobectomy. The major fissure *(arrows)* is visible on cuts through the upper and midlung fields. The middle lobe occupies the anterior portion of the chest, and the lower lobe has elevated to occupy the posterior portion.

plains the normal postoperative radiographic appearance and allows one to localize recurrent disease (Malamed et al., 1977; Pitha and Drapelova, 1970) (Fig. 6–2).

Segmental or Lesser Resections

The postoperative radiograph is similar to that seen after lobectomy, with several important differences. These resections involve cutting across pulmonary parenchyma and require suturing of lung where there is no visceral pleural cover. Therefore, postoperative air leaks from the parenchymal surface are quite common, and a persistent pneumothorax requiring prolonged tube drainage is not uncommon. Postoperative infiltrates in the involved lobe are frequent and represent a combination of hemorrhage, contusion, and atelectasis. These infiltrates usually resolve over days to weeks. A parenchymal scar or pseudotumor from a focal fluid collection may persist (Malamed et al., 1977; Pitha and Drapelova, 1970; Silver et al., 1966). Any postoperative shift of the mediastinum or diaphragm indicates atelectasis since there should be little parenchymal rearrangement due to the resection itself.

As with lobectomy, segmental rearrangement occurs in a predictable pattern if the rest of the lung is normal and there are no adhesions. The more ventral segments tend to shift to fill voids (Malamed et al., 1977; Pitha and Drapelova, 1970).

Bronchoscopy—Mediastinoscopy

Complications of diagnostic bronchoscopy are uncommon, and are usually due to trauma to the upper airway, trachea, or bronchi (Ferguson, 1979). Upper airway trauma includes broken teeth, which may be aspirated, or lacerations of the pharynx, which may present as deep cervical emphysema or as a mass from bleeding or infection. Injury to the tracheobronchial tree is most often due to the biopsy forceps or brush. Endobronchial bleeding may present as local parenchymal opacification, and bronchial perforation as a pneumothorax or pneumomediastinum.

Mediastinoscopy, in experienced hands, carries a 2 per cent complication rate. Bleeding, the most frequent problem, is usually diagnosed and treated at the time of surgery. Other complications include pneumothorax, mediastinitis, and esophageal perforation (Ferguson, 1979). The immediate postprocedure radiograph often demonstrates slight mediastinal widening and localized mediastinal air. Large or progressive collections suggest one of the above complications (Fig. 6–3*A*).

Complications of Lung Surgery

Postoperative Spaces

BENIGN SPACES. Persistent, pleural air collections are noted in 10 to 20 per cent of lobectomies and a higher percentage of smaller resections. In the vast majority of patients, there is no fever or leukocytosis and the radiograph shows little pleural thickening or effusion. Most of these spaces have a benign, self-limited course (Fig. 6–4*A*); they tend to seal over or are replaced with fluid and fibrosis. On occasion, an air collection may persist for weeks or months without apparent ill effects (Adkins and Slovin, 1975; Barker et al., 1966; Brooks, 1979; Christiansen et al., 1965; Kirsh et al., 1975; Malamed et al., 1977, Silver et al., 1966) (Fig. 6–4*B*).

MALIGNANT SPACES. A small percentage of postoperative air spaces follow a more serious clinical course. These *malignant spaces* are associated with fever, leukocytosis, and a persistent or expanding space with effusions and thickened, irregular pleura. They are most often due to an empyema or bronchopleural fistula. Most

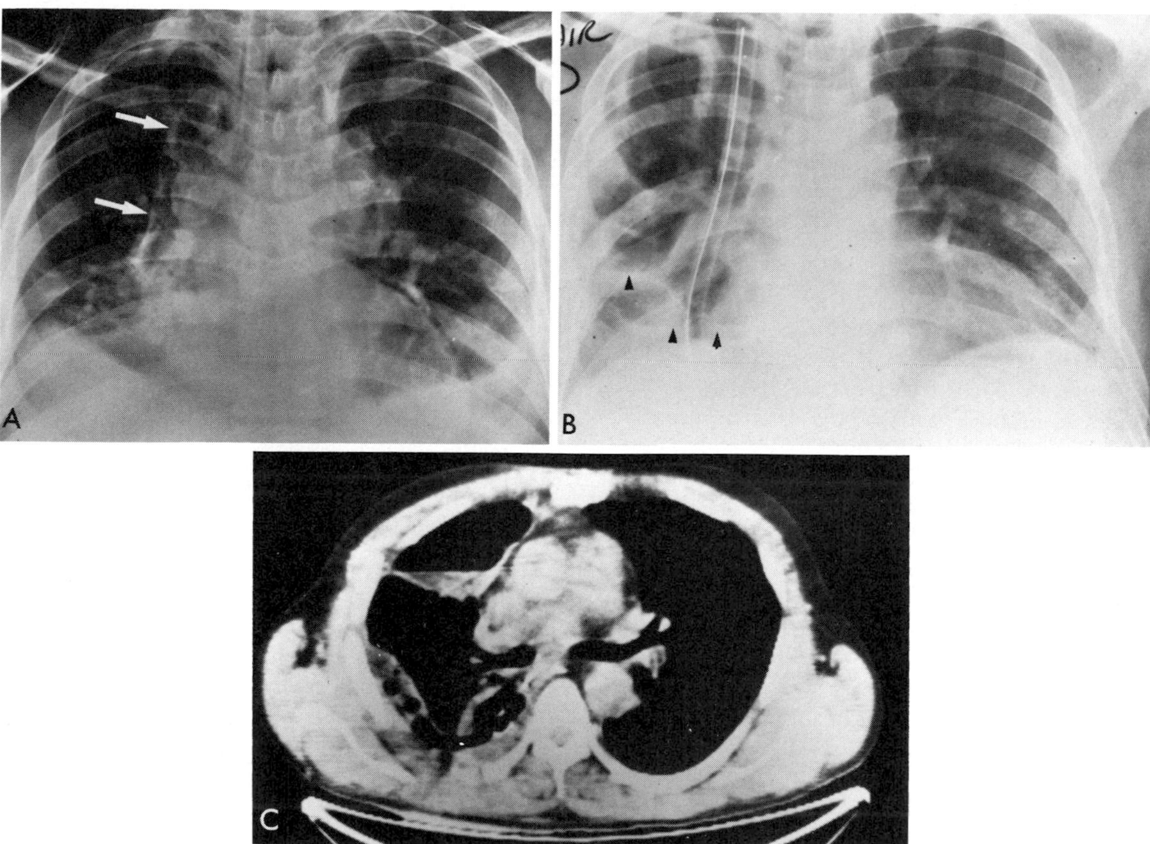

Figure 6–3. Esophageal perforation during mediastinoscopy. *A*, The patient developed marked subcutaneous emphysema following mediastinoscopy for evaluation of adenopathy. The radiograph demonstrates marked subcutaneous emphysema over both shoulders and pneumomediastinum on the right *(arrows)*. The air along the left cardiac border probably represents pneumomediastinum as well; however, a pneumopericardium cannot be excluded. The patient was explored and a rent in the esophagus was repaired. *B*, After several weeks of tube drainage and antibiotic therapy, fever reappeared. The radiograph shows multiple air fluid levels *(arrowheads)* and multiple densities throughout the lung. From the radiographs it could not be determined whether there were lung abscesses as well as pleural loculations. *C*, CT scan below the carina shows two pleural collections, one anteriorly and one posteriorly. No significant parenchymal disease was noted. Based on the CT findings, percutaneous drainage of both collections was instituted. The fever resolved.

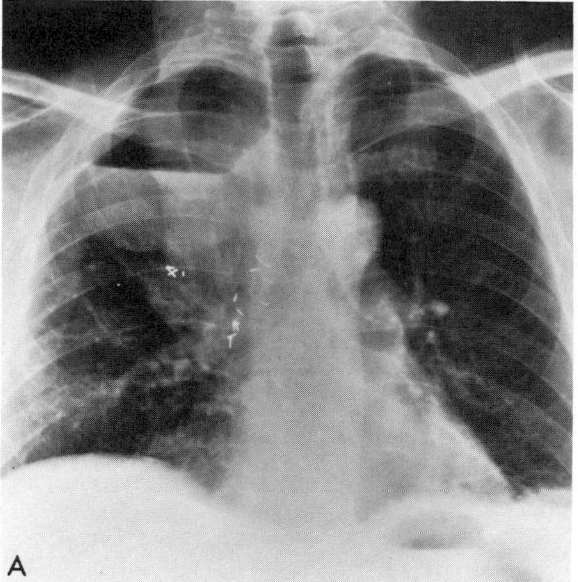

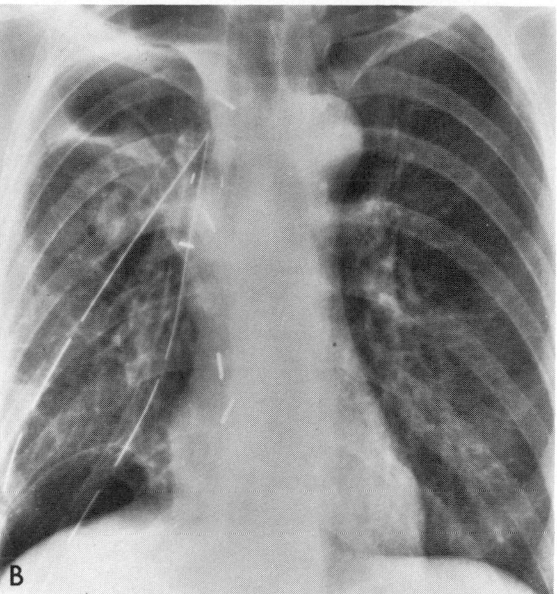

Figure 6–4. Benign postoperative spaces (2 patients). *A*, One week after right upper lobectomy there was a persistent, large air fluid collection at the right apex. The patient was asymptomatic. Over the next few weeks, there was slight further re-expansion of the lung. The remainder of the space filled with fluid. *B*, Following removal of the right upper lobe and the superior segment of the right lower lobe for tuberculosis, the remaining lung never expanded into the apex. This radiograph, approximately eight days post surgery, shows a persistent air collection at the right apex as well as a subpulmonic air collection. The patient was asymptomatic, and the chest tubes were removed two days later without incident.

can still be treated with prolonged chest tube drainage and antibiotics, rather than surgical intervention (Adkins and Slovin, 1975; Barker et al., 1966; Brooks, 1979; Christiansen et al., 1965; Kirsh et al., 1975; Malamed et al., 1977; Silver et al., 1966).

Kirsh et al. in 1975 summarized the current conservative approach to postoperative air spaces as follows: " . . . in the majority of instances, the presence of a persistent post-resection space, with or without fluid (air-fluid level) on the chest radiogram, in an asymptomatic patient implies nothing of dire consequence to the patient. Even enlargement of the space in an asymptomatic space is not an absolute indication for surgical treatment." Postoperative spaces following resection for tuberculous or mycotic infection are usually treated more aggressively.

Empyema

Significant infection of the pleural space occurs in less than 5 per cent of pneumonectomies and a smaller percentage of lesser resections. Empyema may occur alone, may follow a bronchopleural fistula, or may cause a bronchopleural fistula. Most infections occur in the immediate postoperative period, although delayed empyemas may occur years after surgery. *Staphylococcus*, *Pseudomonas*, *Streptococcus*, and *Aerobacter* are the organisms most frequently involved (Brooks, 1979; Young and Perryman, 1979).

There is considerable variation in both the clinical and radiographic appearance of the empyema. Following pneumonectomy, the varied radiographic appearance depends on the state of the hemithorax at the onset of infection: (Adkins and Slovin, 1975; Kerr, 1977; Kirsh et al., 1975; Malamed et al., 1977; Silver et al., 1966):

1. An empty hemithorax may fill very rapidly with fluid.
2. The mediastinum may shift *away from* the surgical side (Fig. 6–5*B*).
3. Air may reappear or the air fluid level in the hemithorax may drop if a communication develops to the outside (Fig. 6–5*C*).
4. Rarely, a gas-forming organism will cause air to reappear in the thorax.

After a lobectomy or lesser resection, empyema is usually suggested by the combination of fever, leukocytosis, pleural thickening, and

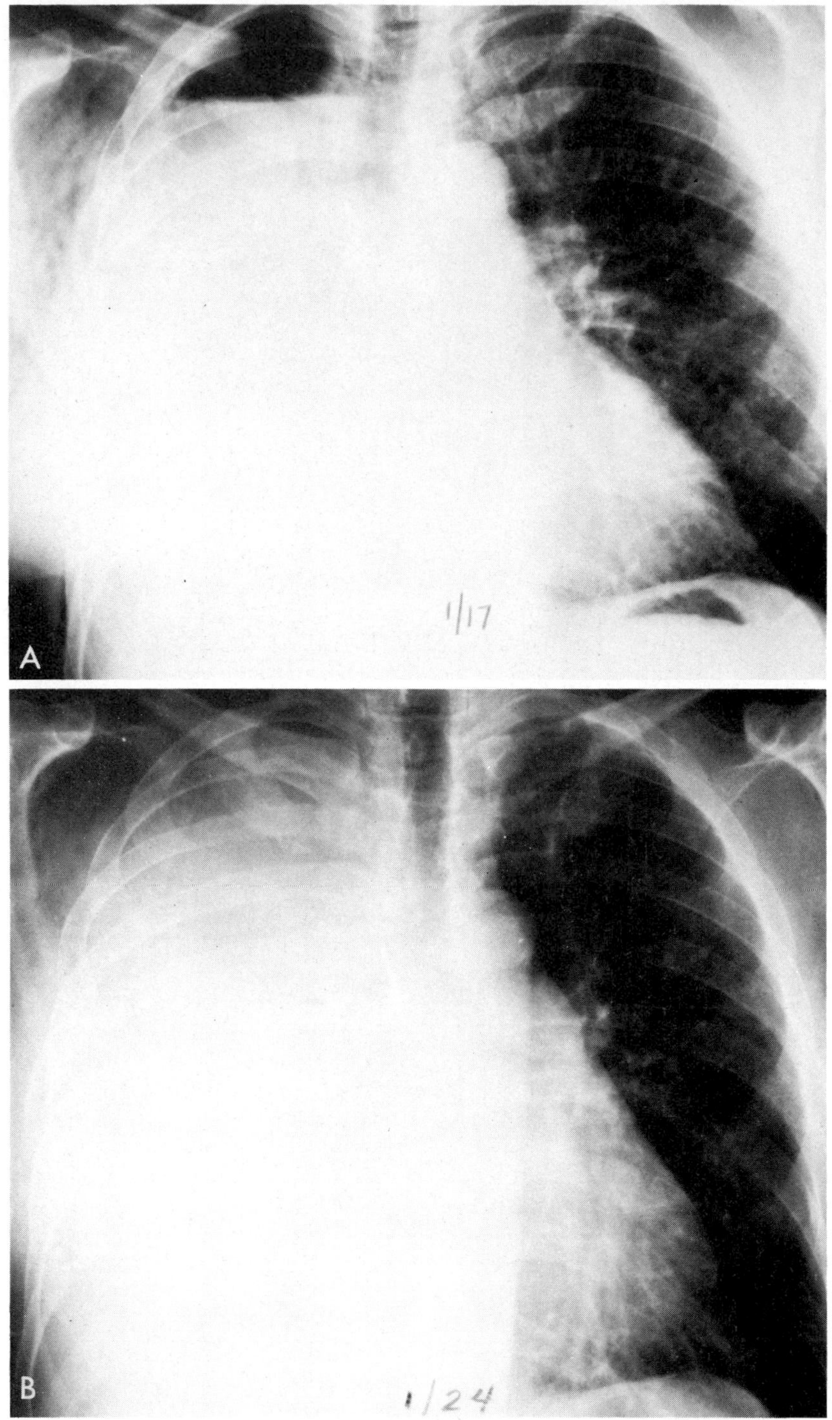

Figure 6–5. Empyema and bronchopleural fistula after pneumonectomy. *A*, Postoperative day 6. The patient is asymptomatic. Fluid occupies most of the right hemithorax, more than is usually found at this stage. However, the mediastinum is shifted slightly to the right and a small amount of subcutaneous air is still present. *B*, Postoperative day 13. The patient developed a mild fever. The entire hemithorax is opaque and the trachea is shifted slightly to the left. The significance of the tracheal shift was not appreciated. During the next ten days the patient's fever persisted without apparent explanation.

Illustration continued on opposite page

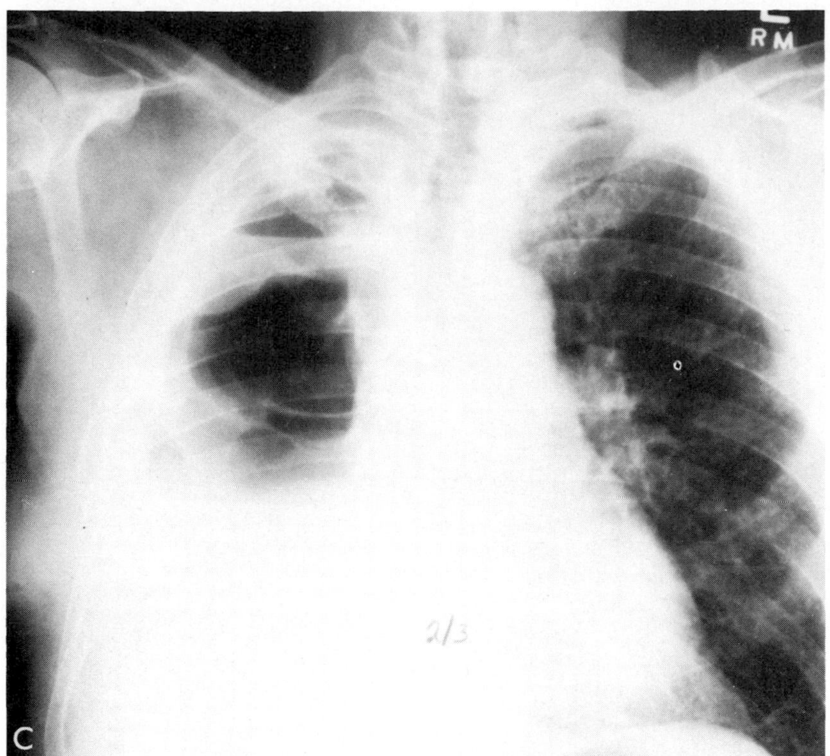

Figure 6–5 *Continued.* *C*, Postoperative day 23. A large quantity of pus drained spontaneously through the original surgical incision. A radiograph shows multiple air fluid levels in the right hemithorax, and the mediastinum is again shifted to the right. The patient was treated with prolonged drainage and antibiotics. Eventually the entire hemithorax was reopacified with fluid. (From Goodman, L. R.: Am. J. Roentgenol. 134:803, 1980. © Copyright 1980, American Roentgen Ray Society.)

fluid accumulation. Multiple loculated pockets are common. Differentiation between a pleural air fluid level and an abscess in the adjacent lung is often difficult both clinically and radiographically. Bronchography, sinography, ultrasonography, ventilation scintigraphy, and computerized tomography may be necessary for further delineation (Kerr, 1977) (see Chapter 4) (Figs. 6–3*B*,*C*, 6–6).

The term "technical empyema" refers to a prolonged external drainage procedure via a tube or surgical flap to vent a persistent air leak, an infected pleural space, or a space created by failure of the remaining lung to re-expand. The tube or flap drains the pleural space to the skin surface until the lung re-expands or the space granulates in. Although not frankly infected, it is assumed to be contaminated. The radiograph usually demonstrates a partially obliterated pleural space with a thickened pleura and a tube in the residual air pocket, or a track in the chest wall (Dorman et al., 1973; Kirsh et al., 1975).

Bronchopleural Fistula

Small air leaks from the cut lung surface or bronchial stump are common in the immediate postoperative period and usually close spontaneously with conservative management. Large or persistent air collections are usually due to bronchopleural fistula. In the immediate post-surgical period, bronchial leaks are rare and usually due to faulty closure of the bronchus. After the first week, bronchopleural fistula is much more common and usually due to infection or residual tumor of the stump (Young and Perryman, 1979); it may even appear years after the surgery (O'Meara and Slade, 1974).

Again, the radiographic changes depend on the state of the hemithorax at the time of the leak (Adkins and Slovin, 1975; Kerr, 1977; Kirsh et al., 1975; Malamed et al., 1977; Padula, 1976). Expected radiographic changes include:

1. A persistent or progressive pneumothorax or pneumomediastinum, despite adequate tube drainage.

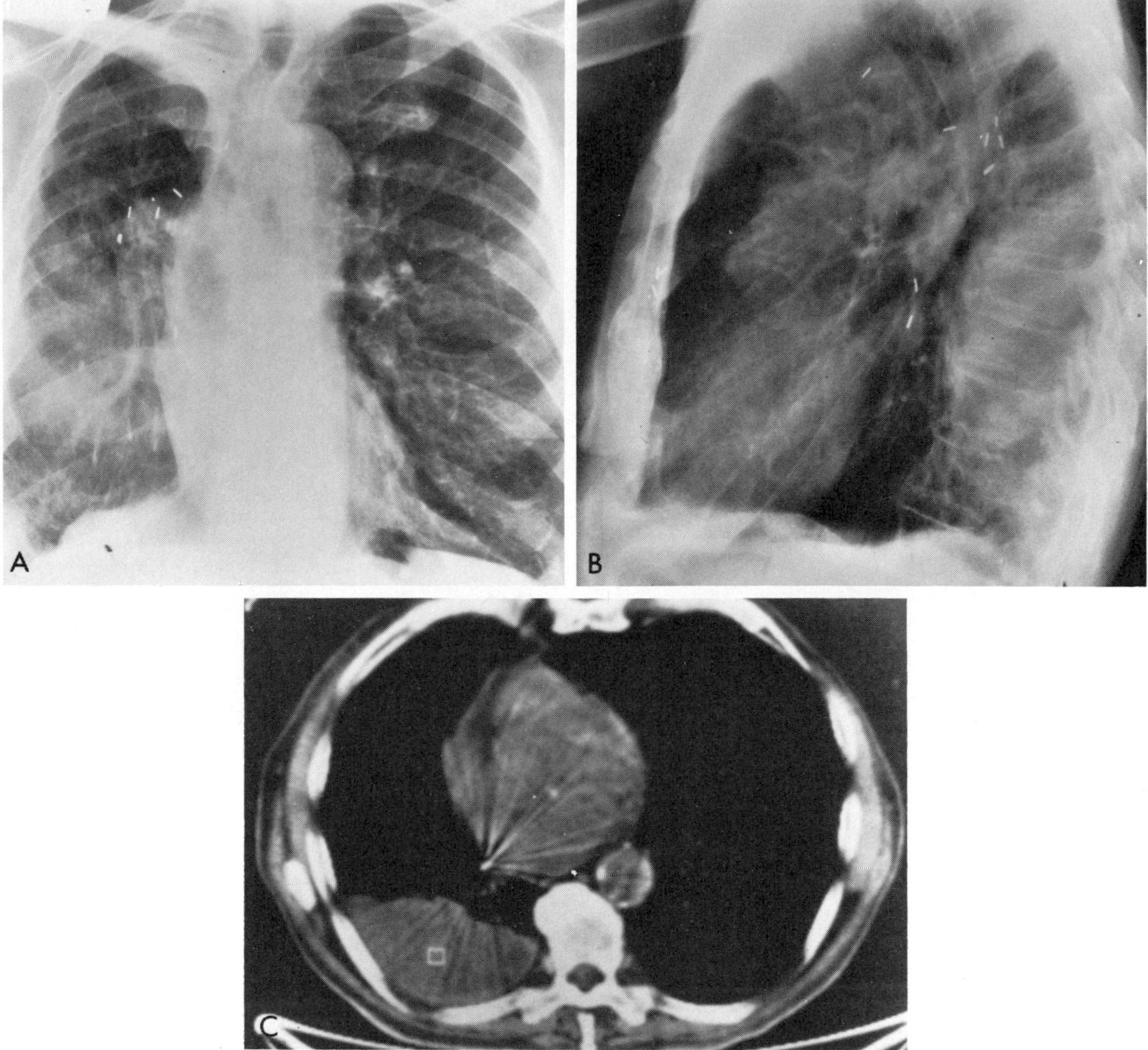

Figure 6–6. Postlobectomy organized fluid collection. *A*, PA radiograph shows a homogeneous radiodensity over the right midlung field. *B*, The lateral radiograph shows an oval homogeneous density posteriorly. *C*, The CT scan demonstrates a homogeneous density conforming to the pleural space. CT numbers were in the midtwenties. Multiple attempts at aspiration yielded no fluid. Cytologic examination of the aspirated material showed amorphous material. This was presumably an organized fluid collection. A follow-up film several months later was unchanged.

2. A 2-cm or more drop of an air fluid level with shift of the mediastinum to the *opposite* side (smaller drops in an air fluid level may be due to many technical factors and do not necessarily indicate a bronchopleural fistula).

3. A sudden pneumothorax or air appearing in a previously fluid-filled area. With a large bronchial connection, the pleural fluid drained via the bronchus may "drown" the opposite lung.

4. The presence of air in the soft tissue as well indicates a bronchopleural cutaneous fistula or an empyema necessitatis (Fig. 6–7).

When a bronchopleural fistula is suspected or when postoperative spaces persist for prolonged periods, radioactive xenon inhalation or evaluation by bronchography or sinography may be helpful. Inhaled xenon will persist in the pleural space during the washout phase. This is particularly valuable in demonstrating a small fistula or confirming the closure of a fistula prior to removing a chest tube (Zelefsky et al., 1977). Bronchography will demonstrate large or moderate leaks, but the viscous oily contrast material will not reveal small leaks. Injection of oily contrast material into the pleural space via the

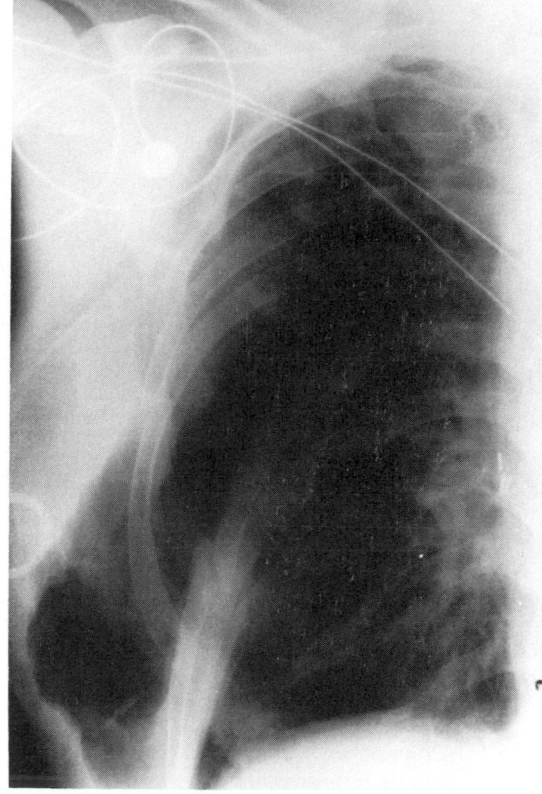

Figure 6–7. Bronchopleural cutaneous fistula. Thoracic dehiscence. Approximately ten days after surgery the patient developed marked subcutaneous emphysema, which is confirmed by the radiograph. The right fifth and sixth ribs are now widely spread; they did not appear that way on earlier radiographs.

chest tube will likewise demonstrate a pleurobronchial connection (Fig. 6–8). In a study of 36 patients with persistent air leaks evaluated by sinography, Andrews et al. (1967) showed that 13 of 20 fistulas demonstrated by contrast material did not close spontaneously; smaller leaks, presumably present but not demonstrable, tended to close by themselves.

Bleeding

Postoperative hemorrhage may be due to slippage of a ligature from a pulmonary vessel, bleeding from intercostal vessels, or lysed adhesions. In the majority, bleeding from the chest tube or the rapid opacification of the hemithorax is usually diagnostic. It is important to emphasize, however, that a large amount of blood can accumulate in the thorax without draining if the tube is obstructed by clot or in a pleural loculation. The radiograph may demonstrate a "hazy" pattern in one area or a loculated pleural collection (McLaughlin and Hankins, 1979). When the patient has had mediastinal surgery, loculated mediastinal or extrapleural collections may be seen (Fig. 6–9).

The differential diagnosis of very rapid fluid accumulation must also include a chylothorax due to thoracic duct injury or the infusion of "intravenous fluid" into the thorax via a wayward catheter (Adkins and Slavin, 1975; Brooks, 1979; Malamed et al., 1977) (see Chapter 3).

Cardiac Herniation

Herniation of the heart through a pericardial defect following intrapericardial pneumonectomy is a rare but often lethal complication. Herniation usually occurs in the immediate postoperative period and presents with signs of obstruction of venous return when herniation is to the right, and hypotension and tachycardia when the heart projects to the left. The radiograph reveals the heart to be shifted to the side of the pneumonectomy. The apex may touch the lateral chest wall, or cardiac rotation may point the apex posteriorly. Air may outline the empty pericardial space. A rapid diagnosis is imperative if surgical reduction is to be successful (Adkins and Slavin, 1975; Arndt et al., 1978; Kirsh et al., 1975).

Esophagopleural Fistula

This rare complication most often occurs following a right pneumonectomy for tuberculosis

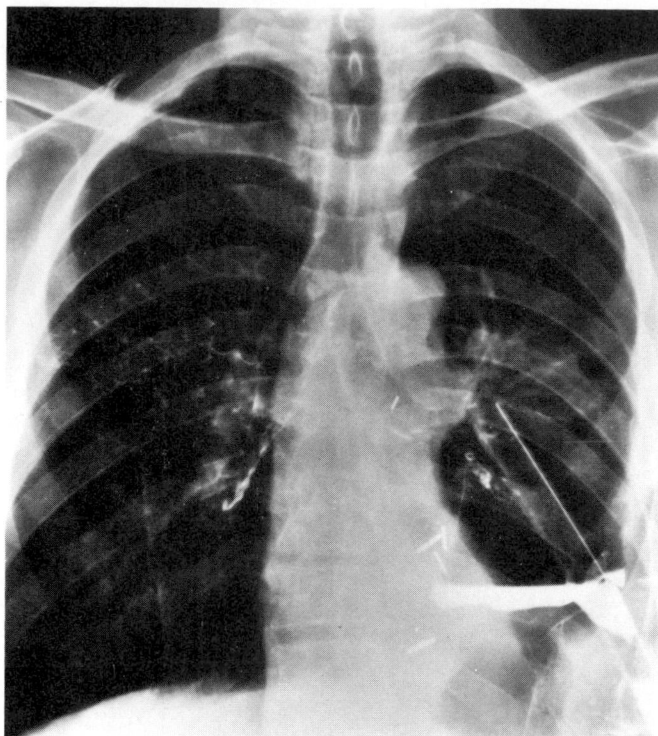

Figure 6–8. Bronchopleural fistula. The patient had thickened pleura stripped to release a trapped left lower lobe. Air persistently drained from the chest tube after surgery. Installation of contrast material into the chest tube demonstrates the residual pleural cavity and also contrast material in the tracheobronchial tree, indicating a pleural parenchymal connection.

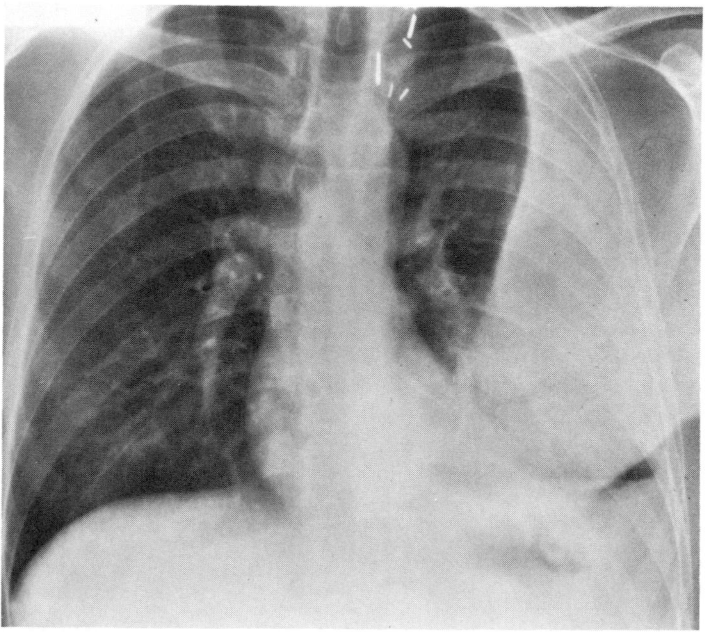

Figure 6–9. Extrapleural hematoma. Following a left sympathectomy, a dense homogeneous opacification was noted lateral to the lung. The opacification did not fill the costophrenic angle and did not shift on decubitus positioning. This extrapleural hematoma gradually shrank over the next ten days.

or cancer. The vast majority arise within six weeks of surgery. During the first two weeks, the fistula is usually secondary to direct esophageal injury or compromise of the blood supply to the lower esophagus at the time of surgery. Late rupture is usually due to adjacent empyema or lymphadenitis, a bronchopleural fistula, or recurrent cancer. The diagnosis is frequently delayed because clinically the picture resembles bronchopleural fistula, empyema, or recurrent tumor. Any patient who develops postoperative dysphagia or a clinical picture of bronchopleural fistula without demonstrable bronchial leak should have an esophagram to rule out an esophageal fistula. The leak is usually in the middle third of the esophagus. Surgical management is complex and mortality is high (Adkins and Slavin, 1975; Kirsh et al., 1975; Sethi and Takaro, 1978).

Lobar Torsion

After lobectomy, an ipsilateral lobe may rotate on its bronchovascular pedicle, compromising its circulation. Initially, venous flow is impeded, causing severe venous engorgement and parenchymal congestion. This rapidly progresses to ischemia and lobar gangrene. This rare complication occurs most often after right upper lobectomy with torsion of the middle lobe. Initially, the middle lobe appears overexpanded yet of increased density. This is followed by volume loss, complete opacification of the lobe, and pleural effusion. The patient is usually gravely ill and the chest tube may drain foul-smelling material. Rapid confirmation by angiography or bronchoscopy may be required before surgical re-exploration. Even with prompt diagnosis, the prognosis is poor (Adkins and Slovin, 1975; Kirsch et al., 1975; Pitha and Drapelova, 1970; Schuler, 1973).

Thoracic Dehiscence

Separation of the posterolateral thoracotomy incision may be complete or may occur with the skin intact. The physiologic changes are those of a flail chest and are potentially lethal (McLaughlin and Hankins, 1979). When the skin is intact, subcutaneous air or herniated lung is visible radiographically. These changes are accentuated by expiration. The radiograph may also show progressive separation of the involved ribs (Fig. 6–7).

CARDIAC SURGERY

Most adult cardiac surgery currently is performed via a median sternotomy, utilizing an extrapleural approach. Although arrhythmias are the most common postoperative clinical problem, postoperative pulmonary infiltrates, edema, and mediastinal hemorrhage are of greatest concern to the radiologist. Specific long-term radiographic alterations following surgery for congenital heart disease, acquired valve disease, and thoracic aortic lesions have been reviewed elsewhere (Hipona, 1971).

The initial postoperative radiograph demonstrates numerous tubes and catheters in the chest. Currently, at our institution, the patient leaves the operating room with the following temporary apparatus in place (Figs. 3–12, 6–10):

1. An anterior mediastinal drainage tube parallel to the sternum.
2. A pericardial drainage tube along the inferior heart border.
3. A central venous pressure (CVP) catheter in the superior vena cava.
4. Epicardial pacer wires and a left atrial catheter exiting via the chest wall.
5. An endotracheal tube in the trachea.
6. An intra-aortic counterpulsation device when circulatory assistance is required (Figs. 3–13, 6–11).

Complications of Cardiac Surgery

Pulmonary Complications

Postoperative atelectasis is noted in the left lower lobe in 75 per cent of patients and bilaterally in another 10 to 20 per cent (Barnhorst, 1973; Benjamin et al., 1982; Gauert et al., 1971; Katzberg et al., 1978.) The densities, especially at the left base, often progress for several days before clearing becomes evident (Fig. 6–10). Despite the relatively slow re-expansion, true postoperative pneumonia is uncommon. The frequent left lower lobe atelectasis may be due to the mechanical manipulation of the lung during surgery, paralysis of the phrenic nerve by the ice used to cool the heart (Benjamin et al., 1982), or mechanical compression of the lower lobe by an enlarged heart.

A mild postoperative pulmonary edema is seen in the first postsurgical day in approximately 25 per cent of patients. In the majority it runs a benign course and responds readily to diuretics (Barnhorst, 1973; Katzberg et al.,

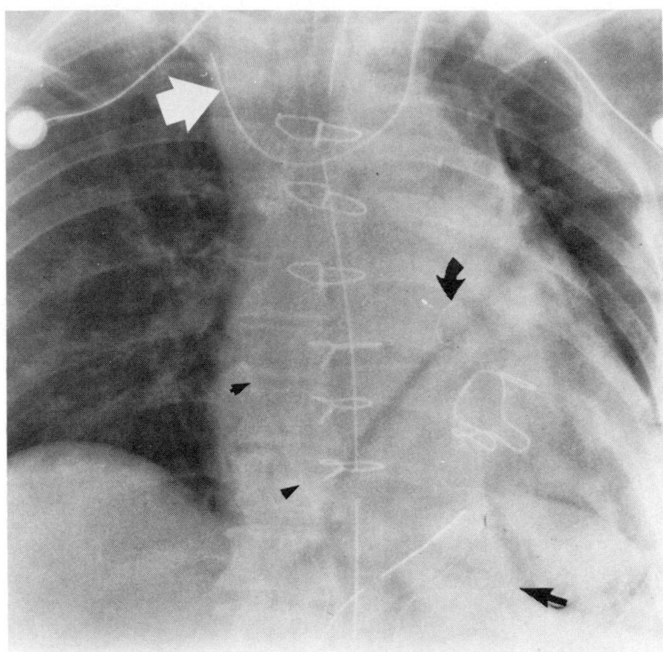

Figure 6–10. Post–mitral valve surgery. The endotracheal tube and the retrosternal and pericardial drainage tubes are in normal position. A left atrial catheter is barely visible over the spine *(arrowheads).* The CVP catheter, inserted via the left jugular vein, is heading cephalad, presumably in the right jugular vein *(white arrow).* The cardiac pacer wires are barely visible over the left hemidiaphragm *(black arrow).* The mitral valve prosthesis is seen in normal position. Incidentally noted above the mitral prosthesis is a curvilinear radiodensity *(curved arrow).* This surgical needle, inadvertently left in the left atrium, eventually embolized to the abdominal aorta. There is also noted moderate widening of the superior mediastinum. The medial half of the left hemidiaphragm and the descending aorta are not visualized owing to adjacent atelectasis.

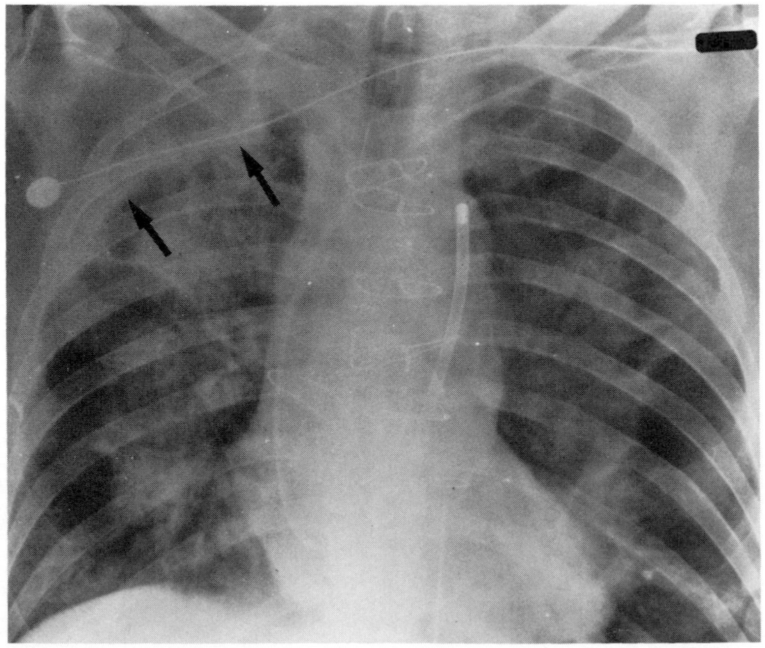

Figure 6–11. Postoperative heart failure. A butterfly pulmonary edema pattern is seen bilaterally. Because of the patient's intractable heart failure, an aortic counterpulsation catheter was inserted. The tip is at the aortic knob. Incidentally noted is a right apical cap indicative of extrapleural bleeding *(arrows).* In addition, there is some mild mediastinal widening. These changes regressed over several days, and repeat surgery was not required.

1978). When failure does not respond to conservative management, an aortic counterpulsation device is usually inserted (Fig. 6–11) (see Chapter 3).

With improved extracorporeal circulation techniques, postoperative respiratory insufficiency is seen less frequently than a decade ago. Originally called "postpump" or "postperfusion" syndrome, it is now recognized as a form of ARDS (see Chapter 5).

Although surgery via the sternotomy is extrapleural, the pleural space (especially the right) is entered in a small percentage of patients. This is usually recognized at the time of surgery and a chest tube inserted. Similarly, a few patients develop a postoperative pneumoperitoneum. Because of the dense adhesions between the inferior parietal pericardium, the diaphragm, and the peritoneum, the abdomen may be entered via the sternotomy. This is a benign mishap, but must not be confused with a perforated abdominal viscus (Glanz et al., 1978; Katzberg et al., 1978). Small amounts of mediastinal and pericardial air are often seen in the immediate postsurgical period and are of no significance.

Small pleural effusions, often bilateral, are frequently seen in the days following surgery. These are usually due to the surgery itself or to mild congestive heart failure, and seldom progress for more than a few days. Effusions due to the postpericardiotomy syndrome are discussed below.

Mediastinal Bleeding

Postoperative mediastinal widening due to bleeding or edema is very frequent following sternotomy, yet only 4 to 14 per cent of patients require reoperation for hemorrhage or tamponade (Fig. 6–11). In the majority, hemodynamic deterioration and prolonged bleeding through the chest tube determine the need for re-exploration (Katzberg et al., 1978; Michaelson et al., 1980). If the chest tube plugs, the radiographic changes become more important in the assessment of postoperative bleeding. Katzberg et al. (1978) tried to relate the postoperative mediastinal width to the severity of bleeding determined clinically. They compared the width of the mediastinum on the posteroanterior presurgical radiograph with the anteroposterior postoperative film, and concluded that:

1. Stable patients without clinical evidence of bleeding widened their mediastinum an average of 35 per cent (Fig. 6–10).
2. Patients with moderate bleeding (30 to 280 ml/hr) who did not require reoperation had a 47 per cent increase in width (Fig. 6–10).
3. Patients requiring re-exploration had a 60 per cent increase in width.
4. All patients with more than a 70 per cent increase in width required surgery.

There was considerable overlap between groups. In the vast majority of patients it is unusual to see progressive enlargement beyond the first day.

Despite the creation of a pericardial window at the time of surgery, approximately 20 per cent of patients requiring reoperation for hemorrhage have cardiac tamponade (Engelman et al., 1970). Clinically, these patients have a low cardiac output syndrome that must be differentiated from a myocardial infarction. In acute cardiac tamponade, there is often *no* radiographic evidence of "cardiac enlargement." Delayed tamponade occurring in the weeks after surgery is often more insidious in onset and is *usually* associated with an enlarging cardiac silhouette (Ellison and Kirsh, 1974; Engelman et al., 1970) (Fig. 6–12).

Postpericardiotomy Syndrome

Postpericardiotomy syndrome is a febrile illness with pericarditis, pleuritis, and often pneumonitis occurring several weeks to several months after surgery (Barnhorst, 1973; Engle et al., 1976). The radiograph usually demonstrates an enlarging cardiac silhouette, a left pleural effusion with or without patchy bibasilar infiltrates. The disease itself is self-limited and does not appear to affect prognosis. Clinically, similar disorders are seen after myocardial infarction (Dressler's syndrome) and cardiac trauma (Barnhorst, 1973; Engle et al., 1976).

Complications of Sternotomy

Fortunately, the complication rate of the median sternotomy itself is less than 2 per cent, since such complications are often serious. Predisposing factors include reoperation for hemorrhage, external cardiac massage, osteoporosis, tracheostomy, and faulty surgical closure.

Sternal or cartilage infection is difficult to document radiographically (Wray et al., 1973). A negative radiographic evaluation does not exclude an established infection. Lateral views of the sternum may show a soft tissue mass or bone destruction, usually around a suture. Lateral tomography or CT scan may be helpful.

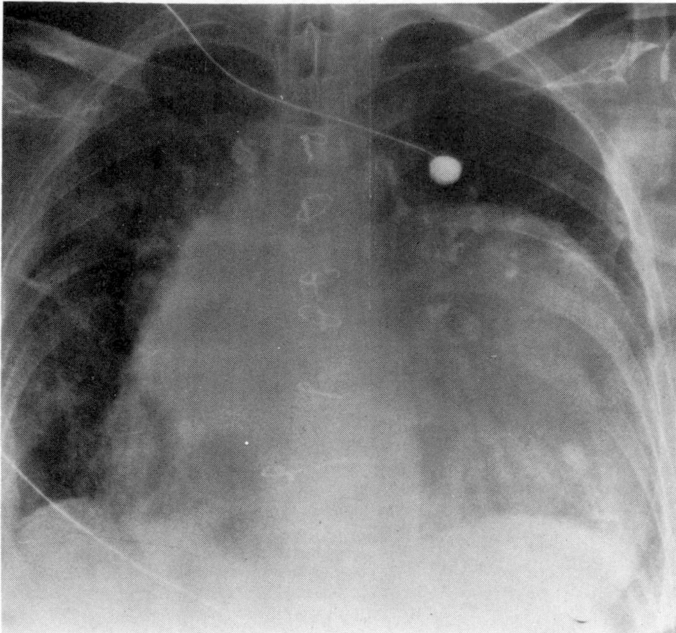

Figure 6–12. Hemopericardium following mitral surgery. The patient returned with severe fatigue following discharge. There were clinical signs of cardiac tamponade. The chest radiograph demonstrates a massive cardiac silhouette, approximately twice the size of the predischarge heart. Laboratory examination revealed the patient to be markedly overanticoagulated. Several hundred milliliters of blood were drained from the pericardial space, resulting in relief of symptoms.

Fractures of the first rib are also an infrequent complication of sternotomy.

Deep wound infections and an unstable sternum are often associated. They may progress to mediastinitis, osteomyelitis, and sternal dehiscence. These problems are usually apparent clinically one to three weeks after surgery (McLaughlin and Hankins, 1979; Michaelson et al., 1980; Sanfelippo and Danielson, 1972; Serry et al., 1980). Again, CT offers an excellent means of evaluating the mediastinum (Fig. 6–13).

A thin (less than 3-mm) lucent cleft in the sternum is seen radiographically during the postoperative period in 30 to 60 per cent of all patients. It is not predictive or indicative of dehiscence unless the cleft progressively widens. The most reliable radiographic sign of

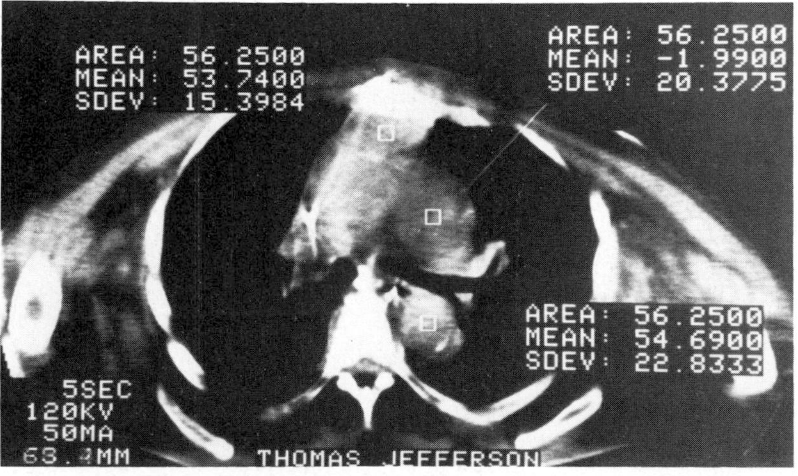

Figure 6–13. Postoperative infection. Following coronary bypass surgery the patient developed a persistent postoperative fever. Some minimal drainage was noted through the anterior chest wall. The chest radiograph *(not shown)* revealed the expected minimal mediastinal widening. This CT examination, at the level of the left main stem bronchus, shows a mediastinal fluid collection anterior to the left main stem bronchus. An infected fluid collection was then drained from this area. (Courtesy of Robert M. Steiner, M.D., Philadelphia, PA.)

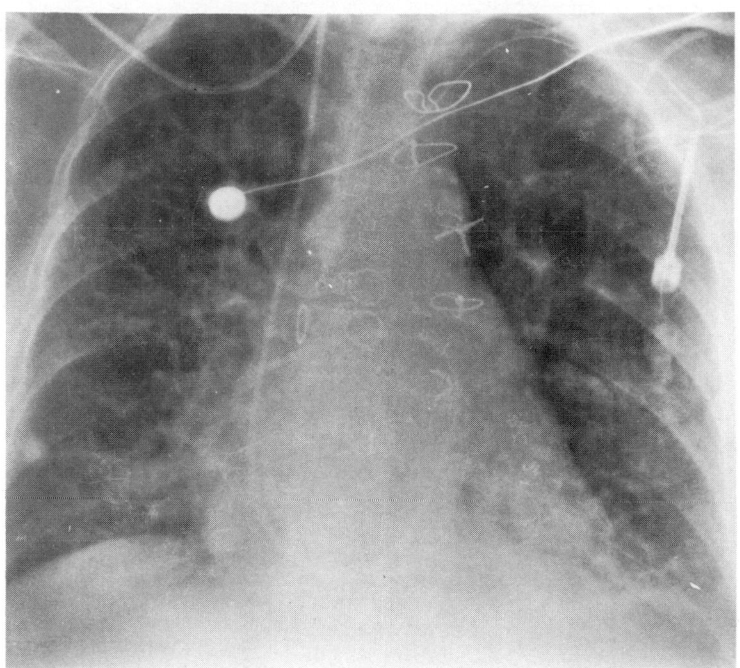

Figure 6–14. Postoperative sternal dehiscence. Sternal infection was noted on clinical examination approximately ten days after surgery. A radiograph several days later reveals that the first suture has unraveled. The upper two sutures are in the midline, and the lower three sutures have migrated to the left (they had all been in line previously). This is definitive evidence of sternal dehiscence (compare with Fig. 3–13). The patient also appears to be in mild congestive heart failure. The Swan-Ganz catheter is in good position.

instability is change in position, shape, or axis of the sutures relative to each other. In complete dehiscence, the sutures usually pull through the bone and migrate with one of the sternal segments (Berkow and Demos, 1976; Ziter, 1977) (Fig. 6–14).

REFERENCES

Adkins, P. C., and Slovin, A. J.: Complications of pulmonary resection. *In* Artz, C. P., and Hardy, J. D. (eds.): Complications in Surgery and Their Management, 3rd ed. Philadelphia, 1975, W. B. Saunders Co., pp. 309–325.

Andrews, N. C., Ver Meulen, V. R., and Christoforidis, A. J.: Injection of contrast media in the post-resection pleural spaces: diagnostic, prognostic and therapeutic value. Dis. Chest 52:656, 1967.

Arndt, R. D., Frank, C. G., Schmitz, A. L., and Haverson, S. B.: Cardiac herniation with volvulus after pneumonectomy. AJR 130:155, 1978.

Barker, W. C., Langston, H. T., and Neffah, E.: Postresectional thoracic spaces. Ann. Thorac. Surg. 2:299, 1966.

Barnhorst, D. A.: Extracardiac thoracic complications of cardiac surgery. Surg. Clin. North Am. 53:937, 1973.

Benjamin, J. J., Cascade, P. N., Rubenferi, M., et al.: Left lower lobe infiltrate following coronary artery by-pass surgery: the effect of topical coding on the phrenic nerve. Radiology 142:11, 1982.

Berkow, A. E., and Demos, T. C.: The mediastinal stripe and its relationship to postoperative sternal dehiscence. Radiology 121:525, 1976.

Brooks, J. W.: Complications following lobectomy. *In* Cordell, A. R., and Ellison, R. G. (eds.): Complications of Intrathoracic Surgery. Boston, 1979, Little, Brown & Co., pp. 235–245.

Christiansen, K. H., Morgan, S. W., Karich, A. F., and Takaro, T.: The pleural space following pneumonectomy. Ann. Thorac. Surg. 1:298, 1965.

Dorman, J. P., Campbell, J. D., Grover, F. L., et al.: Open thoracostomy drainage of post pneumonectomy empyema with bronchopleural fistula. J. Thorac. Cardiovasc. Surg. 66:979, 1973.

Ellison, L. H., and Kirsh, M. M.: Delayed mediastinal tamponade after open-heart surgery. Chest 65:64, 1974.

Engelman, R. M., Spencer, F. C., Reed, G. E., and Tice, D. E.: Cardiac tamponade following open-heart surgery. Circulation 41 (Suppl. 2):165, 1970.

Engle, M. A., Klein, A. A., Hepner, S., and Ehlers, K. H.: The postpericardiotomy and similar syndromes. Cardiovasc. Clin. 7:211, 1976.

Ferguson, T. B.: Complications of bronchoscopy and mediastinoscopy. *In* Cordell, A. R., and Ellison, R. G. (eds.): Complications of Intrathoracic Surgery. Boston, 1979, Little, Brown & Co., pp. 289–293.

Gauert, W. B., Anderson, D. S., Reed, W. A., and Templeton, A. W.: Pulmonary complications following extracorporeal circulation. South. Med. J. 64:697, 1971.

Glanz, S., Ravin, C. E., and Deren, M. M.: Benign pneumoperitoneum following median sternotomy incision. AJR 131:267, 1978.

Goodman, L. R.: Postoperative chest radiograph: II. Alterations after major intrathoracic surgery. AJR 134:803, 1980.

Hipona, F. A.: Cardiac radiology: surgical aspects. Radiol. Clin. North Am., 9:166, 1971.

Katzberg, R. W., Whitehouse, G. H., and DeWeese, J. A.: The early radiologic findings in the adult chest after cardiopulmonary bypass surgery. Cardiovasc. Radiol. 1:205, 1978.

Kerr, W. F.: Late onset post-pneumonectomy empyema. Thorax 32:149, 1977.

Kirsh, M. M., Rotman, H., Behrendt, D. M., et al.: Complications of pulmonary resection. Ann. Thorac. Surg. 20:215, 1975.

Malamed, M., Hipona, F. A., Reynes, C. J., et al.: The Adult Postoperative Chest. Springfield, IL, 1977, Charles C Thomas.

McLaughlin, J. S., and Hankins, J. R.: Wound complications following chest wall incisions. *In* Cordell, A. R., and Ellison, R. G. (eds.): Complications of Intrathoracic Surgery. Boston, 1979, Little, Brown & Co., pp. 333–345.

Michaelson, E. L., Torosian, M., Morganroth, J., and MacVaugh, H.: Early recognition of surgically correctable causes of excessive mediastinal bleeding after coronary artery bypass graft surgery. Am. J. Surg. 139:313, 1980.

O'Meara, J. B., and Slade, P. R.: Disappearance of fluid from the post pneumonectomy space. J. Thorac. Cardiovasc. Surg. 67:621, 1974.

Padula, R. T.: Postoperative management. *In* Sabiston, D. C., Jr., and Spencer, F. C. (eds.): Surgery of the Chest, 3rd ed. Philadelphia, 1976, W. B. Saunders Co., pp. 174–197.

Pitha, F., and Drapelova, D.: Radiographic findings in early stages after operation of the lung. Radiol. Diagn. (Berlin) 11:667, 1970.

Sanfelippo. P. M., and Danielson, G. K.: Complications associated with median sternotomy. J. Thorac. Cardiovasc. Surg. 63:419, 1972.

Schuler, J. G.: Intraoperative lobar torsion producing pulmonary infarction. J. Thorac. Cardiovasc. Surg. 65:951, 1973.

Serry, C., Bleck, P. C., Javid, H., et al.: Sternal wound complications, management and results. J. Thorac. Cardiovasc. Surg. 80:861, 1980.

Sethi, G. K., and Takaro, T.: Esophagopleural fistula following pulmonary resection. Ann. Thorac. Surg. 25:74, 1978.

Silver, A. W., Espinosa, E. E., and Byron, F. X.: The fate of the post-resection space. Ann. Thorac. Surg. 2:311, 1966.

Wray, T. M., Bryant, R. E., and Killen, D. A.: Sternal osteomyelitis and costochondritis after median sternotomy. J. Thorac. Cardiovasc. Surg. 65:227, 1973.

Young, W. G., and Perryman, R. A.: Complications of pneumonectomy. *In* Cordell, A. R., and Ellison, R. G. (eds.): Complications of Intrathoracic Surgery. Boston, 1979, Little, Brown & Co., pp. 257–266.

Zelefsky, M. N., Freeman, L. M., and Stern, H.: A simple approach to the diagnosis of broncho-pleural fistula. Radiology 124:843, 1977.

Ziter, F. M. H.: Major thoracic dehiscence: radiographic considerations. Radiology 122:587, 1977.

Chapter 7

ACUTE THORACIC TRAUMA

by Arl V. Moore, Charles E. Putman, and Carl E. Ravin

TYPES OF TRAUMA

The patient with significant penetrating or blunt thoracic trauma requires intensive medical care from the time he is treated by emergency medical technicians at the trauma scene to the time when he is in stable condition on a hospital ward. The patient with acute chest trauma may require intensive therapy in the emergency room, during surgery if required, and subsequently in the recovery room and intensive care unit (ICU). Portable chest radiographs taken in the emergency room, and subsequently as care and therapy progress, constitute a significant portion of the data base upon which many medical decisions will be made. It is important for the radiologist to be aware of the patient's history and type of trauma in order to interpret the initial and subsequent chest radiographs accurately.

Thoracic trauma is classified into two broad categories, penetrating trauma and blunt trauma. The term "penetrating trauma" encompasses a wide range of injuries in which the physical integrity of the thorax is violated by an object or a missile. Knife and gunshot wounds constitute the majority of penetrating injuries to the thorax.

Blunt chest trauma is frequently thought of as the impact or deceleration and shearing forces sustained in an automobile accident. However, other common forms of blunt trauma such as falls and crush injuries may produce the same types of intrathoracic injuries.

A special form of combined blunt trauma and penetrating injury is seen with the high-velocity bullet wound. High-velocity missiles will cause obvious penetrating trauma to the thorax, but what is not so obvious is the blunt trauma caused by the shock wave generated by the slowing of the bullet. The more the bullet is slowed as it travels through the thorax, the greater is the energy deposited into the soft tissues. The deposited energy is related to the difference in the squares of the incident and exit velocity and is represented mathematically (Moore et al., 1981):

$$E_{deposited} = \frac{1}{2} m(v_1^2 - v_2^2)$$

With low-velocity missiles the associated blunt trauma is usually of no significance because of the low incident energy.

Since the injuries sustained in severe thoracic trauma can be substantial, diagnostic radiographic evaluation depends on reliable interpretation of the anteroposterior (AP) chest radiograph. Many crucial decisions, for example, regarding the need for thoracic aortography, are based on this interpretation. It is mandatory that radiography in this situation be accomplished in an efficient and optimal manner.

The precise role for computerized tomography (CT) and digital subtraction angiography (DSA) in the acutely traumatized patient is yet to be defined. These modalities may replace aortography in part or altogether. CT appeared to provide better definition and understanding of pleural, parenchymal, and mediastinal abnormalities than did other modalities in evaluating the sequalae of thoracic trauma in the cases reviewed by Costin et al. (1981). Until quality prospective studies are available, CT and DSA should remain secondary technologies in the initial evaluation of the trauma patient.

Fractures of the Thoracic Skeleton

The protective nature of the chest wall, including the ribs, sternum, and clavicle, means that these structures are commonly injured. Fractures of certain ribs have a high association with life-threatening injuries to the lungs and mediastinal structures. Because of their relatively protected location, the first and second ribs are less often fractured than are other ribs. Therefore, first- and second-rib fractures may indicate severe cardiovascular, tracheobronchial, and central nervous system injuries. The series of Mattox et al. (1978) indicates that 18 per cent of patients with first-rib fractures and 23 per cent of those with posteriorly displaced clavicle fractures had aortic injuries. In one series of 120 patients the overall morbidity associated with first-rib fractures was 72 per cent, and that with second-rib fractures was 53 per cent (Wilson et al., 1978). In the review by Harrison et al. (1960) of 216 patients with significant blunt chest trauma, the overall mortality was 21 per cent. Of those patients with first-rib fractures the mortality was 36 per cent; with second-rib fractures it was 29 per cent.

Fractures of the lower ribs are often associated with direct blunt injury to the spleen, liver, and retroperitoneal structures. There is also an association of increased abdominal injury with first- and second-rib fractures, again related to the significant degree of blunt trauma required to produce these fractures. Wilson et al. (1978) revealed a slightly greater than 8 per cent incidence of significant abdominal injury associated with both first- and second-rib fractures. Injuries in this series included splenic rupture, liver lacerations, mesenteric tears, retroperitoneal hematomas, and bladder ruptures.

In the severe crushing or deceleration injury, multiple bilateral or unilateral rib fractures may occur. If enough ribs are fractured in one segment of the chest, this segment will no longer move with the rest of the thorax. The "flail segment" will move paradoxically with respiration; if the segment is large enough, respiratory compromise can occur. "Flail" chest is a clinical diagnosis, but the diagnosis may be suggested radiographically by the identification of fractures of numerous contiguous ribs.

The degree of chest trauma a patient receives with external cardiac massage can be significant and can produce bilateral rib fractures, costochondral fractures, and sternal fractures (Lockett et al., 1977). The combination of pain and mechanical impairment from these fractures can produce respiratory embarrassment.

PLEURAL SPACES IN TRAUMATIZED PATIENTS

Pneumothorax

In the acute care setting when the AP chest radiograph is obtained in the supine patient, identification of a pneumothorax may be difficult (Figs. 7–1). This is especially true in patients with small pneumothoraces, because the small amount of air within this pleural cavity is distributed over the ventral aspect of the lung. The only indication of a pneumothorax on this radiograph may be an increased lucency in the costophrenic angle (see Chapter 4).

Since small pneumothoraces can be difficult to detect on the recumbent AP radiograph, the examination obtained employing a horizontal beam will enhance the detection of a pneumothorax. Horizontal beam radiography permits the radiographic beam to be parallel to the visceral pleural–air interface in the nondependent lung. Enhancement of the visceral pleural line can also be accomplished by obtaining the radiograph in the expiratory state. The visibility of the pneumothorax is increased by reducing the volume of the air-containing lung, accentuating the relative amount of air trapped within the pleural space. The combination of the expiratory radiograph with the horizontal beam should optimize the detection of the small pneumothorax.

Pneumothorax is caused most frequently by alveolar disruption and laceration of the visceral pleura, created by shearing forces related to the blunt thoracic trauma (Reynolds and Davis, 1966). Penetrating injuries have two potential sources for air entrance into the pleural cavity. Air may enter directly along the tract of the wound or may enter from an associated pleural laceration. When the wound tract is large, air may enter and leave the pleural space with respiration creating a "sucking chest wound."

Air trapped in the pleural space under considerable pressure creates a special form of pneumothorax, tension pneumothorax (Fig. 7–2A). Substantial intrapleural pressure may produce a collapse of the associated lung, depression of the hemidiaphragm, and a shift of the mediastinum into the opposite hemithorax, creating contralateral lung atelectasis. In the ICU it is important that good lines of communication exist between the radiologist and the referring physician so that therapy can be administered expeditiously. Follow-up chest radiographs in the ICU are valuable in assessing the efficacy of therapy as, for example, in determining

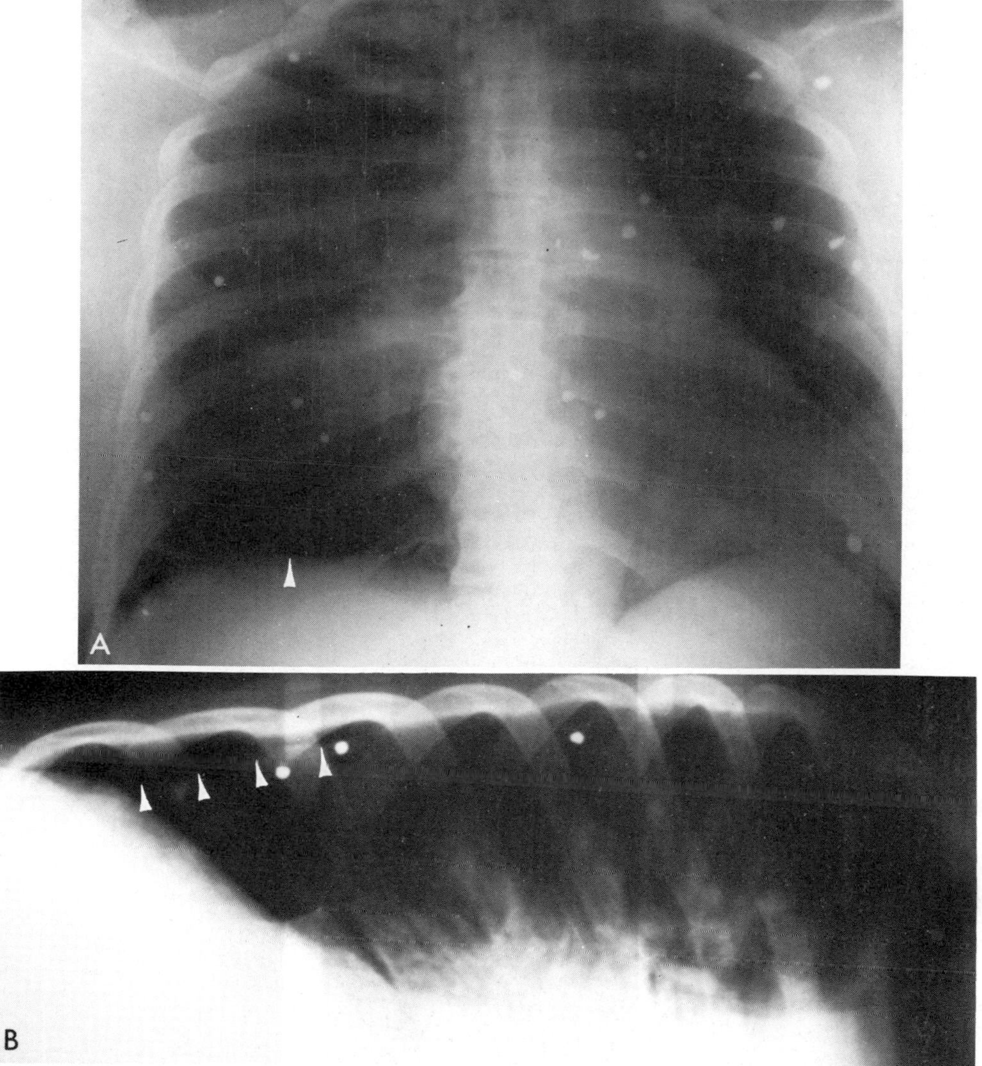

Figure 7–1. *A*, AP chest radiograph, following gunshot, suggests a subpulmonic collection of air on the right *(white arrowhead)*. *B*, Lateral decubitus view with a horizontal beam depicts the pneumothorax *(white arrowheads)*.

chest tube position and evaluating the ability of the chest tube to remove both the air and fluid in the pleural spaces (Fig. 7–2*B*).

Unresponding pneumothorax should suggest a major pulmonary laceration or tracheobronchial, laryngeal, or esophageal laceration, requiring prompt endoscopic evaluation of the airways and esophagus. For definition of the injury and its extent, other imaging modalities such as routine tomography, contrast esophagoscopy, and contrast bronchography are useful, but these require the patient to be physiologically stable. A significant problem in the ICU is the iatrogenic or acquired pneumothorax (barotrauma). Malposition of intravenous lines, difficult endotracheal intubation, and prolonged assisted ventilation can be responsible for abnormal air collections (see Chapter 2).

Hydrothorax

The traumatized patient frequently collects fluid within the pleural spaces. This fluid, often blood, results from tears in the pulmonary parenchyma and the visceral pleura (Fig. 7–3). The bleeding from these small parenchymal lacerations often resolves spontaneously. When the hemothorax is related to significant venous bleeding, the compressive effect from the ex-

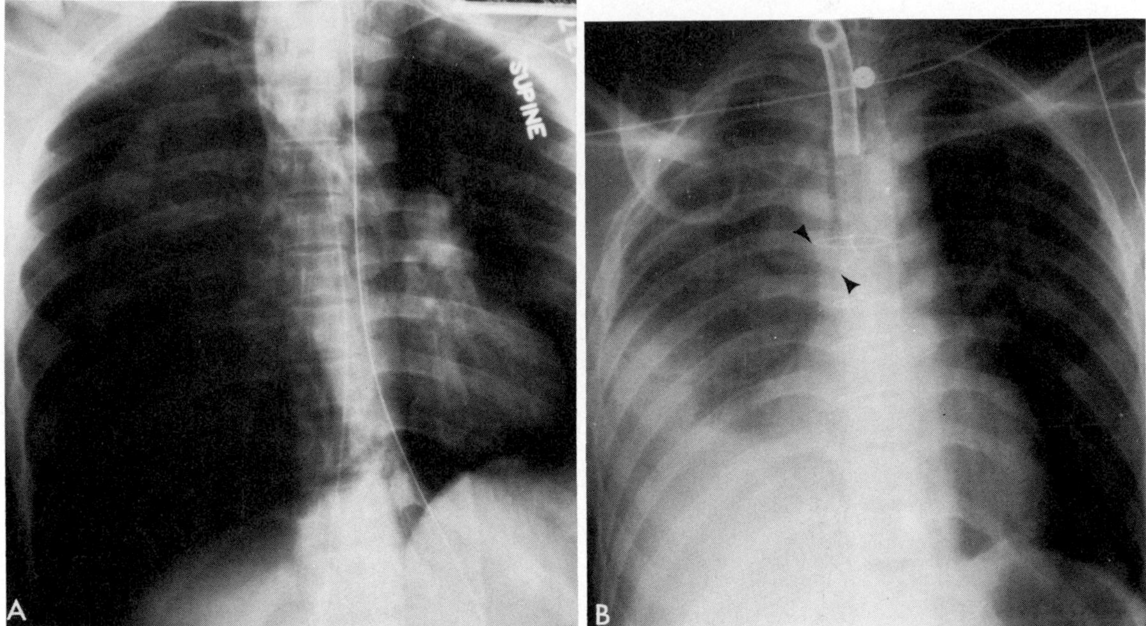

Figure 7–2. *A,* 27-year-old man sustained thoracic injury after an automobile slipped from a jack. AP radiograph revealed a tension pneumothorax. *B,* Follow-up radiographs two weeks later revealed increasing opacification of the right hemithorax. Discontinuity of the right main stem bronchus *(black arrowheads)* suggests bronchial disruption (confirmed at surgery). (From Moore, A. V., Putman, C. E., and Ravin, C. E.: Bull. N.Y. Acad. Med. 57:272, 1981.)

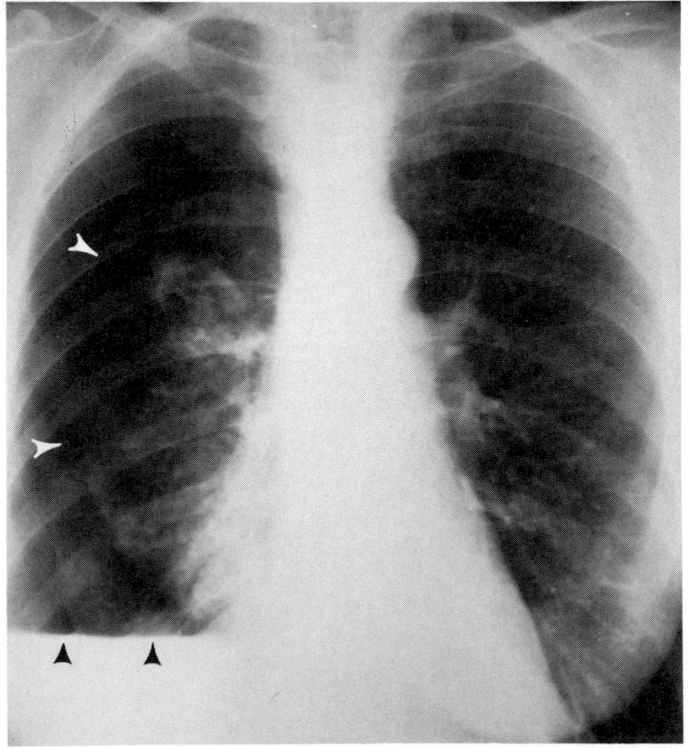

Figure 7–3. PA chest radiograph on a middle-aged woman following right-sided blunt chest trauma. The air fluid level *(black arrowheads)* indicates both fluid (probably blood) and air within the pleural space. The pneumothorax is confirmed by identification of the visceral pleural line *(white arrowheads).* (From Moore, A. V., Putman, C. E., and Ravin, C. E.: Bull. N.Y. Acad. Sci. 57:272, 1981.)

panding blood collection tends to provide hemostasis by its tamponading effect (Doubleday, 1960).

When the hemothorax is seen to be increasing on serial chest radiographs, a more serious vascular injury should be suspected. The injury may be related to a tear in any major mediastinal, pulmonary, or intercostal vessel. With major vessel injury a widened mediastinum is usually present with the hemothorax. When intercostal artery bleeding is suspected as the cause of an expanding hemothorax, bleeding from other sites (for example, the aorta) should also be evaluated (Crawford, 1973). Aortography and selective angiography may be needed to define multiple bleeding sites (see Chapter 9).

PULMONARY PARENCHYMAL TRAUMA

Pulmonary Contusion

The most frequent chest radiographic abnormality in patients suffering major nonpenetrating chest injuries is the pulmonary contusion, which occurs in almost 75 per cent of such patients (Fig. 7–4*A*) (Williams and Bonte, 1963). The contusion is produced by blood or serum accumulating in the alveoli and in the perivascular and peribronchial spaces. Since both spaces are usually involved, the combination of radiographic patterns is identified. The pattern related to bleeding and exudate along the perivascular and peribronchial spaces produces a coarse and linear opacity in the contused area, while alveolar blood and fluid present as a diffuse airspace process.

Characteristically, the radiographic findings of pulmonary contusion appear soon after injury and clear rapidly. Frequently, most of the process will resolve by the third day after the injury. Patients who do not follow this characteristic course should be investigated for other causes, such as infection, endobronchial obstructing lesions, pulmonary emboli, laceration, and recurrent pulmonary hemorrhage (Crawford, 1973). True post-traumatic pneumonias following significant blunt chest trauma are unusual, occurring in only 1.5 per cent of patients in one series (Williams and Bonte, 1963).

Pulmonary Laceration

Pulmonary parenchymal tears, commonly produced by penetrating trauma, are also caused by substantial blunt chest trauma (Hankins et al., 1977; Williams and Bonte, 1961). The large pulmonary laceration becomes a potential space for a pulmonary hematoma. Depending on the amount of transmitted force and the severity of the injury, the laceration may be totally contained within the pulmonary parenchyma or may extend to the visceral pleural surface, causing a hemothorax, a pneumothorax, or a combined hemopneumothorax. Pulmonary lacerations are frequently masked by pulmonary contusions, the laceration often being detected only as the contusion resolves two or three days postinjury (Fig. 7–4*B*) (Williams and Bonte, 1963).

The pulmonary laceration presents radiographically as a spherical or elliptical pulmonary cavity. When both air and blood are present in the space created by the parenchymal tear, the result is an air fluid level. When only blood fills the cavity, it presents as a solid mass or hematoma. Later, as the clot retracts, air may appear within the laceration, producing a crescentic air lucency around the clot. When only air is trapped within the laceration, an enlarging thin-walled lucency may be seen (pneumatocele).

Pulmonary lacerations vary in their course of resolution. Pneumatoceles usually resolve within one to three weeks, but can persist for months. Pulmonary hematomas resolve more slowly. They may resolve completely or may leave a focal scar. On occasion, a hematoma organizes, leaving a permanent "coin lesion" in the lung (Eaton et al., 1973; Williams and Bonte, 1963).

Pulmonary lacerations secondary to penetrating trauma may vary both radiographically and in their clinical course. This is especially true in the lung damaged by the high-velocity missile. When such missiles injure the pulmonary parenchyma, a large amount of tissue necrosis and destruction is created by the shock wave along the bullet path. Morphologically, the path appears as air-filled cavities surrounded by a thick wall of damaged pulmonary parenchyma. These complex lacerations often remain unchanged radiographically for months. Common complications are chronic infection and bronchopleural fistula. Those cavities not responding to conservative medical therapy may ultimately require surgical resection of the involved segment (Spees et al., 1967).

Pulmonary Opacities

Although pulmonary contusion and laceration are causes of pulmonary parenchymal opacity

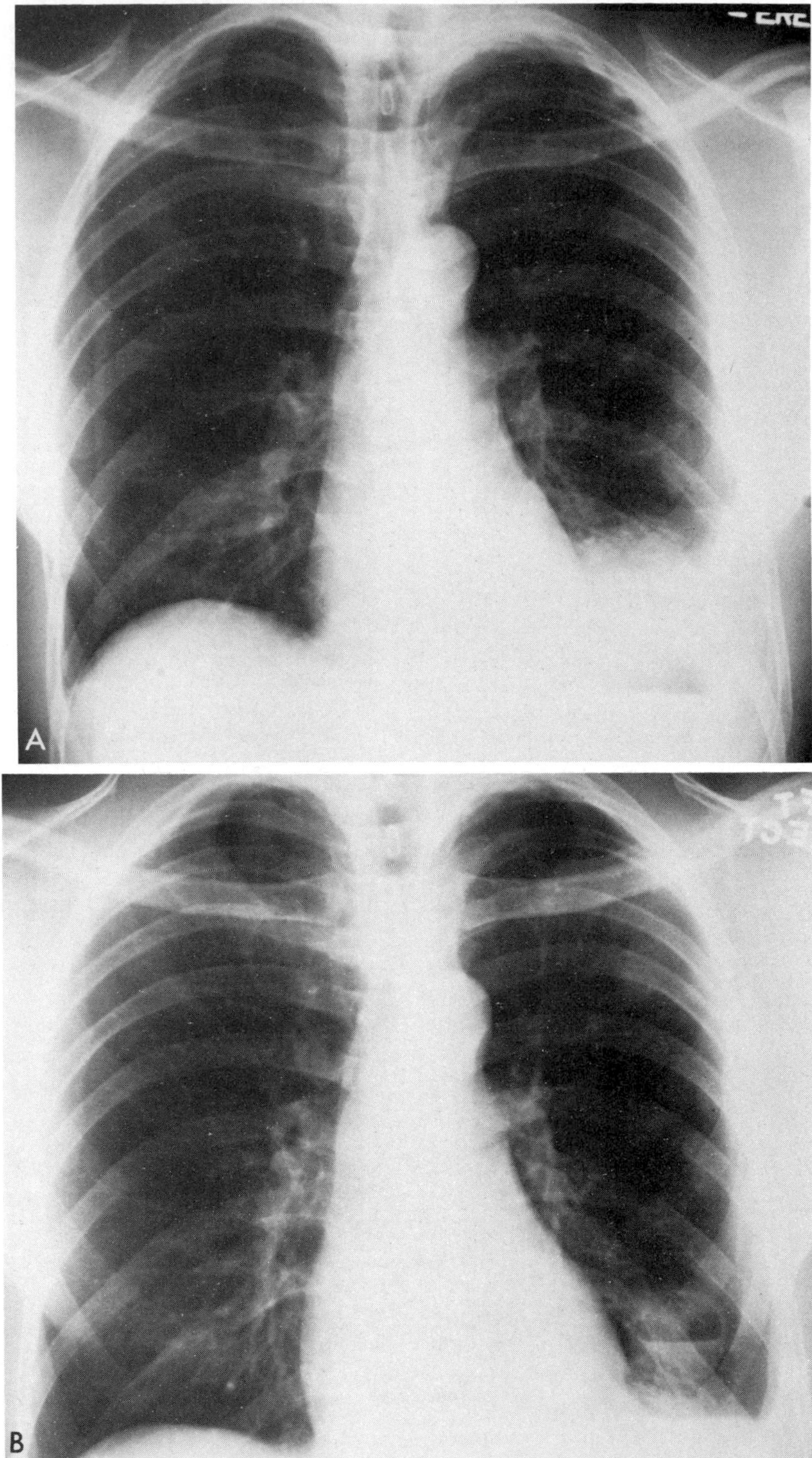

Figure 7–4. *A*, After falling from a ladder, this man presented with a pulmonary contusion and hemothorax on the left. *B*, Approximately one week after the initial chest radiograph, a pulmonary laceration with an air fluid level is demonstrated. Some pleural reaction persists.

that are directly related to thoracic trauma, they are not the only sources of pulmonary opacity in the traumatized patient. Aspiration and atelectasis caused by mucous plugging, or poor ventilation due to splinting from rib fractures, are sources of segmental or subsegmental pulmonary opacity. Diffuse bilateral parenchymal alveolar opacities may be produced by vigorous intravascular volume replacement, by reaction to transfusion products, or by neurogenic pulmonary edema.

ARDS and fat embolism syndrome usually appear 24 hours or more after the injury. The parenchymal airspace opacities usually present as nonspecific patchy areas that can progress to diffuse alveolar opacities indistinguishable from cardiac pulmonary edema. Normal cardiac and pulmonary vessel size are key factors in distinguishing them from cardiac complications. The radiologist should always consider fat embolism or ARDS in the traumatized patient who sustains significant skeletal injury and delayed pulmonary opacities (see Chapter 5).

MEDIASTINAL TRAUMA

Mediastinal Widening

Widening of the mediastinal contour may be due to one or a combination of several significant or insignificant vascular injuries from blunt trauma. The most important cause of a widened mediastinum is aortic or other major vessel laceration. Injuries that may occur concomitantly or as isolated events are esophageal and tracheobronchial disruption, which also can produce mediastinal widening.

VASCULAR INJURY. Traumatic rupture of the aorta is a significant cause of mortality in the clinical setting of nonpenetrating thoracic trauma. The survival rate for those patients sustaining combined thoracic aorta rupture and cardiac injury is the lowest, approximately 4 per cent; for those sustaining isolated aortic rupture, it is approximately 20 per cent (Fig. 7–5). Combining these two groups of patients, those with isolated and those with combined injuries, the overall initial survival rate is approximately 14 per cent (Parmley et al., 1958). Without immediate surgical intervention, approximately 75 per cent of survivors have delayed rupture and die within the first 22 days following the injury (Parmley et al., 1958).

The widened mediastinum is the most important radiographic sign associated with aortic rupture (Fig. 7–5A). Mediastinal widening in the clinical setting of thoracic trauma should suggest the possibility of aortic rupture, and thoracic aortography should be performed. However, in most cases mediastinal widening is not due to a hematoma resulting from extravasation of blood from the aorta. Approximately 60 per cent of patients with aortic rupture will have an intact adventitial tissue layer. Mediastinal widening in this group is caused by tearing of smaller arteries and veins in the mediastinum as a result of the shearing forces and fractures (Ayella et al., 1977).

Evaluation of the chest radiograph should take into account other radiographic findings associated with aortic rupture, which include: tracheal deviation into the right, deviation of the nasogastric tube within the esophagus to the right, loss of sharpness of the aortic knob, left extrapleural cap, left main stem bronchus depression, left-sided hemothorax, and associated thoracic fractures (Flaherty et al., 1969; Gerlock et al., 1980). A possible early sign of a vascular leak is the extrapleural cap, which is produced by fluid or blood dissecting along the potential space created by the parietal pleural and extrapleural soft tissues around the left subclavian artery and vein (Simeone et al., 1975). In some patients the laceration does not involve the adventitial layer, and the chest radiograph may be negative (see Chapter 9).

CARDIAC TRAUMA. Penetrating cardiac injuries rank second to aortic rupture in terms of mortality prior to presentation at the hospital, with a rate approaching 70 per cent (Maynard et al., 1965). Unlike patients with aortic rupture, however, the survival rate of these patients once received by the hospital is lower, with only 40 to 50 per cent of the presenting group surviving. The ability to stabilize patients for surgical therapy upon admission to the hospital is a key factor in their survival (Maynard et al., 1965). The appropriate history, indicating cardiac trauma and laboratory data such as acute electrocardiographic changes that suggest direct myocardial injury, is important in evaluating and accurately interpreting the chest radiograph.

Myocardial injury presents radiographically as a spectrum of findings related to the heart and chest injuries. The cardiac findings may be similar to those seen in acute myocardial infarction: congestive heart failure, ventricular aneurysm, or massive cardiac enlargement. Combined with the appropriate history, a radiologist's index of suspicion for myocardial

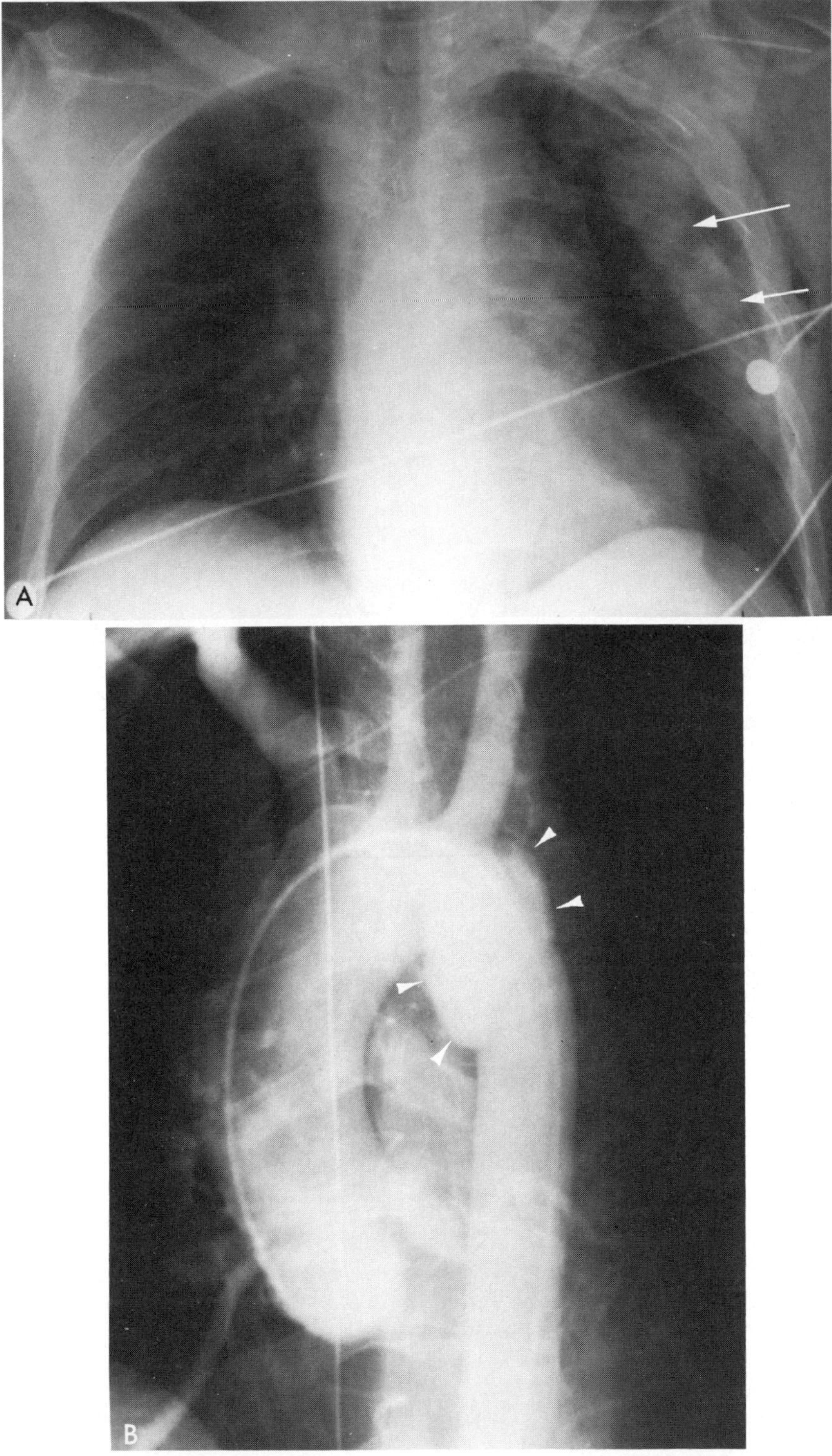

Figure 7–5. *A*, This young man sustained blunt chest trauma in an automobile accident. Note the widened mediastinum and fracture of the first three ribs on the left. There is also subcutaneous air in the left axillary region and subtle left pneumothorax *(arrows)*. *B*, Thoracic aortogram reveals an aortic transection in the region of the aortic isthmus *(arrowheads)*.

injury should be heightened when anterior rib and sternal fractures are associated with a large cardiac shadow and possible pneumopericardium (Bayer and Burdick, 1977).

The diagnosis of myocardial contusion can be difficult. In correlating the clinical data with the radiographic findings, other imaging modalities may assist. The technetium-labeled radionuclide cardiac scan can be very helpful in establishing the diagnosis of cardiac contusion (Bayer and Burdick, 1977). Echocardiographic imaging is useful in the evaluation of pericardial effusions, mitral valve and papillary muscle function, aortic valve and aortic root anatomy, cardiac wall function, and ventricular size. An appropriate indication for echocardiography following trauma is when clinical and radiographic findings do not correlate: for example, when the cardiac silhouette is essentially unchanged radiographically but clinical signs of severe hemodynamic embarrassment are present. Acute cardiac tamponade may occur in the absence of an enlarged cardiac silhouette.

Mediastinal Widening and Mediastinal Air

In addition to the mediastinal widening from bleeding related to esophageal or tracheal bronchial injury, air may be present as well (Fig. 7–6A). A review of 200 cases of significant blunt trauma indicates that either subcutaneous emphysema or pneumomediastinum was identified on the presenting chest radiograph in 40 per cent (Putman). Pneumomediastinum can be an observation unrelated to any apparent intrathoracic injury, or it can represent a life-threatening injury. In a group of 80 patients, 12.5 per cent (10/80) presented with pneumomediastinum as an isolated radiographic finding with no associated etiology. Tension pneumomediastinum, a rare condition in the adult, can produce cardiac and great vessel compromise with a significant reduction in cardiac output.

Esophageal injury. Esophageal rupture rarely occurs as an isolated injury from blunt thoracic trauma. More frequently, it is associated with other thoracic injuries such as aortic rupture and cardiac contusion. When esophageal rupture occurs, the most common complicating factor is an acute mediastinitis with an associated mortality approaching 90 per cent (Worman et al., 1962). Prompt identification and surgical intervention is important for successful treatment. Pneumomediastinum or cervical emphysema is said to be present in approximately 60 per cent of patients who sustain rupture of the esophagus (Heald, 1957). When esophageal rupture is present as an isolated injury in the patient with blunt trauma, a postemetic rupture should be considered (Fig. 7–6A). The air within the mediastinum is usually related to air that leaks from the esophageal lumen, whereas mediastinal widening is usually secondary to soft tissue edema and inflammation from the mediastinitis created by gastric contents.

Diagnosis of the ruptured esophagus is accomplished by contrast esophagoscopy. Water-soluble contrast material will demonstrate 50 per cent of cervical esophageal ruptures and 75 per cent of thoracic esophaageal ruptures (Love and Berkow, 1978). Expected areas of extravasation may be better delineated by subsequent use of barium. Since the site of esophageal rupture may not be identified on the initial esophagram, persistent clinical signs and symptoms may indicate the need for repeat esophagography and esophagoscopy (Fig. 7–7).

The rupture in the esophagus may not necessarily result from the initial trauma. Delayed rupture can occur as a result of segmental esophageal blood supply interruption and subsequent necrosis (Grimes, 1972). In a similarly damaged, but not ruptured, esophagus, iatrogenic manipulation (for example, esophagoscopy, inadvertent esophageal intubation, nasogastric tube insertion) can produce esophageal rupture. Tracheoesophageal fistula can occur as a sequela of acute mediastinitis. Fistula formation may appear as early as three to five days after the injury or may be delayed in presentation for up to three to five months (Love and Berkow, 1978).

Tracheobronchial injury. There are no specific combinations of physical or clinical findings that specifically identify tracheobronchial laceration (Chesterman and Satsangi, 1966; Putman). Certain radiographic findings, however, are highly suggestive. Of those patients with tracheobronchial injury, 10 per cent show no evidence of bronchial injury on the initial chest radiograph. Another 41 per cent have nonspecific radiographic findings such as simple upper rib fractures and uncomplicated pneumothoraces (Burke, 1962). Pneumothorax is seen in approximately two thirds of patients with tracheobronchial injury; 25 per cent of these present with tension pneumothoraces and 5 per cent have bilateral pneumothoraces.

In Burke's series (1962) all patients aged 30 years or over with tracheobronchial injury presented with fractures of one of the first five

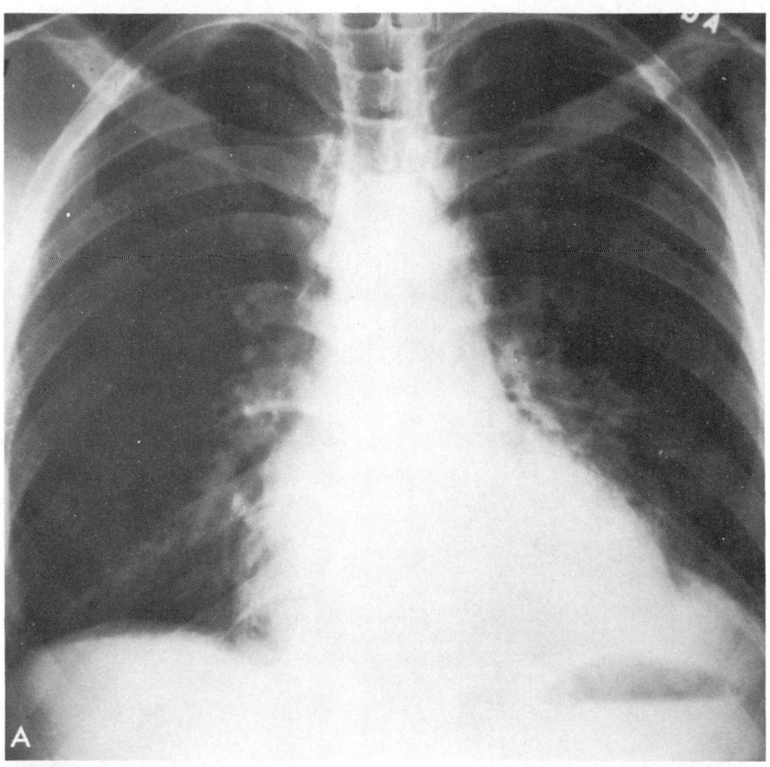

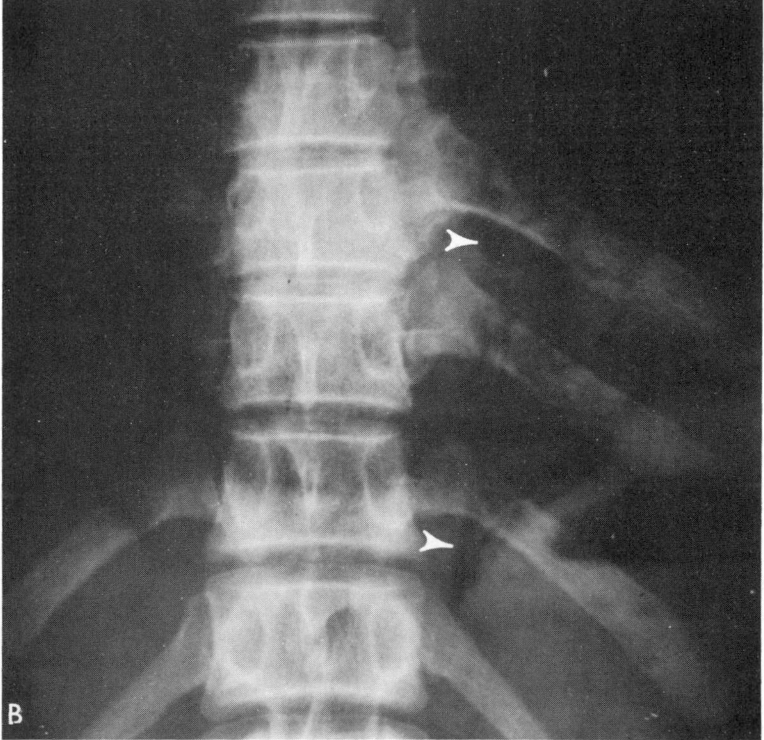

Figure 7–6. *A*, PA chest radiograph of 32-year-old man following an episode of violent vomiting. The radiograph reveals an increased retrocardiac opacity with obliteration of the left hemidiaphragm, and a left subpulmonic effusion. *B*, Overpenetrated view of the left lower lung demonstrates the radiolucent stripe of a pneumomediastinum *(arrowheads)*. Esophageal rupture was confirmed at surgery. (From Moore, A. V., Putman, C. E., and Ravin, C. E.: Bull. N.Y. Acad. Sci. 57:272, 1981.)

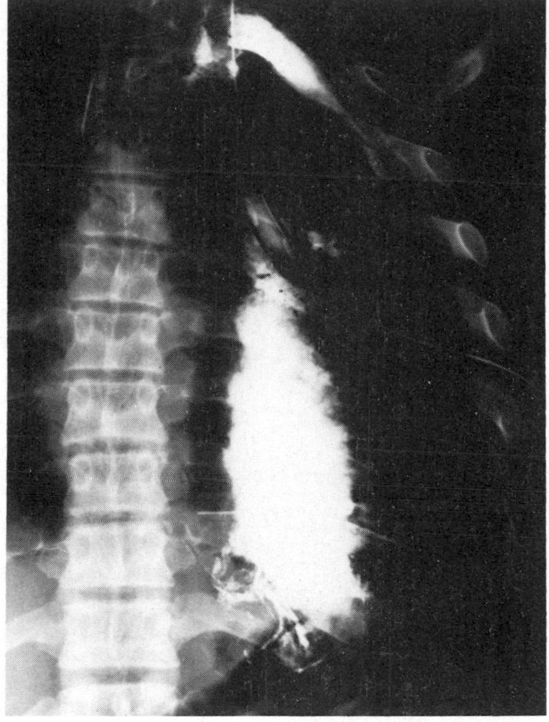

Figure 7–7. Extravasation of oral contrast material is seen in the left hemithorax of a young man who suffered a stab wound in the back. The knife penetrated the diaphragm and gastric fundus, creating a gastropleural communication.

ribs, with over 90 per cent of the fractures occurring within the first three ribs. Those patients without rib fracture and ruptured bronchus were either children or young adults. Rupture of the tracheobronchial tree is most commonly a unilateral injury, with equally frequent involvement of the right and left bronchus, and 80 per cent of disruptions occur within 2.5 cm of the carina (Fig. 7–2*B*) (Burke, 1962).

Atelectasis occurs in the lobe or segment distal to the tracheobronchial injury, and may appear immediately after the injury or be delayed for days. A persistent or recurring pneumothorax, increasing pneumomediastinum, progressive deep cervical emphysema, or progressive atelectasis should signify the need for bronchoscopy.

Age is important from the standpoint of survival. The mortality rate is highest (75 per cent) in the older age group (50 years), and drops impressively (16 per cent) in those from 20 to 50 years of age. For children the mortality rate is somewhat higher (30 per cent) than that for young adults (Burke, 1962). Early identification of the injury is the most significant factor in survival. Incomplete bronchial tears may go unrecognized clinically: injury-related signs may resolve, and the patient may present with bronchial stenosis months or years after the injury (Chesterman and Satsangi, 1966). Surgical correction should therefore be accomplished as soon as is practical in an attempt to prevent chronic pulmonary complications.

DIAPHRAGMATIC INJURY

Both blunt and penetrating trauma may have associated upper abdominal and diaphragmatic injury. Minimal diaphragmatic injuries can occur without escape of abdominal contents into the hemithorax. When this occurs, the only radiographic abnormality may be a slight irregularity in diaphragmatic contour (Minagi et al., 1977). When the diaphragmatic injury is more severe, the identification of gas-containing bowel within the hemithorax often suggests diaphragmatic injury. It is not unusual for severe injuries to the mediastinum, pulmonary parenchyma, chest wall, or abdomen to mask the diaphragmatic rupture, which may not be detected until after stabilization and specific treatment of the other injuries.

Diaphragmatic rupture with visceral herniation has many associated nonspecific signs: pleural effusion, lower lung atelectasis, loss of hemidiaphragm contour, and contralateral mediastinal shift.

More specific means of diagnosing diaphrag-

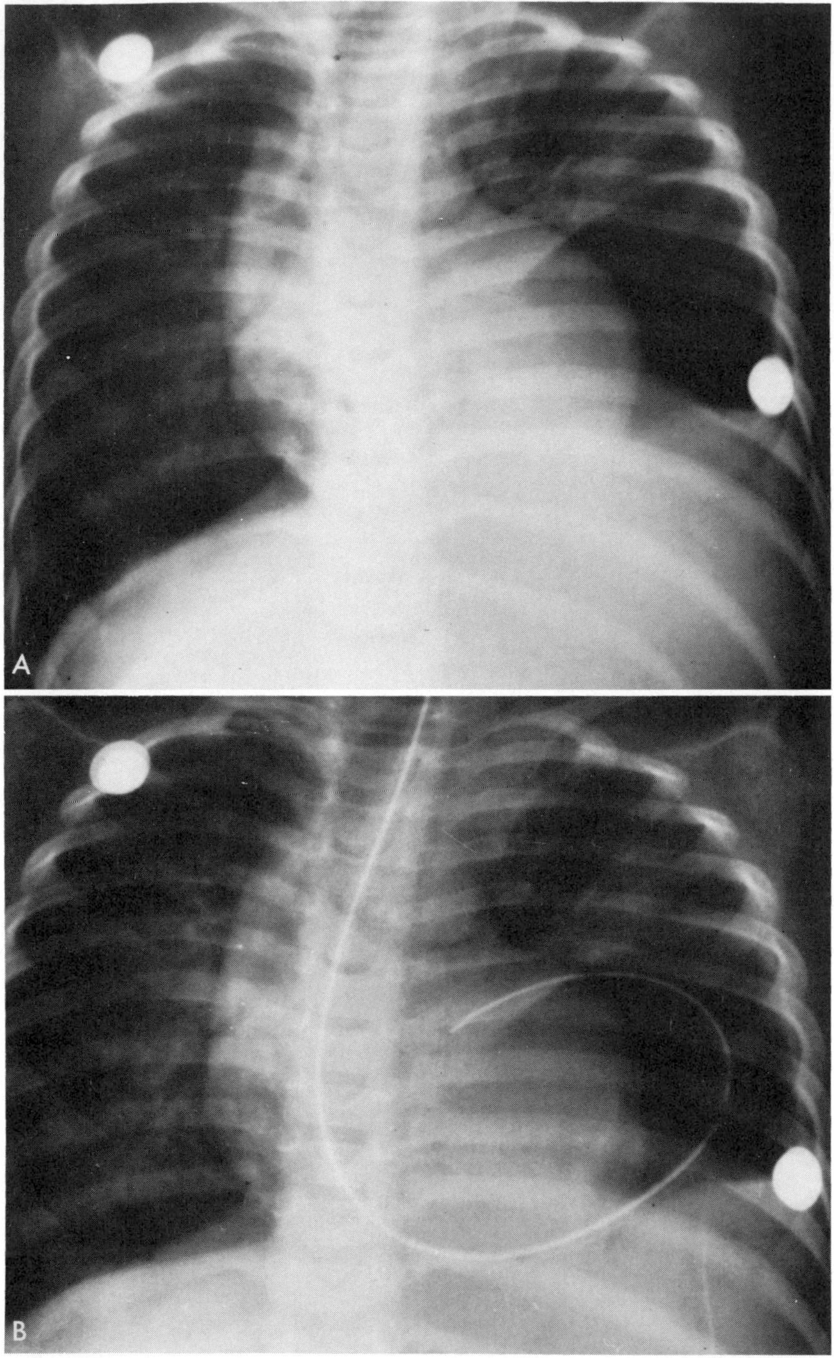

Figure 7–8. *A*, AP radiograph of a 2-year-old boy after he had been struck by an automobile. The admission chest radiograph revealed a large radiolucency at the left lung base. Atelectatic changes in the left upper lung are noted, along with mediastinal shift to the right. *B*, Following passage of a nasogastric tube, a repeat radiograph confirmed the suspected stomach herniation through a ruptured left hemidiaphragm (verified at surgery). (From Moore, A. V., Putman, C. E., and Ravin, C. E.: Bull. N.Y. Acad. Sci. 57:272, 1981.)

matic rupture include the diagnostic pneumoperitoneum (Fig. 7–8). In the acute clinical setting, air may be introduced into the peritoneum under fluoroscopic control, and the diagnosis of diaphragmatic rupture then determined by following the air through the diaphragmatic rent into the hemithorax. Opacification of the stomach or small bowel with orally administered contrast agents may also identify the site of rupture. When oral contrast agents are used, delayed radiographs should be obtained to exclude concomitant or isolated colonic herniation. A liver-spleen scan combined with a perfusion lung scan may also provide diagnostic information.

Diaphragmatic rupture, with associated bowel herniation, occurs on the left in approximately 95 per cent of patients (Hedblom, 1934). Isolated ruptures to the right hemidiaphragm are rarely seen, because visceral herniation is prevented by the liver's protection of the defect. The stomach is the most commonly herniated organ, followed by the colon and omentum in decreasing order of frequency. Other organs or combinations thereof that may herniate include the small intestine, spleen, liver, pancreas, and kidney (Grage et al., 1959; Hedblom, 1934; Keene and Copleman, 1945).

REFERENCES

Ayella, R. J., Hankins, J. R., Turney, S. Z., and Cowley, R. A.: Ruptured thoracic aorta due to blunt trauma. J. Trauma 17:199, 1977.

Bayer, M. J., and Burdick, D.: Diagnosis of myocardial contusion in blunt chest trauma. J.A.C.E.P. 6:238, 1977.

Burke, J. F.: Early diagnosis of traumatic rupture of the bronchus. J.A.M.A. 181:96, 1962.

Chesterman, J. T., and Stasangi, P. N.: Rupture of the trachea and bronchi by closed injury. Thorax 21:21, 1966.

Costin, B. S., Toombs, B., and Rauschkolb, E.: CT in evaluation of sequelae of thoracic trauma. Radiol. Soc. North Am., Chicago, IL, Nov. 1981.

Crawford, W. O., Jr.: Pulmonary injury in thoracic and non-thoracic trauma. Radiol. Clin. North Am. 11:527, 1973.

Doubleday, L. C.: Radiologic aspets of stab wounds of the chest. Radiology 74:26, 1960.

Eaton, R. J., Senior, R. M., and Pierce, J. A.: Aspects of respiratory care pertinent to the radiologist. Radiol. Clin. North Am. 11:93, 1973.

Flaherty, T. T., Wegner, G. P., Crummy, A. B., et al.: Non-penetrating injuries to the thoracic aorta. Radiology 92:541, 1969.

Gerlock, A. J., Jr., Muhletaler, C. A., Coulam, C. M., and Hayes, P. T.: Traumatic aortic aneurysm: validity of esophageal tube displacement sign. AJR 135:713, 1980.

Grage, T. B., MacLean, L. D., and Campbell, G. S.: Traumatic rupture of the diaphragm: a report of 26 cases. Surgery 46:669, 1959.

Grimes, O. F.: Non-penetrating injuries to the chest wall and esophagus. Surg. Clin. North Am. 52:597, 1972.

Hankins, J. R., McAslan, T. C., Shin, B., et al.: Extensive pulmonary laceration caused by blunt trauma. J. Thorac. Cardiovasc. Surg. 519:1977.

Harrison, W. H., Jr., Gray, A. R., Couves, C. M., and Howard J. M.: Severe non-penetrating injuries to the chest: clinical results in the management of 216 patients. Am. J. Surg. 100:715, 1960.

Heald, J. H.: Iatrogenic esophageal perforation. Stanford Med. Bull. 15:202, 1957.

Hedblom, C. A.: Diaphragmatic hernia. Ann. Intern. Med. 8:156, 1934.

Keene, C. H., and Copleman, B.: Traumatic right diaphragmatic hernia: case with delayed herniation of the liver and gallbladder. Ann. Surg. 122:191, 1945.

Lockett, F. C., Rothfeld, B., Meckelnburg, R., and Sagar, V. V.: Detection of bone trauma after cardiopulmonary resuscitation. Md State Med. J. 79:78, 1977.

Love, L., and Berkow, A. E.: Trauma to the esophagus. Gastrointest. Radiol. 2:305, 1978.

Mattox, K. L., Pickard, L., Allen, M. K., and Garcia-Rinaldi, R.: Suspecting thoracic aortic transection. J.A.C.E.P. 7:12, 1978.

Maynard, A. de L., Brooks, H. A., and Froix, C. J. L.: Penetrating wounds of the heart: report on a new series. Arch. Surg. 90:680, 1965.

Minagi, H., Brody, W. R., and Laing, F. C.: The variable roentgen appearance of traumatic diaphragmatic hernia. J. Can. Assoc. Radiol. 28:124, 1977.

Moore, A. V., Putman, C. E., and Ravin, C. E.: The radiology of thoracic trauma. Bull. N.Y. Acad. Med. 57:272, 1981.

Parmley, L. R., Mattingly, T. W., Manion, W. C., and Jahnke, E. J., Jr.: Non penetrating traumatic injury of the aorta. Circulation 17:1086, 1958.

Putman, C. E.: Unpublished data.

Reynolds, J., and Davis, J. T.: Injuries of the chest wall, pleura, pericardium, lungs, bronchi and esophagus. Radiol. Clin. North Am. 4:383, 1966.

Simeone, J. F., Minagi, H., and Putman, C. E.: Traumatic disruption of the thoracic aorta: significance of the left apical extra-pleural cap. Radiology 117:265, 1975.

Spees, E. K., Strevey, T. E., Geiger, J. P., and Aronstam, E. M.: Persistent traumatic lung cavities resulting from medium- and high-velocity missiles. Ann. Thorac. Surg. 4:133, 1967.

Williams. J. R., and Bonte, F. J.: Pulmonary damage in non-penetrating chest injuries. Radiol. Clin. North Am. 1:439, 1963.

Williams, J. R., and Bonte, F. J.: The Roentgenological Aspect of Non-penetrating Chest Injuries. Springfield, IL, 1961, Charles C Thomas.

Wilson, J. M., Thomas, A. N., Goodman, P. C., and Lewis, F. R.: Severe chest trauma: morbidity implication of first and second rib fracture in 120 patients. Arch. Surg. 113:846, 1978.

Worman, L. W., Hurley, J. D., Pemberton, A. H., and Narodick, B. G.: Rupture of the esophagus from external blunt trauma. Arch. Surg. 85:173, 1962.

Chapter 8

THE ABDOMEN—CONVENTIONAL RADIOGRAPHY, ULTRASONOGRAPHY, AND COMPUTERIZED TOMOGRAPHY

by Hideyo Minagi and R. Brooke Jeffrey

Although intra-abdominal complications are far exceeded in number by intrathoracic problems in the critically ill patient, plain films of the abdomen are obtained with some frequency in the intensive care unit (ICU). Abdominal radiographs may be required in the assessment of possible intra-abdominal pathology or in determining the location of support apparatus. Of necessity, the films are usually obtained by means of portable roentgen units at the bedside. Through the use of optimal grid-screen combinations and careful attention to detail by the technologist, satisfactory radiographs can ordinarily be obtained. When the patient's condition permits, however, superior radiographic detail can be obtained in the radiology department.

The advent of ultrasonography and computerized tomography (CT) has greatly altered the diagnostic approach to abdominal disease in critically ill patients. Following a description of traditional plain film findings in abdominal disease, a discussion of these new modalities as applied to the ICU patient will be presented.

RADIOGRAPHIC LOCALIZATION OF SUPPORT APPARATUS

Malposition of any of the variety of tubes placed in the alimentary tract may be disastrous. Since most of the alimentary tubes now in use are radiopaque, their radiographic localization is a relatively simple matter. The radiographic appearance of correctly positioned nasogastric, gastrostomy, small bowel, and rectal tubes is well known to radiologists and requires no discussion. Complications related to the use of these tubes occasionally arise, however, and the role of the radiologist in their recognition may be critical (Figs. 8–1, 8–2).

Balloon tamponade of variceal bleeding is a form of treatment in which the radiologist's role may be critical. The Sengstaken-Blakemore (SB) tube consists of an intragastric balloon, an esophageal balloon, and an intragastric irrigating channel. The round 250-ml intragastric balloon serves to anchor the tube in the cardia of the stomach. The sausage-shaped esophageal balloon is inflated to a pressure of 25 to 45 mm Hg to provide variceal tamponade. The correct position and inflation of the balloons must be verified on each radiograph. Evidence of aspiration pneumonitis or esophageal rupture should be sought. Esophageal laceration or rupture is most often the result of inflation of the gastric balloon within the esophagus, excessive traction on the tube, excessive inflation of the esophageal balloon, or excessively long periods of tamponade. Migration of the esophageal balloon into the hypopharynx, resulting in subsequent suffocation, has also occurred, usually as

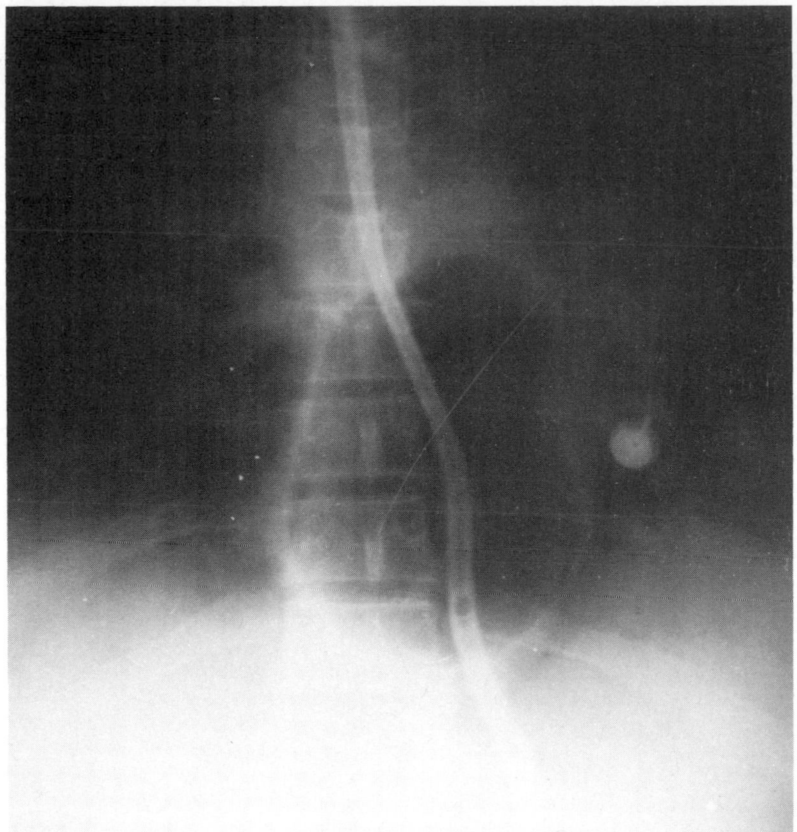

Figure 8–1. Malpositioned Sengstaken-Blakemore (SB) tube. The gastric balloon has been inflated within the distal esophagus rather than in the fundus of the stomach.

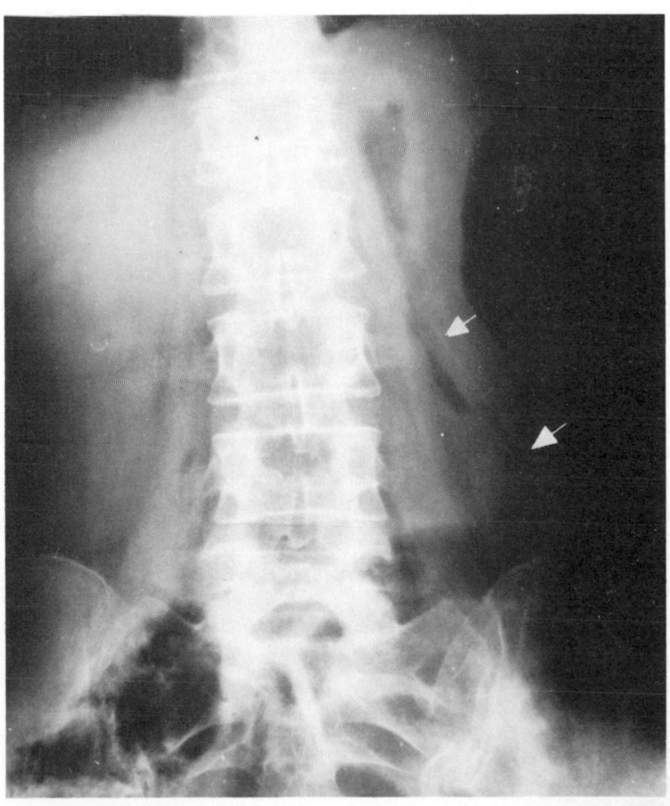

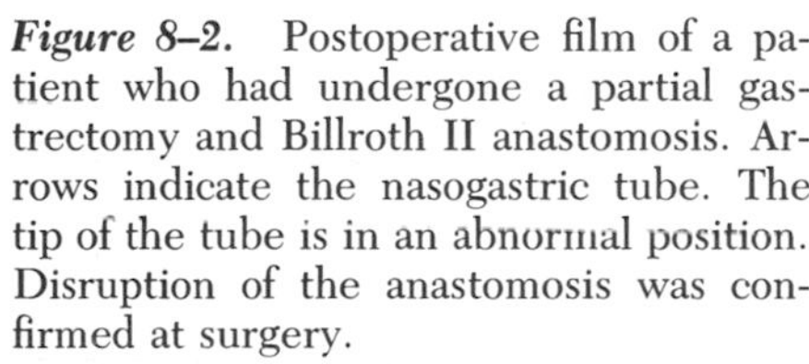

Figure 8–2. Postoperative film of a patient who had undergone a partial gastrectomy and Billroth II anastomosis. Arrows indicate the nasogastric tube. The tip of the tube is in an abnormal position. Disruption of the anastomosis was confirmed at surgery.

the result of inadequate anchoring of the tube by the gastric balloon (Pitcher, 1971; Wechsler et al., 1982).

The Linton tube consists of a single 800-ml intragastric balloon with two additional channels for esophageal and gastric aspiration. The large intragastric balloon has a tamponading effect, which obviates the need for an esophageal balloon (Linton, 1966).

ABDOMINAL PATHOLOGY

Radiographic findings of intra-abdominal pathology in the ICU patient are relatively limited. They may be categorized as abnormal gas collections, abnormal bowel gas patterns, and abnormal calcifications.

Abnormal Gas Collections

The classic radiographic finding of free intraperitoneal gas, gas trapped by the inferior aspect of a hemidiaphragm, is most often noted on an upright chest film. Miller and Nelson (1971) have pointed out the importance of beam diversion and film exposure as factors in demonstrating small degrees of pneumoperitoneum.

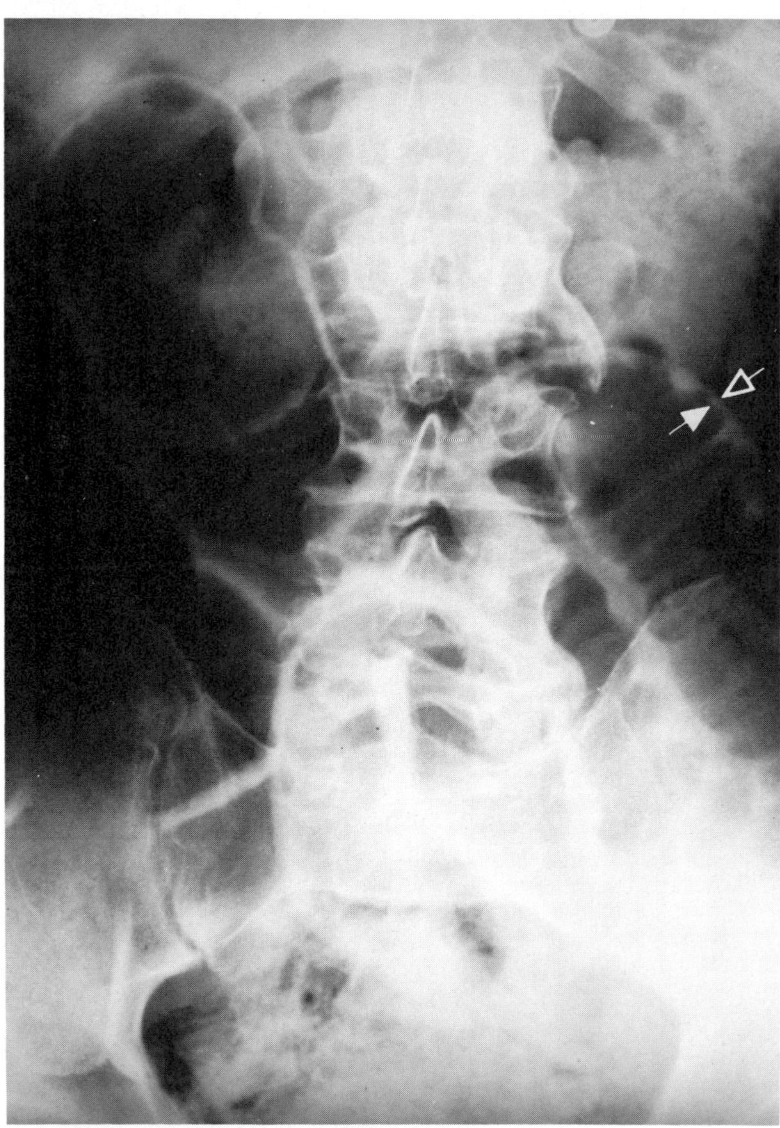

Figure 8–3. Pneumoperitoneum. The mucosal surface of the bowel is outlined by intraluminal gas *(solid arrow)*. The serosal surface of the bowel, normally not visualized, is outlined by intraperitoneal gas *(open arrow)*. Identical findings are present in the right upper quadrant.

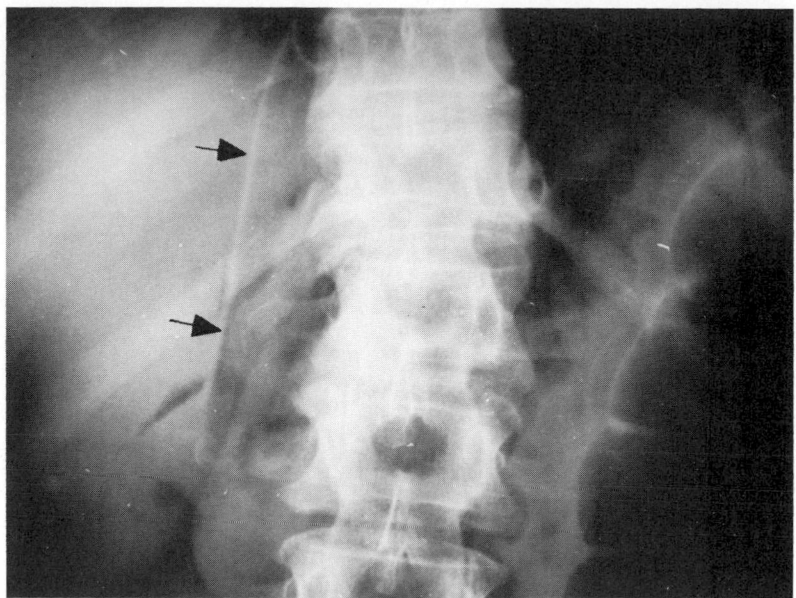

Figure 8–4. Pneumoperitoneum. Free air surrounds the falciform ligament, rendering it visible *(arrows)*. Air outlines the inner and outer wall of the colon.

They recommend placing the patient in the left lateral decubitus position for 10 to 20 minutes and making the exposure in that position, using ordinary chest x-ray exposure techniques. When possible, according to them, the patient should then be tilted to an upright position for an exposure of the chest in order to reveal air beneath the right hemidiaphragm. Using this sequence, they were able to demonstrate as little as 1 ml of intraperitoneal air with consistency. For a variety of reasons, however, such positioning ordinarily is not feasible within the ICU. Supine films of the abdomen may establish the presence of pneumoperitoneum by the demonstration of both sides of the wall of a gas-filled viscus (Fig. 8–3). Intraperitoneal air surrounding the falciform ligament may occasionally render that structure visible (Fig. 8–4). However, the radiographic demonstration of pneumoperitoneum usually requires horizontal beam radiographs. When upright films cannot be obtained, left lateral decubitus films often demonstrate air over the surface of the liver (Fig. 8–5).

Retroperitoneal gas collections may be seen in cases of retroperitoneal bowel perforation (Fig. 8–6) or in retroperitoneal infections by gas-forming organisms. Retroperitoneal gas dissects along fascia or muscle planes, producing a characteristic streaky lucency. Air may also surround the kidney, making it clearly visible on the abdominal radiograph. Retroperitoneal gas does not change with varying patient positions, unlike intraperitoneal gas.

Intra-abdominal abscesses due to gas-forming organisms are sometimes demonstrable by supine radiographs. The radiologist must scrutinize each abdominal film critically in order to recognize extraintestinal gas collections (Figs. 8–7, 8–8). Serial films are often helpful in demonstrating fixed collections of air.

Intramural gas, as in the gallbladder (Fig. 8–9) or urinary bladder (Fig. 8–10), may reflect infection by a gas-forming organism. Intramural gas within the bowel wall is often evidence of bowel infarction (Fig. 8–11), although a benign form of intramural bowel gas, pneumatosis cystoides intestinalis, is encountered on rare occasions. In these cases, the intramural gas collections are generally spherical and well defined, and often limited to the colon. The intramural gas seen in a necrotic bowel appears as curvilinear lucencies that circumscribe a bowel loop when observed front on, or parallel a long segment when seen lengthwise (Kleinman et al., 1976). The clinical evaluation of the patient with intramural intestinal gas usually provides ready distinction between benign pneumatosis and that associated with bowel necrosis.

Retroperitoneal and intraperitoneal air associated with ventilator therapy is being encountered with increasing frequency (Fig. 8–12). High ventilator pressures result in breakdown

Text continued on page 161

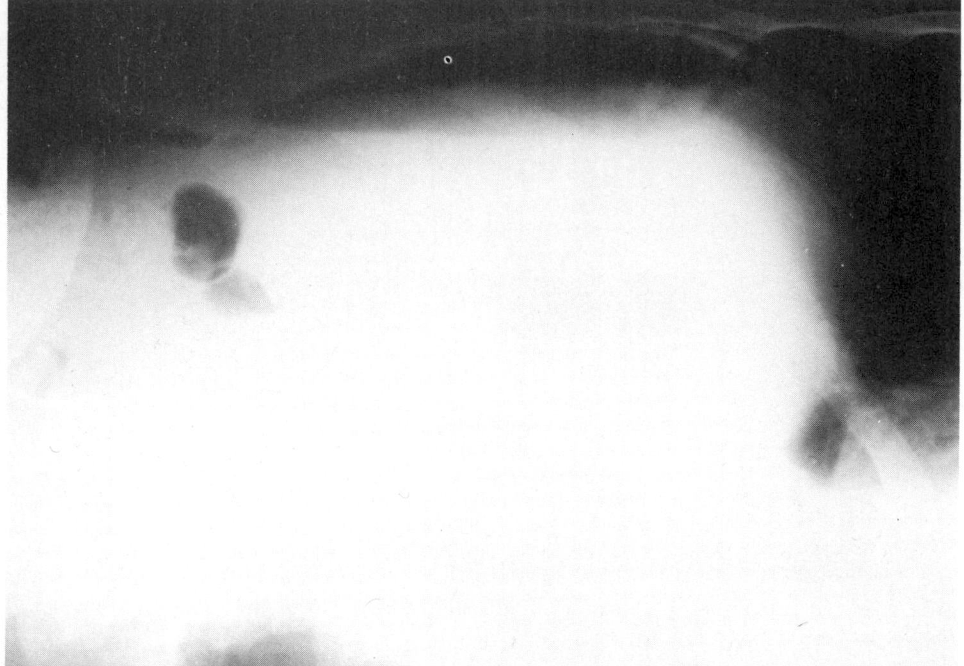

Figure 8–5. Pneumoperitoneum. Left lateral decubitus film demonstrates free air over the lateral surface of the liver.

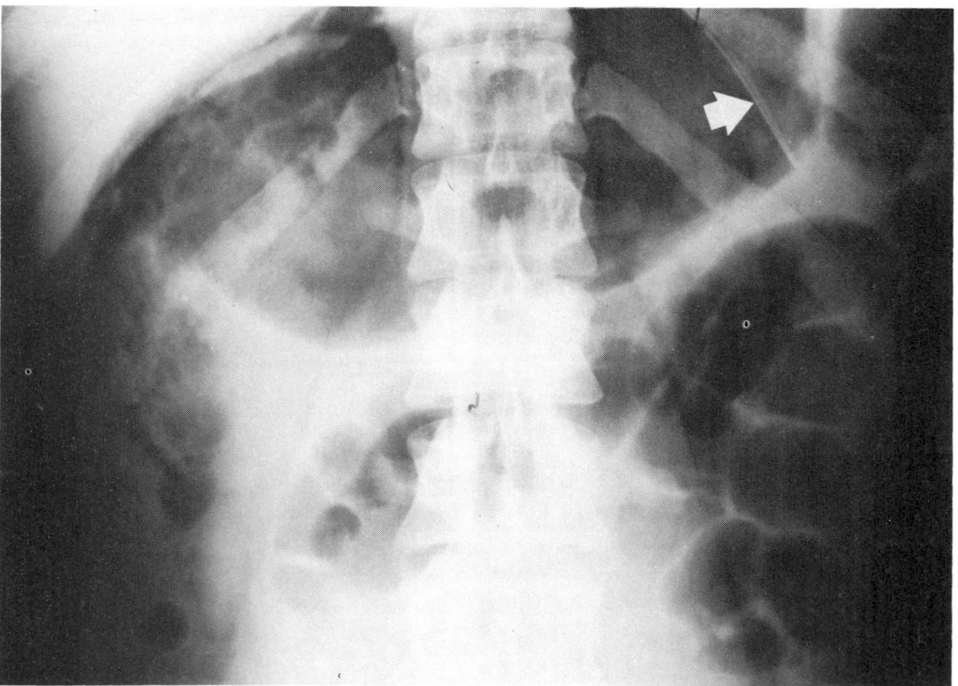

Figure 8–6. Retroperitoneal perforation of a duodenal ulcer. Gas from the duodenal lumen has dissected around the right kidney, resulting in a streaky and bubbly lucency. A nasogastric tube *(arrow)* is in the dilated stomach.

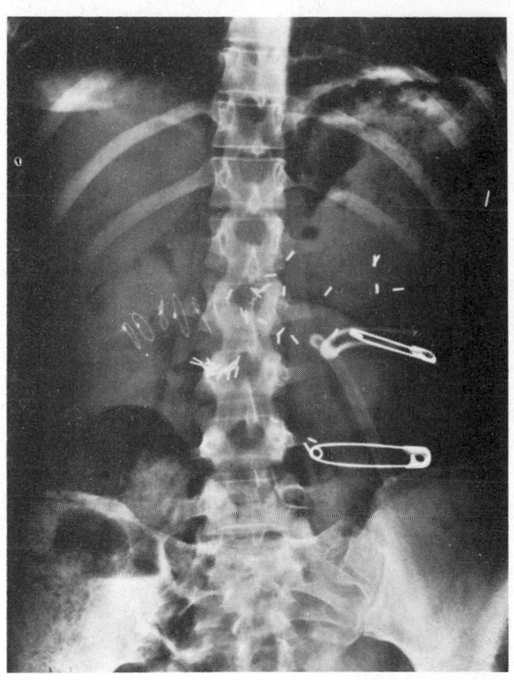

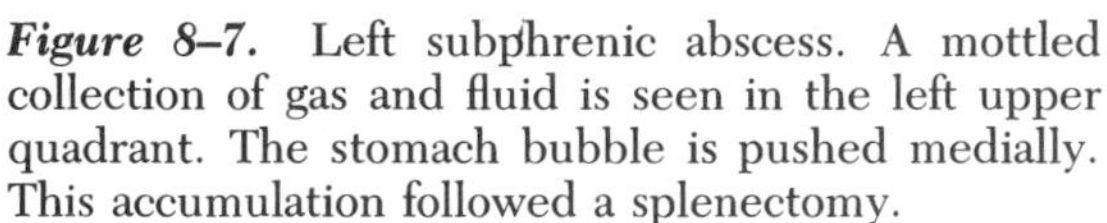

Figure 8–7. Left subphrenic abscess. A mottled collection of gas and fluid is seen in the left upper quadrant. The stomach bubble is pushed medially. This accumulation followed a splenectomy.

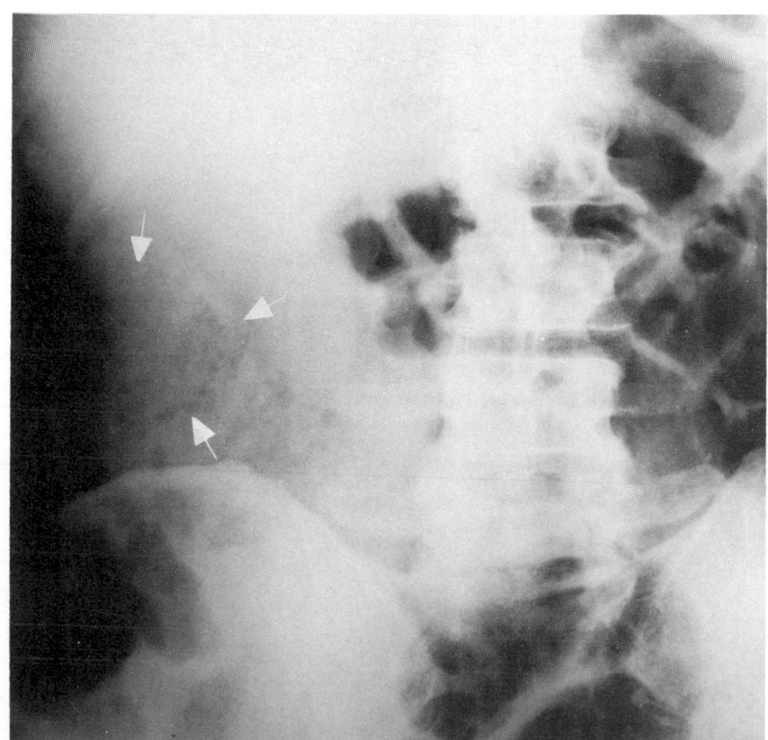

Figure 8–8. Right flank abscess due to a perforated carcinoma of the ascending colon. A mottled or bubbly gas collection is present in the right flank *(arrows)*. Such collections may be difficult to distinguish from normal intraluminal stool.

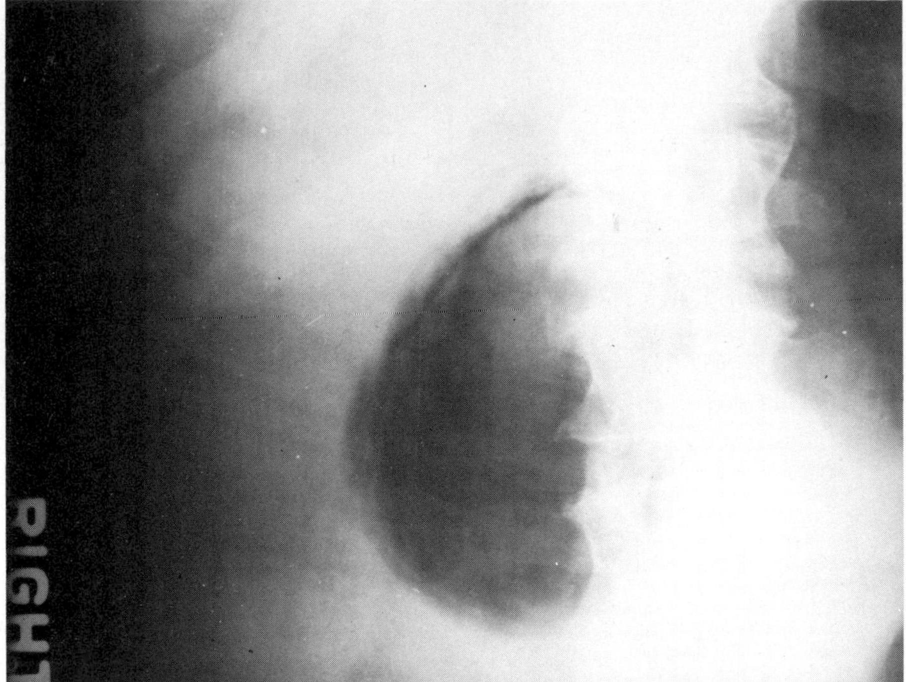

Figure 8–9. Emphysematous cholecystitis. Intramural and intraluminal gas outlines the gallbladder.

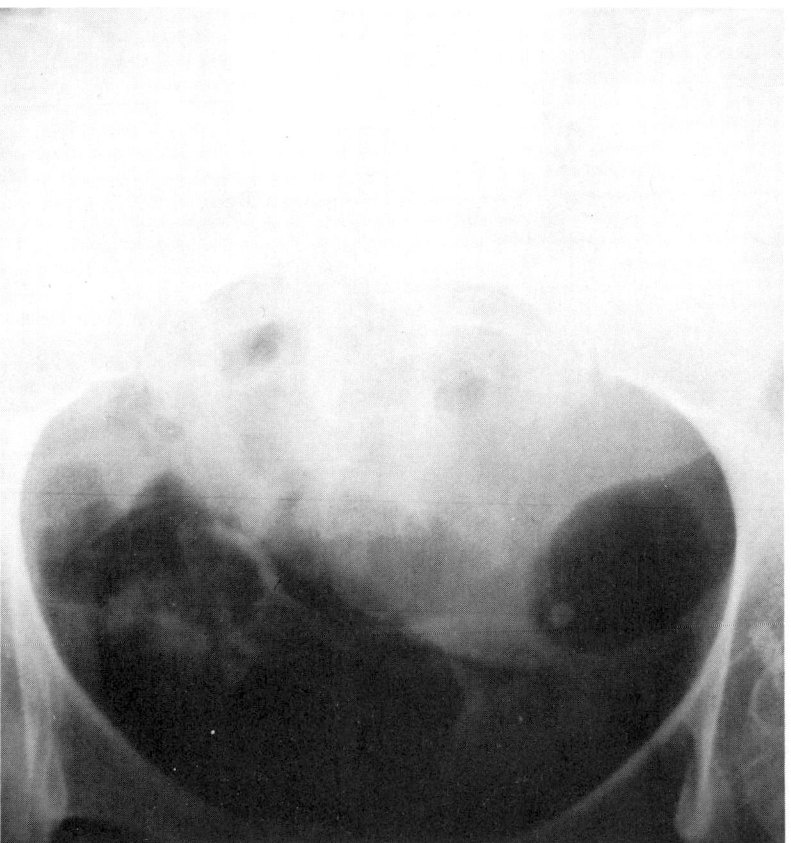

Figure 8–10. Emphysematous cystitis. Intramural and intraluminal gas outlines the urinary bladder.

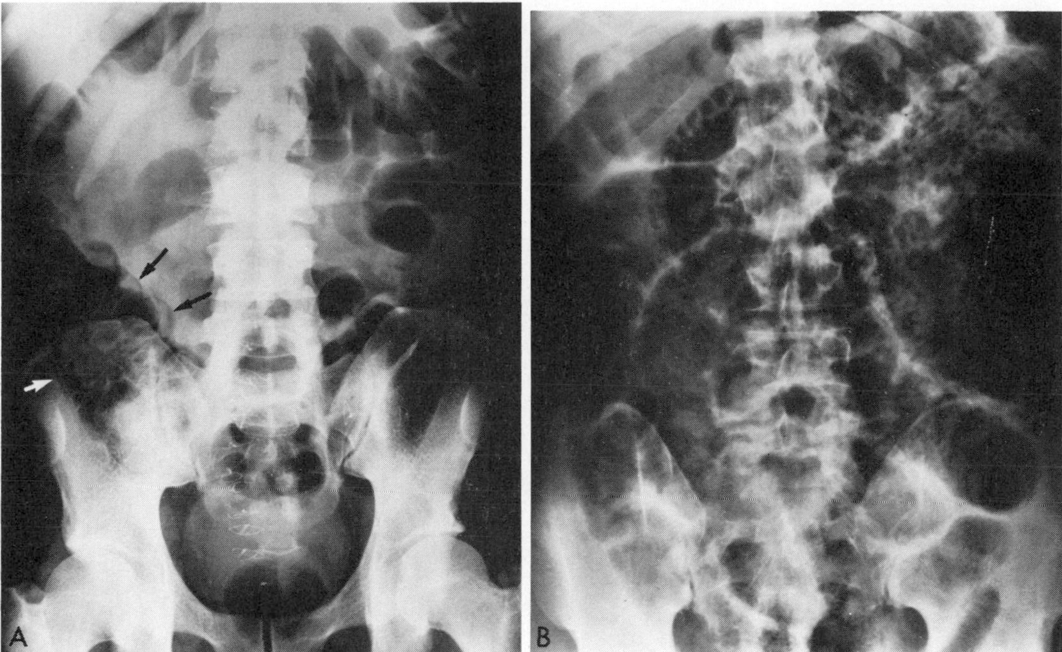

Figure 8–11. Air in the bowel wall (2 patients). *A*, Gas is present within the wall of the cecum and ascending colon *(arrows)* of a man with necrotizing colitis and acute myelogenous leukemia. *B*, A young patient with severe viral gastroenteritis and pancreatitis developed extensive gas collections throughout the gastrointestinal tract, which were confirmed at autopsy.

of alveolar walls and subsequent dissection of air along the bronchovascular sheaths into the mediastinum. The pneumomediastinum may dissect along structures traversing the diaphragm from the thoracic to the abdominal cavities, resulting in the radiographic visualization of retroperitoneal air. Rupture of this air into the peritoneal cavity results in pneumoperitoneum. In the context of the critically ill patient, distinction between air from a perforated viscus and iatrogenic air resulting from ventilator therapy may be impossible on the basis of plain films alone. Rohlfing et al. (1976) noted that pneumoperitoneum and pneumoretroperitoneum related to ventilator therapy (in the absence of perforated viscus) was invariably accompanied by pneumomediastinum on chest radiographs.

Branching streaks of air over the liver may be due to air within the biliary tree or air within the portal venous system. Ordinarily reflecting the presence of a fistulous communication between the bowel and the biliary drainage system, air within the biliary tree is a widely recognized sign of intra-abdominal pathology (Fig. 8–13). When it is seen following bile duct surgery or following biliary enteric surgical drainage, it is of no clinical significance.

The presence of gas within the portal venous system is a grave prognostic radiographic sign; it usually reflects bowel necrosis with subsequent passage of gas from the venous system of the involved bowel to the portal vein (Fig. 8–14). Portal vein gas may be distinguished radiographically from gas within the biliary tree. Portal vein gas demonstrates a finer branching pattern and extends to the periphery of the liver. Gas in the biliary tree demonstrates a more centrally located arborizing air pattern with wider tubular structures, and never reaches the periphery of the liver.

Abnormal Bowel Gas Patterns

In the critically ill patient, abdominal distention is a disturbing clinical finding. Acute gastric dilatation (Fig. 8–15) is a potentially lethal complication often encountered following abdominal surgery. It may also result from aerophagia stimulated by the placement of an intratracheal tube, by the presence of an endotracheal tube in the esophagus, or by a tracheoesophageal fistula. The early radiographic recognition of gastric dilatation makes possible prompt naso-

Text continued on page 164

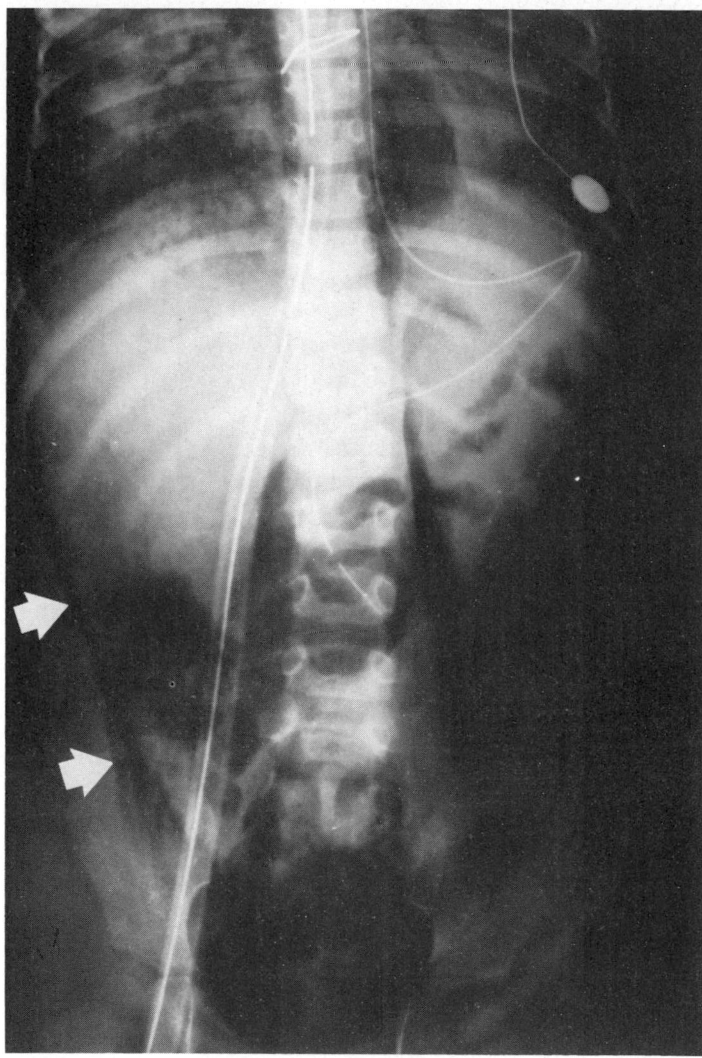

Figure 8–12. Extensive retroperitoneal air associated with ventilator therapy in a child. Note the long streaks of air parallel to the psoas muscles and the flank stripes *(arrows)*. There is also a right pneumothorax, a pneumomediastinum, and bilateral interstitial emphysema. A mediastinal drainage tube is in place.

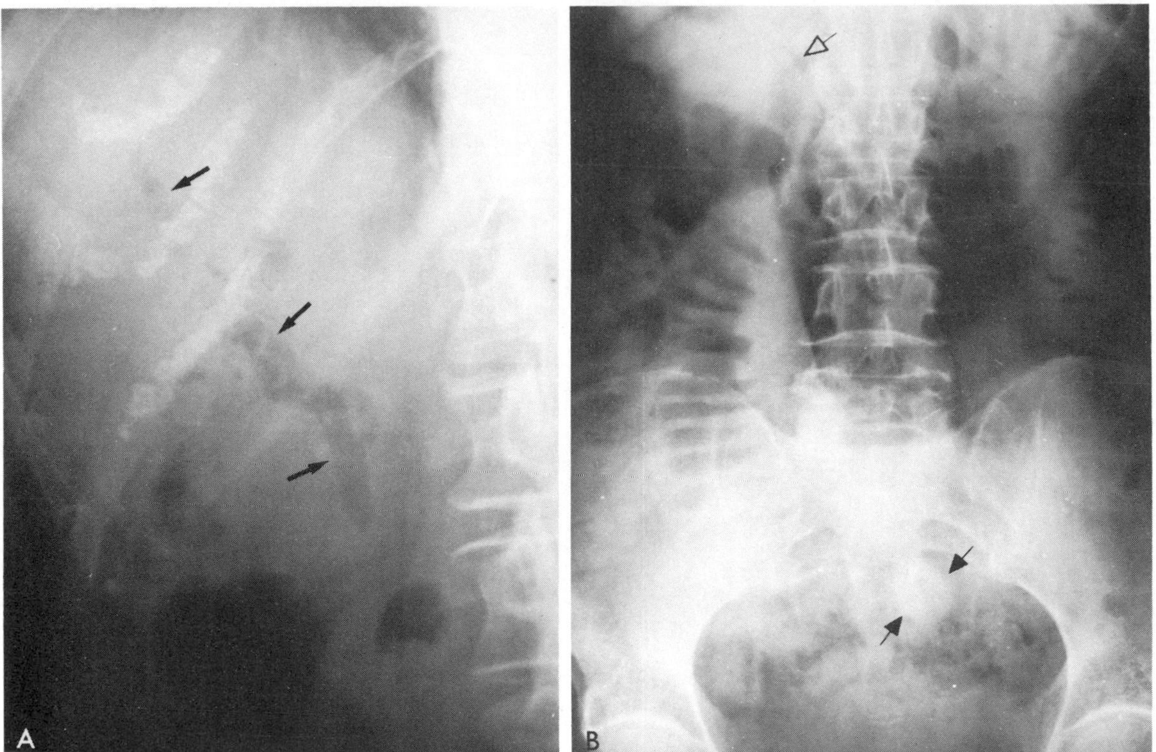

Figure 8–13. Gas in the biliary tree (2 patients). *A*, Biliary-enteric fistula. The gas *(arrows)* is confined to the central area of the liver. *B*, Gallstone ileus. A large, opaque gallstone is impacted in the small bowel *(solid arrows)*. Note the obstructive small bowel gas pattern and air within the biliary tree *(open arrow)*.

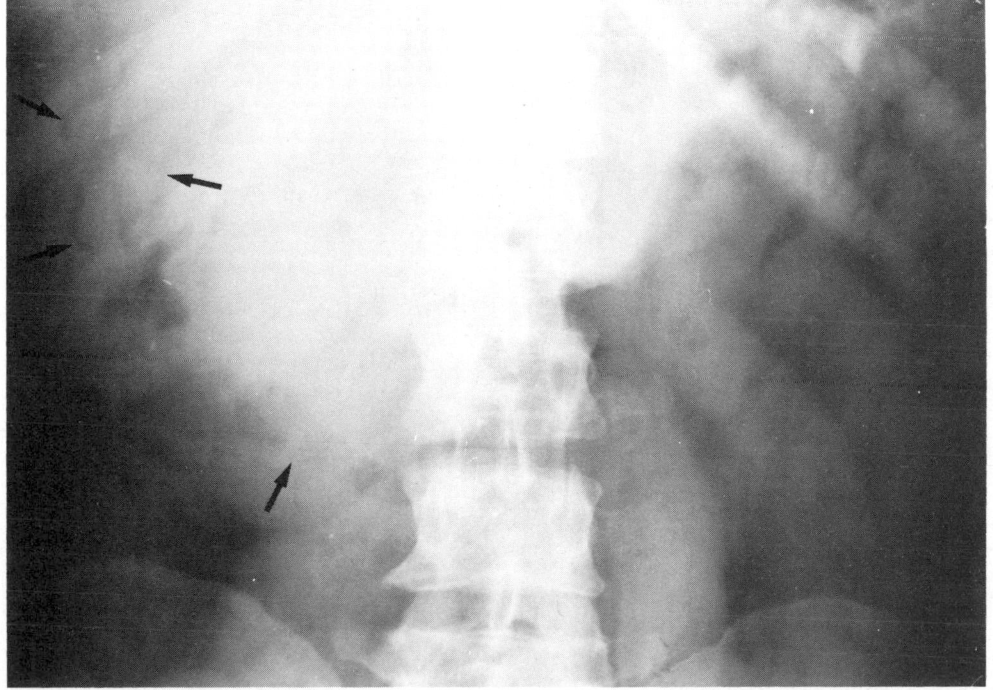

Figure 8–14. Portal vein gas *(arrows)* secondary to an infarcted bowel. The gas lucencies are thinner and more peripheral than with biliary air.

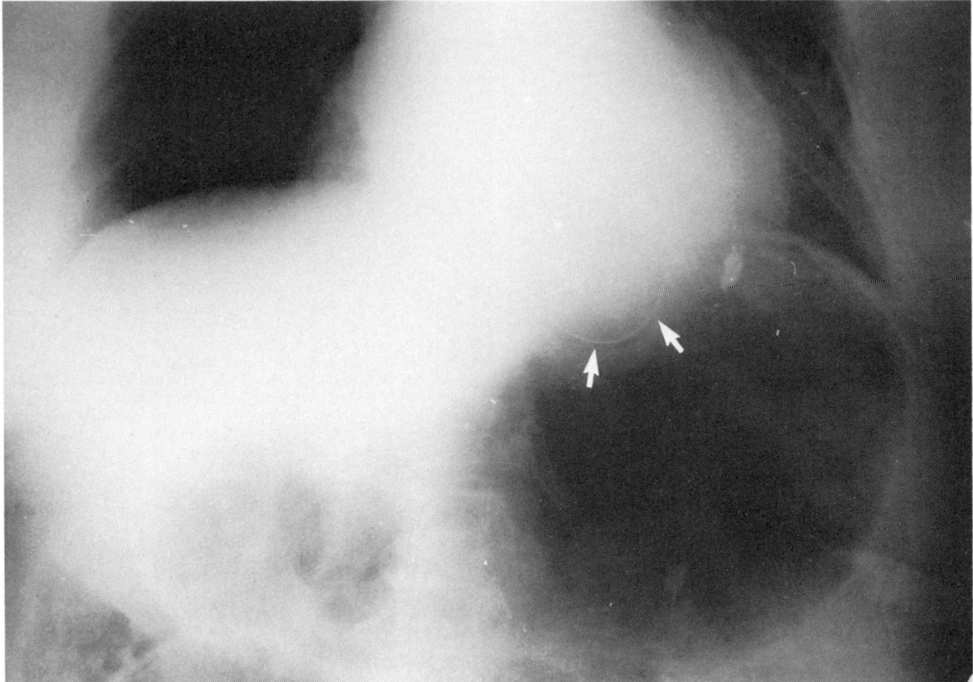

Figure 8–15. Acute gastric dilatation. The nasogastric tube is coiled within a hiatus hernia *(arrows)*. Repositioning of the tube led to prompt decompression, resolution of abdominal distention, and improvement in respiratory status.

gastric decompression and the initiation of the appropriate diagnostic studies.

In most cases of abdominal distention within the ICU, the principal differential diagnosis both clinically and radiographically is that of adynamic ileus and mechanical bowel obstruction. The radiographic hallmark of mechanical small bowel obstruction is dilatation of the small bowel disproportionate to colonic dilatation (Figs. 8–13*B*, 8–16*A*). On horizontal beam films, a relatively large amount of intraluminal fluid may be noted within the obstructed bowel (Fig. 8–16*B*). Adynamic ileus, on the other hand, is typically characterized by proportionate small and large bowel gaseous distention (Fig. 8–17). Although air fluid levels are often noted on horizontal beam films, the amount of intraluminal fluid is relatively small.

The above characterizations are very useful, but in actual practice plain films, particularly when only supine filming is possible, sometimes do not permit definitive diagnosis. In such cases, opaque contrast material may be administered by mouth or tube and followed by serial films. Both barium sulfate and water-soluble agents have been advocated for this purpose (Heinz et al., 1971). Barium has been recommended as the agent of choice because of its superior definition of bowel detail. Water-soluble agents, on the other hand, traverse the gut more quickly, sometimes permitting a more expeditious diagnosis of obstruction or adynamic ileus. Adding 10 ml of a water-soluble agent to the barium mixture decreases transit time by approximately 50 per cent without degrading the superior definition obtained with barium (Goldstein et al., 1971).

Gaseous distention of the colon is also a source of diagnostic difficulty; it is a reflection of either adynamic ileus or mechanical colonic obstruction. In either case, small bowel distention may also be apparent. In colonic obstruction, distention of the colon proximal to the level of obstruction and relative collapse distally are typical findings (Fig. 8–18).

The use of mechanical ventilators has been linked with isolated colonic ileus, particularly in patients with chronic obstructive pulmonary disease (COPD) (Golden and Chandler, 1975). Radiographically, remarkable degrees of cecal dilatation may be noted (Fig. 8–19). In severe cases, cecostomy may be indicated to circumvent possible cecal perforation. Laufer (1976) has emphasized the value of the left lateral view of the rectum (with the patient lying left side down) in differentiating colonic ileus from me-

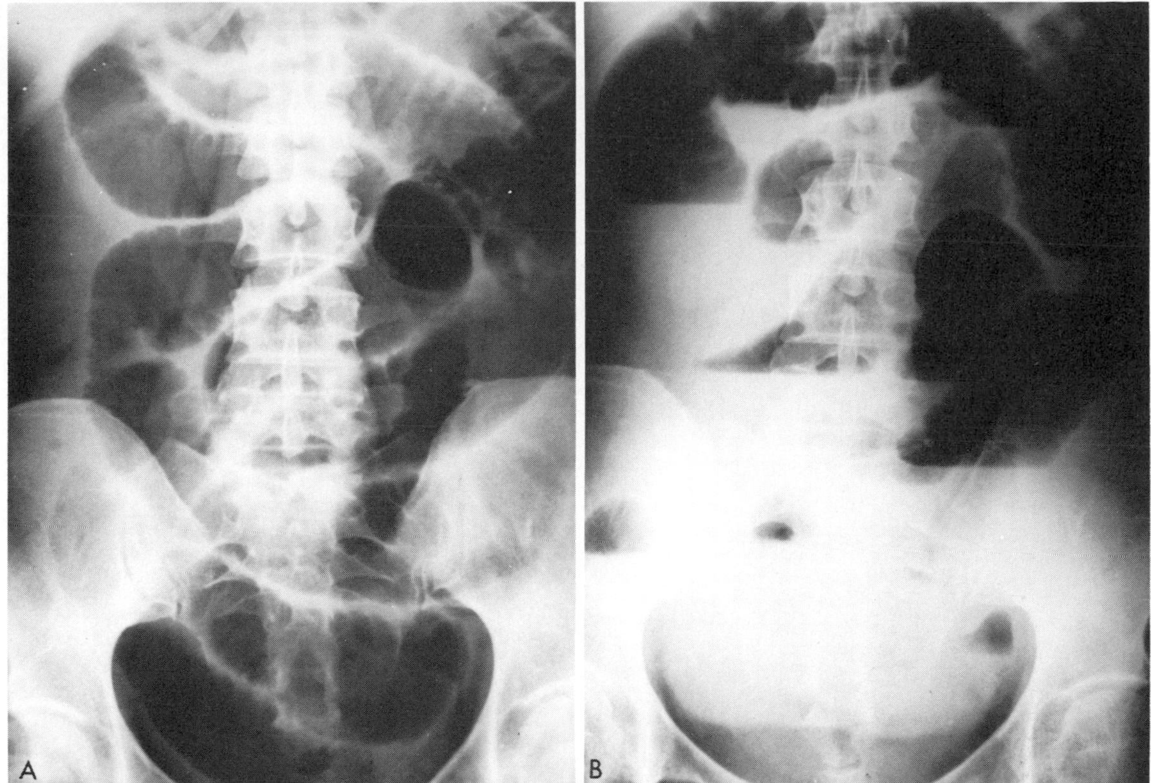

Figure 8–16. Mechanical small bowel obstruction. *A*, Disproportionate dilatation of the small bowel with no dilatation of the colon. *B*, Horizontal beam (upright) film demonstrates the presence of copious intraluminal fluid.

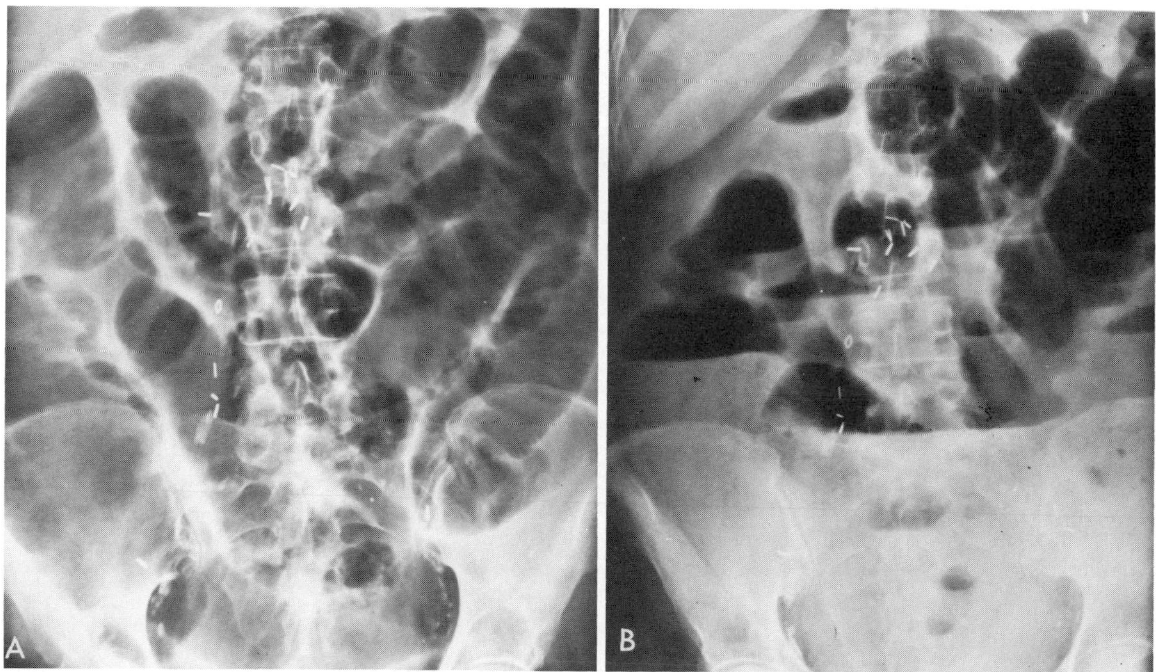

Figure 8–17. Severe adynamic ileus. This middle-aged man with lymphoma developed severe abdominal distention while being treated with vincristine. *A*, Supine radiograph shows extensive dilatation of the large and small bowel. *B*, Upright radiograph shows multiple air fluid levels. In spite of a normal barium enema the patient was taken to surgery. No obstruction was found.

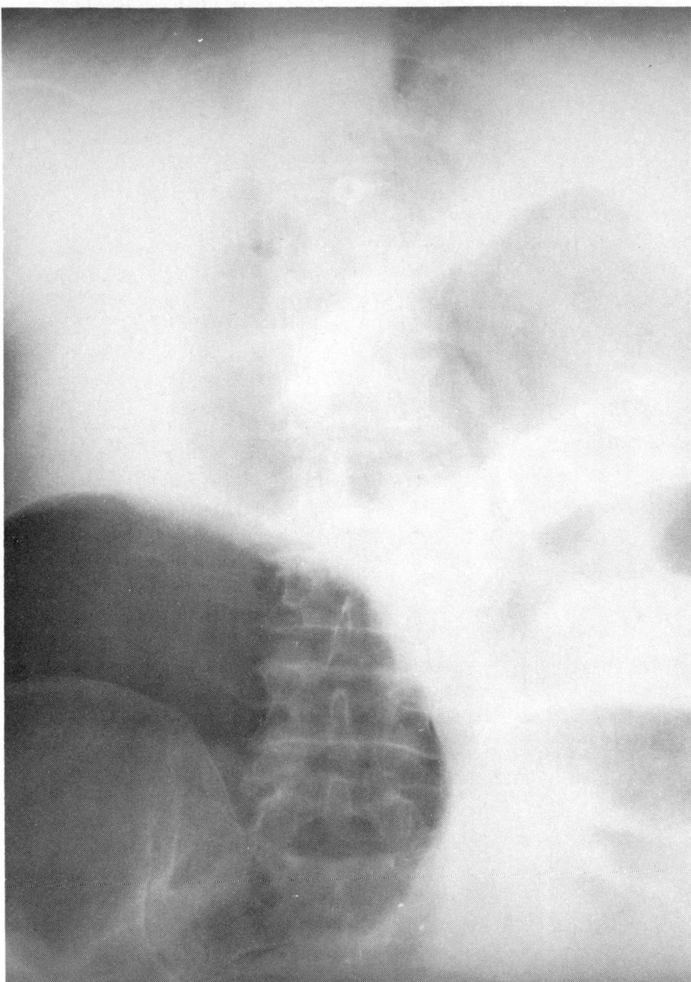

Figure 8–18. Colonic obstruction due to carcinoma of the splenic flexure. Note marked distention of the cecum.

chanical low colonic obstruction. Gaseous distention of the rectum on this view indicates that there is no mechanical obstruction.

Bowel infarction is a relatively common and often fatal occurrence in the ICU. In patients with an infarcted bowel, plain abdominal films are seldom diagnostic. Rarely, however, gas in the bowel wall or portal venous system, or both, may indicate the correct diagnosis (Figs. 8–11, 8–14). More often, the radiographic findings are nonspecific. Tomchik and associates (1970), in their review of 67 patients with proved bowel infarction, found a pseudo-obstructed small bowel pattern in 39 per cent, a combination of small bowel and transverse colon dilatation in 17 per cent, and a splenic flexure cut-off pattern in 16 per cent. They also noted that a large fecal residue was present in the colon in a surprisingly small number of patients (5 per cent); four fifths of the patients demonstrated no feces or only a small residue. Thickening of the bowel wall in the presence of an abnormal gas pattern is suggestive of bowel infarction, but may be seen with bowel hemorrhage or edema from any cause (Fig. 8–20). Tomchik and associates found nonocclusive infarction to be the commonest type of bowel infarction in their series, accounting for one half of all bowel infarctions. Plain abdominal films were suggestive or diagnostic in 8 per cent of these patients. Radiographic findings were present in 46 per cent of patients with embolic infarction, in 30 per cent of those with venous thrombosis, and in 11 per cent of those with infarctions attributed to arterial thrombosis (see Chapter 9).

Abnormal Calcifications

The various forms of abnormal intra-abdominal calcifications are encountered with sufficient

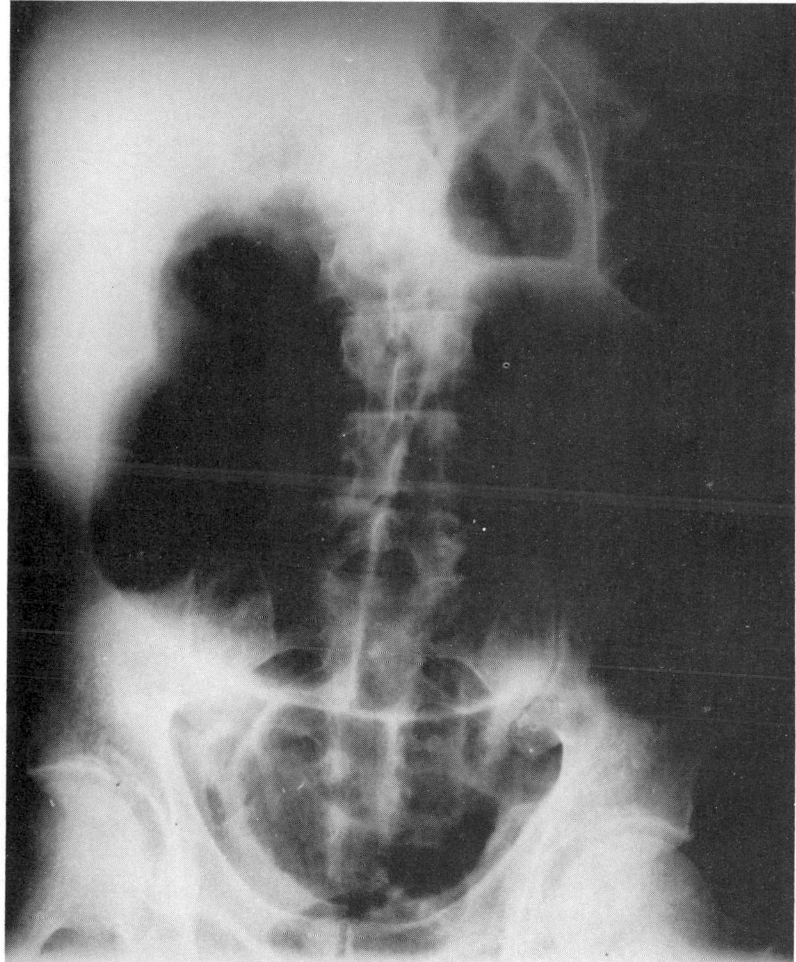

Figure 8–19. Colonic ileus. Marked dilatation of the cecum and ascending colon. No obstruction was found at surgery. Serosal tears were noted over the cecum, indicating impending cecal perforation.

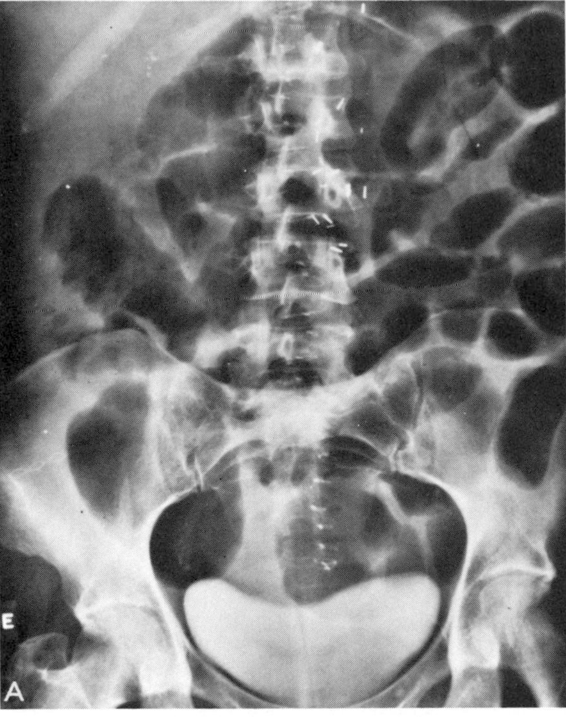

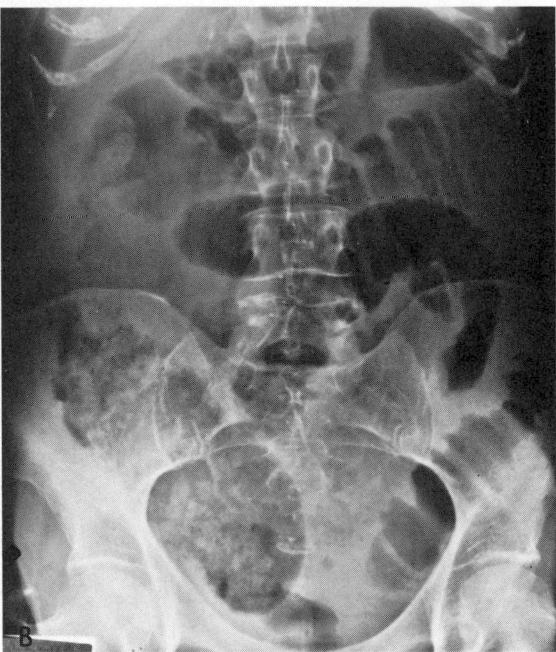

Figure 8–20. Bowel ischemia (2 patients). *A*, Several days after abdominal aortic graft surgery the patient developed abdominal pain and diarrhea. The AP radiograph shows several thickened loops of small bowel in the left upper quadrant. Gangrenous small bowel and peritonitis was found at surgery. *B*, A 66-year-old woman with a two-day history of abdominal pain and vomiting, and a previous history of diverticulitis and postoperative adhesions. Supine radiograph shows three dilated loops of small bowel to the left of midline. The wall of the lowest loop is markedly thickened and irregular. At surgery there were multiple dilated loops of small bowel due to adhesions. A 20-cm segment of gangrenous jejunum was removed.

frequency by the practicing radiologist that an exhaustive review of such calcifications appears to be unwarranted in this chapter. Suffice it to say that the radiographic findings of such calcifications may have the same clinical importance in the ICU patient as in the patient who is not in the ICU (Figs. 8–13*B*, 8–21, 8–22).

ABDOMINAL CT AND ULTRASOUND

Computerized tomography and ultrasonography are important adjuncts to conventional radiologic methods of abdominal imaging. Both are noninvasive techniques that can directly image both intra- and extraperitoneal structures and are particularly useful in diagnosing abnormal fluid collections, such as abdominal abscesses (Korobkin et al., 1978; McNeil et al., 1981; Wolverson et al., 1976), hemorrhage (Sagel et al., 1977), or other cystic collections. In addition, both can be utilized for either diagnostic aspiration of suspected abscesses or percutaneous catheter drainage (Gerzoff et al., 1979, Gronvall et al., 1977; Haaga and Weinstein, 1980) (see Chapter 9). The following discussion is an overview of the role of abdominal CT and ultrasound in the evaluation of the intensive care patient.

In addition to the lack of ionizing radiation, one of the principal advantages of ultrasound is that portable real-time examinations can be performed at the bedside. This avoids the difficult and often hazardous transportation of the patient with multiple life support systems. Real-time scanning can be performed significantly faster than B-mode ultrasound and enables the examiner to make a rapid survey of the entire abdomen. The liver and urine-filled bladder provide acoustic windows and make ultrasound particularly helpful in imaging the right upper quadrant and pelvis.

The major limitations of abdominal ultrasound in the ICU patient are twofold: (1) over-

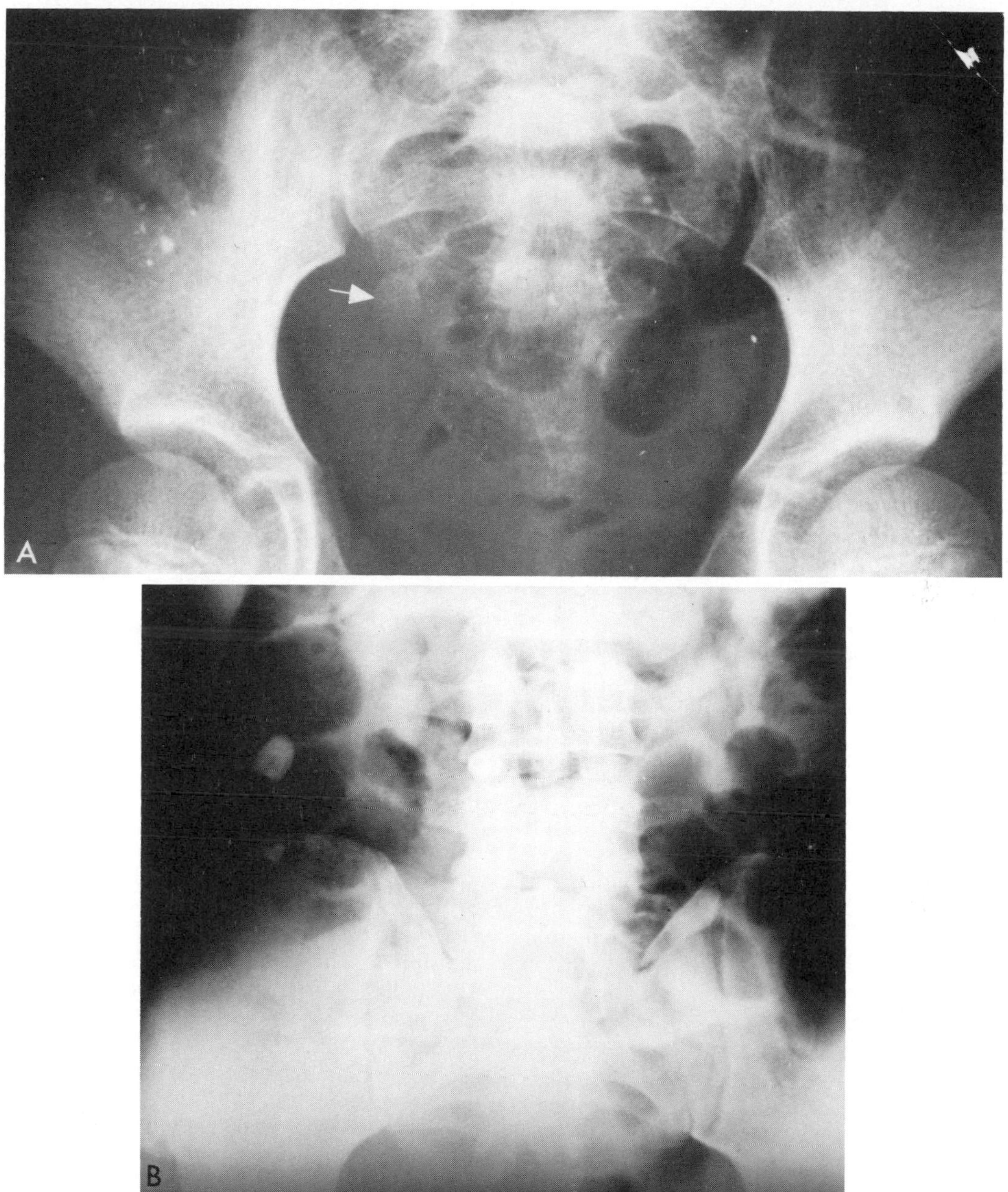

Figure 8–21. Appendicolithiasis. Such calcifications may be spherical or ovoid *(arrow)*, *A*, or faceted, *B*. The stones seen in *B* were contained within an abscess cavity following perforation of the appendix.

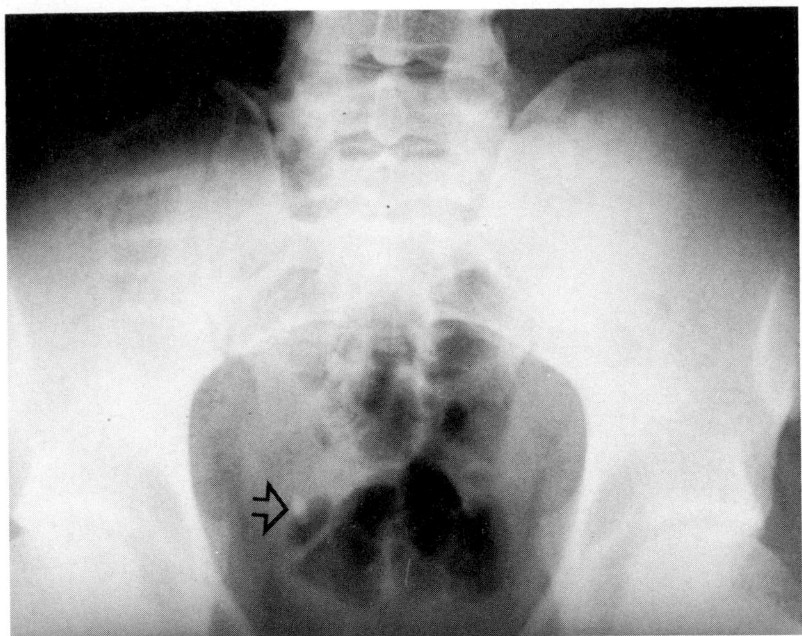

Figure 8–22. Right ureteral calculus. An opaque calculus *(arrow)* is lodged near the right ureterovesical junction. Ureteral calculi are generally ovoid, with their long axes in the longitudinal axis of the ureter.

lying bowel gas and (2) the lack of adequate skin surface for the transducer because of open wounds or drains. Either may preclude an adequate examination. Evaluation of retroperitoneum is particularly difficult in patients with abdominal ileus. Nevertheless, abdominal ultrasound is often the first diagnostic study performed after plain films of the abdomen. It is the screening method of choice in the diagnosis of renal or biliary obstruction, in the evaluation of ascites, and in the diagnosis of abscesses located in the right upper quadrant or pelvis (Figs. 8–23, 8–24).

Despite the effort required to transport the patient for abdominal CT scanning, computerized tomography continues to be an increasingly important mode of abdominal imaging in critically ill patients. Unlike ultrasound, CT is not limited by overlying bowel gas or lack of skin contact. In most patients it can reliably image both intra- and extraperitoneal organs. CT image quality may be degraded by patient motion, or by high-density materials such as residual barium, vascular clips, or drains. Nevertheless, when CT is technically adequate, no other study can afford the degree of anatomic precision that it provides.

One of the major contributions of abdominal CT and ultrasound has been in the diagnosis of intra-abdominal abscess, which continues to be a leading cause of morbidity in the postoperative patient (Connell et al., 1980). Ultrasound is particularly helpful in diagnosing abscesses in the right upper quadrant, either intrahepatic or in the subphrenic space (Figs. 8–23, 8–24). Pelvic abscesses are also readily demonstrated by ultrasound. Sonographically, abscesses appear as complex fluid collections containing multiple low-level internal echoes. Microbubbles with acoustic shadowing may be seen in gas-containing abscesses (Kressel and Filly, 1978). The most specific CT features of an abscess are an encapsulated fluid collection containing multiple gas bubbles (Figs. 8–25, 8–26).

Ultrasound, CT, and gallium-67 imaging are often complementary and increase the likelihood of abscess detection. In addition, CT or ultrasound are of great value as guides for diagnostic percutaneous needle aspiration of abnormal fluid collections. Percutaneous abscess drainage techniques have been quite useful in cases of unilocular abscesses that can be safely approached and adequately aspirated via a catheter (Haaga and Weinstein, 1980) (see Chapter 9).

Intra-abdominal and retroperitoneal hemor-

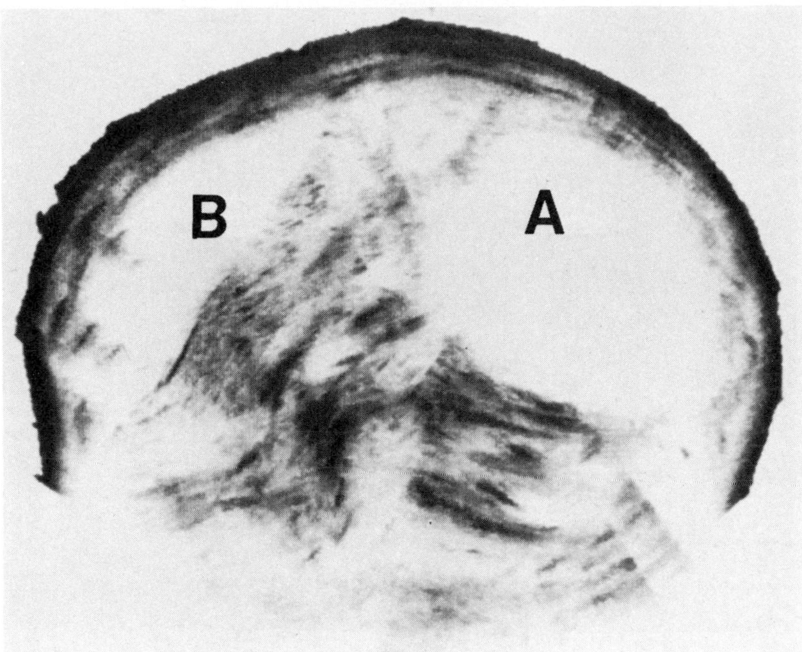

Figure 8–23. Gunshot wound to the porta hepatis. Three weeks postoperatively, the sonogram demonstrates a subcapsular hepatic fluid collection (B = biloma) and a larger fluid collection to the left of midline (A = abscess within lesser sac at surgery). Prior to surgical drainage, diagnostic needle aspiration established both diagnoses.

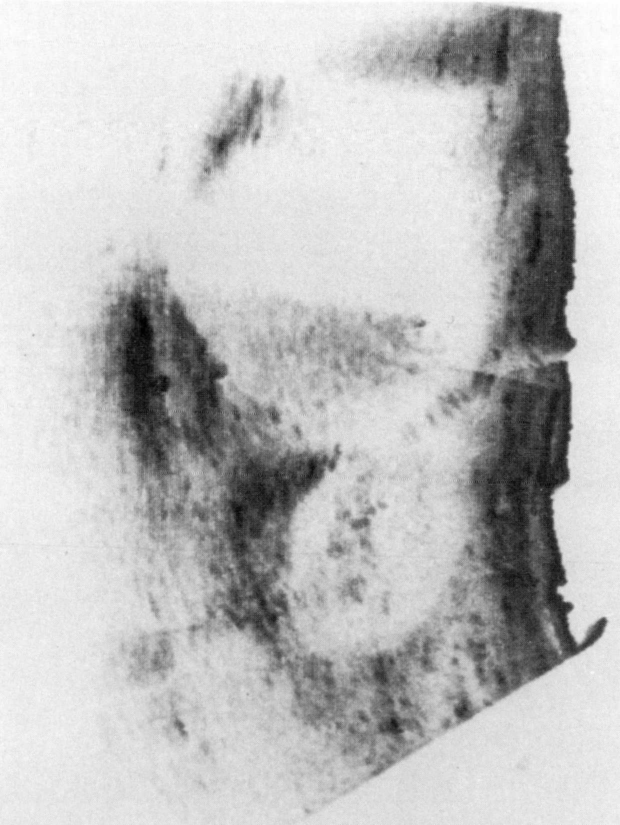

Figure 8–24. Echogenic debris layers within a pseudocyst in the tail of the pancreas.

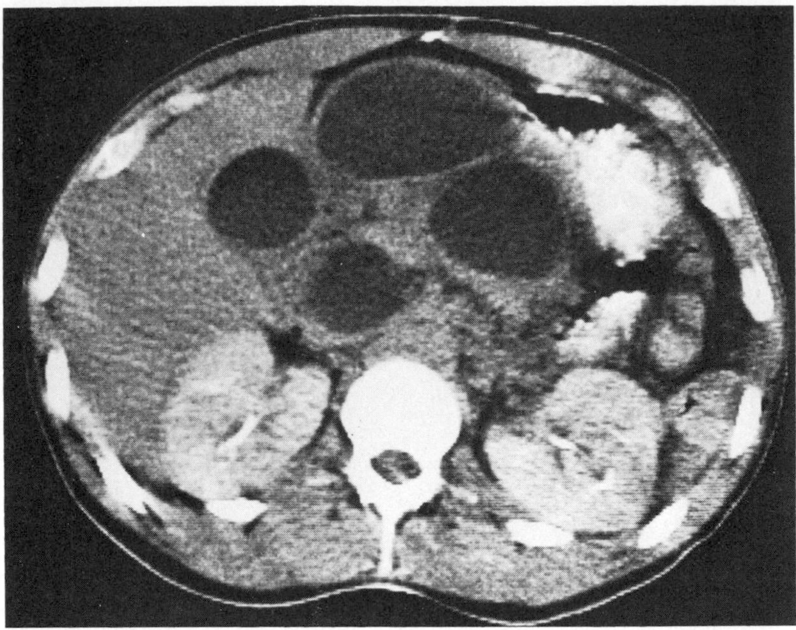

Figure 8–25. Acute pancreatitis. Multiple intrapancreatic and lesser sac fluid collections are demonstrated.

rhage, particularly in patients receiving anticoagulation, is a common clinical problem in the ICU. Ultrasound may demonstrate a sonolucent mass with low-level echoes that has a similar appearance to that of an abdominal abscess (Wicks et al., 1978).The relatively high CT number of freshly extravasated blood (above 40 Hounsfield units) is useful in the CT diagnosis of acute hemorrhage (Fig. 8–27) (Sagel et al., 1977).

REFERENCES

Connell, T. R., Stephens, D. H., Carlson, H. C., and Brown, M. L.: Upper abdominal abscess: a continuing and deadly problem. Am. J. Roentgenol. 134:759, 1980.

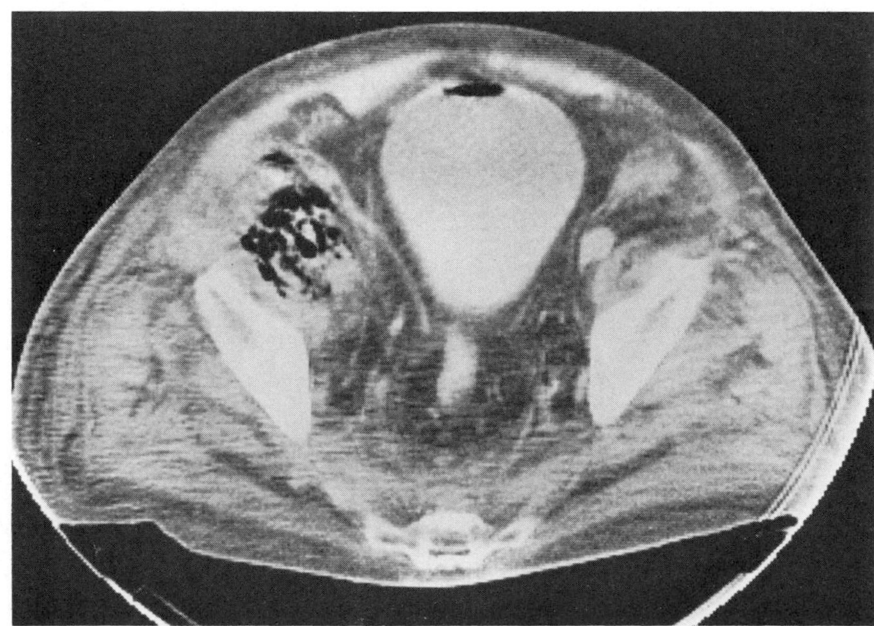

Figure 8–26. Gas-forming abscess within the right iliopsoas muscle. Direct extension from a chronically infected right femoral venous catheter.

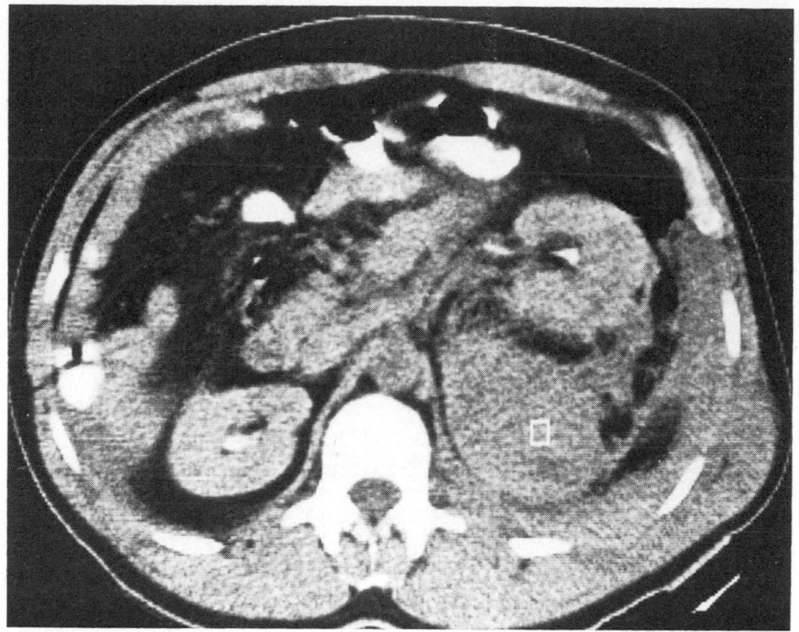

Figure 8–27. Spontaneous retroperitoneal hemorrhage secondary to excessive anticoagulation. The left kidney is displaced anteriorly by a high-density area (with cursor) in the posterior pararenal space representing an acute hematoma.

Gerzoff, S. G., Robbins, A. H., Birkett, D. H., et al.: Percutaneous catheter drainage of abdominal abscesses guided by ultrasound and computed tomography. Am. J. Roentgenol. 133:1, 1979.

Golden, G. T., and Chandler, J. G.: Colonic ileus and cecal perforation in patients requiring mechanical ventilatory support. Chest 68:661, 1975.

Goldstein, H. M., Poole, G. J., Rosenquist, C. J., et al.: Comparison of methods for acceleration of small intestinal radiographic examination. Radiology 98:519, 1971.

Gronvall, J., Gronvall, S., and Hegedus, V.: Ultrasound-guided drainage of fluid-containing masses using angiographic catheterization techniques. Am. J. Roentgenol. 129:997, 1977.

Haaga, J. R., and Weinstein, A. J.: CT-guided percutaneous aspiration and drainage of abscesses. Am. J. Roentgenol. 135:1187, 1980.

Heinz, E. R., Peters, H. E., Jr., Tucker, D., et al.: Forum: Which oral contrast media may be used in x-ray evaluation of a suspected small bowel obstruction? Mod. Med. 39:202, 1971.

Kleinman, P., Meyers, M. A., Abbott, G., and Kazam, E.: Necrotizing enterocolitis with pneumatosis intestinalis in systemic lupus erythematosus and polyarteritis. Radiology 121:595, 1976.

Korobkin, M., Callen, P.W., Filly, R. A., et al.: Comparison of computed tomography, ultrasonography, and gallium-67 scanning in the evaluation of suspected abdominal abscess. Radiology 129:89, 1978.

Kressel, H. Y., and Filly, R. A.: Ultrasonographic appearance of gas-containing abscesses in the abdomen. Am. J. Roentgenol. 130:71, 1978.

Laufer, I.: The left lateral view in the plain-film assessment of abdominal distension. Radiology 119:265, 1976.

Linton, R. R.: The treatment of esophageal varices. Surg. Clin. North Am. 46:485, 1966.

McNeil, B. J., Sanders, R., Alderson, P. O., et al.: A prospective study of computed tomography, ultrasound and gallium imaging in patients with fever. Radiology 139:647, 1981.

Miller, R. E., and Nelson, S. W.: The roentgenologic demonstration of tiny amounts of free intraperitoneal gas; experimental and clinical studies. Am. J. Roentgenol. 112:574, 1971.

Pitcher, J. L.: Safety and effectiveness of the modified Sengstaken-Blakemore tube: a prospective study. Gastroenterology 61:291, 1971.

Rohlfing, B. M., Webb, W. R., and Schlobohm, R. M.: Ventilator-related extra-alveolar air in adults. Radiology 121:25, 1976.

Sagel, S. S., Seigel, M. J., Stanley, R. J., and Jost, R. G.: Detection of retroperitoneal hemorrhage by computed tomography. Am. J. Roentgenol. 129:403, 1977.

Tomchik, F. S., Wittenberg, J., and Ottinger, L. W.: The roentgenographic spectrum of bowel infarction. Radiology 96:249, 1970.

Wechsler, R. J., Steener, R. M., Goodman, L. R., et al.: Iatrogenic esophageal-pleural fistula: subtlety of diagnosis in the absence of mediastinitis. Radiology 144:239, 1982.

Wicks, J. D., Silver, T. M., and Bree, R. L.: Gray scale features of hematomas: an ultrasonic spectrum. Am. J. Roentgenol. 131:977, 1978.

Wolverson, M. K., Jagannadharao, B., Sundarum, M., et al.: CT as the primary diagnostic method in evaluating intra-abdominal abscess. Am. J. Roentgenol. 133:1089, 1976.

Chapter 9

INVASIVE DIAGNOSTIC AND THERAPEUTIC PROCEDURES IN THE CRITICALLY ILL

by Morton G. Glickman

All special procedures require prior consultation between the radiologist and the patient's physician. A special procedure should be considered only if it can reasonably be expected to provide a definitive answer to a clinically important problem. Careful planning minimizes the time and instrumentation required for the procedure. Whenever possible, these studies should be performed at the bedside, since it is safer and frequently simpler to move even cumbersome radiographic equipment than to mobilize the patient. These factors must be weighed against the decreased diagnostic quality of some bedside procedures and the increased exposure of patients and personnel to radiation from bedside radiographic examination.

Nuclear medicine examinations often can be performed at the bedside without significant loss of diagnostic quality and without significant exposure of others to radiation. Portable scanners or cameras are commercially available, and their purchase should be considered in hospitals that have heavily populated intensive care units (ICUs).

Ultrasonography is simple, painless, and safe, and it does not require premedication. In many situations it provides information not available by other means. Bedside examination can be performed when necessary using portable ultrasound machines without hazard to ICU patients or personnel.

Gray-scale ultrasonography records anatomic images of two-dimensional sections through soft tissues. Fluid can be distinguished from solid tissue, and characteristic sound wave reflection patterns from the parenchyma of solid organs often permit recognition of diseases affecting viscera such as the liver, kidneys, and pancreas. Real-time ultrasonography generates and displays rapid, sequential images at a rate of up to 1000 per second, effectively demonstrating motion of pulsatile organs. Currently available gray-scale ultrasound provides highly detailed images of organs and tissue planes in the abdomen, and real-time ultrasound permits detailed examination of the heart. Bedside ultrasound examination in many instances provides more definitive diagnostic information than do bedside radiography or fluoroscopy.

Portable fluoroscopic equipment is available, but is cumbersome, and radiation shielding of other patients and ICU personnel is impractical. Procedures, such as angiography, that require fluoroscopy must be performed in the radiology department. Angiography and other invasive catheter procedures are potentially hazardous, especially to seriously ill patients. The risk of these procedures is minimized if they are performed with specialized equipment not available at the bedside.

If angiography or percutaneous drainage procedures become necessary, the inconvenience, discomfort, and risk of transportation to the radiology department are justified in most instances. Procedures that ought to be simple may be complicated by unanticipated problems, such as an anatomic variant. Sophisticated radiographic equipment capable of producing optimal radiographic quality and demonstrating the maximal diagnostic information is often critically important to the solution of the complex clinical problems that arise in the very ill.

There are no absolute contraindications to angiography, but there are numerous *relative* contraindications. These include impaired renal function, pulmonary edema, recent myocardial infarction, severely impaired respiratory function, and previous anaphylactic reaction to contrast medium. When contrast medium must be injected into patients with borderline pulmonary edema or decreased renal function, intravenous (IV) administration of fluids should be carefully limited. The blood pressure and central venous pressure (CVP) should be monitored carefully, and adequate time should be taken between injections to permit partial diuresis of the previous bolus. With these precautions, doses of up to 200 ml of contrast medium given over a one- or two-hour period are usually tolerated well. In selected patients with myocardial infarction, angiography may be performed with similar precautions, plus continuous ECG monitoring and the provision of reassurance and medication for pain and anxiety. The systemic effects of radiographic procedures are discussed in detail in Chapter 10.

Every attempt should be made to reduce the dose of the contrast medium without sacrificing diagnostic information. This is best accomplished by avoiding aortography, by utilizing only selective or superselective injections, and by use of biplane filming. If the films in each plane are exposed alternatively rather than simultaneously, scattered radiation is reduced and film quality is diagnostically adequate.

Anticoagulation therapy or clotting deficiencies should not be considered contraindications to angiography. The only breach of a vessel wall during angiography occurs at the site of catheter insertion, and hemorrhage can be controlled by manual compression. In anticoagulated patients prolonged compression may be necessary, but this should not preclude a clinically indicated procedure.

Local complications may occur at the site of catheter insertion. The frequency of thrombosis of the catheterized vessel is related to the size of the catheter, perhaps to the length of the procedure, and to the techniques used for obtaining hemostasis following catheter removal. As a general rule, the catheter used for angiography should have the smallest possible outer diameter. Ultra–thin-walled polyethylene catheters should be used whenever possible for selective injections. These catheters are not appropriate for aortography, since they frequently cannot withstand the pressure required to deliver a bolus of contrast medium adequate to opacify the aorta. Teflon is a much stronger material than polyethylene, and a thin-walled Teflon catheter with a No. 6 French outer diameter can be safely and effectively used for aortography.

Following removal of the catheter, compression over the puncture site should not obliterate the distal pulse. Compression should be no stronger than that necessary to prevent bleeding. A Doppler ultrasound probe taped over the pedal pulse allows continuous monitoring of the blood flow peripheral to the arterial compression site during compression. When these precautions are taken, thrombosis at the puncture site rarely occurs. Recurrent bleeding from the puncture site can always be controlled by compression.

ABSCESS: DIAGNOSTIC PROCEDURES

The site of infection in a febrile patient is usually clear because of localizing symptoms or physical signs. If these suggest abdominal abscess, ultrasonography or computerized tomography (CT) can demonstrate the presence or absence of an abscess and the anatomic relationship of an abscess to surrounding viscera (see Chapter 8). In the absence of localizing symptoms or signs, radionuclide scanning following injection of gallium-67 citrate is the diagnostic procedure of choice.

Gallium-67 has similar properties to ferric iron. At sites of inflammation gallium-67 is bound to iron-binding proteins such as lactoferrin, which in turn are bound to local inflammatory cells (Hoffer, 1981). Thus, gallium-67 is selectively concentrated at sites of inflammation, and gallium-67 scanning is highly sensitive in localizing occult abscesses and in documenting diffuse infections such as peritonitis or cellulitis (Fig. 9–1) (Hoffer, 1980).

Gallium-67 scans may be performed at the bedside; they may be positive as early as six hours after IV injection, but a period of 24 hours is usually required for localization. Al-

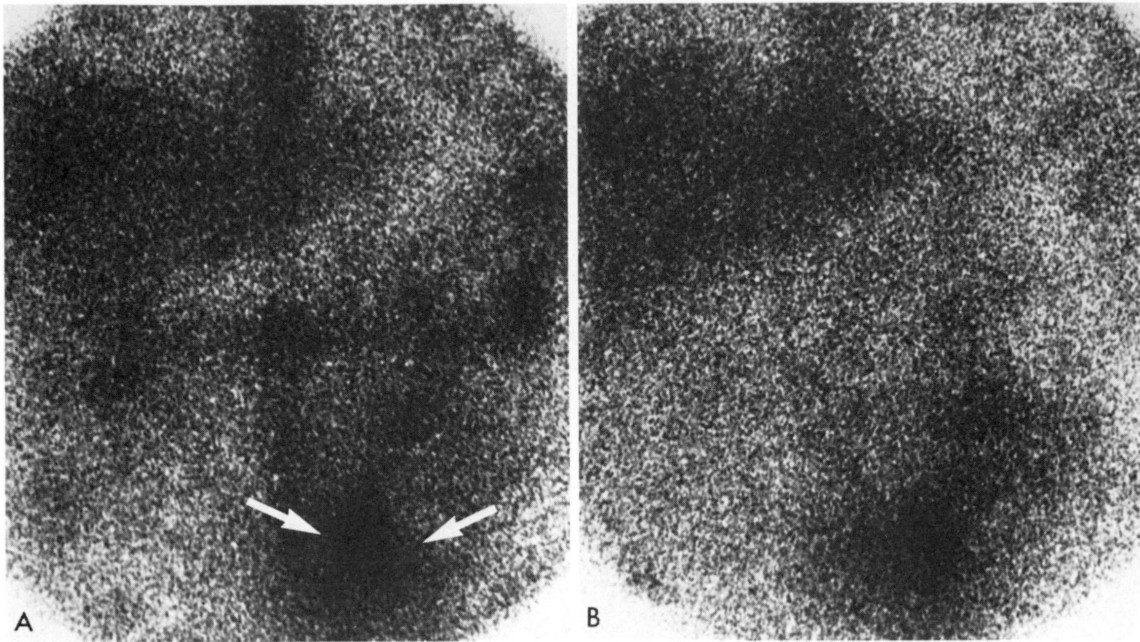

Figure 9–1. Psoas abscess in a 45-year-old man with a fever of unknown origin. *A*, Scan obtained 48 hours after injection of gallium-67 demonstrates uptake in the liver, spine, and colon. In addition, a large, round, dense gallium-67 concentration is present in the lower abdomen *(arrows)*. *B*, Ninety-six hours after injection, the isotope, which had been excreted into the bowel, has been passed. The mass in the left lower abdomen remains present. It is denser than the liver and unchanged from its earlier appearance. Oblique projections demonstrated that the mass was posterior and therefore retroperitoneal. A left psoas abscess was subsequently identified and drained.

though gallium-67 activity accumulates in the normal liver and in the skeleton, the density of gallium-67 uptake at sites of infection in liver and bone is greater than in the uninvolved areas (Fig. 9–2). Correlation of the gallium-67 scan with a radionuclide liver or bone scan can minimize the frequency of error caused by normal uptake of gallium-67 by these organs.

During the first 24 hours following injection, gallium-67 is excreted primarily by the kidneys and thereafter predominantly by the gastrointestinal (GI) tract. The bladder may be recognized on scans obtained during the first 12 hours. Delayed scanning, 48 to 72 hours after injection, permits diagnosis of renal and perirenal inflammatory disease. Subtraction scans may be performed by injecting either ^{99m}Tc-sulfur colloid (liver-spleen scan) or ^{99m}Tc-glucoheptonate (renal scan) after the gallium-67 scan has been completed. These images may then be subtracted from the gallium-67 image to improve detection of intra-abdominal abscesses. Since gallium-67 is excreted into the GI tract, bowel cleansing with cathartics or enemas is useful to avoid false-positive interpretations.

ABSCESS: PERCUTANEOUS DRAINAGE

Traditional surgical management of abscesses involves incision, removal of all purulent material, and subsequent maintenance of a drainage tract until the infection has resolved and healing begins. Surgical exploration has been necessary in order to identify the most direct route for drainage and to avoid, where possible, contamination of uninfected organs, tissue planes, and potential spaces. However, modern gallium scanning, ultrasonography, and CT diagnose abscesses with a high degree of accuracy, and permit selection of the most direct routes for drainage of an intrathoracic or intra-abdominal abscess. Demonstration of the relationship of an abscess to surrounding viscera, tissue planes, and major vessels permits safe percutaneous needle insertion. Catheterization techniques developed for angiography are employed for replacement of the needle with a wide-bore catheter to remove purulent material and drainage until the infection resolves.

These techniques are particularly useful for

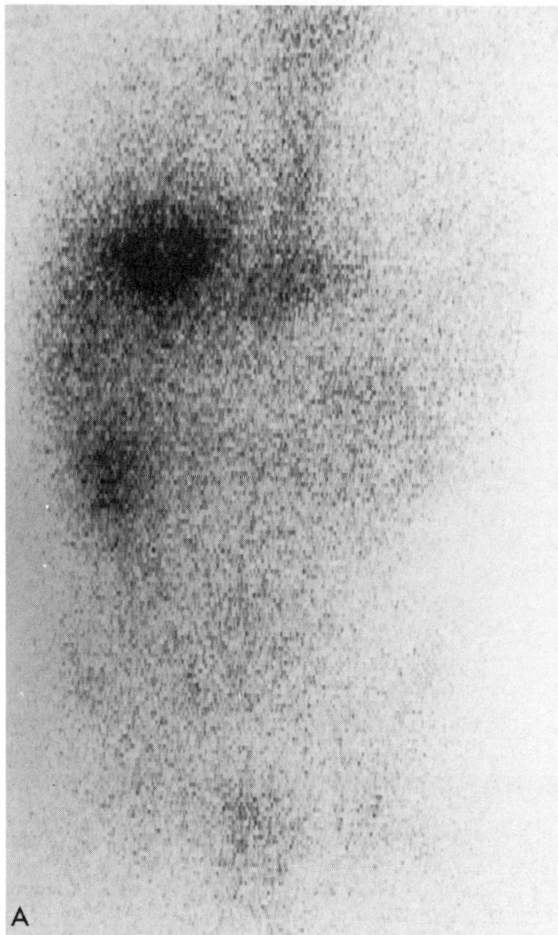

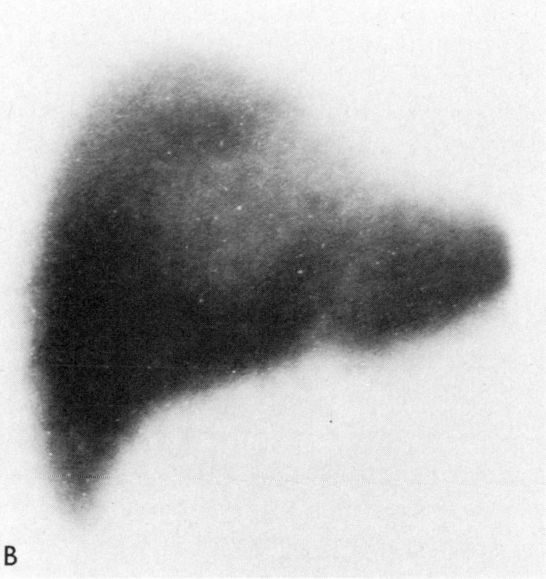

Figure 9–2. Hepatic abscesses in a 57-year-old man with nonlocalizing abdominal pain and fever. *A*, Scan obtained 72 hours after injection of gallium-67 shows normal uptake in the liver, thoracic spine, and bladder but dense, abnormal concentration in two nodules within the liver, one adjacent to the diaphragm and the other at the tip of the right lobe. *B*, Technetium 99m colloid liver scan shows defects corresponding to the areas of gallium-67 concentration.

patients in the ICU, since general anesthesia and surgical exploration can be avoided. If cross-sectional imaging can demonstrate a safe route of access, the needle is inserted using either CT, ultrasound, or fluoroscopy for guidance. Initial puncture can be made with a thin-walled, flexible 22-gauge needle, which is unlikely to cause clinically significant visceral injury or hemorrhage, even if the needle is misdirected (Haaga et al., 1979). Use of a 22-gauge needle that has a removable hub simplifies subsequent catheter insertion (Hawkins, 1979). Once the needle enters the abscess cavity, its position is verified by aspiration of purulent material and introduction of contrast medium if fluoroscopy or CT is used, or air if ultrasound is used (Fig. 9–3*A*). A guidewire is inserted through the needle, the hub of the needle is removed, and a catheter is introduced as a sheath over the needle-guidewire assembly into the abscess cavity. Progressively larger guidewires and catheters are then inserted until the tract is large enough to accommodate a wide-bore drainage catheter. An 8 French catheter is usually sufficient for most abscesses, but catheters as large as 16 French may be necessary if the contents of the abscess are particularly viscous. More than one catheter may be necessary if the abscess if loculated. Broad-spectrum antibiotics should be initiated prior to the procedure. Gram stain and culture of the aspirated material will then permit more specific antibiotic selection.

The most commonly used abscess drainage catheters are pre-curved to assume a coiled shape within the abscess cavity (Fig. 9–3*B*). Multiple side-holes are made along the coil to ensure adequate drainage even if some of the side-holes become obstructed by purulent material. The lumen of the catheter can be kept patent with occasional irrigation or insertion of a guidewire. If a double-lumen balloon catheter is used, the balloon is inflated within the abscess cavity to prevent inadvertent withdrawal of the

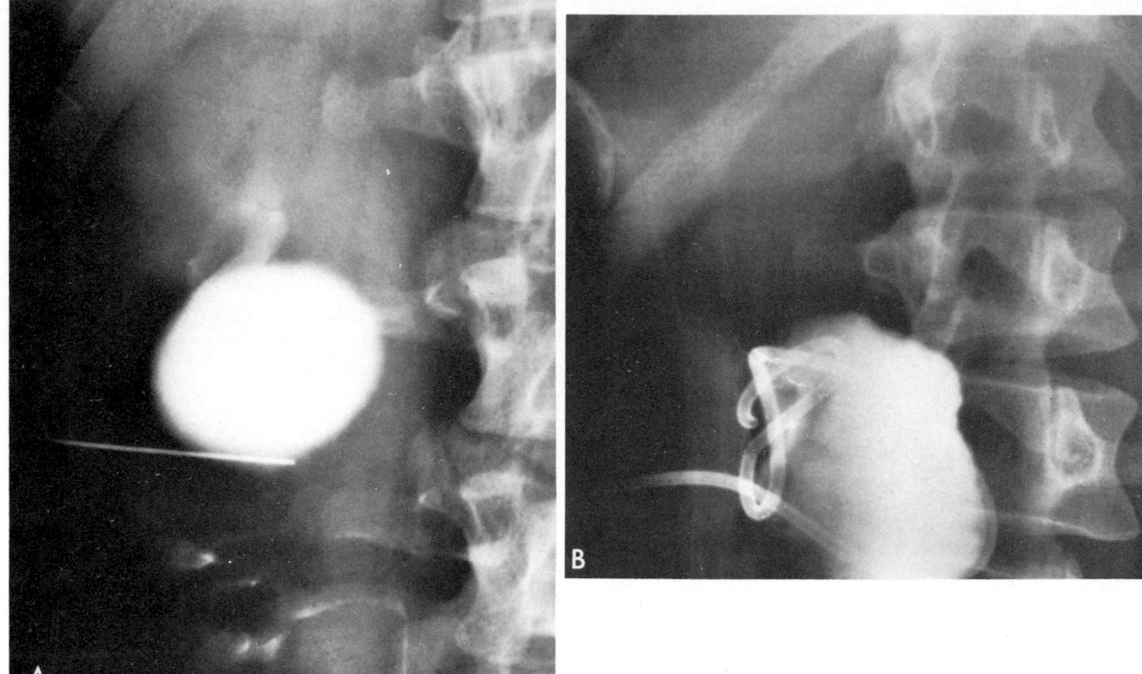

Figure 9–3. Intrarenal abscess in a 30-year-old woman with right flank pain and fever. IVP and ultrasound showed a round, fluid-filled mass in the midportion of the right kidney. *A*, A 22-gauge needle has been inserted through the flank into the lesion under fluoroscopy. After aspiration of purulent material, which documented the diagnosis of abscess, contrast medium has been injected to demonstrate the size and shape of the abscess cavity. *B*, After introduction of the guidewire and dilating catheters, an 8.3 French drainage catheter has been inserted and coiled within the abscess cavity. Multiple side-holes along the coil ensure drainage. Within 24 hours the patient became afebrile, and the catheter was removed 14 days after insertion. The catheter tract healed and there has been no recurrence of symptoms.

catheter. The catheter is sutured to the skin at the insertion site. Catheter drainage is maintained until drainage ceases, after which the catheter is removed.

In the two largest series reported to date, 22 of 24 and 28 of 33 abdominal abscesses, respectively, were successfully drained by this technique (Gerzof et al., 1979; Haaga and Weinstein, 1980). Failure of this technique has resulted from incomplete drainage of highly viscous material, loculation within the abscess cavity or unrecognized satellite abscesses, and continued internal contamination, for example, by a leaking bowel anastomosis. If percutaneous drainage fails to resolve the infection, the procedure does not complicate subsequent surgical management or increase the surgical risk. Rather, incomplete drainage is often temporarily effective, permitting improvement of the patient's general condition and thereby reducing the risk of surgery (Gerzof et al., 1979). Although this procedure is relatively new and no large series have so far been reported, the complication rate appears to be low, and those that have occurred have been surgically treatable (Gerzof et al., 1979; Haaga and Weinstein, 1980; Haaga et al., 1979).

Depending on the location of the lesion and the potential risk to surrounding structures, percutaneous abscess drainage can occasionally be performed as a bedside procedure under ultrasound guidance. However, most abscess drainage procedures are probably more efficiently performed in the x-ray department where multiple imaging modes are available.

PERCUTANEOUS BIOPSY

Because of the fine anatomic and structural detail provided by ultrasound, CT, and angiography, masses in previously hidden sites can be identified and characterized without surgical exploration. This diagnostic information also makes percutaneous biopsy for cytologic, histologic, or bacteriologic examination applicable to a wide variety of clinical problems. Percutaneous biopsy may obviate the necessity for surgery by confirming metastasis or by documenting that a mass is benign or malignant. Previous cytologic diagnosis of a potentially resectable malignancy permits surgical preplanning, thereby saving time in the operating room.

Once a suspicious mass is demonstrated, the biopsy is performed using CT, ultrasound, or fluoroscopy for needle guidance. CT provides elegant cross-sectional images that permit accurate needle placement into even very small masses (Ferrucci and Wittenberg, 1978). Since CT also demonstrates tissue planes and adjacent viscera, puncture of structures such as bowel or major vessels can be avoided. The route for needle placement is chosen on the basis of initial CT images. The needle is then advanced into subcutaneous tissue and an image is obtained to ensure that the direction of the needle precisely traverses the planned route. The needle is advanced into the mass, its proper position is confirmed, and the specimen is obtained (Fig. 9–4*A*, *B*). In view of the limited availability of CT, needle placement under fluoroscopic or ultrasound guidance is preferable, unless the lesion biopsied is small or in a dangerous location (Fig. 9–4*C*, *D*) (Ferrucci and Wittenberg, 1979; McLoughlin et al., 1979).

Ultrasound machinery is more widely available and permits percutaneous biopsy at the bedside if necessary. Fluoroscopy must be performed in the x-ray department, but needle placement under fluoroscopic guidance may be simpler and more accurate than with ultrasound, especially if the mass is adjacent to radiopaque structures such as a biliary or ureteral drainage tube (Pereiras et al., 1978). Fluoroscopy is the method of choice if biopsy can be performed at the time when a suspicious mass is identified during a diagnostic radiographic procedure such as intravenous pyelography (IVP), arteriography, or lymphangiography.

The choice of needle size and design varies with the anatomic location of the lesion and with the probable diagnosis. Thin-walled 22-gauge needles are most appropriate for biopsy of deep seated lesions. The small caliber and flexibility of these needles minimize the likelihood of damage to viscera or hemorrhage. In large published series, complications such as hemorrhage, infection, fistula formation, or tumor seeding along the needle tract occurred rarely when fine needles were used, although some authors reported that arteries and contaminated organs such as the colon were punctured during some of these biopsies (Pereiras et al., 1978; Prando et al., 1979; Smith et al., 1975). Although the risk of fine needle biopsy is very low, the size of the needle lumen frequently precludes aspiration of a tissue core, and the diagnosis must be established by cytologic examination. Cytologic smears are considerably more difficult to interpret than histologic sections; therefore, fine needle aspiration biopsy should be attempted only if an experienced cytopathologist is available (Otis, 1980; Tao et al., 1980). In experienced hands, however, fine needle biopsy accurately identifies the disease in 80 to 90 per cent of patients (Ferrucci and Wittenberg, 1979; Pereiras et al., 1978). Large-bore needles capable of obtaining a tissue core increase the accuracy of percutaneous biopsy procedures, but also increase the hazard of the procedure. Their use should therefore be restricted to superficial lesions or lesions whose location poses little risk of puncturing arteries or contaminated viscera (see also lung aspiration in Chapter 4).

BILIARY SYSTEM OBSTRUCTION

Obstructive jaundice can be distinguished from jaundice due to hepatocellular disease or other nonobstructive diseases simply, and with a high degree of accuracy, by ultrasound or nuclear medicine. Biliary tract obstruction results from a wide range of diseases including benign, curable problems such as choledocholithiasis as well as malignant, incurable diseases such as metastatic gallbladder carcinoma. Regardless of the underlying disease, obstructive jaundice requires prompt drainage in order to avoid or to treat cholangitis and the absorptive abnormalities and fluid imbalances that result from exclusion of bile salts from the GI tract.

Until recently, relief of biliary tract obstruction has been possible only by means of surgery, but a newly developed nonsurgical technique for decompression of the obstructed biliary tract in the high-risk ICU patient has now gained widespread acceptance. Transhepatic cholangiography is used to opacify the biliary tract and identify the site of obstruction. In most cases the radiographic appearance of the obstruction permits diagnosis of its cause.

If a surgically treatable lesion such as choledocholithiasis is demonstrated, a percutaneous biliary drainage catheter can be inserted to

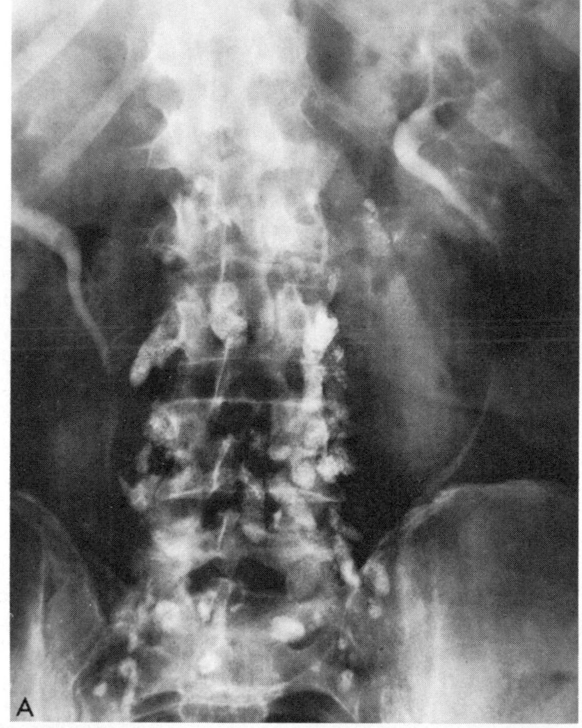

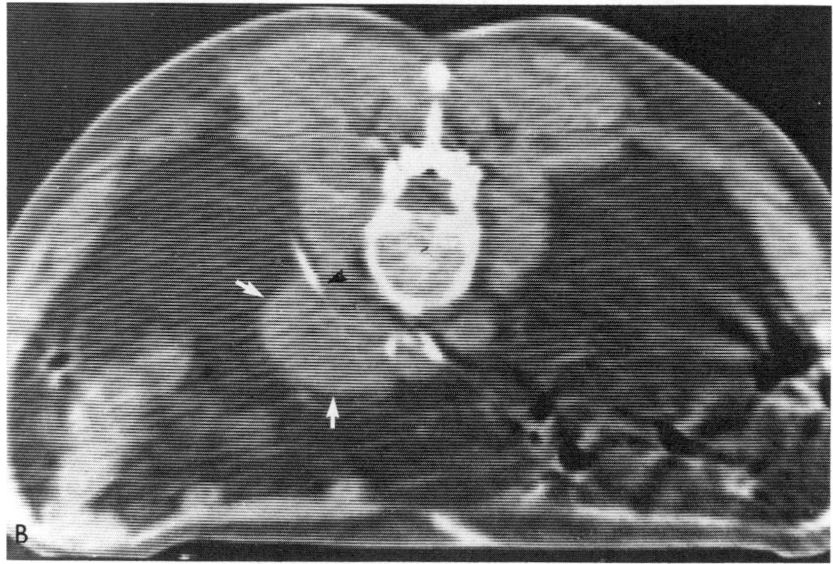

Figure 9–4. Large, asymptomatic retroperitoneal mass in an elderly man. *A*, The size and extent of the mass are shown by lateral displacement of the left ureter. *B*, Needle biopsy was performed using computerized tomography for guidance. In this image, the patient is lying prone and the tip of the biopsy needle (*arrowhead*) is demonstrated within the mass (*white arrows*). Aspirated material documented malignancy but the specimen was insufficient for a more specific diagnosis. The biopsy was repeated using fluoroscopy for guidance. Frontal projection (*C*) shows the tip of the needle within the mass (*arrow*). The appropriate depth for needle insertion was determined by reference to the computerized tomographic image. The lateral radiograph (*D*) demonstrates that the needle is at the desired depth, 2 cm anterior to the vertebral body (*arrow*). The cytologic diagnosis was adenocarcinoma, most likely metastatic from the prostate. Immunohistochemical analysis of the cell block for prostatic acid phosphatase documented the prostatic origin of the tumor.

Illustration continued on opposite page

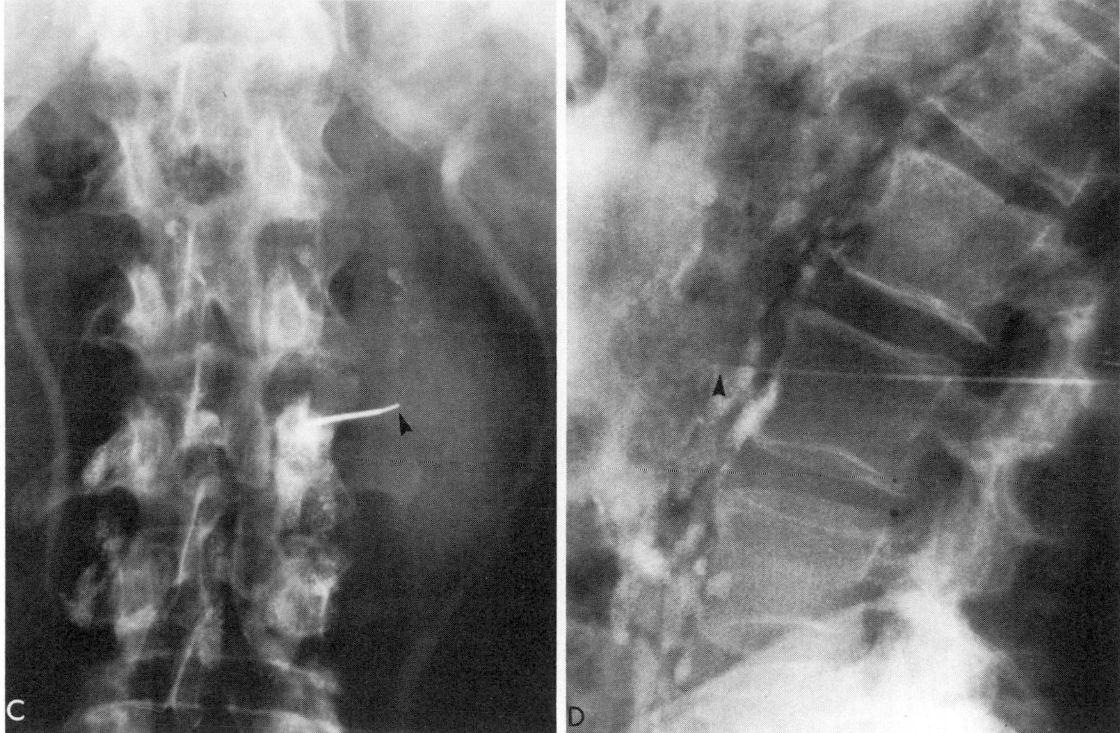

Figure 9–4 *Continued.*

temporarily decompress the system while the patient's other medical conditions are being treated. If surgery is not feasible, palliative percutaneous biliary drainage offers relief and a possible route for the chemical dissolution of or percutaneous removal of the calculi.

If the obstruction is thought to be due to malignancy, percutaneous aspiration biopsy can be performed using the drainage catheter as a radiographic landmark for the biopsy needle. Diagnostic evaluation can then be instituted to demonstrate the extent and potential resectability of the tumor. If the tumor is resectable, the optimal surgical procedure can be planned. If it is unresectable, percutaneous drainage may be continued indefinitely (Fig. 9–5).

Percutaneous transhepatic drainage of an obstructed biliary system is well tolerated, even by severely ill, unstable patients. Using local anesthesia, fluoroscopic control, and sterile technique, a thin-walled, flexible 22-gauge needle is advanced into the hepatic parenchyma. Incremental injections of small volumes of contrast medium are made under fluoroscopy as the needle is gradually withdrawn. Opacification of a bile duct indicates that the tip of the needle is within the biliary system. At that point, bile is aspirated and is replaced with contrast medium. By changing the patient's position, the contrast medium, which has a higher specific gravity than bile, is moved to the point of obstruction; radiographs are then obtained.

Because of the small bore and the flexibility of the fine needle used for puncture, complications rarely occur. In a series of 314 patients examined by this technique, Okuda et al. (1974) reported bile peritonitis in 0.64 per cent and clinically significant hemorrhage in 0.64 per cent. In a series of 140 patients reported by Ferrucci (1978), bile peritonitis resulted in one patient (0.7 per cent) and clinically significant hemorrhage did not occur.

The drainage catheter is inserted by a second percutaneous puncture, using an 18-gauge needle within a thin-walled polyethylene sheath directed by fluoroscopy into a previously demonstrated dilated duct. In patients with compromised clotting systems, a second puncture can sometimes be avoided if the initial puncture is made with a modified 22-gauge needle that has a removable hub (Hawkins, 1979). After a bile duct is cannulated, a flexible angiographic guidewire is threaded through the needle and

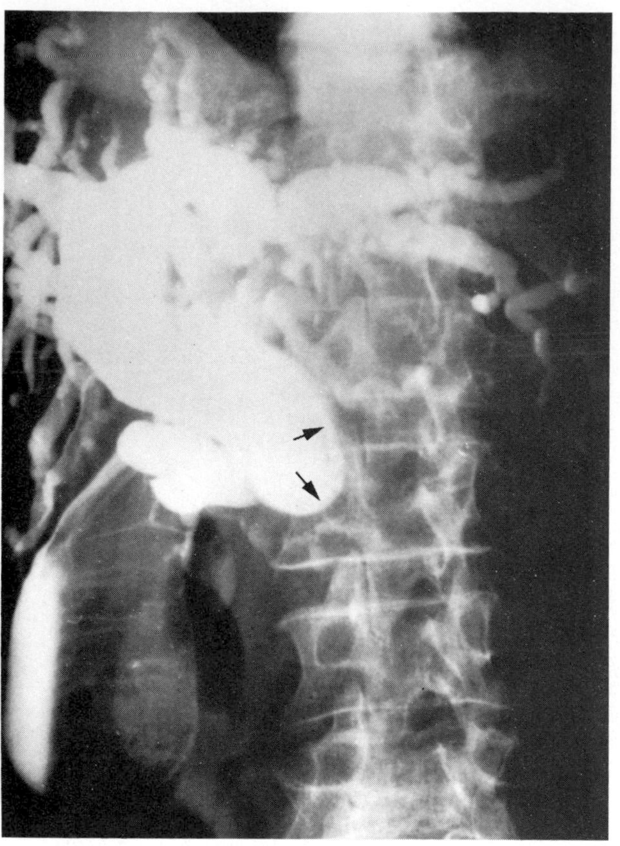

Figure 9–5. Obstruction of the common bile duct in an 80-year-old woman with painless jaundice. The bile ducts were punctured percutaneously and, after introduction of a guidewire and dilating catheters, a drainage catheter has been inserted and permitted to coil in the common bile duct just above the point of obstruction (*arrows*). Contrast medium injection shows marked dilation of the intrahepatic bile ducts, the gallbladder, and the common bile duct. Using the radiopaque drainage catheter as a landmark, a 22-gauge needle was inserted under fluoroscopy to the site of obstruction, and aspiration biopsy performed. Cytologic examination confirmed the diagnosis of cholangiocarcinoma. External drainage was maintained until further diagnostic examination documented the extent of the local disease and the absence of metastases, and definitive surgical resection was performed.

advanced several centimeters into the biliary system to maintain position during catheter manipulation. The polyethylene sheath is advanced over the needle-guidewire assembly into the bile duct. Progressively larger-diameter catheters are introduced until a catheter large enough to drain even viscous, infected bile is in place. The catheter should contain multiple side-holes as well as an end-hole to ensure adequate drainage. After satisfactory position is documented, the catheter is sutured to the skin.

Long-term catheter drainage may be indicated in patients with inoperable, malignant diseases or in those whose concurrent disease precludes surgery. If long-term catheter drainage is necessary, the catheter should be advanced across the site of obstruction and fixed in a position that permits bile drainage into the duodenum. This allows normal flow of bile salts into the GI tract and eliminates the necessity for external drainage. Internal drainage is possible in most patients, even in the presence of apparently complete bile duct obstruction (Fig. 9–6). In cases of high-grade obstruction or cholangitis, external drainage for several days is prudent to minimize the risk of sepsis before attempts are made to manipulate the catheter past the obstruction. Under fluoroscopy, the obstructed lumen of the bile duct is gently probed with a small, soft catheter or guidewire. Once the obstruction is traversed, the lumen is dilated with progressively larger catheters until the drainage catheter can be advanced into the duodenum.

The catheter used for internal drainage is fashioned specifically for each patient. The length of the common duct from the site of obstruction to the duodenum, and the length of the bile duct from the site of entry of the catheter from the liver parenchyma to the site of obstruction, are carefully measured. Side-holes are cut in appropriate locations along the catheter, which is positioned so that no side-holes are present in the segment of the catheter that is outside the biliary system. Thus, bile that enters the catheter peripheral to the obstruction can traverse the obstruction within the catheter and drain into the distal common bile duct or directly into the duodenum. Although external drainage is not necessary once internal drainage is established, a segment of the catheter is maintained external to the skin

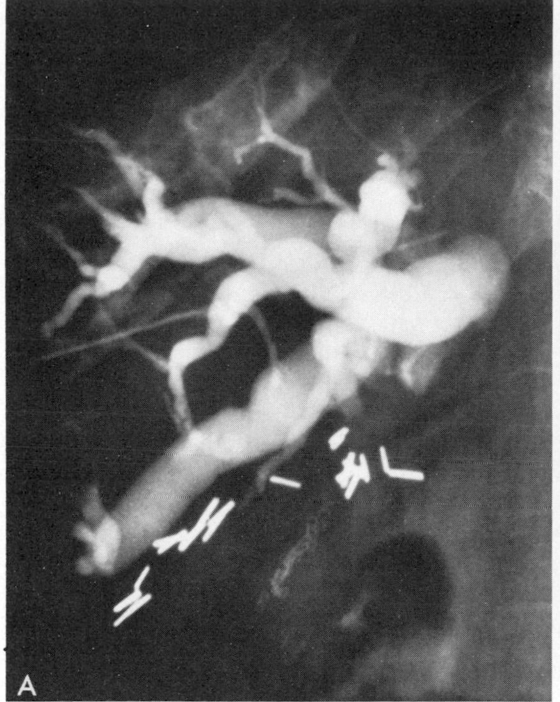

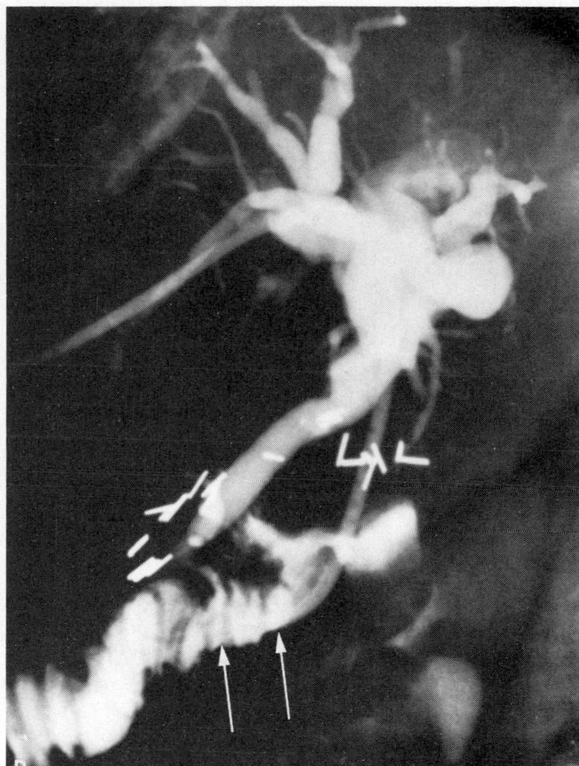

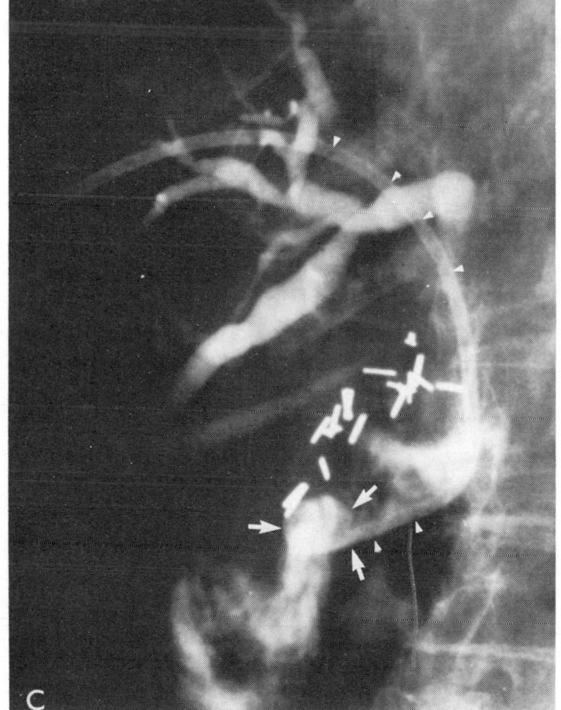

Figure 9–6. Internal drainage of obstructed bile duct in an 82-year-old woman with carcinoma of the ampulla of Vater bypassed surgically one year previously. She now presents with painless jaundice. *A*, The intrahepatic bile ducts were punctured percutaneously by a 22-gauge needle. Contrast medium has been injected and demonstrates dilated right hepatic ducts that are completely obstructed near the porta hepatis. Neither the left hepatic duct nor the common bile duct is opacified. After insertion of a guidewire and dilating catheters, a drainage catheter was advanced into the right hepatic ducts. With careful manipulation under fluoroscopy, the guidewire was directed through the apparently obstructed segment of the bile duct and through the choledochojejunostomy into the jejunum. *B*, The drainage catheter has been advanced over the guidewire through the obstruction, and the guidewire has been removed. Contrast medium injected through the catheter has further opacified the right hepatic ducts and has passed through the catheter into the jejunum (*white arrows*), documenting that the side-holes are properly placed for internal drainage. *C*, Ten minutes later most of the contrast medium has passed further distally into the jejunum, permitting visualization of the entire length of the radiopaque catheter. The central end of the catheter is coiled (*white arrows*) in the jejunum to minimize the likelihood of accidental withdrawal. Side-holes are visible (*arrowheads*) in the segments of the catheter that are within the jejunum and within the intrahepatic ducts. Internal drainage was maintained for six months until the patient's death from metastases. During that time the bilirubin levels remained within normal limits.

to permit easy access in case the catheter becomes obstructed or it becomes necessary to change its position.

Long-term maintenance of internal biliary drainage catheters is well tolerated (Pollock et al., 1979). Catheter lavage two or three times a week is usually sufficient to maintain long-term patency. The catheters may deteriorate with time and should be changed at intervals of three or four months, a simple procedure once the percutaneous tract is established. Procedures for catheter placement that leave the catheter entirely within the liver have been devised and can be simply performed, but their value for long-term drainage is questionable because of limited access if they become obstructed.

The major complication of percutaneous biliary drainage is sepsis (Clark et al., 1981). Broad-spectrum antibiotics should be administered for 24 hours prior to the procedure and continued for three or four days thereafter. Long-term antibiotic coverage is not necessary. The patient should be well hydrated before the procedure, and clotting factors should be evaluated to assess the risk of hemorrhage. In patients with pre-existing infection, continuous CVP monitoring is useful for 24 to 48 hours following the procedure so that hypotension associated with gram-negative sepsis can be immediately recognized and intensively treated (Pollock et al., 1979).

URINARY TRACT OBSTRUCTION

Urinary tract obstruction, hitherto a problem soluble only by surgery, can be treated by percutaneous catheterization and drainage in patients in whom surgery is contraindicated. Although this procedure can be performed at the bedside, using ultrasound for needle guidance, catheter manipulation is more simply and accurately performed under fluoroscopic guidance.

The renal pelvis is identified by injecting contrast medium intravenously. If the pelvis is not visualized, a flexible 22-gauge needle is inserted into the anticipated location of the dilated renal pelvis until urine is aspirated. Contrast medium is then injected to opacify the system. Because of the fine caliber and flexibility of the needle, the risk of renal injury or of clinically significant hemorrhage is very small.

Once the collecting system is visualized, the optimal route for catheter insertion is selected. The posterolateral approach to the kidney minimizes the risk of injuring abdominal viscera or contaminating the peritoneal cavity with infected urine. The catheter is inserted in the posterior axillary line, so that the large paraspinous muscles are avoided and only fascial planes are traversed by the catheter. This lessens patient discomfort during respiration and reduces the likelihood of kinking of the catheter when the patient lies supine. The catheter enters the kidney through the renal cortex, which helps to anchor it and avoids the major renal vessels, which are centrally located in the kidney. An 18-gauge needle ensheathed by a 5 French Teflon catheter is inserted into the renal collecting system, urine aspirated, and the inner needle is removed. A guidewire is inserted and the Teflon catheter is removed. Progressively larger catheters are advanced over the guidewire to dilate the tract. In most cases an 8 French catheter provides sufficient drainage. If the aspirated urine is viscous owing to infection, 10 or 12 French catheters may be necessary.

If the patient is clinically unstable or if the urine is infected, external drainage should be established. A drainage catheter that assumes a coiled shape within the renal pelvis is inserted (Fig. 9–7). Multiple side-holes are present in the coiled segment of the catheter. The catheter is sutured to the skin, and the aspirated urine is examined by Gram stain and sent for culture. Nephrostomy drainage catheters can also be

Figure 9–7. Percutaneous nephrostomy in a 70-year-old woman with unresectable carcinoma of the cervix obstructing both ureters. *A*, An 8.3 French Pigtail drainage catheter has coiled within each renal pelvis, providing bilateral external drainage. Ten days later the left nephrostomy was converted to an internal drainage system. *B*, A straight catheter has been inserted into the collecting system of the left kidney and manipulated to the distal left ureter. Injection of contrast medium shows marked narrowing of the distal ureter at the ureterovesical junction (*arrow*). *C*, After manipulation of the guidewire through the ureterovesical junction, an internal drainage catheter has been advanced into the bladder. Its coiled shape within the bladder minimizes the likelihood of accidental withdrawal. Numerous side-holes are present in the segment of the catheter within the ureter, and also within the bladder, to permit passage of urine from the kidney past the obstruction. Subsequently, the right nephrostomy was also converted to internal drainage. Over a follow-up period of ten months, creatinine levels have remained normal and the patient has had normal bladder function. The catheters have been changed at intervals of three months.

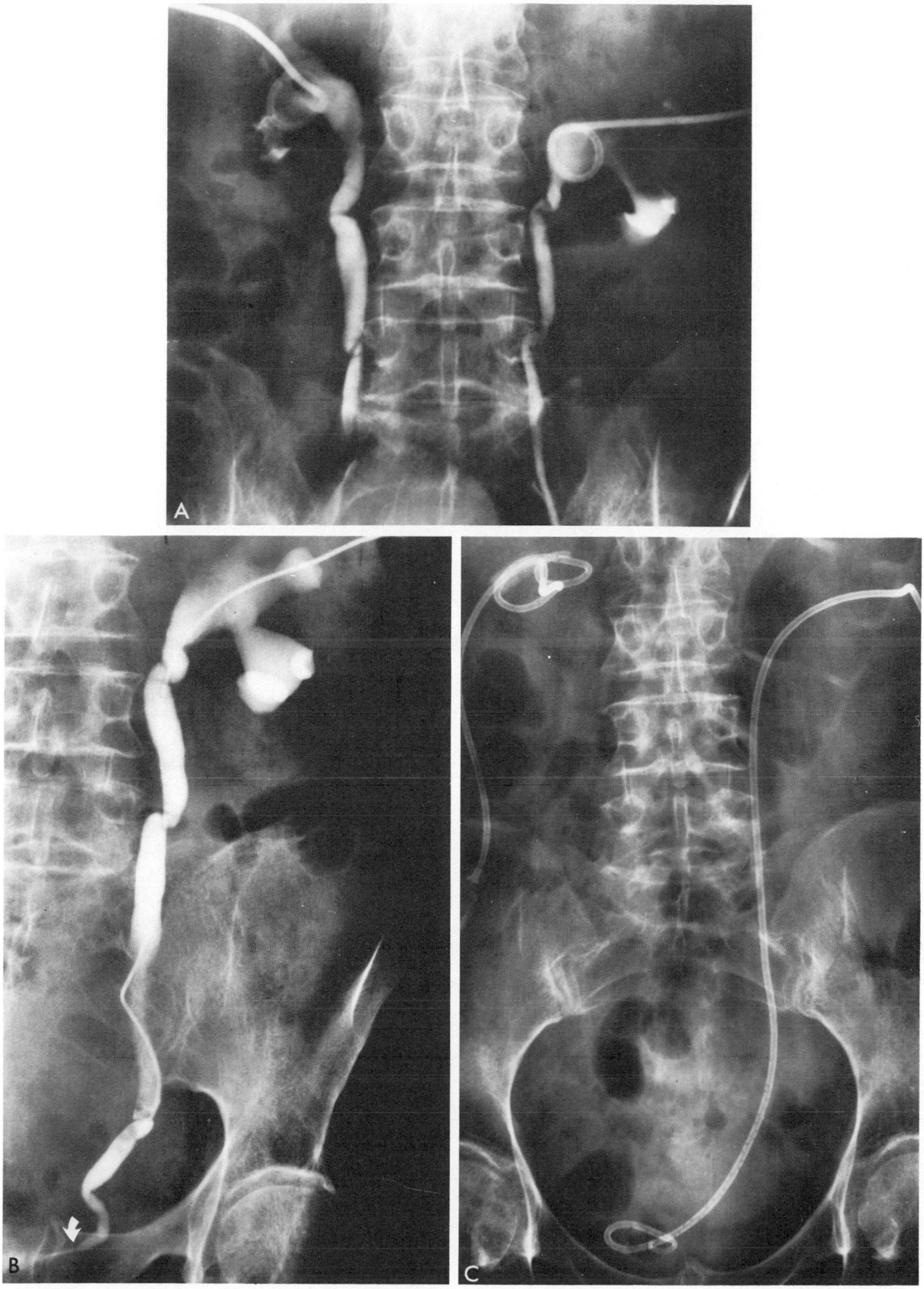

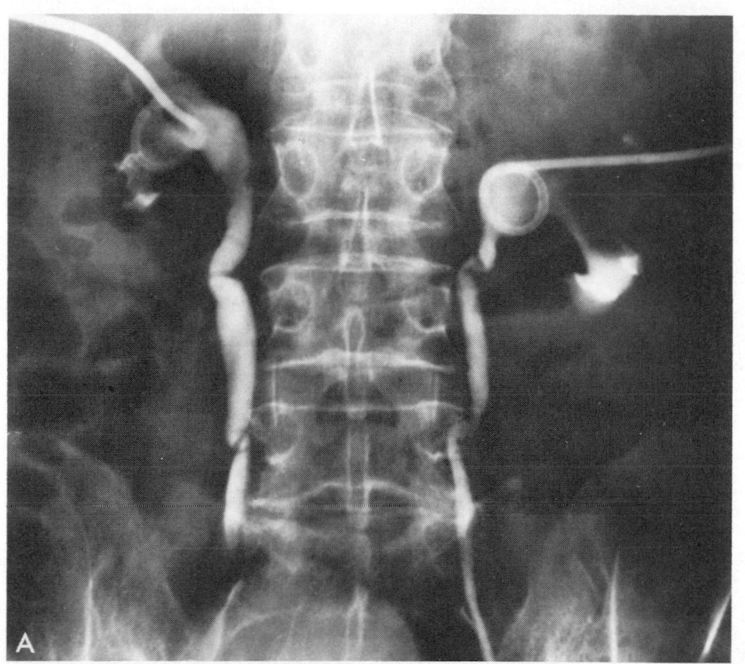
A
B
C

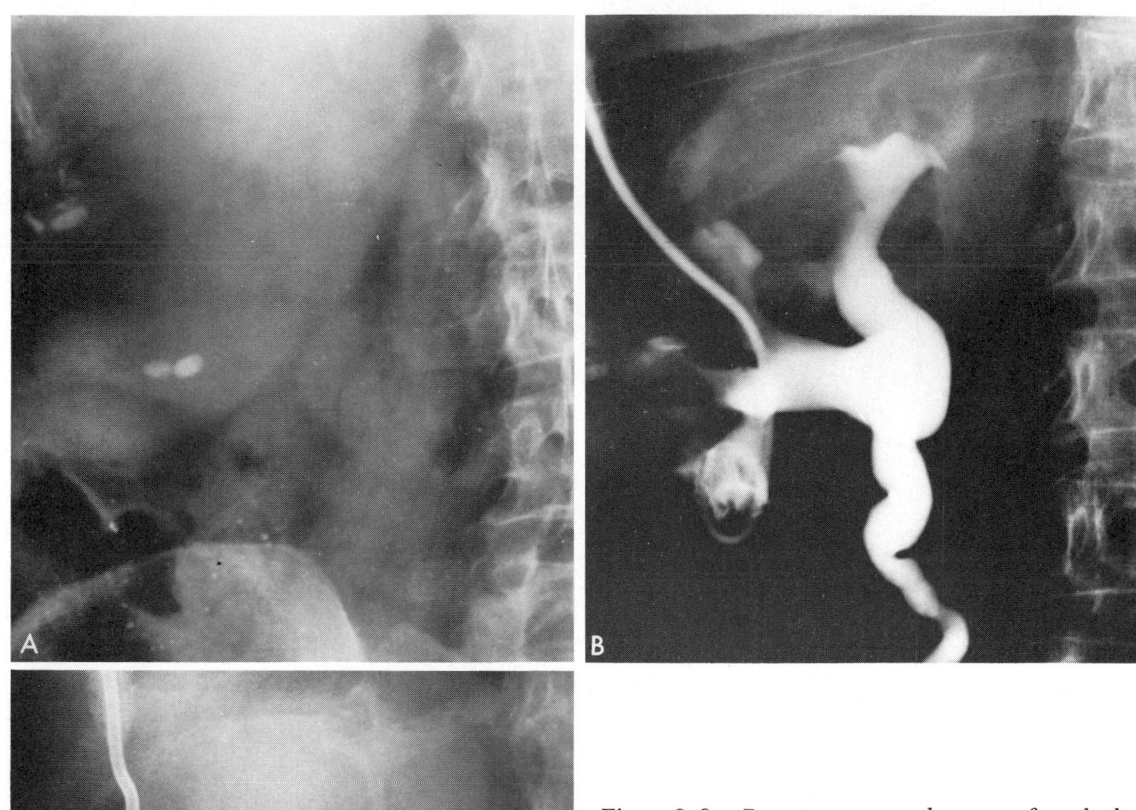

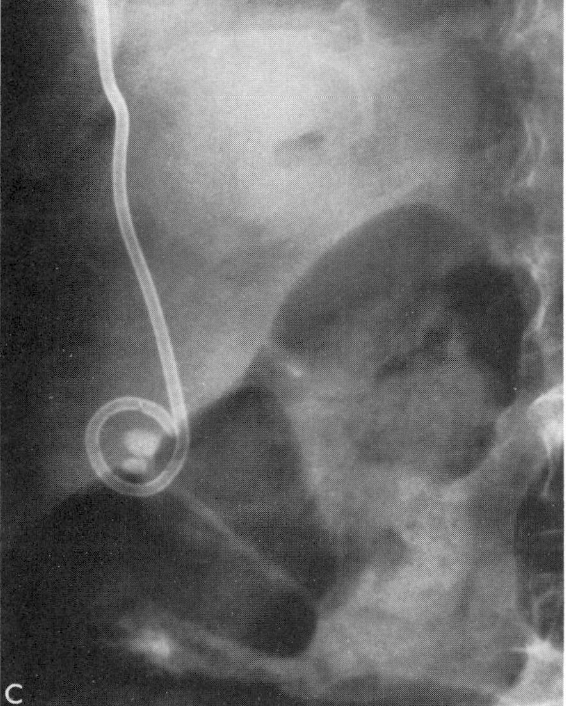

Figure 9–8. Percutaneous nephrostomy for calculus dissolution in a 71-year-old woman with renal calculi in a solitary kidney. The contralateral kidney was previously removed for unrelated disease. *A*, Plain film shows two opaque calculi in the right midabdomen. *B*, A nephrostomy catheter has been inserted through a calix in the midportion of the right kidney and manipulated through the lower pole and fundibulum into the lower pole calix, which contains the calculi. *C*, After drainage of the contrast medium, the position of the catheter in the lower pole calix can be clearly seen. The coiled end surrounds the calculi and is in excellent position for injection of dissolving agents.

used as a direct conduit for insertion of superficial biopsy brushes, for installation of stone-dissolving chemicals (Fig. 9–8), and for manipulation of stone removal baskets.

Internal drainage into the bladder avoids the necessity of external drainage apparatus. In a clinically stable patient, internal drainage can be established at the time of initial nephrostomy catheter insertion. If the patient's condition requires temporary external drainage, internal drainage can be established as his condition improves. Under fluoroscopic control, the guidewire is manipulated through the nephrostomy catheter, down the ureter, and through the site of obstruction. Even when the obstruction appears complete radiographically, the guidewire can usually locate the lumen and traverse the obstruction. Catheters are then advanced over the guidewire to dilate the obstructed segment, and a drainage catheter is positioned so that side-holes are present in the ureter above the obstruction and in the bladder below the obstruction (Fig. 9–7*C*). The catheter is then sutured to the skin and the external end of the catheter is capped.

Systemic antibiotics are a useful precaution before the procedure, but may be discontinued after 24 to 48 hours. The catheter should be flushed with a few milliliters of sterile saline twice a week to maintain patency. Although these catheters are well tolerated by most patients, the external catheter can be easily changed to an internal system (Bragongiari et al., 1980) using fluoroscopy. A guidewire is inserted through the internal drainage catheter into the bladder, and the catheter is removed. A polyethylene catheter preshaped to form coils at both ends is advanced over the guidewire and permitted to coil in the bladder. A second catheter is advanced over the guidewire, pushing the drainage catheter ahead of it until the tip of the drainage catheter is entirely contained within the renal pelvis. The guidewire is removed, and the catheter assumes its coiled shape at both ends with one coil in the bladder and the other in the renal pelvis. Side-holes along both coils permit drainage from the kidney to the bladder. If the catheter needs to be repositioned or replaced, it can be reached from the bladder by a cystoscope.

In a review of 516 percutaneous nephrostomies, a drainage catheter was reported to be successfully placed in 94 per cent (Stables et al., 1978). Complications such as sepsis, exacerbation of pyonephrosis, severe hematuria requiring transfusion, and perirenal hematoma occurred in 4 per cent of these cases. No mortality was reported. Since this review, catheter techniques have been refined, and the frequency of some of these complications may be lower (Ho et al., 1980). Transient, mild hematuria can be anticipated for 24 to 48 hours after catheter insertion. Clinically significant damage to the renal cortex as a result of catheterization has not been reported. Severe hemorrhagic diathesis is the only contraindication to the procedure.

ABDOMINAL TRAUMA

The most common clinically significant intra-abdominal injury following blunt trauma is rupture of the spleen. Hepatic lacerations occur less frequently, but pose a similar diagnostic and therapeutic problem. Injuries to the spleen or liver are usually apparent in the emergency room, and the appropriate diagnostic procedure is generally performed before the patient reaches the ICU. However, if the capsule of the injured organ remains intact or if the laceration occurs at a point where the rib cage or retroperitoneal tissues produce tamponade, signs of intra-abdominal hemorrhage may be delayed. Severe or prolonged pain in the left or right upper quadrant, reduction of the hematocrit value, or hypotension should raise the possibility of abdominal visceral injury.

Radiographic signs of splenic laceration include fracture of the lower left ribs, elevation of the left hemidiaphragm, displacement of the gastric air shadow toward the right, enlargement of the splenic shadow, and obliteration of some or all of the adjacent retroperitoneal or properitoneal fat lines. Hepatic injury may be suspected if right-sided rib fractures are present or if perihepatic fat lines are obliterated on radiographs of the abdomen. Since both the liver and the spleen are predominantly intraperitoneal structures, peritoneal lavage provides a rapid, simple, and safe means of supporting or excluding the diagnosis of visceral injury (Ahmad and Polk, 1976).

Hepatic and splenic lacerations can be demonstrated by radionuclide scanning. Transection of the spleen causes a transverse linear or wedge-shaped defect (Gilday and Alderson, 1974). A radioactive marker placed at the level of the lateral abdominal wall permits detection of displacement of the liver or spleen (Fig. 9–9). Since both organs normally lie against the lateral abdominal wall, displacement suggests

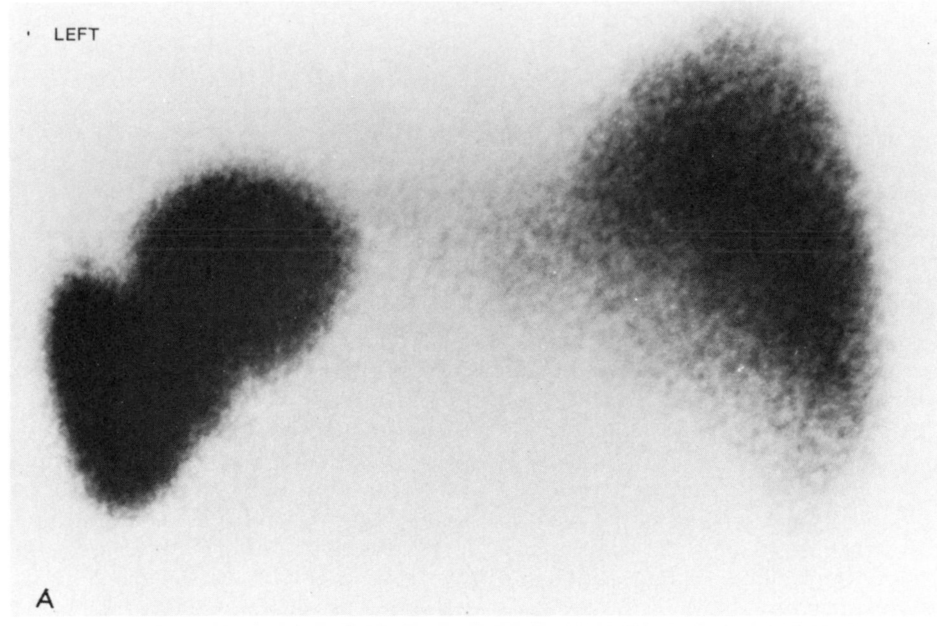

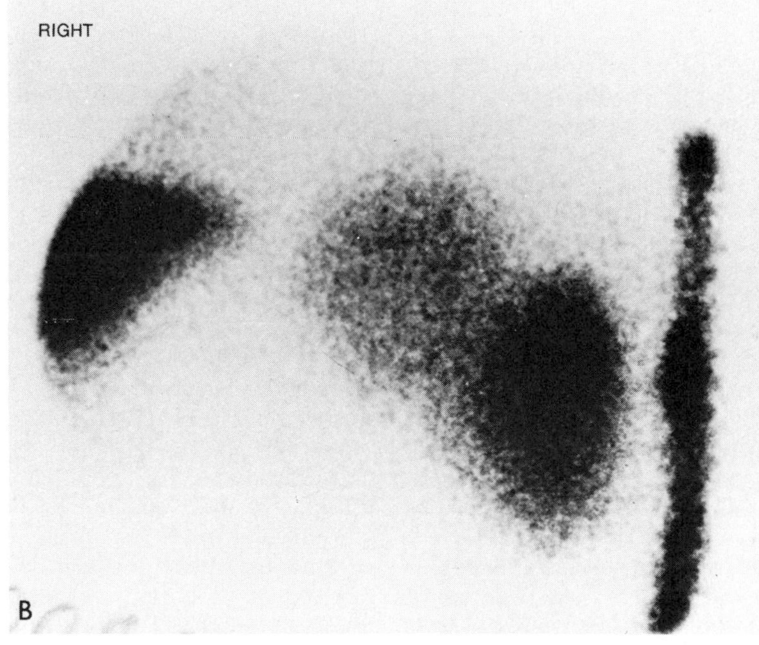

Figure 9–9. Splenic laceration in a 24-year-old man with left upper quadrant pain following an auto accident. *A*, Technetium 99m colloid scan obtained posteriorly with the patient lying on his left side shows irregularity in the lateral contour of the spleen. *B*, Anterior scan with the patient supine and with a linear radioactive marker over the lateral abdominal wall shows diminished activity in the superior half of the spleen and displacement of the superior half of the spleen away from the lateral abdominal wall. At surgery a laceration was present, coursing obliquely through the midportion of the spleen. The superior half of the spleen was contused and surrounded by a subcapsular hematoma.

the presence of a hematoma, either beneath the capsule or outside the capsule in the peritoneal cavity. Intrasplenic or intrahepatic hematoma can be identified as a round area of absent activity within the organ. Contusion causes diminished activity in the affected portion of the organ.

Radionuclide scanning of the liver and spleen is a highly accurate means of identifying clinically significant injuries, if the patient is sufficiently mobile to be scanned in multiple projections. In a review of 162 patients examined for possible liver injuries, Gilday and Alderson (1974) reported no known false-negative scans, although two of the 17 positive scans were false-positive. In the same review, of 136 negative spleen scans, only two were proved to be false-negative, and of 69 positive scans, five were false-positive.

Selective hepatic or splenic angiography should be considered if the radionuclide scan is inconclusive or conflicts with clinical findings. The most specific angiographic sign of splenic or hepatic injury is extravasation of contrast medium (Fig. 9–10). Other signs include: (1) single or multiple irregular lucencies in the parenchymal phase of the arteriogram, (2) stretching and displacement of intrasplenic or intrahepatic arteries, (3) premature venous opacification, and (4) discontinuity of the hepatic or splenic contour (Lim et al., 1972). Normal splenic lobulations due to invagination of the capsule may produce irregularity of the splenic contour and simulate splenic laceration on a radionuclide scan or an arteriogram. However, lobulation can be distinguished by arteriography, since the splenic parenchyma is dense and sharply marginated on both sides of the capsular invagination, whereas the margins of the spleen adjacent to a laceration are irregular and lack sharp definition.

Subcapsular hematomas displace the liver or the spleen away from the lateral or posterior abdominal wall. This may be the only angiographic sign of injury, especially if angiography is delayed beyond the first few days after injury (Fig. 9–11). When no abnormality is identified in the frontal projection, angiographic injection should be repeated in the right posterior oblique projection if splenic injury is suspected, and in the left posterior oblique projection if hepatic injury is suspected (Lepasoon and Olin, 1971).

Computerized tomography had only limited application in the evaluation of thoracic and abdominal trauma patients until the recent introduction of a new-generation machine with scanning times of only a few seconds. Since prolonged suspension of respiration is not necessary with short scan times, highly detailed and accurate CT images of thoracic and abdominal viscera have radically altered the diagnostic approach to traumatized patients. CT permits examination of multiple organs including the brain, spine, and viscera of the thorax, abdomen, and pelvis within a relatively short time. In a recent retrospective analysis of 250 patients with abdominal trauma examined by CT, injuries to the spleen, liver, pancreas, and kidneys were demonstrated with greater accuracy and better anatomic detail than by radionuclide scan, and without the discomfort and potential morbidity of angiography (Federle, 1981). CT clearly demonstrates intraperitoneal or retroperitoneal hematomas, which may be difficult to diagnose by angiography or radionuclide scanning (Mall and Kaiser, 1980). Prospective studies of the efficacy of CT in patients with abdominal trauma are under way, but results to date suggest that CT should be the primary diagnostic procedure in patients with abdominal trauma whose clinical condition does not require immediate surgical intervention, or in patients who, following surgery, have evidence of undetected injury. The results of CT examination may alter the surgical approach, may direct exploration toward the most severe or clinically significant injury, or may indicate the absence of significant injury, thus rendering exploratory surgery unnecessary.

UPPER GASTROINTESTINAL HEMORRHAGE

Gastrointestinal hemorrhage is a severe, frequently lethal complication that occurs with dismaying frequency in the ICU. Massive, life-threatening hemorrhage from acute gastritis has a reported incidence of 5 per cent among patients in surgical ICUs (Bogoch, 1976; Skillman et al., 1969). Gastrointestinal bleeding occurs in 20 to 25 per cent of patients with acute respiratory failure (Harris et al., 1976; Khan and Seriff, 1976). Approximately one half require at least two unit transfusions, and this group has a mortality greater than 50 per cent.

Severe upper gastrointestinal hemorrhage may also result from esophagitis, gastric or duodenal ulcer, and esophageal varices. Acute gastritis and esophagitis are diffuse mucosal diseases that cause arterial bleeding from multiple sites of surface inflammation. These lesions are associated with increased acid levels and

Text continued on page 192

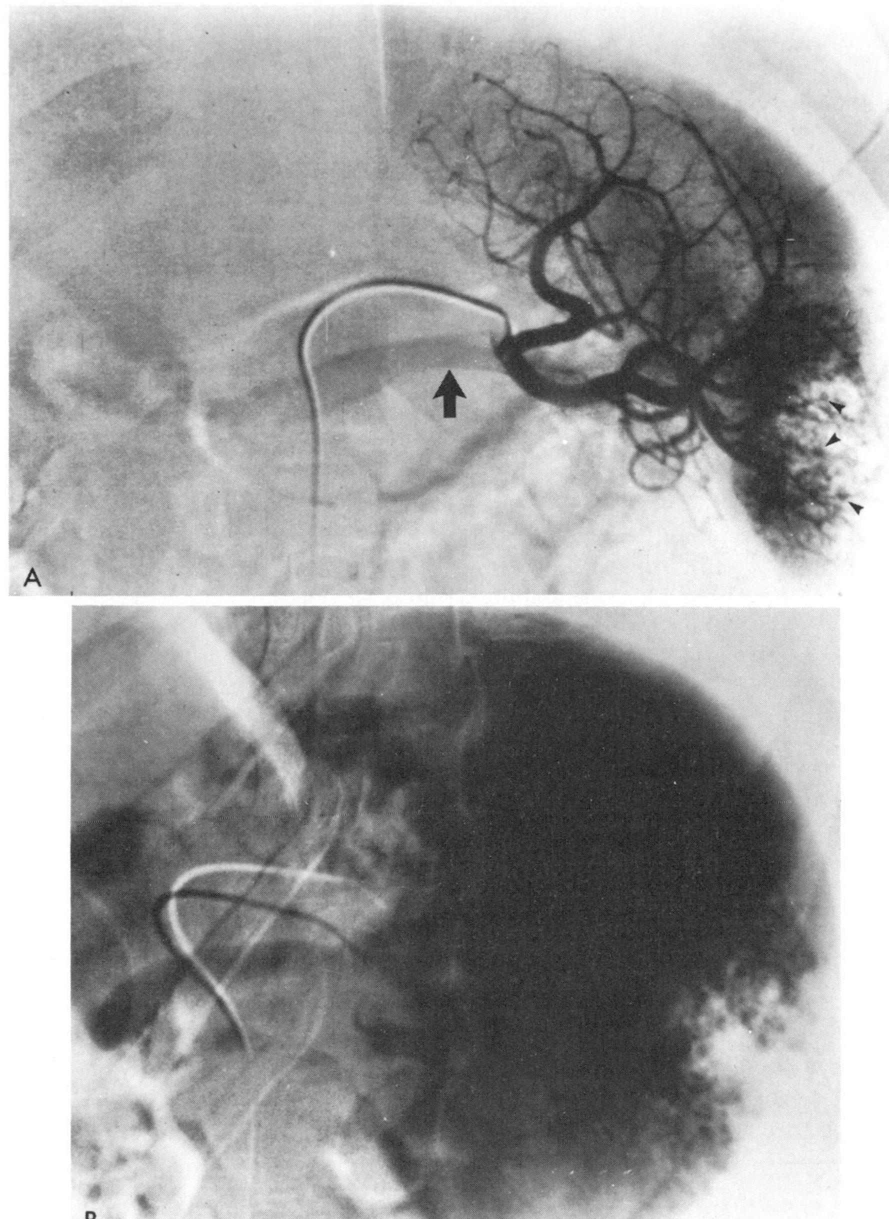

Figure 9–10. Splenic laceration in a 17-year-old boy who was involved in a motorcycle accident. Vital signs were stable. The patient had left upper quadrant pain and tenderness. Plain abdominal radiography showed a posterolateral fracture of the left tenth rib. *A*, Splenic arteriogram in the frontal projection shows punctate sites of active extravasation of contrast medium (*arrowheads*) in the lower pole of the spleen. Parenchymal lucency in the same area represents an intrasplenic hematoma. Premature opacification of the splenic vein (*arrow*) indicates intrasplenic arteriovenous communication. *B*, Subtraction print from the parenchymal phase in the right posterior oblique projection again shows the rounded intrasplenic hematoma. In this projection the x-ray beam is tangent to the hematoma, and the contour of the hematoma appears to extend beyond the capsule of the spleen, suggesting that the capsule may have ruptured. Arteriovenous communication and probable rupture through the splenic capsule precluded conservative therapy, and splenectomy was performed.

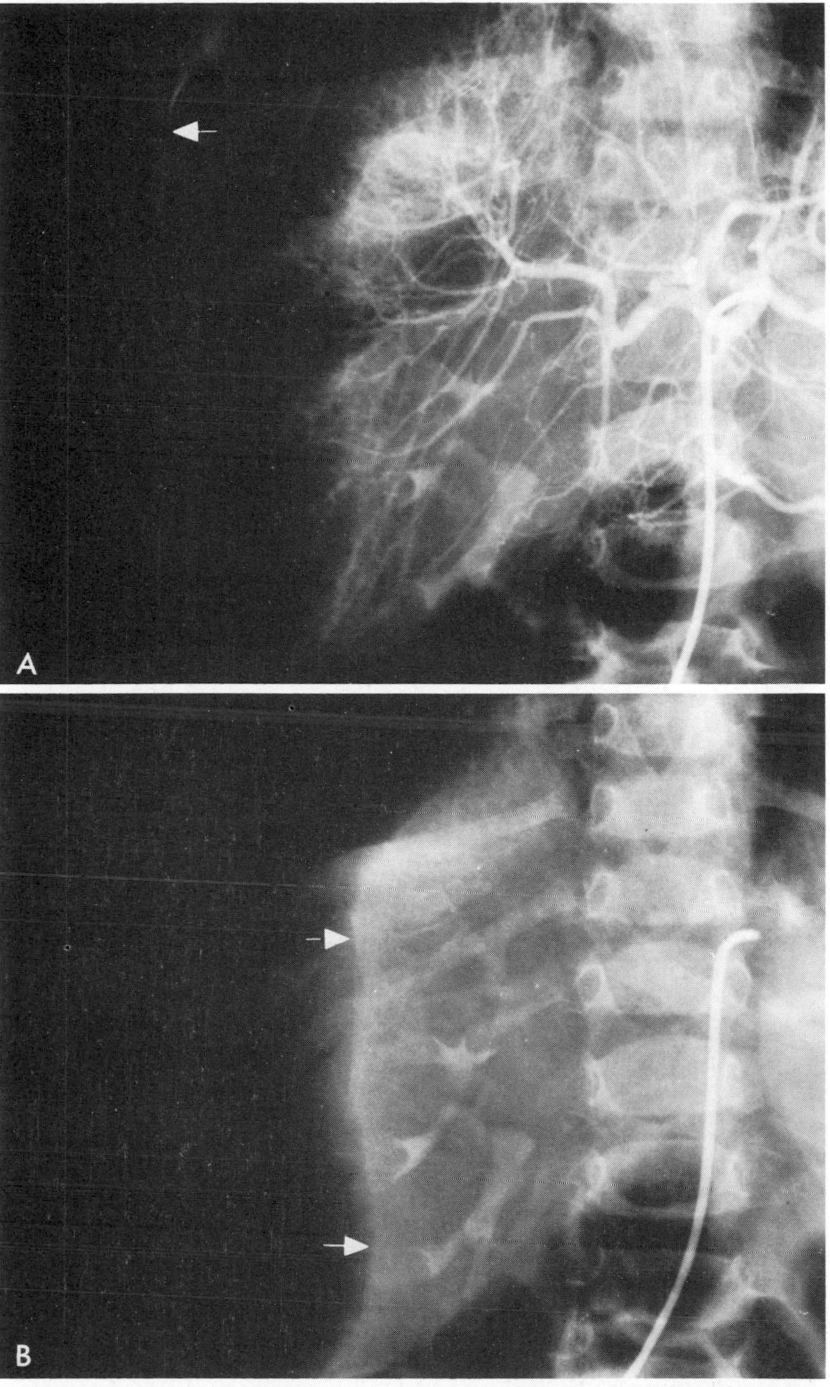

Figure 9–11. Subcapsular hematoma of the liver in a 13-month-old battered child with a palpable right upper quadrant mass. *A*, Celiac axis arteriogram shows displacement of the hepatic arteries from the right flank (*arrow*) by an avascular mass. *B*, In the parenchymal phase, the margin of the opacified liver (*arrows*) can be identified. There is no evidence of an intrahepatic hematoma. The sharp edge of the periphery of the liver indicates that the mass is subcapsular or extracapsular rather than intrahepatic. At surgery a large subcapsular hematoma was evacuated.

may result from physiologic stress (Valencia-Parparcen, 1976). Penetrating gastric and duodenal ulcers bleed massively when large submucosal arteries are eroded, and local, noninvasive measures are seldom effective in controlling such hemorrhage. Varices that bleed are located in the submucosa of the stomach and esophagus. Although venous, the large volume of blood and the high pressure within the varices frequently preclude local control by ice water lavage or compression with a Sengstaken-Blakemore tube.

Since each of these lesions may require a different form of therapy, the cause and the site of bleeding must be established. Direct visualization of the mucosal surface of the esophagus, stomach, and duodenum by means of endoscopy is the most effective first step in obtaining this information. Endoscopy in experienced hands can be performed safely and rapidly. In most cases, the endoscopist can precisely localize the source of bleeding and can differentiate between mucosal erosion, penetrating peptic ulcer, and esophageal varices. Even when endoscopy is unsuccessful in identifying the specific cause and site of bleeding, the endoscopist can usually localize the bleeding to the distribution of a single artery, simplifying subsequent angiography.

If endoscopy fails to document the cause and site of bleeding, angiography should be performed for definitive diagnosis. Angiographic demonstration of contrast medium extravasation identifies arterial bleeding. Extravasated contrast medium appears in the arterial phase, and on serial films remains opaque through the parenchymal and venous phases of the arteriogram. The location of the extravasation, the site of the vessel from which extravasation arises, and the number of sites of extravasation all provide information on the nature of the lesion. Hemorrhage from chronic, penetrating ulcer arises from a single large artery, and extravasation accumulates within the crater. The extravasated contrast medium assumes the shape of the ulcer crater, and is most commonly on the lesser curvature of the gastric antrum or in the duodenum (Fig. 9–12). In acute mucosal dis-

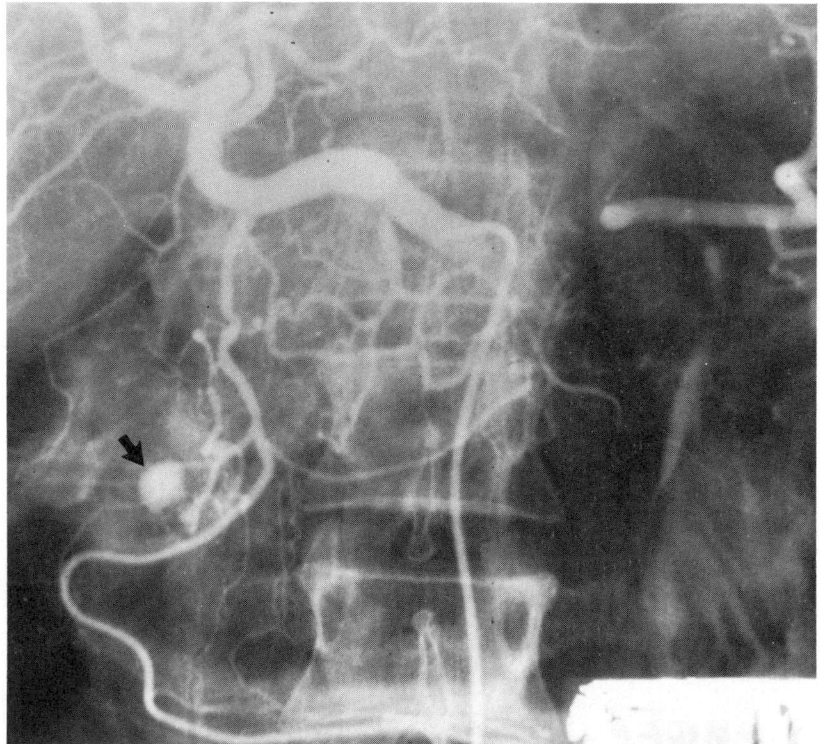

Figure 9–12. Penetrating duodenal ulcer in a 48-year-old man with acute upper gastrointestinal hemorrhage. Endoscopy could not be performed. In the early arterial phase of a common hepatic artery injection, extravasation (*arrow*) is present in the descending portion of the duodenum. The extravasation arises from a primary branch of the gastroduodenal artery. Only a single site of extravasation is present. The extravasation is dense and round, suggesting accumulation within an ulcer crater. The patient was taken to surgery, where the ulcer was oversewn and pyloroplasty and vagotomy were performed.

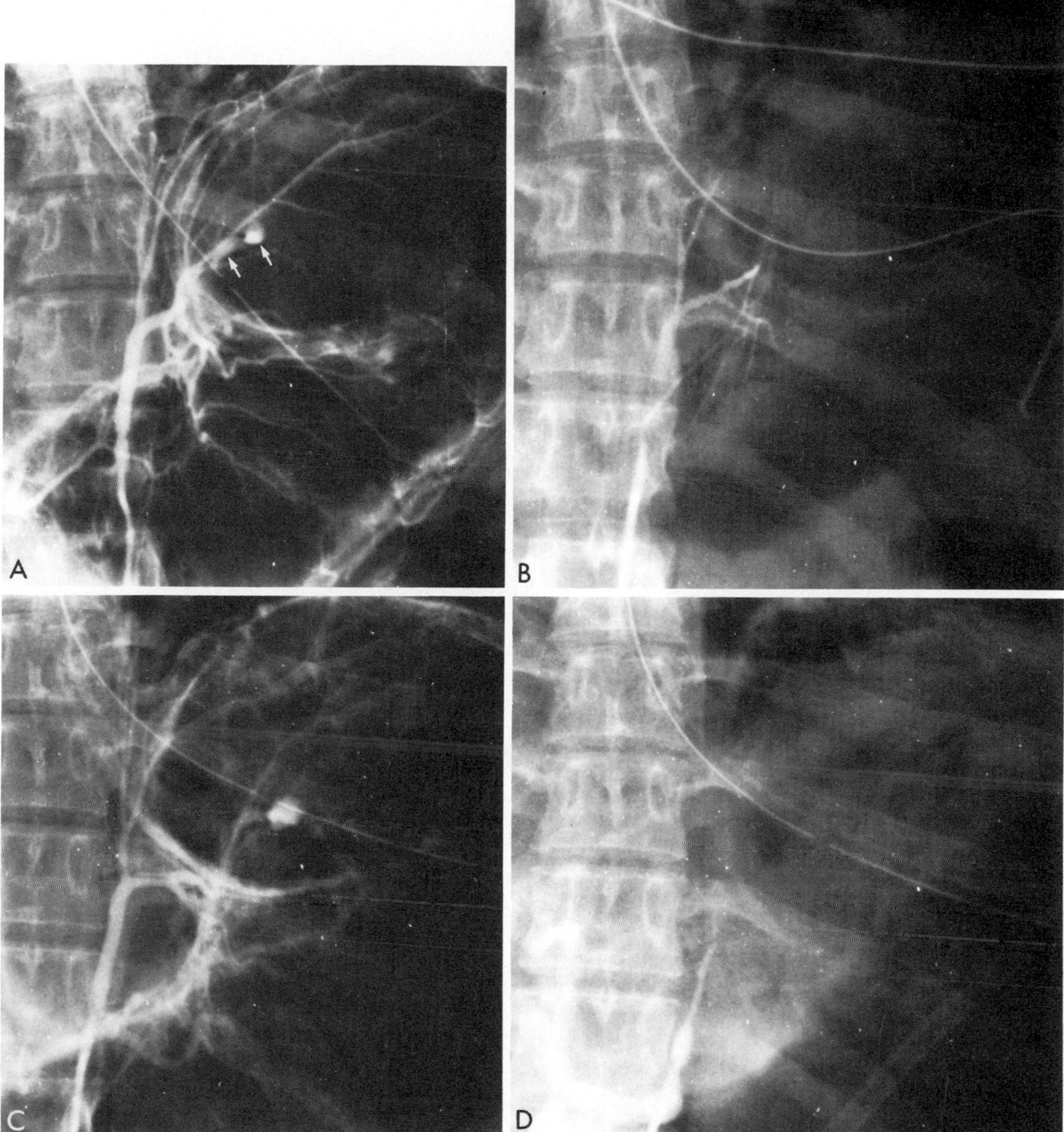

Figure 9–13. Stress ulcer in a 24-year-old woman in the surgical ICU under therapy for ascending cholangitis following cholecystectomy. Sudden, massive upper gastrointestinal hemorrhage developed. Endoscopy documented acute gastritis in the fundus of the stomach. *A*, Selective left gastric arteriography shows extravasation (*arrows*) into the fundus of the stomach in the midarterial phase. The absence of sharp margins in the extravasated contrast medium suggests that the contrast medium is not collecting within ulcer craters. These findings support the endoscopic diagnosis of gastritis. Vasopressin was infused into the left gastric artery at a rate of 0.2 units per minute. *B*, After 30 minutes, a repeat left gastric arteriogram shows intense constriction of the left gastric artery and its branches and no further extravasation. The nasogastric aspirate demonstrated that the gastric bleeding had ceased, and vasopressin infusion was continued. Twenty-four hours later, gastric hemorrhage recurred and was not controlled, even though the infusion rate of vasopressin was increased to 0.4 units per minute. *C*, Arteriographic injection shows that the left gastric artery and its branches have returned to their normal caliber in spite of the continued vasopressin infusion, and contrast medium again extravasates in the fundus. Small emboli were then injected through the arterial catheter. *D*, Following embolization, the left gastric artery and its branches have been obstructed. No further contrast medium extravasates. At this time the nasogastric aspirate confirmed that bleeding had stopped. Gastroscopy seven days later documented that the gastritis had healed. No mucosal abnormality was present to suggest either inflammation or ischemia.

Text continued on page 196

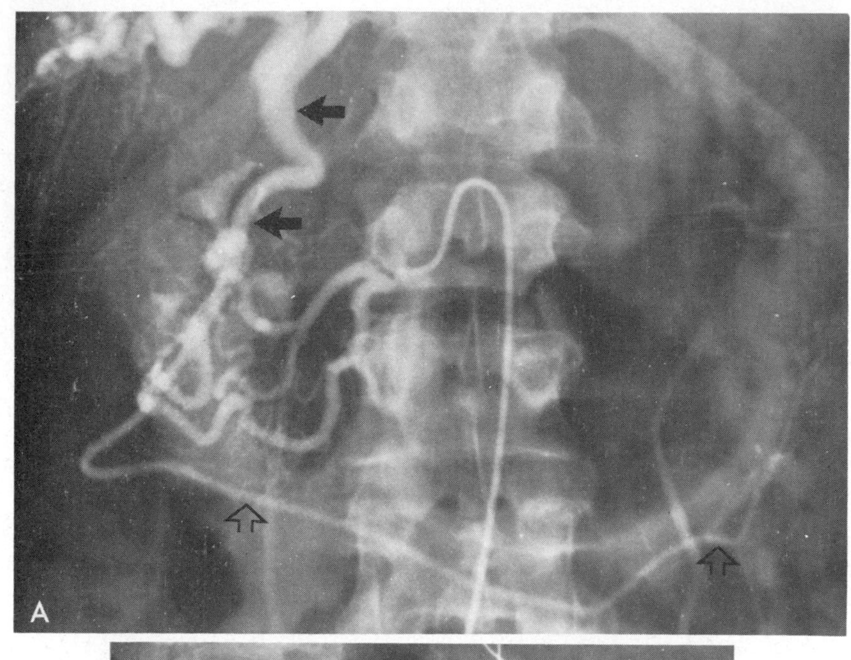
A

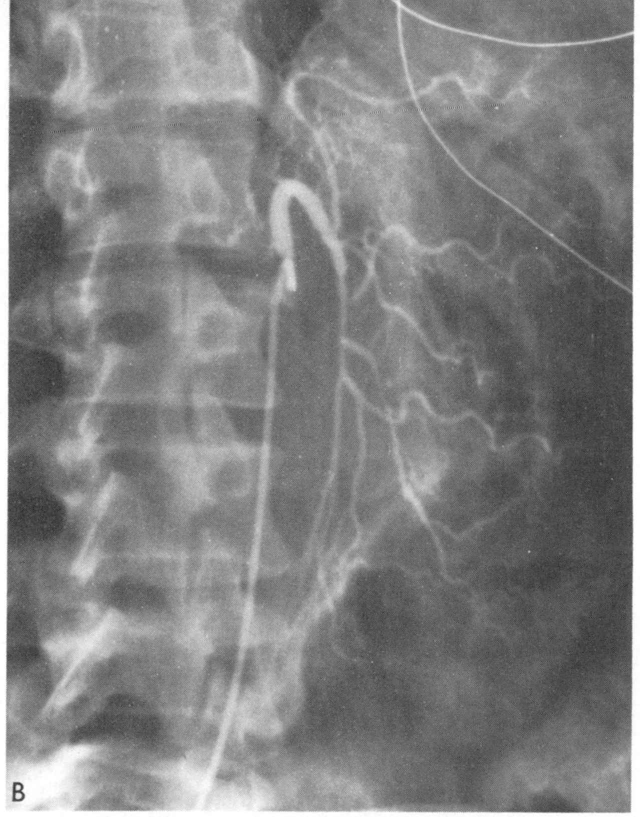
B

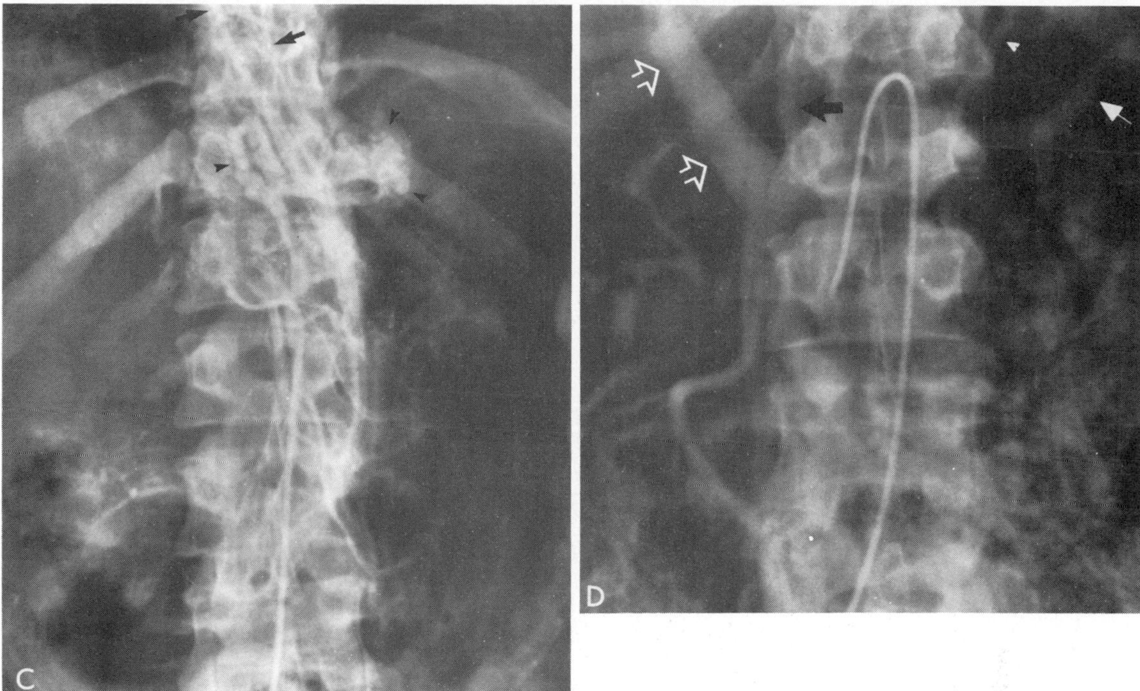

Figure 9–14. Angiographic diagnosis of portal hypertension and bleeding from esophageal varices. A 34-year-old chronic alcoholic presented with massive upper gastrointestinal hemorrhage. Neither cirrhosis nor portal hypertension had been previously documented, and on physical examination neither the liver nor the spleen was enlarged. Endoscopy was unsuccessful because of the patient's inability to cooperate. *A*, The arteries that supply the duodenum were selectively injected to exclude the possibility of a hemorrhagic duodenal ulcer. The arteries that supply the greater curvature of the stomach and the duodenum can be selectively injected by catheterization from above via the hepatic artery, or from below via the superior mesenteric artery. In this case, the inferior pancreatic arcade was catheterized via the superior mesenteric artery. Injection opacifies the gastroduodenal artery (*solid arrows*), which supplies the duodenum, and the right gastroepiploic artery (*open arrows*), which supplies the greater curvature of the stomach. No extravasation is present. *B*, Selective injection of the left gastric artery opacifies the arterial supply to the lesser curvature and fundus of the stomach and to the distal esophagus. Again, no extravasation is present, although nasogastric aspiration immediately after the injection documented that active hemorrhage was continuing. The absence of extravasation in the presence of demonstrated active bleeding indicates that the cause of bleeding is not arterial hemorrhage from gastritis, esophagitis, a gastric ulcer, or a mucosal tear. *C*, Venous phase of the selective left gastric arteriogram shows gastric varices (*arrowheads*). In the absence of portal hypertension, gastric veins drain inferiorly to opacify the portal vein. In this case the portal vein is not opacified. Instead, contrast medium in the gastric veins crosses superiorly to opacify the esophageal venous plexus (*arrows*). Reverse flow in the gastric veins indicates portal hypertension. The portal and mesenteric venous system was then investigated by selectively injecting the superior mesenteric artery. *D*, Venous phase of the superior mesenteric arteriogram shows the splenic vein (*white arrow*), a short gastric vein (*white arrowhead*), and the coronary vein (*black arrow*), as well as the portal vein (*white open arrows*). Contrast medium injected into the superior mesenteric artery should opacify only the superior mesenteric veins and their normal drainage pathway, the portal vein. Opacification of the splenic, short gastric, and coronary veins indicates that some of the mesenteric venous blood is being diverted away from the liver and into the azygous venous system by way of splenic, gastric, and esophageal collaterals. Diversion of blood from the portal vein occurs only in portal hypertension. The absence of arterial extravasation, the documentation of portal hypertension, and the demonstration of gastric and esophageal varices during an episode of active, massive bleeding indicates that the hemorrhage arises from gastric or esophageal varices. Vasopressin was infused into the superior mesenteric artery, and within 30 minutes the nasogastric aspirate cleared. Three weeks later a portacaval shunt was surgically created to decompress the portal system and prevent recurrence of variceal hemorrhage.

eases, hemorrhage arises from more peripheral arteries in single or multiple sites, usually in the distal esophagus or the gastric fundus (Fig. 9–13). The number of extravasation sites and the location of the extravasation suggest the underlying disease. Since no ulcer crater is present in these superficial diseases, the contrast medium that extravasates does not have a rounded, sharply marginated contour. Thus, the appearance of extravasated contrast medium distinguishes mucosal diseases that are associated with stress from other causes of bleeding. If extravasation is not identified, the diagnosis of gastritis can be suggested by a dense mucosal blush (Athanasoulis et al., 1974).

Extravasation from a single, large, submucosal artery due to erosion by a penetrating gastric or duodenal ulcer may be identified on aortic injections, and is nearly always identified on celiac artery injections. Since extravasation due to esophagitis, gastritis, or mucosal laceration (Mallory-Weiss tear) arises from more peripheral vessels and is less well localized, selective left gastric or gastroduodenal artery injections are frequently necessary. If the nasogastric tube is not returning bright-red blood at the time of the arteriogram, it is unlikely that extravasation will be demonstrated.

If no arterial extravasation is present during selective injections, and yet the nasogastric tube demonstrates that the patient is still actively bleeding during the injection, venous bleeding must be considered. Since venous extravasation is rarely recognized angiographically, the diagnosis of bleeding esophageal varices can be made only indirectly by angiography. The diagnosis is assumed if, while the nasogastric aspirate documents continued active upper gastrointestinal tract hemorrhage, gastric or esophageal varices are demonstrated and no extravasation occurs during selective injection of the appropriate artery (Fig. 9–14) (Baum and Nusbaum, 1971; Rosch et al., 1971).

Once the diagnosis is established, several therapeutic alternatives are available for each type of lesion. Vasoconstrictor infusion or embolization is preferable to surgery for hemorrhage resulting from mucosal lesions such as gastritis and esophagitis. Mortality of 30 to 50 per cent has been reported following emergency surgery for these lesions, and the incidence of recurrent bleeding following surgery is high (Byrne and Guardione, 1973; Drapanas et al., 1971; Welch, 1973). Left gastric artery catheterization and vasopressin infusion have controlled arterial hemorrhage resulting from gastritis and esophagitis in 80 to 85 per cent of cases (Athanasoulis et al., 1974; White et al., 1974). Intravenous vasopressin infusion, although much simpler than arterial infusion, frequently fails to control arterial hemorrhage (Thomson and Goldin, 1979). For those patients in whom selective arterial vasoconstrictor infusion is not successful, the bleeding can be controlled by embolization of the left gastric artery through the arterial catheter (Reuter et al., 1975).

The most commonly used vasoconstrictor for intra-arterial infusion is vasopressin. A dose of 0.1 to 0.4 unit per minute is infused. In arterial bleeding, vasopressin infusion is most reliable when the catheter is selectively placed in the artery from which extravasation arises, usually the left gastric artery or the gastroduodenal artery (Fig. 9–13*B*). If these arteries cannot be selectively catheterized, less selective infusion into the celiac axis may be successful. Laboratory and clinical investigations have shown that vasopressin infused into the celiac axis does not compromise hepatic arterial blood flow (White et al., 1974).

Following a 10- to 20-minute intra-arterial vasopressin infusion, the arteriogram is repeated. The arterial and parenchymal phases are carefully analyzed, and the infusion rate is adjusted to a dosage level at which there is no further arterial extravasation but at which the parenchymal blush of the stomach is preserved. At this infusion rate, hemorrhage usually remains controlled and the likelihood of ischemic complications is minimized. The infusion rate should not exceed 0.4 unit of vasopressin per minute. Higher rates of infusion are seldom effective in controlling hemorrhage that cannot be controlled by a lower infusion rate, and the frequency of ischemic complications is considerably increased (Athanasoulis et al., 1976).

Systemic effects of vasopressin infusion at these dosage levels seldom present a serious problem if blood pressure, electrocardiogram (ECG), and urinary output are carefully monitored and if systemic side effects are promptly treated. Arterial infusion of vasopressin should be continued for 48 hours. If the bleeding remains controlled, the initial infusion rate should be continued for 12 hours and then reduced by 50 per cent. The infusion rate is then gradually reduced to zero by 48 hours. The catheter is left in place for an additional 24 hours and is kept open with D5W or saline solution. If no further bleeding occurs, the catheter can then be removed.

Systemic blood levels gradually rise during intra-arterial infusion, and cardiac output is reduced by an average of 15 to 20 per cent (Athanasoulis et al., 1976). The infusion should be slowed or stopped if ECG changes, bradycardia, hypertension, or signs of visceral ischemia occur. In most cases, these changes are rapidly reversible and the infusion can be restarted at a lower dosage level in 30 to 60 minutes. Decreased urinary output or electrolyte imbalance due to the antidiuretic hormone (ADH) effect of vasopressin is treated with diuretics (Athanasoulis et al., 1976). A tunnel device should be placed beneath the ICU patient in his bed to permit portable radiographs of the abdomen to be taken without moving the patient. In this way, the position of the catheter can be documented frequently during the infusion by injecting a few milliliters of contrast medium while a portable radiograph is exposed.

The most serious complication of intra-arterial vasoconstrictor infusion is bowel infarction. Several cases have been reported of infarction of the entire small bowel following vasopressin infusion into the superior mesenteric artery. However, in these cases, the vasoconstrictor infusion was not initiated until late in the course of the hemorrhage, and infarction was probably influenced by prolonged splanchnic shock as well as vasopressin infusion (Renert et al., 1972). The frequency of this complication can be minimized by instituting diagnostic and therapeutic procedures as soon as possible after the onset of bleeding.

Arterial embolization for control of hemorrhage should be reserved for those patients in whom arterial vasopressin infusion fails (Figs. 9–13, 9–15). A number of embolic agents may be effective, depending on the specific problem, but the simplest and safest material for most clinical problems is surgical gelatin (Gelfoam). This material, used safely for many years during surgical procedures, is cut into tiny pledgets, which are injected through a selectively placed arteriographic catheter to obstruct the bleeding artery and achieve hemostasis. Although limited mucosal sloughing is frequently visible by endoscopy following embolization of arteries in the stomach or duodenum, the incidence of clinically significant infarction is low (Bookstein et al., 1974; Reuter et al., 1975). Nonetheless, the frequency of ischemic complications is probably higher than with vasoconstrictor infusion, since embolization completely removes the local arterial supply.

Surgery is the treatment of choice for hemorrhage from peptic ulcers. Surgical therapy controls hemorrhage, provides long-term control of gastric hyperacidity, and offers an acceptably low mortality. If surgery is contraindicated because of concurrent disease, angiographic therapy may be attempted. Intra-arterial infusion of vasoconstrictors is successful in controlling hemorrhage in only about half of the patients with peptic ulcer (Athanasoulis et al., 1976; Brant et al., 1972). Selective injection of emboli through the angiographic catheter into the bleeding artery is more often successful (Fig. 9–15), but has greater risk (Bookstein et al., 1974; Prochaska et al., 1973). Therefore, as with gastritis, arterial embolization should be reserved for those patients in whom hemorrhage does not respond to vasoconstrictor infusion.

Hemorrhage from gastric or esophageal varices is definitively treated by the surgical creation of a portal-to-systemic venous shunt. When shunt procedures are performed as an emergency, however, mortality is prohibitively high (Edmondson et al., 1971; Welch, 1973). Several techniques have proved useful for arresting hemorrhage from varices, providing time for therapy of concurrent disease so that definitive surgery can be performed as an elective procedure, with a considerably reduced mortality rate (Welch, 1973). The simplest of these is intravenous infusion of vasopressin. In clinical trials, this technique has achieved a success rate comparable to that of intra-arterial infusion (Athanasoulis et al., 1976; Chojkier et al., 1979; Conn et al., 1972). If the diagnosis of variceal bleeding can be established by endoscopy, no further diagnostic procedure is necessary.

The dosage for IV infusion in cases of hemorrhage from gastric or esophageal varices, is 0.2 to 0.4 unit per minute. At this low dose, continuous IV infusion is not associated with tachyphylaxis and the systemic side effects are usually well tolerated. The systemic vasopressin levels are similar to those measured during intra-arterial infusion, and the decrease in cardiac output is also similar. Superior mesenteric arterial blood flow and portal pressure are both reduced by an average of 50 per cent, which is close to the reduction achieved by the same dose of vasopressin in the superior mesenteric artery (Athanasoulis et al., 1976).

Occasionally, hemorrhage from varices that cannot be controlled by IV vasoconstrictor infusion does respond to direct intra-arterial infusion, presumably because the drug reaching the peripheral mesenteric arteries is more concentrated (Athanasoulis et al., 1976). Infusion of vasopressin into the superior mesenteric artery via an angiographic catheter controls bleeding in 50 to 75 per cent of patients (Athanasoulis

Text continued on page 200

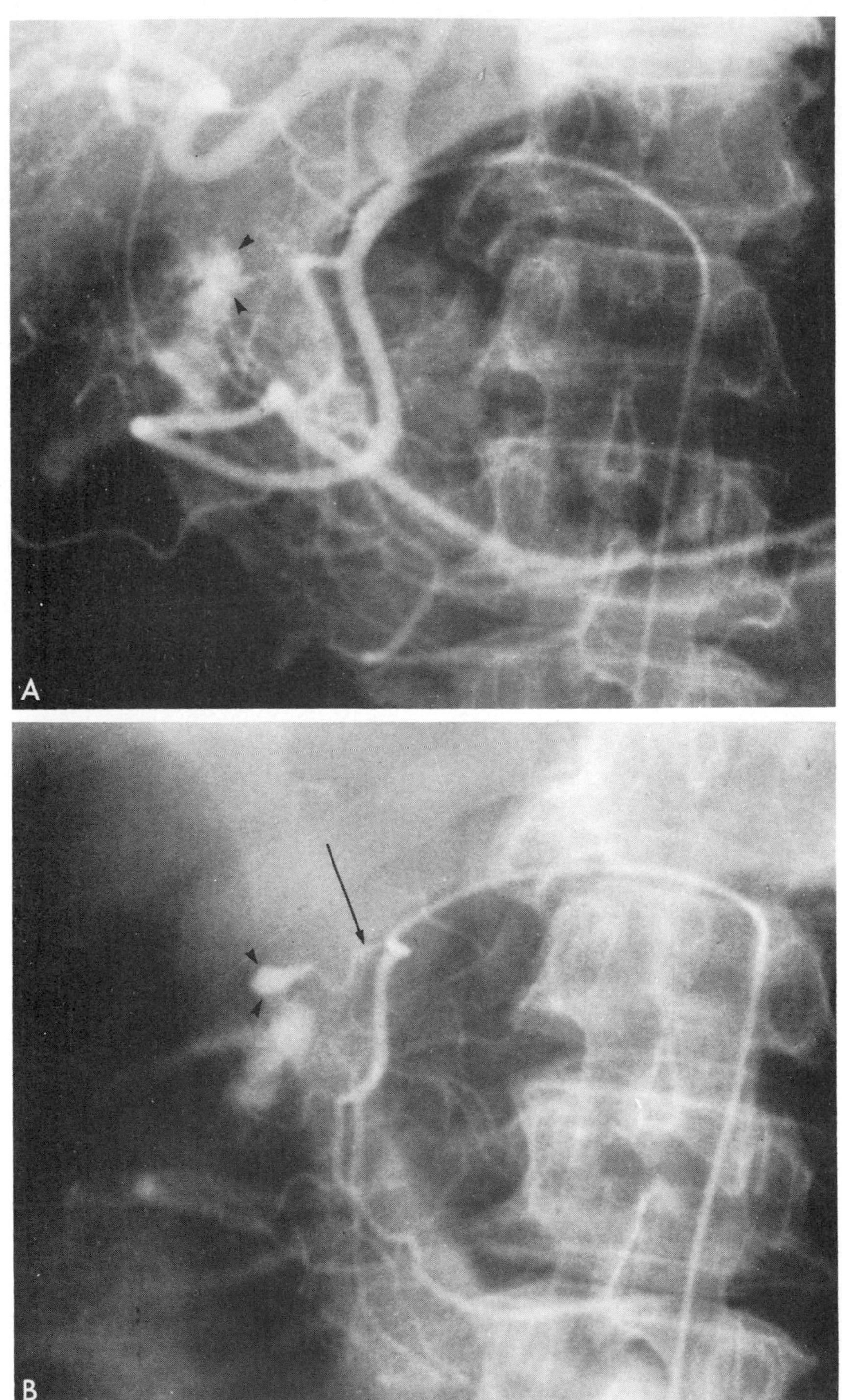
A
B

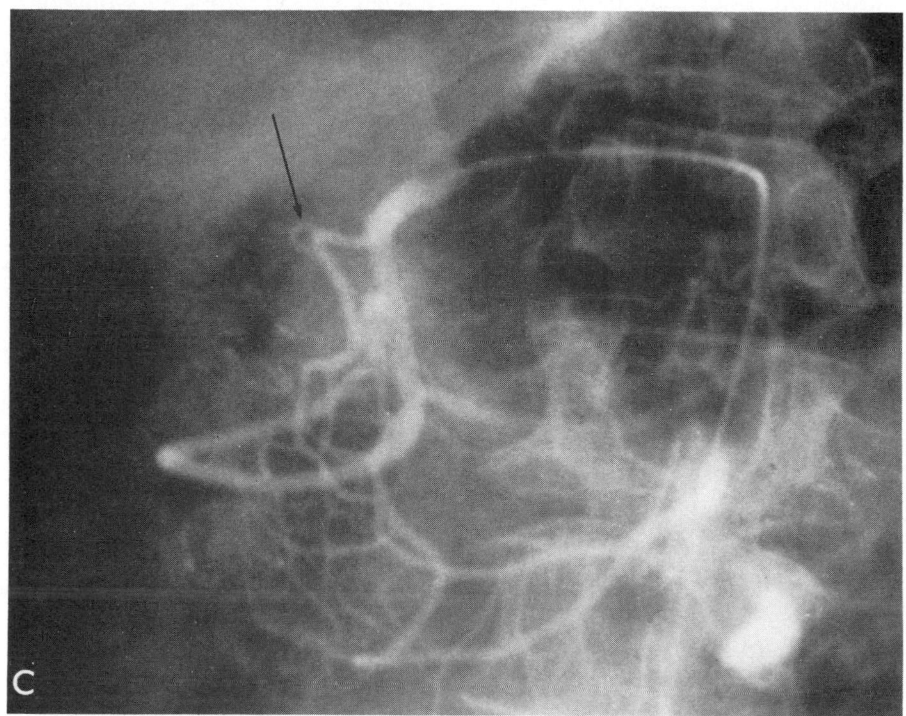

Figure 9–15. Angiographic control of hemorrhage arising from a duodenal ulcer in a 59-year-old man with hepatitis and respiratory distress syndrome. Endoscopy was performed shortly after the onset of hematemesis. Endoscopic lavage cleared the esophagus of blood sufficiently to permit visualization of normal esophageal mucosa and documentation of the absence of esophageal varices. Large clots and rapidly accumulating fresh blood precluded endoscopic visualization of the mucosa in the gastric antrum and duodenum, but the gastric fundus and body were more readily cleared by lavage, and the mucosa was normal. Thus, although endoscopy could not establish the diagnosis, endoscopic examination suggested that the hemorrhage probably originated from the distribution of the gastroduodenal artery. *A*, Via hepatic artery catheterization, a selective gastroduodenal arteriogram shows extravasation in the descending duodenum (*arrowheads*). The location of the hemorrhage and the appearance of the extravasation in subsequent radiographs suggest the diagnosis of peptic ulcer. Surgery was contraindicated because of concurrent disease. *B*, Vasopressin was infused into the gastroduodenal artery, but a repeat arteriogram after 30 minutes shows persistent extravasation (*arrowheads*) although the arteries have become markedly constricted. The catheter was then advanced into the small duodenal branch from which the hemorrhage arose (*arrow*) and a small Gelfoam pledget was injected. *C*, The catheter was withdrawn into the gastroduodenal artery and injection shows no further extravasation. Only a small proximal segment of the artery from which the hemorrhage arose is opacified (*arrow*). The remainder of the artery has been obstructed by the embolus. Because the embolus was selectively placed into the bleeding artery, the uninvolved gastroduodenal artery branches remain intact. The nasogastric aspirate promptly cleared. Medical therapy for peptic ulcer disease was initiated, and no further gastrointestinal hemorrhage occurred during the patient's hospitalization.

et al., 1976; Chojkier et al., 1979; Conn et al., 1972). Since the superior mesenteric artery is the arterial source of more than half of the blood flow that reaches the portal vein, reduction of the superior mesenteric arterial flow decreases the volume of blood reaching the portal circulation and lowers the portal pressure. Vasoconstrictor infusion into the superior mesenteric artery reduces portal pressure by approximately 50 per cent without critically compromising circulation to the bowel (Athanasoulis et al., 1976). For superior mesenteric arterial infusion in variceal bleeding, vasopressin is infused at the same rate as in arterial bleeding—0.1 to 0.4 unit per minute. Gastric lavage is performed after 30 minutes of infusion to document that hemorrhage has stopped. The arteriogram is repeated to demonstrate that arterial constriction has indeed been accomplished and that the mucosal blush of the bowel is preserved at the chosen infusion rate.

Hemorrhage from varices can also be controlled by direct embolization or sclerosis of the bleeding veins. Although this technique is newer and less widely used than arterial or venous vasopressin infusion, results to date suggest that obliteration of varices controls bleeding even in patients in whom vasopressin therapy has failed, and also reduces the frequency of early rebleeding (Pereiras et al., 1977).

Two nonsurgical methods are available by which varices can be directly obliterated. By means of an endoscope, submucosal injection of a sclerosing agent into the esophagus near the visible bleeding varix results in immediate obstruction of the varix and development of fibrosis of the esophageal wall. When feasible, the method in experienced hands is safe, rapid, and effective (Terblanche et al., 1979). It may not be feasible if the rate and volume of bleeding preclude adequate visualization of the esophageal wall or if bleeding arises from gastric varices.

The other method requires transhepatic catheterization of the portal vein, using the fluoroscopic and needle-guidewire catheter techniques described earlier for catheterization of the intrahepatic biliary system. Once the catheter enters the portal system, it is manipulated through the portal vein into the splenic vein. Contrast medium injection and serial, rapid-sequence filming demonstrate the coronary vein, short gastric veins, and all other portal-systemic venous collaterals, and document the degree to which portal venous flow to the liver is compromised. Direct portal, splenic, and mesenteric pressure measurements also provide helpful prognostic information. Some or all of the varices, depending on joint surgical, medical, and radiologic judgment, are selectively embolized (Fig. 9–16).

Transhepatic embolization of varices, although a more time-consuming and more complex procedure than endoscopic sclerosis of varices, provides considerable diagnostic information that is not otherwise available and permits more complete obliteration of the network of varices (Widrich et al., 1978). Demonstration of the size and location of the splenic, portal, and mesenteric veins; demonstration of the collateral flow patterns before and after embolization; and measurement of pressure contribute significantly to analysis of the potential risks and benefits of surgical creation of a portal-systemic shunt in each patient, and to the choice of the most appropriate shunt procedure.

MESENTERIC INFARCTION

Acute mesenteric ischemia is a major complication of cardiac, vascular, and systemic diseases associated with hypotension. Improvements in the therapy of critically ill patients have prolonged survival and led to an increase in the frequency of this and other complications. In spite of significant advances in our understanding of mesenteric ischemia, the diagnosis frequently remains elusive until infarction is manifest (Boley et al., 1973; Britt and Cheek, 1969). Reduction of the incidence of bowel infarction and associated mortality can be anticipated only if the complication is suspected early in its course; once suspicion has been raised, an aggressive diagnostic approach is required.

Mesenteric ischemia that results from mechanical occlusion of an artery is a well-known complication of atrial fibrillation, bacterial endocarditis, and other cardiac and arterial disorders. The frequency of mesenteric ischemia resulting from a low-flow syndrome without arterial or venous occlusion has only in recent years been appreciated. This mechanism may account for up to half of mesenteric vascular complications (Williams, 1971).

Nonocclusive mesenteric ischemia is believed to result from splanchnic vasoconstriction in response to decreased cardiac output, hypovolemia, vasopressor administration, or shock. Splanchnic vasoconstriction permits maximal perfusion of vital organs such as the heart,

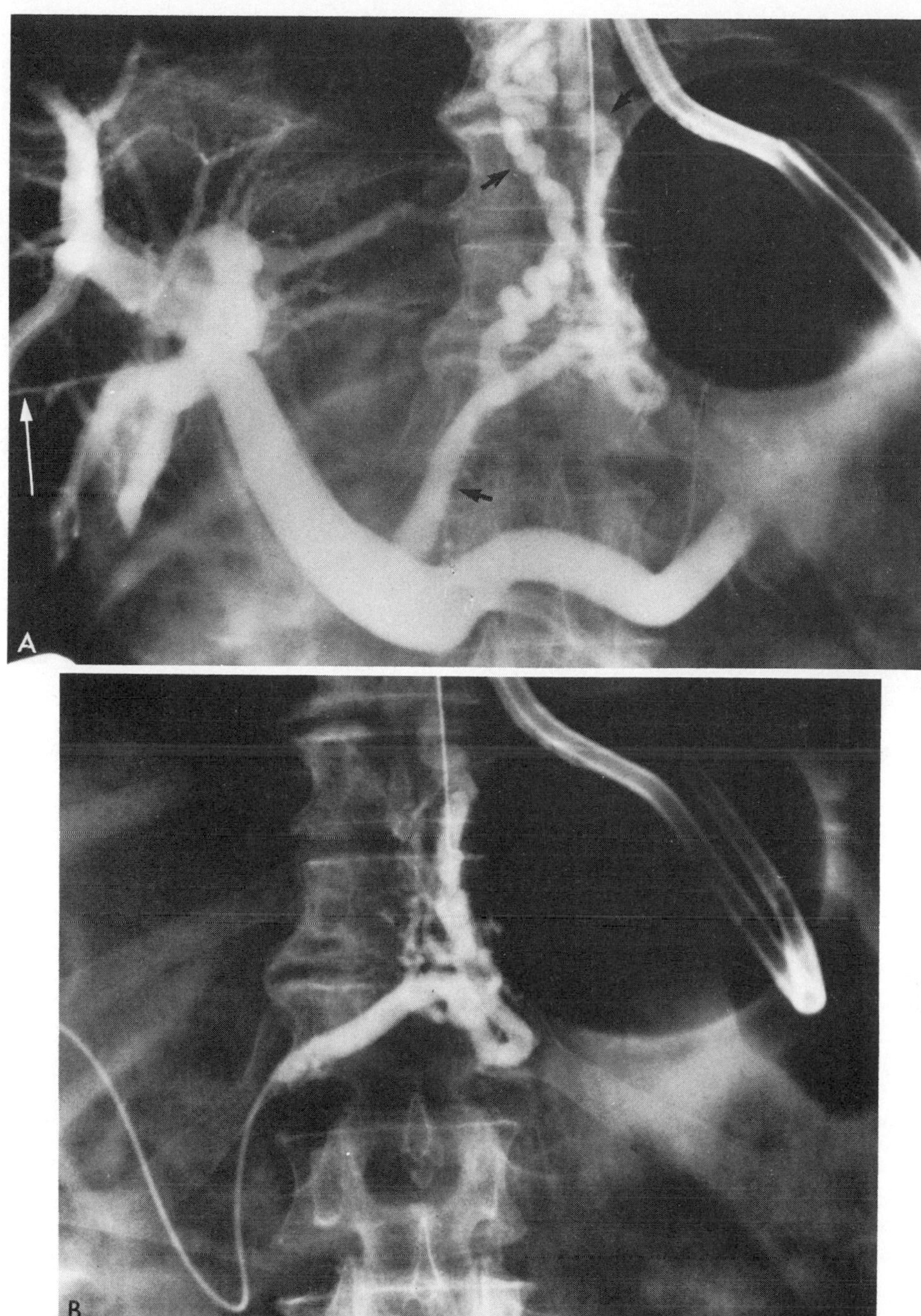

Figure 9–16. Esophageal varices in a chronic alcoholic with massive upper gastrointestinal hemorrhage. Endoscopy diagnosed bleeding from esophageal varices. The bleeding was controlled with intravenous vasopressin infusion, and a decision was made, following diagnostic angiography, to perform a splenorenal shunt. However, prior to surgery esophageal hemorrhage recurred and could no longer be controlled with IV vasopressin infusion. The portal vein was catheterized via transhepatic puncture in an attempt to control hemorrhage preoperatively and to preclude the necessity of ligating the coronary vein surgically. *A*, The catheter (*white arrow*) traverses the liver parenchyma to enter the portal vein. Injection with the catheter tip in the splenic vein demonstrates a large coronary vein and gastric and esophageal varices (*black arrows*). *B*, The catheter has been selectively placed in the coronary vein.

Illustration continued on following page

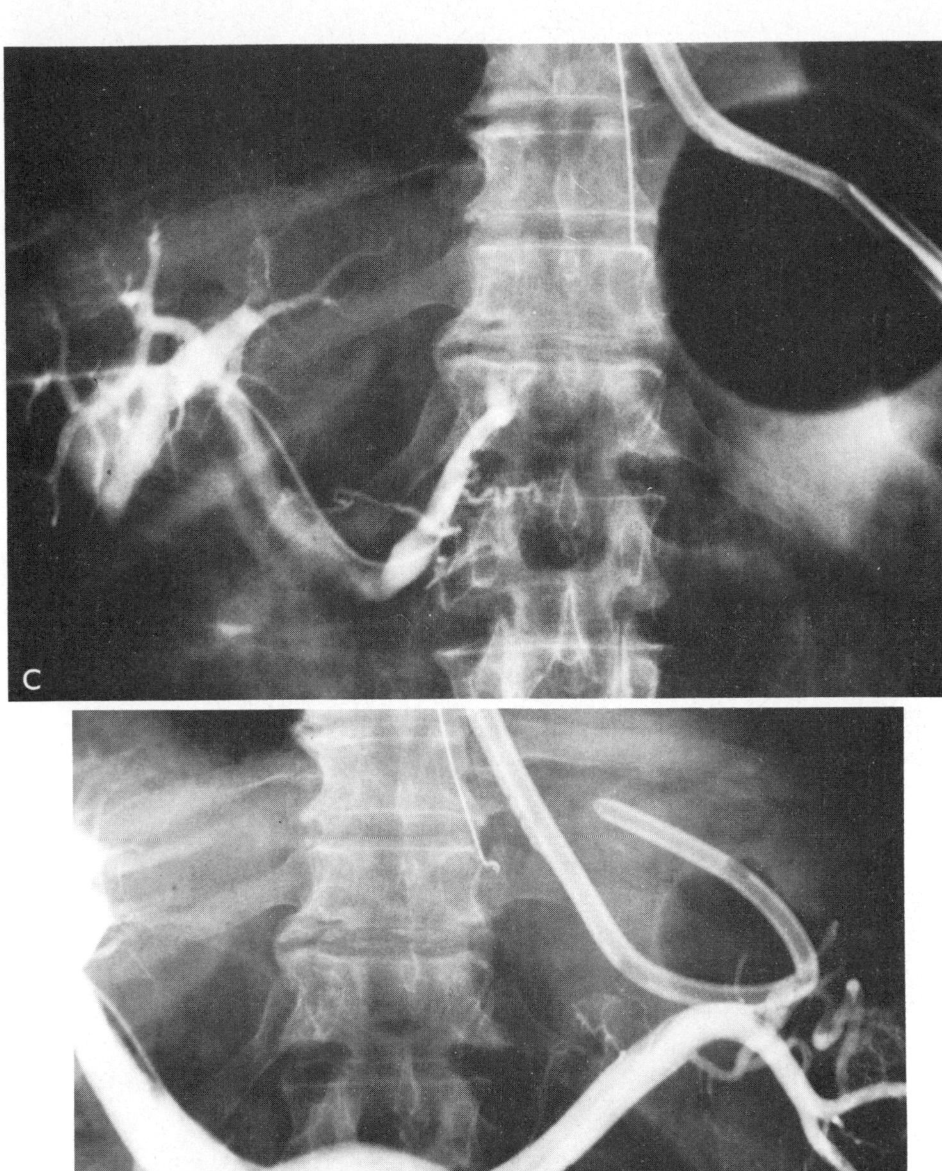

Figure 9–16 *Continued.* *C*, After slowly injecting 8 ml of 95 per cent alcohol into the coronary vein, injection shows complete obliteration of the varices and stasis within the coronary vein. *D*, Splenic vein injection 15 minutes later, with the gastric balloon deflated, shows complete occlusion of the coronary vein and no patent gastric or esophageal varices. Upper gastrointestinal hemorrhage abruptly ceased, and two days later a splenorenal shunt was surgically created.

brain, and kidneys during low-flow states. Effective treatment of systemic low-flow states, however, does not necessarily improve bowel circulation. Prolonged splanchnic vasoconstriction states may irreversibly jeopardize perfusion of the bowel. Experimental animal studies have demonstrated that splanchnic vasoconstriction may persist for several hours after correction of the systemic low-flow state (Boley et al., 1973). Digitalis improves cardiac output and systemic perfusion, but it may contribute to the persistence of mesenteric ischemia, since digitialis has a direct vasoconstrictor effect on superior mesenteric arterial smooth muscle (Ferrer et al., 1965).

Occlusive mesenteric ischemia results from in situ thrombosis or from embolization of the superior or inferior mesenteric arteries. Thrombosis commonly occurs in advanced atherosclerotic disease. Mesenteric emboli arise from atrial thrombi in patients with atrial fibrillation of rheumatic heart disease, and from ventricular thrombi associated with scars or aneurysms following myocardial infarction. Since the bowel is supplied by the celiac artery, the superior mesenteric artery, and the inferior mesenteric artery, and since abundant collateral circulation exists among these three arteries, thrombosis or embolization of one of them seldom results in mesenteric ischemia. However, mesenteric ischemia can be anticipated if thrombosis of one of the mesenteric arteries is superimposed on previously compromised mesenteric flow owing to aneurysm or dissection of the aorta or to atherosclerotic stenosis of other mesenteric arteries (Fig. 9–17).

Abdominal symptoms should be carefully evaluated in patients with cardiac disease, in postoperative patients, and in patients with hypotension due to burns, sepsis, pancreatitis, or hemorrhage. Unexplained abdominal pain or distention should raise the suspicion of mesenteric ischemia. Melena is also a common presenting sign. A characteristic clinical presentation consists of severe, unrelenting pain in the absence of abdominal findings on physical examination. As ischemia progresses, nausea, vomiting, and diarrhea may occur. Intestinal infarction results in leukocytosis, fever, and peritoneal signs.

Abdominal radiographs are helpful to exclude free air or other causes of pain. In mesenteric ischemia without infarction, abdominal radiographs may be normal or may demonstrate intestinal distention and air fluid levels. Thickening of the bowel wall and valvulae conniventes, functional intestinal obstruction, and air in the portal vein or bowel wall usually indicate infarction (see Chapter 8).

Although symptoms and radiographic signs are largely nonspecific, the high mortality from untreated mesenteric ischemia justifies an aggressive diagnostic evaluation in high-risk patients as soon as the diagnosis is suspected. Angiography permits definitive diagnosis. Aortography in both the frontal and lateral projections evaluates the status of the aorta and the origins of the celiac, superior mesenteric, and inferior mesenteric arteries. In the presence of longstanding thrombosis of a major mesenteric artery, collateral circulation may be evident. Recent emboli produce a crescentic cut-off of the artery and proximal stasis of contrast medium. The renal arteries should also be carefully evaluated by aortography, since renal infarction may produce similar abdominal symptoms.

If no vascular obstruction is demonstrated, the superior mesenteric artery should be selectively catheterized and injected for demonstration of the peripheral mesenteric branches, the mucosal blush, and the mesenteric veins. In the absence of arterial or venous obstruction, the following angiographic criteria suggest a diagnosis of nonocclusive mesenteric ischemia: (1) diffuse or segmental constriction of the superior mesenteric artery and its branches, (2) irregularity in the contour and occasionally a beaded appearance of spastic mesenteric arterial branches, (3) slower-than-normal appearance of the mucosal blush of the bowel, and (4) a patchy diminution of the mucosal blush of the bowel (Fig. 9–18).

The diagnosis is established if these abnormalities are improved or reversed by vasodilator infusion. A dose of 3 mg papaverine per minute is infused for 15 minutes and is followed by a bolus injection of 30 mg papaverine. The arteriogram is then repeated to document mesenteric arterial dilatation, and to verify an increase in the rapidity of development and in the density of the mucosal blush (Siegelman et al., 1974).

Embolic occlusion of the proximal portion of the superior mesenteric artery requires surgical embolectomy or a bypass. Thrombotic occlusion may also require surgery unless well-established collateral circulation is present. Nonocclusive mesenteric ischemia can be treated by the selective intra-arterial infusion of vasodilators. Since splanchnic vasoconstriction frequently accompanies mesenteric arterial obstruction, vasodilator infusion may be indicated in patients with arterial occlusion who are treated surgically (Boley et al., 1973).

Text continued on page 206

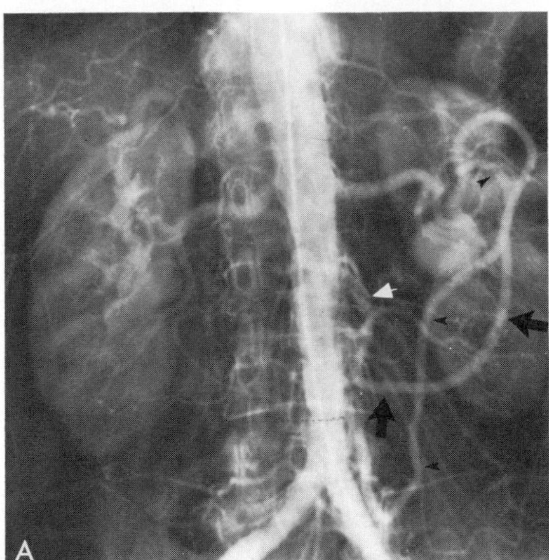

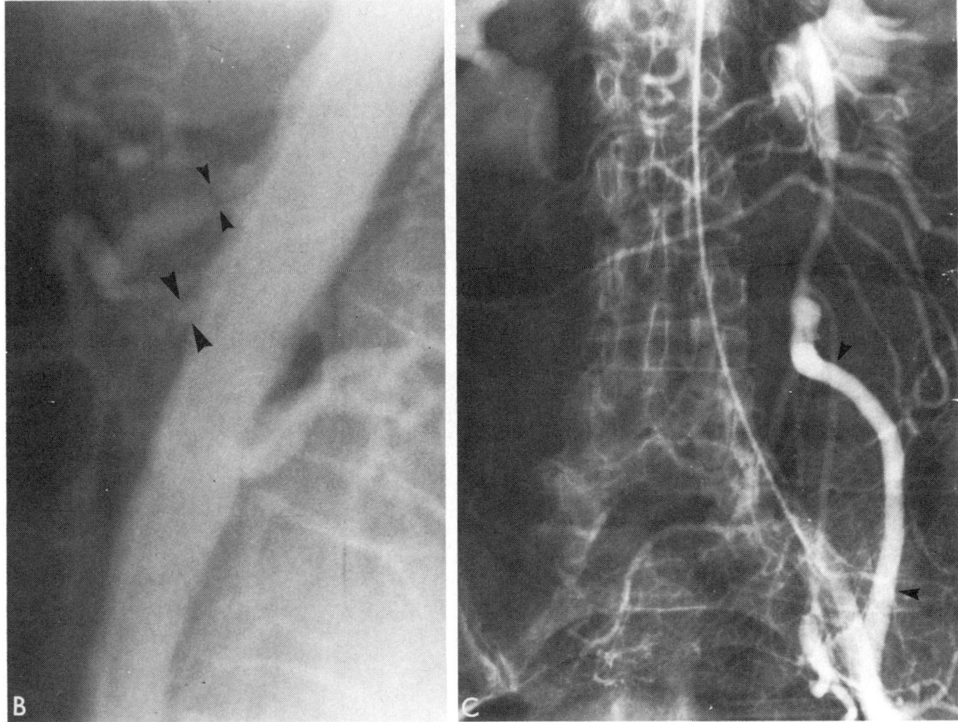

Figure 9–17. Mesenteric ischemia secondary to superior mesenteric artery thrombosis in a 59-year-old woman. *A*, Aortogram shows obstruction of the superior mesenteric artery and marked enlargement of the main trunk of the inferior mesenteric artery. Through enlargement of an anastomotic branch of the inferior mesenteric artery (*arrowheads*), the middle colic artery is opacified (*black arrows*) and reconstitutes the superior mesenteric artery (*white arrow*) near its origin. *B*, In the lateral projection, the stump of the obstructed superior mesenteric artery is identified (*large arrowheads*). The celiac axis, which is a potential source of collateral circulation to the superior mesenteric artery, is tightly stenotic near its origin (*small arrowheads*). At surgery a graft was placed between the left external iliac artery and the superior mesenteric artery. *C*, Postoperative transaxillary catheterization of the left external iliac artery opacifies the graft (*arrowheads*) and the superior mesenteric artery and its branches.

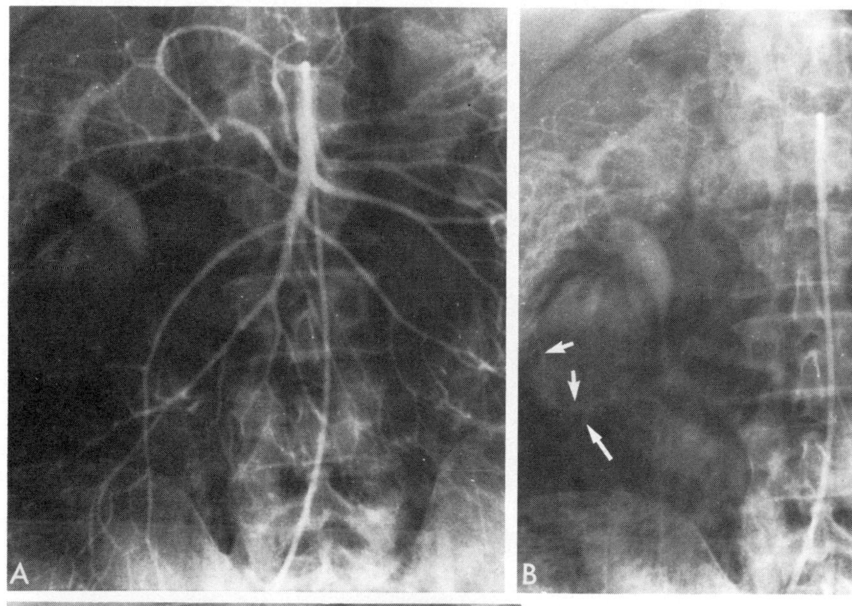

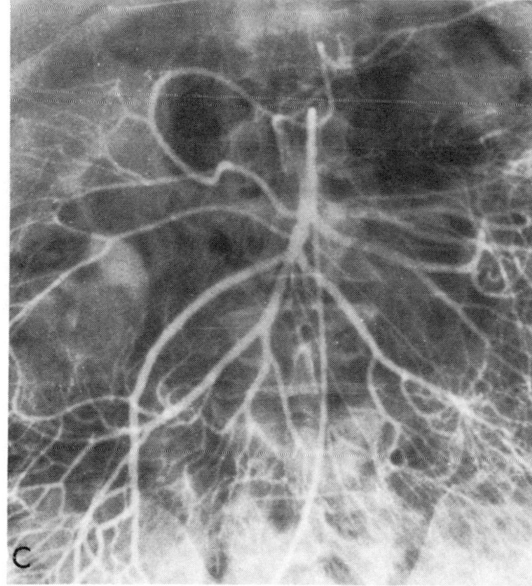

Figure 9–18. Nonocclusive mesenteric ischemia in a 54-year-old man with congestive heart failure (CHF) and a 12-hour history of increasing abdominal pain and distention. *A*, Superior mesenteric arteriogram shows constriction of most of the branches of the superior mesenteric artery. Peripheral branches that supply the midportion of the ileum, superimposed on the spine, and the ascending colon are especially sparse. *B*, In the parenchymal phase, the mucosal blush of the jejunum in the left upper quadrant and of the transverse colon are well preserved. The mucosal blush of the ileum is patchy. Arterial flow to the cecum is retarded (*arrows*) and mucosal blush is virtually absent. Papaverine was infused through the arterial catheter. *C*, Twenty-four hours after the beginning of papaverine infusion, repeat injection shows the normal size of the superior mesenteric arterial branches and excellent flow to all parts of the bowel.

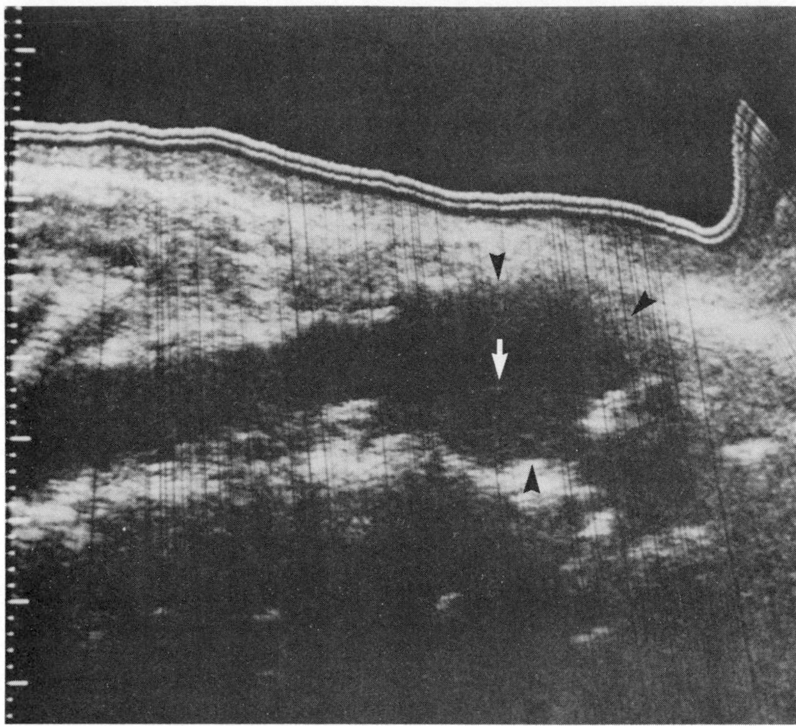

Figure 9–19. Abdominal aortic aneurysm in an elderly man with a pulsatile abdominal mass. Ultrasound examination in the sagittal plane (midline) demonstrates saccular dilatation of the distal abdominal aorta (*arrowheads*). Low-level intraluminal echoes (*white arrow*) represent a posteriorly located mural thrombus.

In the absence of a prospective randomized trial in a large group of patients, the efficacy of intra-arterial vasodilator infusion in treating nonocclusive mesenteric ischemia remains controversial. However, several published series report angiographically demonstrated reversal of mesenteric vasoconstriction and no progression to infarction. The disappearance of abdominal symptoms, the excellent survival rates, and the absence of complications in these series seem to justify this aggressive angiographic diagnostic and therapeutic approach (Boley et al., 1973).

Papaverine, tolazoline hydrochloride (Priscoline), and prostaglandin E have been used successfully for mesenteric vasodilation by intra-arterial administration (Davis et al., 1975). Prostaglandin E remains an experimental drug. Tolazoline hydrochloride may be more hazardous than papaverine, since it causes coronary arterial vasoconstriction (Habboushe et al., 1974). Papaverine produces demonstrable mesenteric vasodilation and is metabolized by the liver, a property that minimizes the systemic effects of the drug when it is administered selectively into a mesenteric artery (Boley et al., 1973).

Prior to intra-arterial vasodilator infusion, efforts should be made to reverse congestive heart failure (CHF), cardiac arrhythmia, hypotension, and hypovolemia, since pharmacologic mesenteric vasodilation may compromise cerebral, cardiac, and renal perfusion (Siegelman et al., 1974). For therapeutic infusion, papaverine is delivered into the superior mesenteric artery at a dose of 35 mg per hour for 24 hours (Boley et al., 1973; Siegelman et al., 1974).

AORTA

Abdominal Aortic Aneurysms

Abdominal aortic aneurysms may be asymptomatic or may present with life-threatening complications that require emergency surgery. Aneurysms less than 6 cm in their largest diameter are unlikely to rupture and may be treated conservatively if followed closely (Gliedman et al., 1957; Klippel and Butcher, 1966). Aneurysms larger than 6 cm in diameter require prophylactic resection. Ruptured aneurysms may bleed massively or leak slowly. In either case, a ruptured aneurysm is invariably fatal and requires emergency diagnosis and immediate surgery (Eastcott, 1973). Lesser complications, such as duodenal obstruction or obstruction of the left ureter, compression of paravertebral nerve roots, or distal embolization of cholesterol fragments or thrombi, should also be considered indications for resection (Eastcott, 1973; Sondheimer and Steinberg, 1964).

Most aneurysms are palpable, and the diagnosis can frequently be made or strongly suspected by physical examination. Most aortic aneurysms that are large enough to be clinically significant contain calcification that can be recognized on frontal, oblique, or lateral films of the abdomen. Ultrasonography provides a simple, painless means of establishing a definitive diagnosis in the ICU patient. The entire length of the abdominal aorta can be visualized in most patients (Fig. 9–19). The size of the aortic lumen can be measured, and in most cases the outer wall of the aorta is also demonstrated; thus, the amount of thrombus within the aneurysm and the thickness of the wall can be determined (Goldberg and Lehman, 1970). In patients who cannot be transported from the ICU, portable ultrasonography can be used at the bedside.

Angiography is indicated following diagnosis by ultrasonography if additional anatomic information is required, or if ultrasonography is unsatisfactory (air in the overlying bowel) or inconsistent with the clinical picture. Angiography demonstrates the rate and pattern of blood flow and whether it is laminar or turbulent (Fig. 9–20*A*, *B*). The relationship of the aneurysm to the renal arteries and the status of the aortic wall between the aneurysm and renal arteries determine whether the aorta can be effectively clamped proximal to the aneurysm and whether reconstruction by a graft is feasible (Fig. 9–20*C*). Demonstration of the presence or absence of aneurysm extension beyond the aortic bifurcation or of stenosis in the iliac arteries aids in determining where the distal end of a graft should be placed (Eastcott, 1973).

The thickness of the wall of the aneurysm can be determined by angiography even though only the lumen is opacified, because superior mesenteric arterial branches that cross the midline are stretched across the anterior wall of the aneurysm (Fig. 9–21). In the lateral projection, measurement of the amount of anterior displacement of these branches permits measurement of the anteroposterior (AP) diameter of the outer wall of the aneurysm. In the frontal projection, the displaced superior mesenteric arterial branches are stretched and attenuated. The length of the stretched segments permits measurement of the lateral diameter of the aneurysm.

Thoracic Aortic Dissection

Aortic dissection most commonly occurs in hypertensive patients. The most prominent symptom is pain, which may simulate a myocardial infarction. Once myocardial infarction is excluded (see Chapter 11), the diagnosis of aortic dissection can be suggested by chest radiography and established by angiography or CT.

Radiographs of the chest usually show an elongated or tortuous aorta, but since dissection occurs within the lumen of the aorta, the aortic diameter may be normal (Fig. 9–22). The only definitive, although rare, radiographic sign of aortic dissection is displacement of calcified plaques of the aortic intima away from the border of the aortic shadow (Fig. 9–23). The heart may or may not be enlarged, depending on the severity of the hypertension and on whether the dissection results in aortic valve insufficiency.

Approximately 75 per cent of dissections involve the ascending aorta (Eastcott, 1973). Although surgery in this area is hazardous, the high incidence of lethal rupture into the pericardium makes operative repair mandatory. Emergency surgery has a higher mortality than surgery performed in a stabilized patient. During the acute phase, medical therapy directed toward a gradual reduction of blood pressure over one or two weeks before surgery is helpful in selected patients (Thompson et al., 1969).

Computerized tomography can accurately demonstrate or exclude aortic dissection in many cases and can document whether or not the ascending aorta is affected. This information is often sufficient to direct therapeutic decisions and may obviate the necessity for angiography in many or most patients (Heiberg et al., 1981). Angiography, however, remains useful if the results of the CT examination are equivocal or at variance with the clinical signs. Angiography may be more sensitive than CT in demonstrating the distal extent of the dissection, and it provides information not available from CT, such as evaluation of the patency of essential aortic branches and of the function of the aortic valve. Further investigation will be necessary to determine the extent to which CT can replace angiography in the evaluation of patients with suspected aortic dissection.

Angiographic catheter manipulation and in-

Text continued on page 213

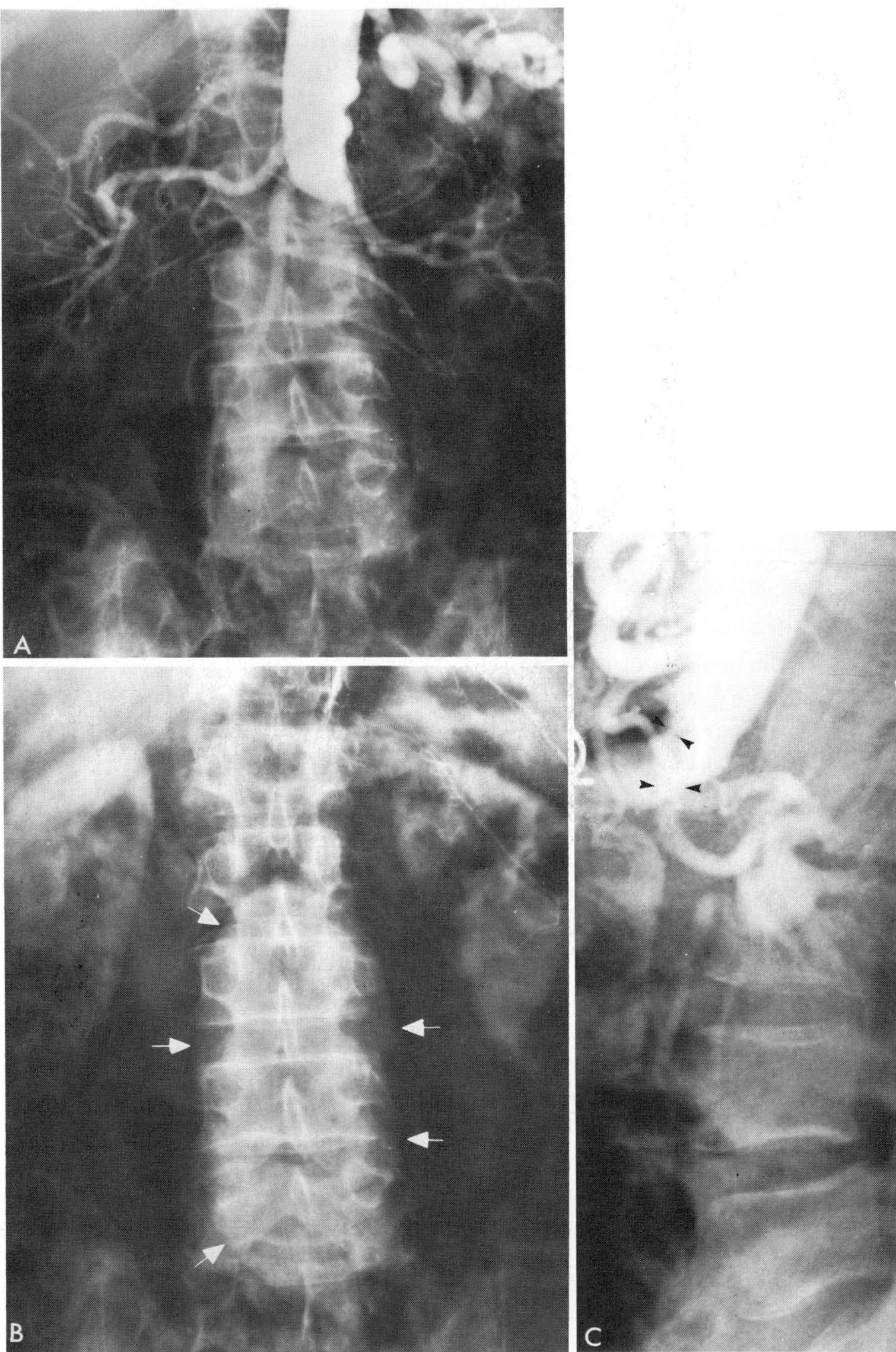

Figure 9–20 *See legend on opposite page.*

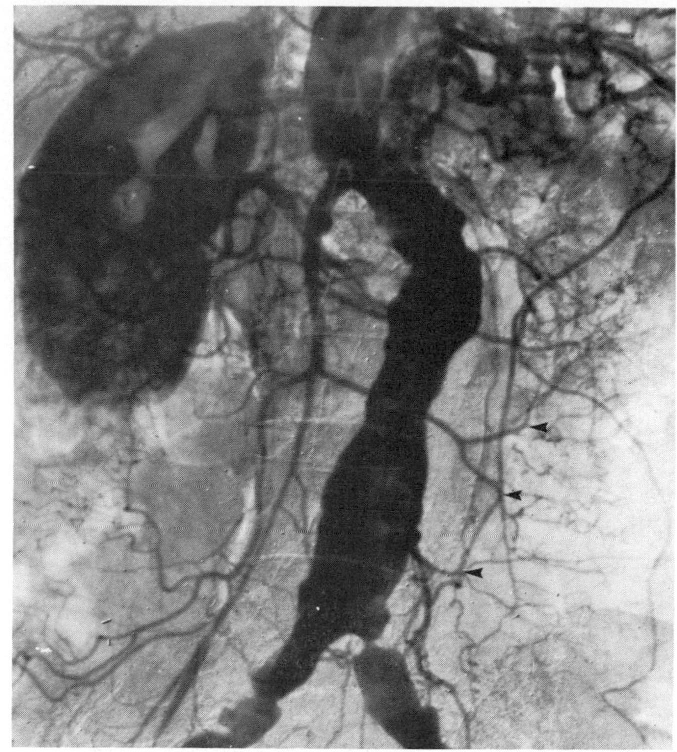

Figure 9–21. Abdominal aortic aneurysm in a 68-year-old woman with a large, pulsating abdominal mass. Aortogram shows tortuosity of the aorta and irregularity of the lumen, but the lumen is only mildly dilated. Large amounts of thrombus in the wall of the aneurysm maintain an approximately normal-caliber lumen and permit linear, rather than turbulent, blood flow. Thus, flow remains rapid, and perfusion of the extremities is excellent in spite of tight stenosis at the origin of the left common iliac artery. Although the opacified lumen is only mildly dilated, the diagnosis of aortic aneurysm can be established because of straightening and displacement of superior mesenteric arterial branches that cross the midline over the anterior surface of the aorta. The left lateral margin of the aneurysm can be identified by angulation of the superior mesenteric arterial branches as they are reflected off the edges of the aneurysm and into the paravertebral gutter (*arrowheads*). Note absence of left renal blood flow because of atherosclerotic obstruction of the left renal artery.

Figure 9–20. Abdominal aortic aneurysm in a 65-year-old man with a pulsating abdominal mass. Ultrasound documented that the mass was an aneurysm, but the relationship of the aneurysm to the origins of the renal arteries could not be ascertained. *A*, Aortogram shows marked diminution of blood flow through the aneurysm. The celiac, superior mesenteric, and renal arteries are opacified through several orders of branching, but no contrast medium is yet visible in the aneurysm. The origin of the right renal artery appears to be approximately 1 cm proximal to the aneurysm, but the origin of the left renal artery appears to be much closer to the origin of the aneurysm. *B*, After the proximal aorta and visceral arteries have lost their opacification, the aneurysm (*arrows*) remains opacified. Thus, the levels of origin and termination of the aneurysm are clearly identifiable because of differential flow rate within the aneurysm, and within the aorta proximal and distal to the aneurysm. *C*, Only on the lateral projection can the actual relationship of the renal arteries to the aneurysm be clearly seen. Proximal to the aneurysm the aorta is abruptly angulated anteriorly, so that a segment of aorta crosses almost horizontally before entering the aneurysm. The origins of both renal arteries can be identified (*arrowheads*) superimposed on the aortic lumen. A segment of aorta approximately 2 cm in length is present between the margins of the renal arteries and the aneurysm. This is a sufficient length of aorta to permit insertion of a infrarenal aortic graft. The patient was taken to surgery, where the aneurysm was resected and a Dacron graft successfully placed.

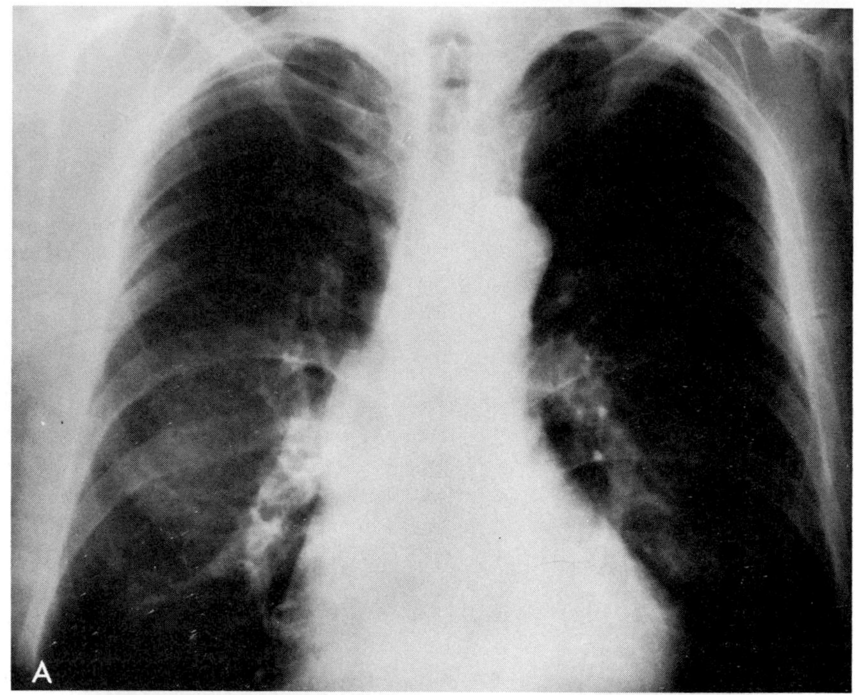
A

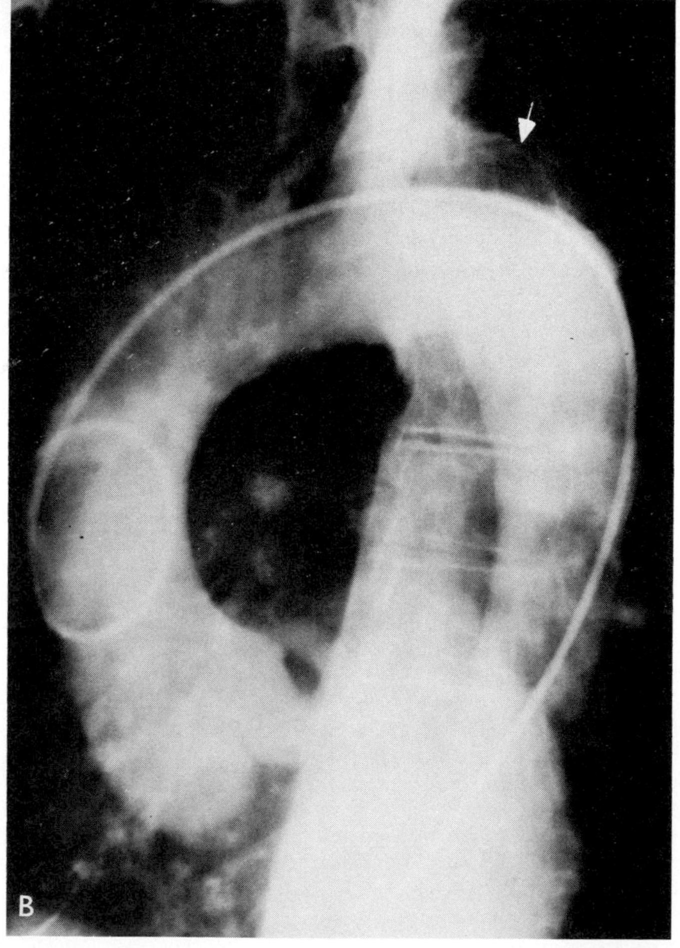
B

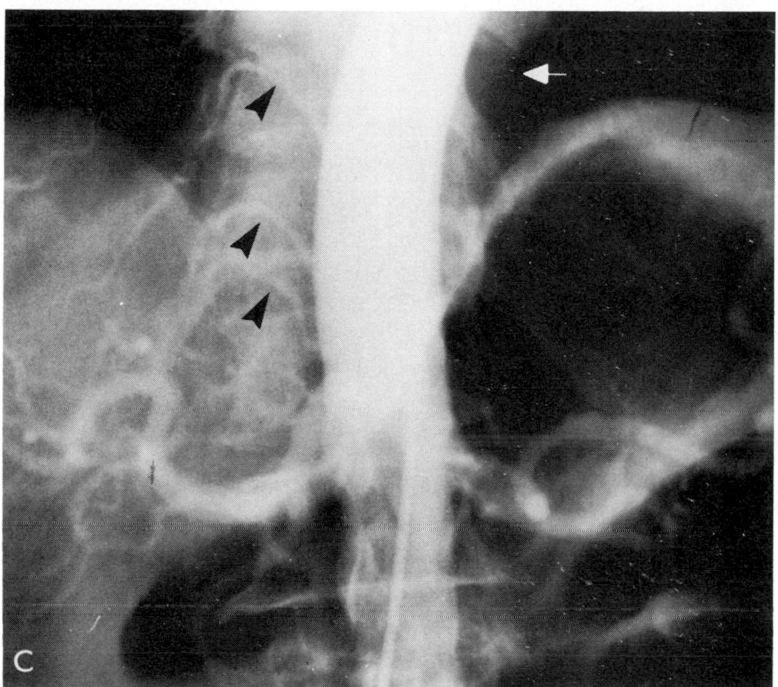

Figure 9–22. Aortic dissection beginning distal to the left subclavian artery in a 76-year-old man with long-standing hypertension and a history of aortic dissection discovered three years previously, which was treated with antihypertensive medication. His current admission was prompted by a sudden onset of paraplegia. *A*, Chest radiograph shows left ventricular enlargement and prominent aortic knob. Both findings are consistent with a history of hypertension. There are no specific signs that suggest aortic dissection. *B*, At aortography the diagnosis of aortic dissection is established by a wide, unopacified soft tissue shadow at the aortic knob (*arrow*), which represents the false lumen. *C*, Injection of the descending aorta also shows the unopacified false lumen (*white arrow*). Lower intercostal arteries on the right side are normal (*arrowheads*) but are absent on the left side. Paraplegia resulted from extension of the dissection into the distal thoracic aorta, causing obstruction of the left intercostal arteries that supply the thoracic spinal cord.

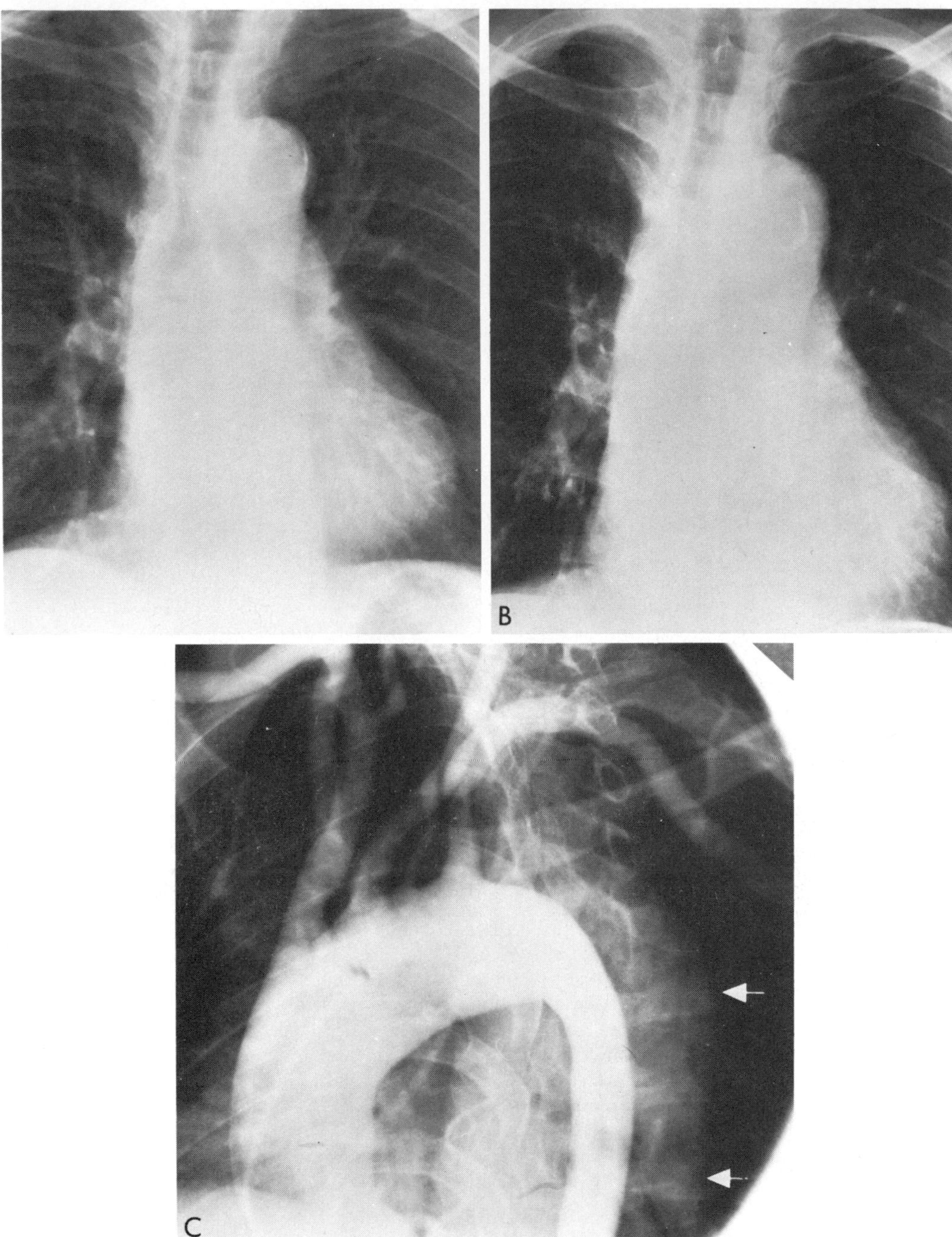

Figure 9–23. Aortic dissection beginning distal to the left subclavian artery in a 62-year-old man with a history of hypertension and sudden onset of severe chest pain. ECG and enzyme studies excluded myocardial infarction. *A*, Chest radiograph obtained one year earlier shows calcification in the aortic knob separated from the lateral edge of the aortic shadow by only 1 mm. *B*, Chest radiograph taken on current admission shows medial displacement of the calcification in the aortic knob. *C*, Aortogram shows a small-caliber, opacified descending aorta (true lumen) and a wide, parallel soft tissue shadow (*arrows*), which represent the unopacified false lumen.

jection require the utmost care in patients with dissection, since the dissected aortic wall is easily traumatized and since aortic flow and pressure vary in the true and false lumina. Useful precautions include: (1) use of a soft, J-shaped guidewire, carefully monitored fluoroscopically whenever the catheter is advanced; (2) fluoroscopically monitored, low-pressure, manual injection of contrast medium in order to estimate the aortic flow rate before each pressure injection; and (3) measurement of intra-aortic pressure at the catheter tip.

Angiographic diagnosis of aortic dissection relies on the demonstration of two lumina in the aorta. If contrast medium enters both lumina, differential rates of flow can often be demonstrated during serial filming. When a portion of the dissected intima is positioned parallel to the x-ray beam, it is visualized as a lucent stripe between the contrast medium in the true and false lumina, a definitive sign of aortic dissection (Fig. 9–24). If flow is very slow in the false lumen or if thrombosis has obliterated the false lumen, narrowing of the true lumen and marked thickening of the aortic wall are sufficient for a diagnosis of dissection (Figs. 9–22*B*, 9–23*C*). Since the dissection may involve only a small portion of the circumference of the aorta, oblique and lateral projections are frequently necessary for a positive diagnosis. If the dissection extends into the abdomen, the abdominal aorta should be examined.

In addition to the diagnosis of dissection, attention should be paid to evaluation of the

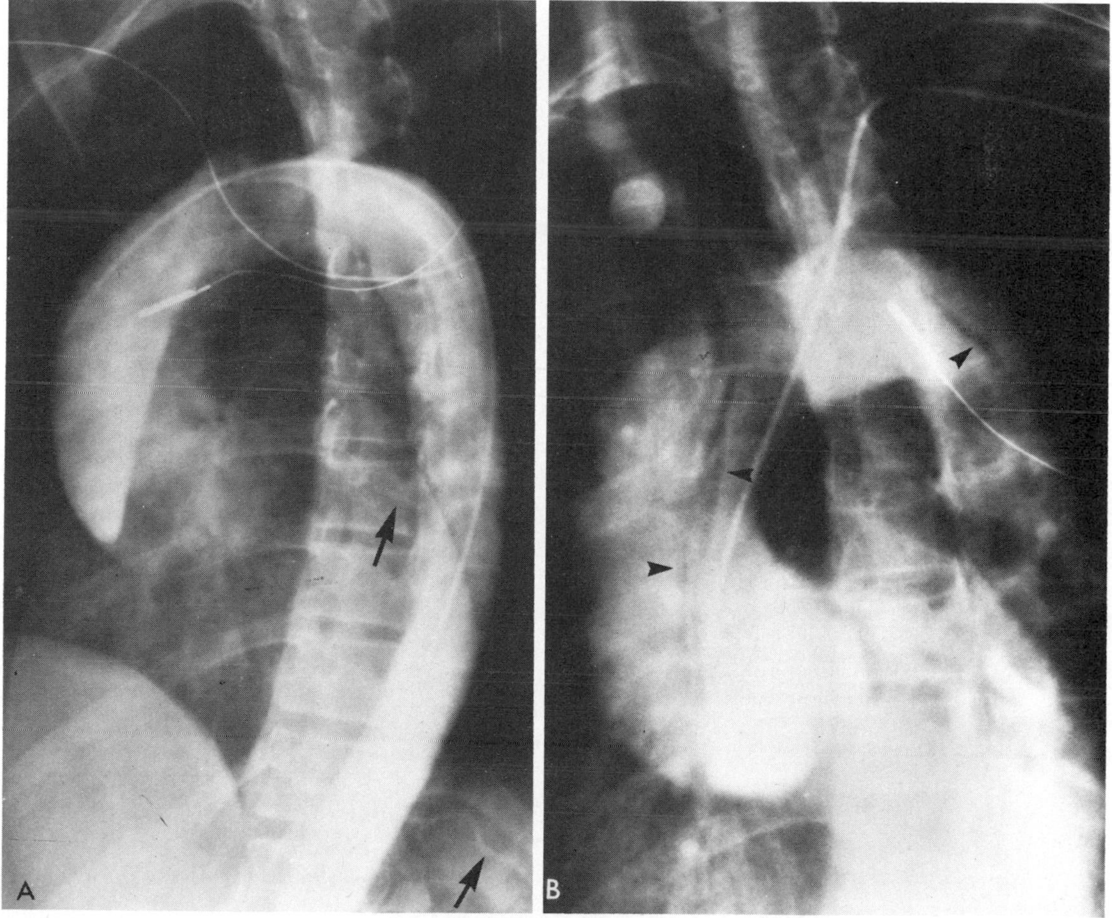

Figure 9–24. Aortic dissection beginning at the aortic valve in a 35-year-old woman with severe hypertension and recent onset of chest and abdominal pain. *A*, Aortic arch arteriogram performed via the left femoral artery opacifies a large compartment, the false lumen, that begins within 1 cm of the aortic valve and extends into the abdominal aorta. The only thoracic branches that arise from this lumen are two intercostal arteries (*arrows*). *B*, Aortic arch arteriogram via the left axillary artery opacifies the true lumen. No aortic regurgitation is present. Contrast medium opacifies the false lumen as well, and lucent stripes (*arrowheads*) in both the ascending and descending portions of the aorta represent the dissected intima that separates the two lumina.

rate of flow in the false lumen and of the patency of aortic branches. If there is little or no blood flow through the false lumen of the dissection, it is unlikely that the dissection will progress (McFarland et al., 1972). In such a patient, antihypertensive medical therapy has a greater chance of success than in patients with free communication of blood between the true and false lumina and rapid flow in the false lumen. Obstruction of essential aortic branches requires immediate surgical correction. Obstruction of intercostal or lumbar arteries should be carefully looked for, since occlusion of these arteries may jeopardize the viability of the spinal cord (Fig. 9–22*C*).

Aortic Laceration

Motion and torsion of the aorta, the heart, and the pulmonary artery following sudden deceleration produce traction and frequently disruption of the aorta at points of fixation. Laceration at the root of the aorta occurs relatively often, but this injury usually is rapidly fatal. The most common site of treatable aortic disruption is at the attachment of the ligamentum arteriosum.

Physical examination may be misleading (Figs. 9–25, 9–26). In over one third of patients with aortic laceration, physical examination gives no evidence of significant internal injury (Kirsh et al., 1976). Therefore, the diagnosis often depends heavily on radiographic examination. Chest radiographs are mandatory in patients who have sustained deceleration injury, and must be carefully evaluated. In a review of a large series of patients who were not treated surgically, Parmley et al. (1958) found that, of those who survived for at least one hour, 49 per cent died within 24 hours and 90 per cent died within four months of injury.

Several radiographic signs suggest the diagnosis of aortic laceration:

1. *Left apical extrapleural cap:* A potential space exists between the aortic arch and the parietal pleura on the left side into which blood may dissect, producing a smooth thickening of the pleural shadow at the apex of the lung (Simeone et al., 1975). This sign may be present prior to widening of the mediastinum. However, patients with upper rib fractures or small vessel bleeding may also have an apical cap (Figs. 9–25*A*, 9–26*A*).

2. *Mediastinal widening:* Extravasation initially accumulates adjacent to the descending aorta immediately inferior to the aortic knob, between the aorta and the parietal pleura. A hematoma in this area widens the mediastinal shadow (Figs. 9–25*A*, 9–26*A*).

3. *Obscured or abnormal aortic contour:* Hematoma adjacent to the descending aorta may enlarge the aortic knob on a chest radiograph and may compress the contiguous lung parenchyma enough to obscure the shadow of the aortic knob or descending aorta (Figs. 9–25*A*, 9–26*A*).

4. *Displacement of the trachea and/or esophagus:* The trachea and esophagus are closely associated with the aorta in the middle mediastinum. Even very small para-aortic hematomas often displace these structures to the right. If a nasogastric tube is present, displacement of the radiopaque tube or of the trachea to the right of the spinous process of the fourth thoracic vertebra on a nonrotated chest radiograph is a sensitive and relatively specific sign of aortic injury (Fig. 9–25*A*) (Gerlock et al., 1980).

5. *Hemothorax:* If the parietal pleura is disrupted during injury, mediastinal hemorrhage may accumulate within the pleural space. The presence of pleural fluid, especially on the left, suggests an aortic laceration (Fig. 9–26*B*).

6. *Fracture of the first or second rib:* Fractures of these ribs are uncommon unless there has been severe trauma. If the trauma was severe enough to fracture the first or second rib, injury to the aorta should be considered (see also Chapter 7).

Patients with hemodynamic instability following a deceleration injury require emergency exploratory thoracotomy. If chest radiographic signs suggest aortic disruption, thoracotomy without previous angiographic confirmation is appropriate. If the patient's clinical condition is stable, angiography should be done to reliably document or exclude aortic laceration (Lim et al., 1972).

Aortic laceration is manifested angiographically by extravasation of contrast medium into a false aneurysm (Figs. 9–25*B*, 9–27). The distinction between a false aneurysm produced by aortic laceration and a true or mycotic aneurysm may not be possible in every case, but in a patient who has sustained a deceleration injury, one must assume that the lesion is traumatic. If the aortic adventitia remains intact, the only abnormality may be irregularity of the lumen of the aorta. Therefore, at least two projections should be obtained in order to exclude the diagnosis of aortic laceration. The intercostal arteries should be carefully studied to exclude intercostal avulsion as a possible source of hem-

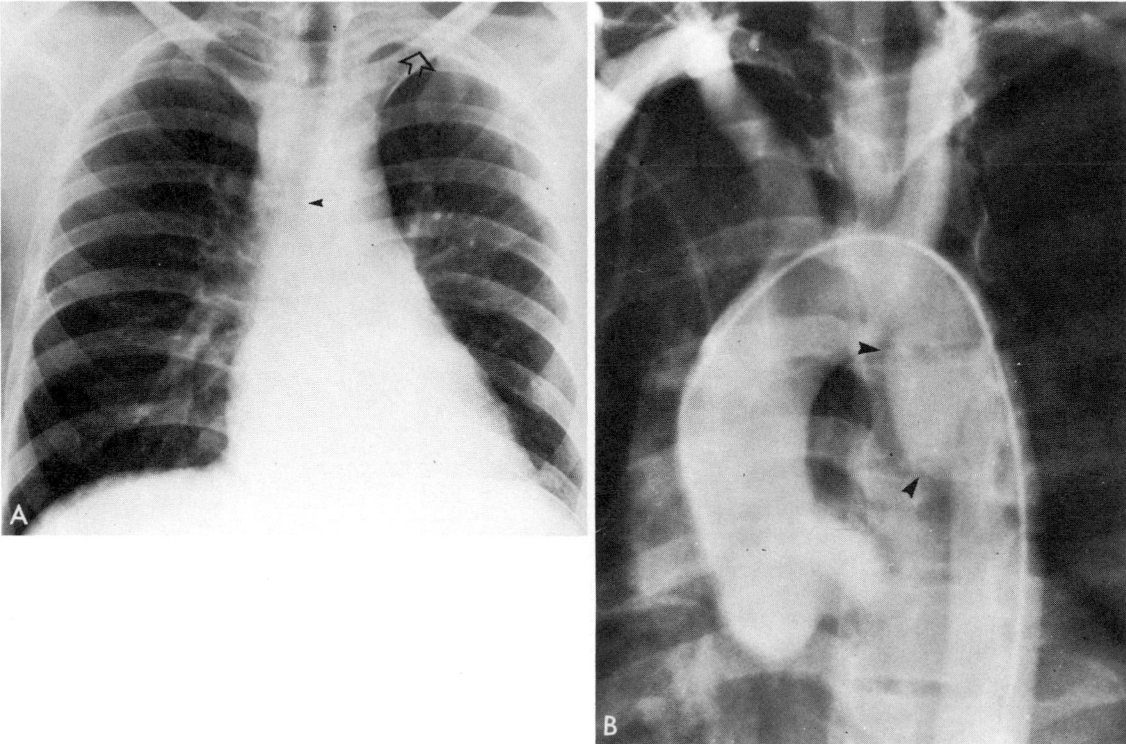

Figure 9–25 Aortic laceration in a 26-year-old man who suffered a deceleration injury in an automobile accident. Vital signs were stable and physical examination was normal. *A*, PA chest radiograph shows possible mediastinal widening. The shadow of the aortic knob is obscured and the distal portion of the trachea is displaced to the right (*arrowhead*). Pleural thickening at the left pulmonary apex (*open arrow*) suggests extrapleural blood collection. *B*, Aortogram in the right posterior oblique projection shows a false aneurysm (*arrowheads*) on the undersurface of the aortic arch just distal to the left subclavian artery; this is characteristic of aortic laceration.

orrhage (Fig. 9–26*C*, *D*). In deceleration injuries the great vessels are seldom injured, since they are sufficiently redundant to move with the aorta. However, in patients with crush injuries or sternal fractures, these vessels should be carefully evaluated at the time of aortography (Fig. 9–28).

RETRIEVAL OF BROKEN CATHETERS

A most vexing complication in the ICU is loss of a portion of an IV catheter. Radiopaque catheters can be localized by means of chest radiography, and in most cases broken catheters can be removed nonoperatively. Venography should be performed to verify that the catheter lies within the lumen of a vein and to demonstrate the potential access routes to that vein (Fig. 9–29). A simple snare inserted percutaneously into the femoral vein permits retrieval of the broken catheter under fluoroscopic control (Fisher and Ferreyro, 1978).

Although commercially prepared snares are available, a snare is easily made with materials commonly stocked in the angiographic department. A No. 7 or 8 French catheter without a tapered tip is used. The catheter may be curved as necessary, depending on the location of the broken catheter. The core of an angiographic guidewire is removed from the guidewire, kinked in the middle, and folded in half (Fig. 9–30). The kinked end of the doubled-over guidewire core is inserted through the angiographic catheter. The length of the catheter is adjusted so that the doubled-over guidewire core can be advanced at least 2 cm beyond the tip of the catheter As the guidewire core is advanced beyond the tip of the catheter, the kink straightens to form an open loop. The snaring procedure is simplified if the distal 2 cm of this loop is bent 90 degrees, so that the opening of the loop is oriented vertically (Fig. 9–30*B*).

Text continued on page 222

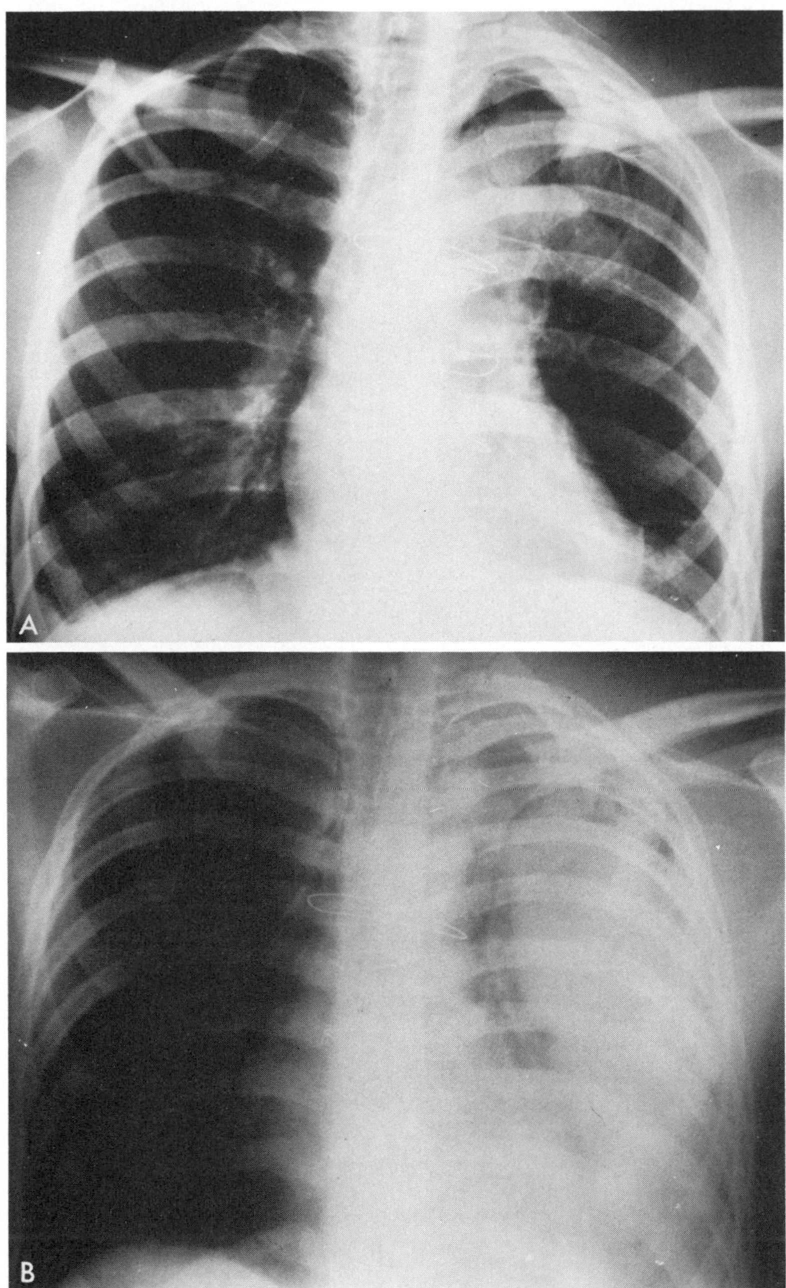

Figure 9–26. Intercostal artery transection in a 20-year-old man who was stabbed in the posterior left upper thorax. Thoracotomy was performed shortly after admission without preoperative angiography. Exploration of the aortic arch and left subclavian artery showed no vascular injury. *A*, Chest radiograph, five days postoperatively. The mediastinum is widened. The aortic knob and descending aortic shadows have been obscured. An apical extrapleural cap is present in the left hemithorax. *B*, The following day the patient became dyspneic; the chest radiograph shows virtually complete opacification of the left hemithorax.

Illustration continued on opposite page

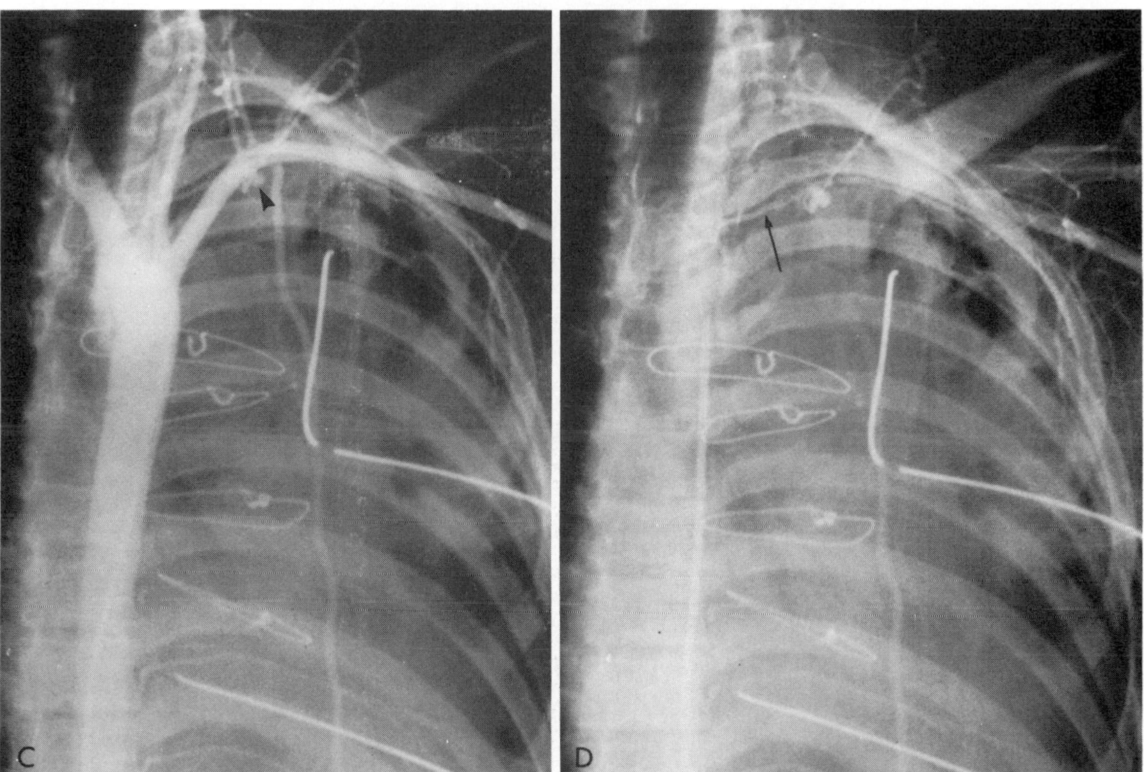

Figure 9–26 *Continued* *C*, Emergency aortogram demonstrates extravasation (*arrowhead*) superimposed on the left subclavian artery. *D*, In the late arterial phase, when the left subclavian artery is no longer opacified, the third intercostal artery remains opacified (*arrow*). Irregularities along its course and persistent arterial opacification indicate that the third intercostal artery, rather than the subclavian artery, is the injured vessel. This was confirmed at surgery.

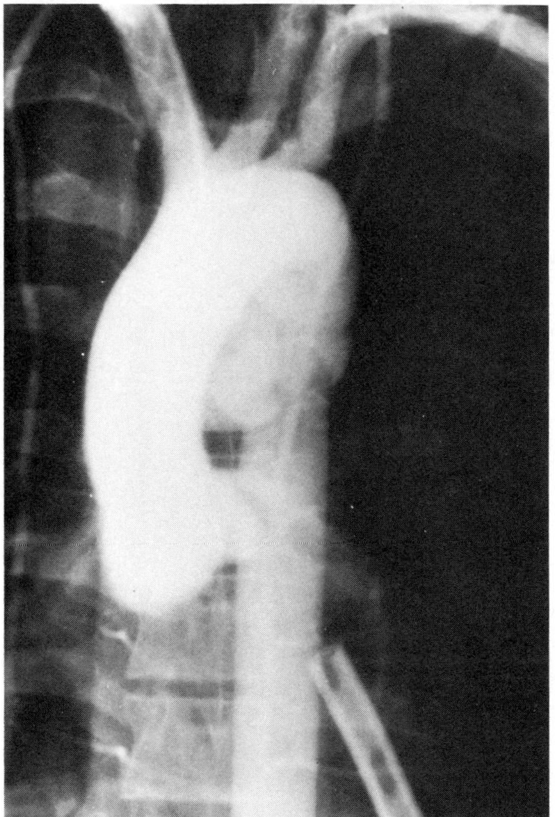

Figure 9–27. Aortic laceration in a 24-year-old man admitted after a motorcycle accident. Several left-sided ribs were fractured. In the emergency room a chest tube was inserted because of a hemopneumothorax. Although the patient was hypotensive, the vital signs were stable. Aortogram shows disruption of the aorta just distal to the left subclavian artery. The false aneurysm, which extends toward the right, is large and contains several compartments.

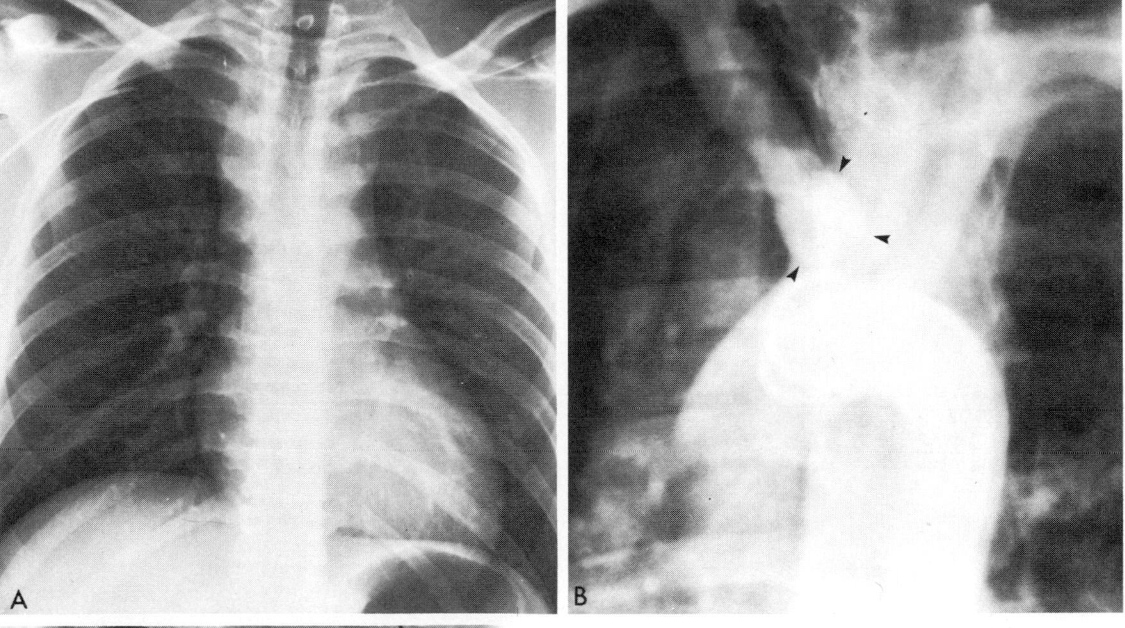

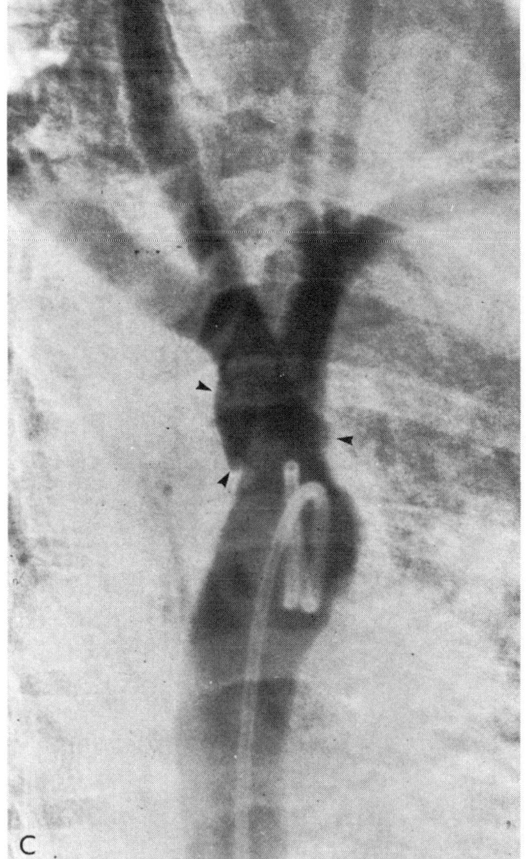

Figure 9–28. Partial avulsion of the brachiocephalic artery in a 21-year-old man who sustained a crush injury to the chest. On admission vital signs were normal, and physical examination, including a complete neurologic examination, was normal except for a mild superficial anterior chest wall contusion. *A*, AP chest radiograph was considered normal. Possible widening of the mediastinal shadow was not considered significant because of the AP position. Eighteen hours after admission a bruit became audible, and aortography was performed. *B*, Right posterior oblique projection shows a small fusiform false aneurysm superimposed on the brachiocephalic artery (*arrowheads*). *C*, In the left posterior oblique projection, the false aneurysm is bell-shaped (*arrowheads*). At surgery the brachiocephalic artery was partially avulsed from the aorta. An aortobrachiocephalic artery bypass graft re-established vascular continuity.

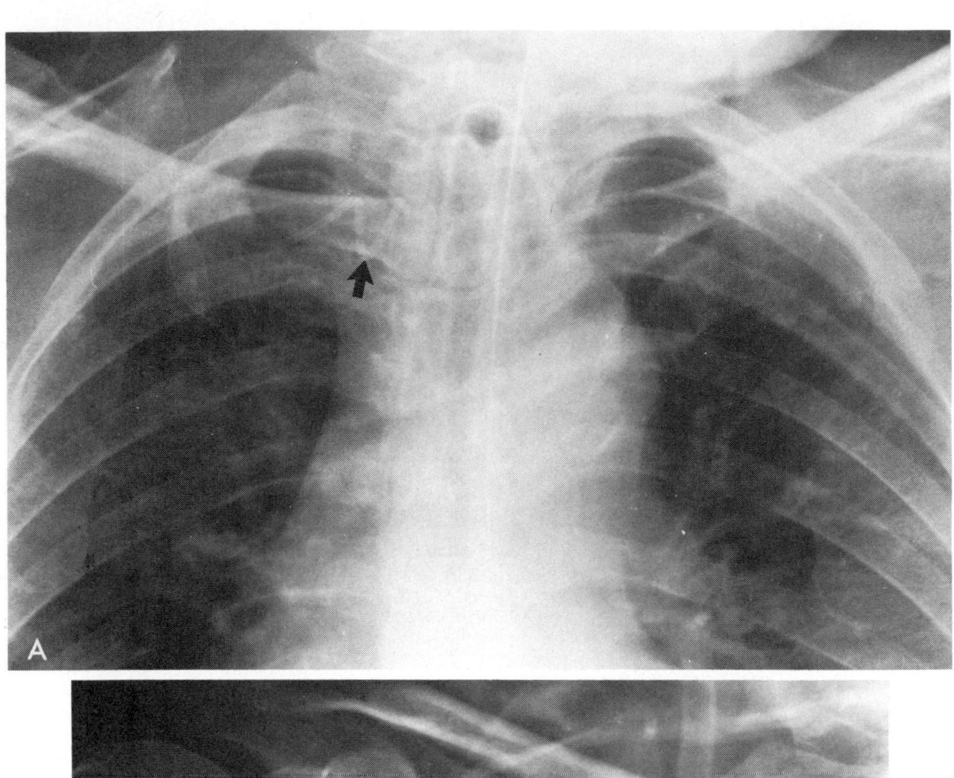

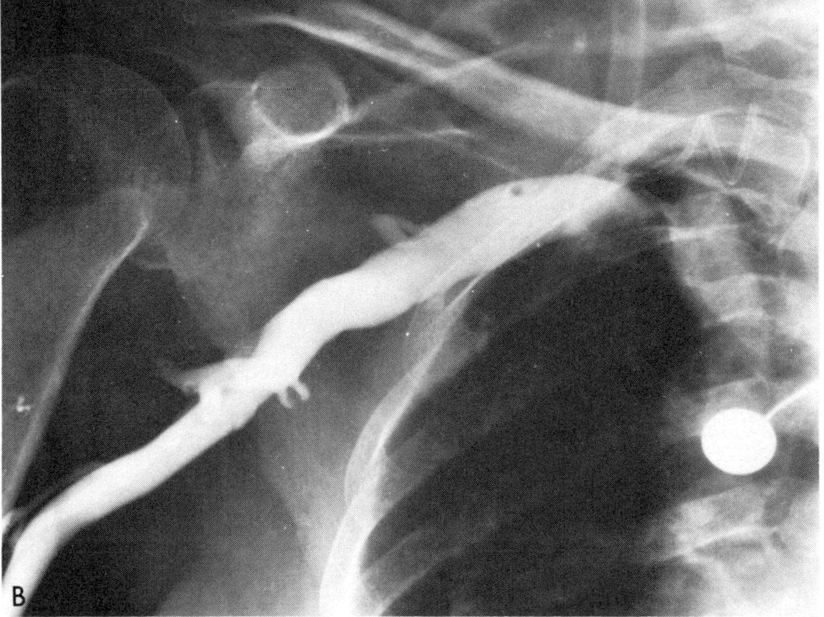

Figure 9–29. Catheterization of the right subclavian vein was attempted, but no blood could be aspirated and the catheter was torn during withdrawal. *A*, Chest radiograph shows the radiopaque catheter superimposed on the right clavicle (*arrow*). *B*, Venogram opacifies the right subclavian vein. The catheter fragment lies outside the vein. (Courtesy of B. Rubin, M.D., Washington, DC.)

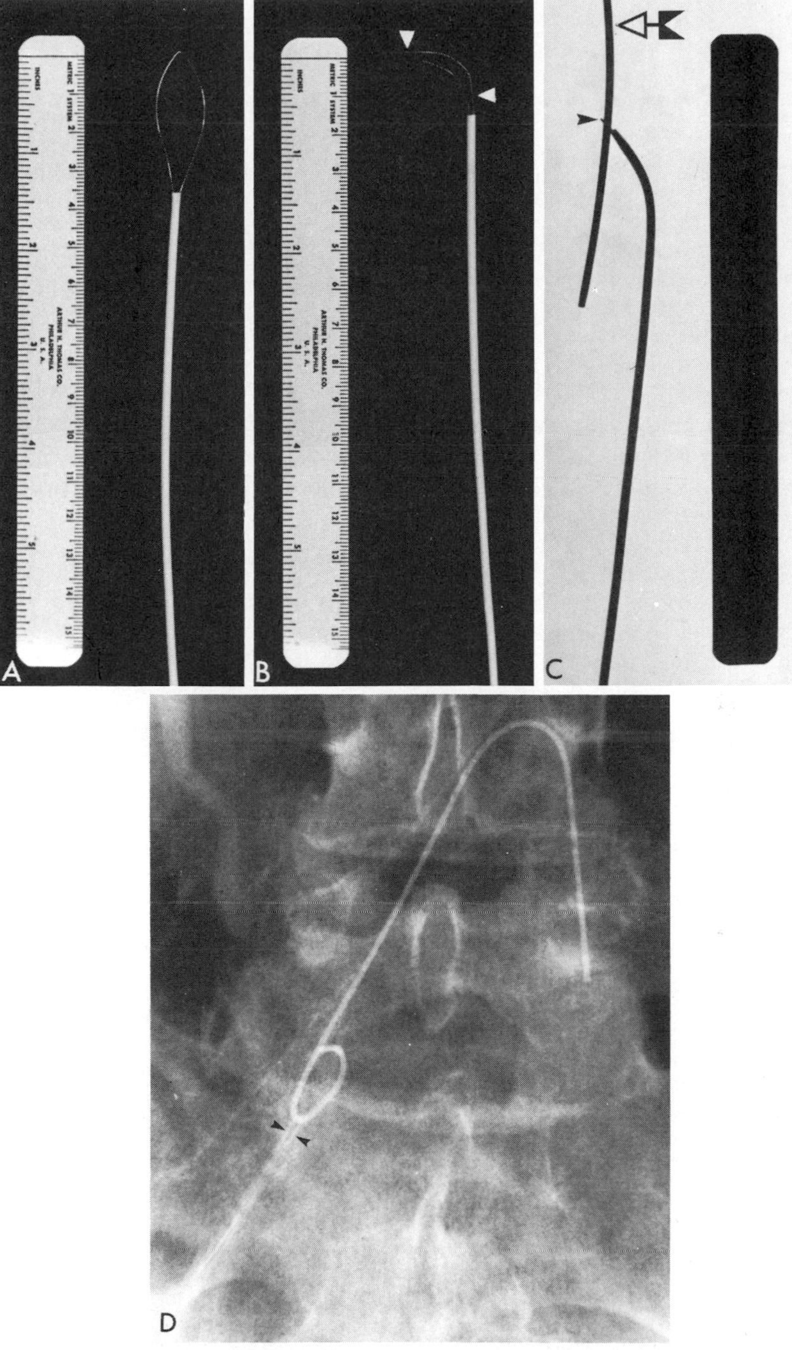

Figure 9–30. Retrieval of a broken catheter. *A*, A doubled-over guidewire core protrudes 3 cm beyond the tip of a nontapered No. 7 French catheter. *B*, The guidewire core is bent 90° (*arrowheads*) in order to engage the longitudinally oriented free end of the broken catheter. *C*, The doubled-over guidewire core is then withdrawn slowly in order to tighten the snare (*arrowhead*) around the broken catheter (*arrow*). *D*, Spot film obtained during retrieval of a broken angiographic guidewire from the aortic bifurcation. The snare (*arrowheads*) has been tightened around the broken guidewire, permitting removal of the snare and the broken wire through the femoral artery puncture site.

The angiographic catheter is manipulated so that it is parallel to one end of the broken catheter, and is advanced until the end of the broken catheter enters the loop formed by the guidewire core. The guidewire core is then gently pulled back through the angiographic catheter, reducing the size of the loop, until the broken catheter is firmly grasped within the snare. That point can be identified fluoroscopically since, when firmly snared, the broken catheter moves with movement of the angiographic catheter. The angiographic catheter is then withdrawn from the femoral vein, pulling with it the broken catheter.

Femoral puncture is preferable to brachial or jugular vein puncture, especially if the broken catheter is in the heart or pulmonary artery. Fewer curves are encountered in the venous system and the broken catheter is withdrawn across fewer venous bifurcations. Each bifurcating vein encountered during withdrawal presents a surface irregularity that can potentially dislodge the snared catheter. If the brachial vein is used for insertion, the 270-degree curve between the catheter insertion site and the pulmonary artery makes manipulation of the snare difficult. A femoral approach is preferable, even if a broken catheter is in the subclavian vein, since the wider caliber of the superior vena cava and the proximal subclavian vein permit more accurate snare manipulation than the smaller distal subclavian vein.

REFERENCES

Ahmad, W., and Polk, H. C., Jr.: Blunt abdominal trauma. Arch. Surg. 111:489, 1976.

Athanasoulis, C. A., Baum, S., Waltman, A. C., et al.: Intra-arterial posterior pituitary extract for acute gastric mucosal hemorrhage. N. Engl. J. Med. 290:597, 1974.

Athanasoulis, C. A., Waltman, A. C., Novelline, R. A., et al.: Angiography: its contribution to the emergency management of gastrointestinal hemorrhage. Radiol. Clin. North Am. 14:265, 1976.

Baum, S., and Nusbaum, N.: Control of gastrointestinal hemorrhage by selective mesenteric artery infusion of vasopressin. Radiology 98:497, 1971.

Bogoch, A.: Hematemesis and melena. *In* Bockus, H. L. (ed.): Gastroenterology, 3rd ed. Philadelphia, 1976, W. B. Saunders Co.

Boley, S. J., Sprayregen, S., Veith, F. J., and Siegelman, S. S.: An aggressive roentgenologic and surgical approach to acute mesenteric ischemia. Surg. Annu. 5:355, 1973.

Bookstein, J. J., Chlosta, E. M., Foley, D., and Walter, J. F.: Transcatheter hemostasis of gastrointestinal bleeding using modified autogenous clot. Radiology 113:277, 1974.

Bragongiari, L. R., Lee, K. R., Moffat, R. E., et al.: Conversion of percutaneous ureteral stent to indwelling pigtail stent over guidewire. Urology 15:461, 1980.

Brant, B., Rosch, J., and Krippaehne, W. W.: Experiences with angiography in the diagnosis and treatment of acute gastrointestinal bleeding of various etiologies. Ann. Surg. 176:419, 1972.

Britt, L. G., and Cheek, R. C.: Nonocclusive mesenteric vascular disease. Ann. Surg. 169:704, 1969.

Byrne, J. J., and Guardione, V. A.: Surgical treatment of stress ulcers. Am. J. Surg. 125:464, 1973.

Chojkier, M., Groszmann, R. J., Atterbury, C. E., et al.: A controlled comparison of continuous intra-arterial and intravenous infusions of vasopressin in hemorrhage from esophageal varices. Gastroenterology 77:540, 1979.

Clark, R. A., Mitchell, S. E., Colley, D. P., and Alexander, E.: Percutaneous catheter biliary decompression. Am. J. Roentgenol. 137:503, 1981.

Conn, H. O., Ramsby, G. R., and Storer, E. H.: Selective intra-arterial vasopressin in the treatment of upper gastrointestinal hemorrhage. Gastroenterology 63:634, 1972.

Davis, L. J., Anderson, J., Wallace, S., and Jacobson, E. D.: Experimental use of prostaglandin E_1 in nonocclusive mesenteric ischemia. Am. J. Roentgenol. 125:99, 1975.

Drapanas, T., Woolverton, W. C., Reeder, J. W., et al.: Experiences with surgical management of acute gastric mucosal hemorrhage. Ann. Surg. 173:628, 1971.

Eastcott, H. H. G.: Arterial surgery, 2nd ed. Philadelphia, 1973, J. B. Lippincott Co.

Edmondson, H. T., Jackson, F. C., Juler, G. L., et al.: Clinical investigation of portacaval shunt. Ann. Surg. 173:372, 1971.

Federle, M. P.: Abdominal trauma: the role and impact of computed tomography. Invest. Radiol. 16:260, 1981.

Ferrer, M. I., Bradley, S. E., Wheeler, H. O., et al.: The effect of digoxin in the splanchnic circulation in ventricular failure. Circulation 32:524, 1965.

Ferrucci, J. T., Jr.: Diagnostic imaging of the liver and bile ducts. Invest. Radiol. 13:269, 1978.

Ferrucci, J. T., Jr., and Wittenberg, J.: CT biopsy of abdominal tumors: aids for lesion localization. Radiology 129:739, 1978.

Ferrucci, J. T., Jr., and Wittenberg, J.: Reply. Radiology 131:800, 1979.

Fisher, R. G., and Ferreyro, R.: Evaluation of current techniques for nonsurgical removal of intravascular iatrogenic foreign bodies. Am. J. Roentgenol. 130:541, 1978.

Gerlock, A. J., Jr., Muhletaler, C. A., Coulam, C. M., and Hayes, P. T.: Traumatic aortic aneurysms: validity of esophageal tube displacement sign. Am. J. Roentgenol. 135:713, 1980.

Gerzof, S. G., Robbins, A. H., Birkett, D. H., et al.: Percutaneous catheter drainage of abdominal abscesses guided by ultrasound and computed tomography. Am. J. Roentgenol. 133:1, 1979.

Gilday, D. L., and Alderson, P. O.: Scintigraphic evaluation of liver and spleen injury. Semin. Nucl. Med. 4:357, 1974.

Gliedman, M. L., Ayers, W. B., and Vestal, B. L.: Aneurysms of the abdominal aorta and its branches: a study of untreated patients. Ann. Surg. 146:207, 1957.

Goldberg, B. B., and Lehman, J. S.: Aortosonography: ultrasound measurement of the abdominal and thoracic aorta. Arch. Surg. 100:652, 1970.

Haaga, J. R., Craig, G., Weinstein, A. J., and Cooperman, A. M.: New interventional techniques in inflammatory abdominal disease. Radiol. Clin. North Am. 17:485, 1979.

Haaga, J. R., and Weinstein, A. J.: CT-guided percutaneous aspiration and drainage of abscesses. Am. J. Roentgenol. 135:1187, 1980.

Habboushe, F., Wallace, H. W., Nusbaum, M., et al.: Nonocclusive mesenteric vascular insufficiency. Ann Surg. 180:819, 1974.

Harris, S. K., Bone, R. C., and Ruth, W. E.: Gastrointestinal hemorrhage in a respiratory intensive care unit (abstr.). Am. Rev. Respir. Dis. 113:178, 1976.

Hawkins, I. F.: New fine needle for cholangiography with optional sheath for decompression. Radiology 131:252, 1979.

Heiberg, E., Wolverson, M., Sundaram, M., et al.: CT findings in thoracic aortic dissection. Am. J. Roentgenol. 136:13, 1981.

Ho, P. C., Talner, L. B., Parsons, C. L., and Schmidt, J. D.: Percutaneous nephrostomy: experience in 107 kidneys. Urology 16:532, 1980.

Hoffer, P. B.: Gallium and infection. J. Nucl. Med. 21:484, 1980.

Hoffer, P. B.: Use of gallium-67 in the diagnosis of occult infections. Conn. Med 45:288, 1981.

Khan, F., and Seriff, N. S.: Stress ulcer bleeding as a major cause of death in patients undergoing treatment for acute respiratory failure. (abstr.).. Am. Rev. Respir. Dis. 113:180, 1976.

Kirsch, M. M., Behrendt, D. M., Orringer, M. B., et al.: The treatment of acute rupture of the aorta: a 10-year experience. Ann. Surg. 184:308, 1976.

Klippel, A. P., and Butcher, H. R., Jr.: The unoperated abdominal aortic aneurysm. Am. J. Surg 111:629, 1966.

Lepasoon, J., and Olin, T.: Angiographic diagnosis of splenic lesions following blunt abdominal trauma. Acta Radiol. (Diagn.) 11:257, 1971.

Lim, R. C., Jr., Glickman, M. G., and Hunt, T. K.: Angiography in patients with blunt trauma to the chest and abdomen. Surg. Clin. North Am. 52:551, 1972.

Mall, J. C., and Kaiser, J. A.: CT diagnosis of splenic laceration. Am. J. Roentgenol. 134:265, 1980.

McFarland, J., Willerson, J. T., Dinsmore, R. E., et al.: The medical treatment of dissecting aortic aneurysms. N. Engl. J. Med. 286:115, 1972.

McLoughlin, M. J., Ho, C.-S., and Tao, L.-C.: Computed tomography biopsy of abdominal tumors (letter). Radiology 131:800, 1979.

Okuda, K., Tanikawa, K., Emura, T., et al.: Nonsurgical percutaneous transhepatic cholangiography—diagnostic significance in medical problems of the liver. Dig. Dis. 19:21, 1974.

Otis, R. D.: Fine needle aspiration of lung lesions: observations by a pathologist. Conn. Med. 44:471, 1980.

Parmley, L. F., Mattingly, T. W., Manron, W. C., and Jahnke, E. J., Jr.: Nonpenetrating traumatic injury of the aorta. Circulation 17:1086, 1958.

Pereiras, R., Viamonte, M., Jr., Russell, E., et al.: New techniques for interruption of gastroesophageal venous blood flow. Radiology 124:313, 1977.

Pereiras, R. V., Meiers, W., Kunhardt, B., et al.: Fluoroscopically guided thin needle aspiration biopsy of the abdomen and retroperitoneum. Am. J. Roentgenol. 131:197, 1978.

Pollock, T. W., Ring, E. R., Oleaga, J. A., et al.: Percutaneous decompression of benign and malignant biliary obstruction. Arch. Surg. 114:148, 1979.

Prando, A., Wallace, S., Von Eschenbach, A. C., et al.: Lymphangiography in staging of carcinoma of the prostate. Radiology 131:641, 1979.

Prochaska, J. M., Flye, M. W., and Johnsrude, I. S.: Left gastric artery embolization for control of gastric bleeding: a complication. Radiology 107:521, 1973.

Renert, W. A., Button, K. E., Field, S. L., and Casarella, W. J.: Mesenteric venous thrombosis and small bowel infarction following infusion of vasopressin into the superior mesenteric artery. Radiology 102:299, 1972.

Reuter, S. R., Chuang, V. P., and Bree, R. L.: Selective arterial embolization for control of massive upper gastrointestinal bleeding. Am. J. Roentgenol. 125:119, 1975.

Rosch, J., Dotter, C. T., and Rose, R. W.: Selective arterial infusions of vasoconstrictors in acute gastrointestinal bleeding. Radiology 99:27, 1971.

Siegelman, S. S., Sprayragen, S., and Boley, S. J.: Angiographic diagnosis of mesenteric arterial vasoconstriction. Radiology 112:533, 1974.

Simeone, J. F., Minagi, H., and Putman, C. E.: Traumatic disruption of the thoracic aorta: significance of the left apical extrapleural cap. Radiology 117:265, 1975.

Skillman, J. J., Bushnell, L. S., Goldman, H., and Silen, W.: Respiratory failure, hypotension, sepsis, and jaundice, a clinical syndrome associated with lethal hemorrhage from acute stress ulceration of the stomach. Am. J. Surg. 117:523, 1969.

Smith, E. H., Bartrum, R. J., Chang, Y. C., et al.: Percutaneous aspiration biopsy of the pancreas under ultrasonic guidance. N. Engl. J. Med. 292:825, 1975.

Sondheimer, F. K., and Steinberg, I.: Gastrointestinal manifestations of abdominal aortic aneurysms. Am. J. Roentgenol. 92:1110, 1964.

Stables, D. P., Ginsberg, M. J., and Johnson, M. L.: Percutaneous nephrostomy: a series and review of the literature. Am. J. Roentgenol. 130:75, 1978.

Tao, L.-C., Sanders, D. E., McLoughlin, M. J., et al.: Current concepts in fine needle aspiration biopsy cytology. Hum. Pathol. 2:94, 1980.

Terblanche, J., Northover, J. M. A., Bornman, P., et al.: A prospective controlled trial of sclerotherapy in the long-term management of patients after esophageal variceal bleeding. Surg. Gynecol. Obstet. 148:323, 1979.

Thompson, A. E., Spracklen, F. H. N., Besterman, E. M. N., and Bromley, L. L.: Recognition and management of dissecting aneurysms of the aorta. Br. Med. J. 4:134, 1969.

Thomson, K. R., and Goldin, A. R.: Angiographic techniques in interventional radiology. Radiol. Clin. North Am. 17:375, 1979.

Valencia-Parparcen, J.: Acute gastritis. *In* Bockus, H. L. (ed.): Gastroenterology, 3rd ed. Philadelphia, 1976, W. B. Saunders Co.

Welch, C. E.: Abdominal surgery, part I. N. Engl. J. Med. 288:609, 1973.

White, R, I., Jr., Harrington, D. P., Novac, G., et al.: Pharmacologic control of hemorrhagic gastritis: clinical and experimental results. Radiology 111:549, 1974.

Widrich, W. C., Robbins, A. H., Nabseth, D. C., et al.: Pitfalls of transhepatic portal venography in therapeutic coronary vein occlusion. Am. J. Roentgenol. 131:637, 1978.

Williams, L. F.: Vascular insufficiency of the intestines. Gastroenterology 61:757, 1971.

Chapter 10

SYSTEMIC EFFECTS OF INVASIVE RADIOGRAPHIC STUDIES—IMPLICATIONS FOR PATIENT MANAGEMENT

by H. Joel Gorfinkel

Since the advent of intensive care facilities, the radiologist has become an important member of the team caring for the critically ill patient. Invasive diagnostic studies involving the heart and vascular system are frequently indicated in these acutely ill patients. Therefore, it is essential for the radiologist and intensivist (intensive care specialist) to be familiar with the consequences and complications of radiographic contrast studies and with the methods of treatment used to handle these problems.

This chapter is divided into three sections. The first section deals with the techniques for electrocardiographic (ECG) and hemodynamic monitoring during angiography. The second section describes the rhythm disturbances associated with catheter manipulations within the vascular system. The final section discusses the pharmacologic and pathophysiologic effects of contrast media on certain organ systems and the complications that may occur. The more common complications of catheterization itself (perforation, extravasation, hemorrhage, thrombosis, and embolism) are discussed briefly in Chapter 9. The basics of cardiopulmonary resuscitation (CPR) are discussed in the appendix.

TECHNIQUES, EQUIPMENT, AND INDICATIONS FOR CARDIOVASCULAR MONITORING

Critically ill patients frequently have an unstable cardiovascular status. They may have preexistent cardiac arrhythmias and may be undergoing procedures, such as pulmonary angiography, that predispose them to arrhythmias. It is essential that the angiographic laboratory be equipped with specific monitoring and life support equipment to follow and treat such patients.

An absolute necessity is an ECG machine that incorporates a strip chart recorder and oscilloscopic display of the ECG. The next item needed is a hemodynamic pressure module and transducer system to measure and record intravascular pressures. Compact systems incorporating an ECG module, pressure modules, an oscilloscopic display, and a strip chart recorder are available from many manufacturers.

The next essential item is a direct-current (DC) defibrillator—one that delivers both a synchronized countershock (for cardioversion of atrial and ventricular tachyarrhythmias) and a nonsynchronized countershock (for treatment of ventricular fibrillation).

Finally, the angiographic laboratory must be equipped with suctioning apparatus, an oxygen delivery system, and an emergency "crash" cart containing all the essential drugs and accessories necessary for treatment of cardiopulmonary arrest and other emergencies. Table 10–1 lists the items that should be contained in the crash cart. The number of items and drugs in this list has been pared down to the few essential ones needed to make a resuscitative effort. Those drugs and materials necessary for prolonged resuscitation or advanced life support will be brought to the scene by the hospital cardiac arrest team and need not be part of the angiographic laboratory's crash cart.

ECG Monitoring

Patients undergoing pulmonary, cardiac, or aortic root angiography or high-risk patients receiving any type of intravascular contrast material should be monitored electrocardiographically, since these procedures may produce ventricular arrhythmias. The patient should be connected to the ECG machine with the conventional four limb leads. The chest lead need not be connected to the patient, but should be kept available in case an arrhythmia develops that requires analysis of the precordial leads to enhance diagnostic accuracy. Electrode jelly or paste should be applied generously to the leads to ensure optimal contact and thereby minimize the likelihood of artifacts. The lead that displays

TABLE 10–1. Essential Items for a Basic Life Support Crash Cart*

I. Respiratory management
   A. Oxygen supply with reducing valves capable of delivering 15 liters/min with mask and reservoir bag
   B. Oropharyngeal airway
   C. Laryngoscope with blades
   D. Assorted adult-size (cuffed) endotracheal tubes
   E. Syringe with clamps for endotracheal tube cuffs
   F. Bag with valve and manually triggered, oxygen-powered resuscitator
II. Circulatory management
   A. Venous infusion sets (micro- and macro-)
   B. Indwelling venous catheters
      1. Catheter outside needle (size 14 to 22)
      2. Catheter inside needle (size 14 to 22)
      3. Central venous pressure (CVP) catheters
   C. Intravenous (IV) setup and solutions (D5W and Ringer's lactate solution)
      1. Cutdown set
      2. Sterile gloves
      3. Assorted syringes (5, 10, and 20 ml), needles, stopcocks, and venous extension tubes
   D. Intracardiac needles
   E. Tourniquets, adhesive tape, and 4 × 4 inch gauze pads
      Essential drugs
      1. Sodium bicarbonate
         a. Prefilled syringes: 50 ml, 7.5% solution (44.6 mEq)
         b. Ampules: 50 ml, 7.5% solution (44.6 mEq)
      2. Epinephrine
         a. Prefilled syringes: 10 ml (1.0 mg in 1:10,000 dilution)
         b. Ampules: 1 ml (1.0 mg in 1:1000 dilution)
      3. Atropine
         a. Prefilled syringes: 10 ml, 1.0 mg/10 ml (0.1 mg/ml)
         b. Vials: 20 ml (0.4 mg/ml)
      4. Lidocaine hydrochloride
         a. Prefilled syringes: 10 ml, 100 mg/10 ml (1% solution)
         b. Vials or ampules: 50 ml, 1.0 gm/vial (20 mg/ml)
      5. Calcium chloride
         a. Prefilled syringes: 10 ml calcium chloride (10%), 1.0 gm
         b. Ampules: 10 ml calcium chloride, 10%; 10 ml calcium gluconate, 10%
   G. Drugs for treatment of allergic reactions
      1. Epinephrine, as above
      2. Diphenhydramine hydrochloride (Benadryl); ampules: 50 mg
      3. Hydrocortisone vials: 1.0 gm

*Adapted from Standards and Guidelines for Cardiopulmonary Resuscitation (CPR) and Emergency Cardiac Care (ECC), J.A.M.A. (Suppl.)244:453, 1980.

the tallest P and QRS complexes should be chosen. This is usually lead II, but the lead needs to be determined in each patient. Intracardiac manipulation of catheters and injection of contrast material into the heart or pulmonary arteries should never be conducted without observation of a high-quality, artifact-free ECG signal.

Defibrillator

The defibrillator should be turned on in the nonsynchronized mode (defibrillating mode) and tested to ensure that it is in proper working order. The electrodes should be easily accessible and should be prepared with generous amounts of electrode paste or with pads fully soaked in normal saline solution. However, in order to protect the circulating personnel from obtaining an accidental shock, the defibrillator should not be energized with a charge. If needed, it may be energized to full capacity within seconds.

Hemodynamic Monitoring

Monitoring of the right-sided cardiac and pulmonary arterial pressures is required whenever pulmonary angiography is performed. Anyone performing pulmonary angiography should be familiar with the proper use of the pressure transducer system. Data concerning these pressures are extremely useful in helping to assess the pathophysiologic severity of a pulmonary embolus in a patient suspected of having this diagnosis. In patients without complicating diseases that elevate the pulmonary arterial pressure (such as chronic severe left ventricular failure, chronic obstructive pulmonary disease [COPD], or mitral stenosis), the higher the pulmonary arterial pressure, the more severe the embolus (McIntyre and Sarahara, 1974). In addition, the risks involved in angiography in patients with severe elevation of the pulmonary arterial pressure (above 50 mm Hg) increase. In such patients, selective injections should be performed with smaller quantities of contrast material at lower injection pressures, in order to help prevent serious hemodynamic complications such as an abrupt drop in cardiac output accompanied by shock. In technically difficult arteriographic cases, in which the catheter cannot be advanced easily to the proper position, it is useful to follow the hemodynamic waveform. In this manner, catheter entrapment can be quickly identified by damping of the characteristic arterial pulse waveform. When this occurs, the catheter should be immediately withdrawn several centimeters and redirected in order to prevent dissection or perforation of the vessel wall.

Every patient should have an easily accessible, widely patent intravenous (IV) line functioning before the procedure is started. This ensures the prompt administration of emergency drugs should the need arise. The angiographic catheter will not suffice for this purpose, since a complication may occur before the catheter has been inserted. Similarly, arterial catheters should never be used for drug administration, because of the local toxic effects produced by agents such as barbiturates, tranquilizers, and sympathomimetic amines (Gould and Lingon, 1977; Klatte et al., 1969).

RHYTHM DISTURBANCES ASSOCIATED WITH INTRAVASCULAR CATHETER MANIPULATION

Most patients tolerate the introduction of angiographic catheters into the circulatory system without difficulty. Infrequently, patients may develop profound sinus bradycardia, occasionally accompanied by significant hypotension, as the venous cutdown is being performed or as a vein or artery is punctured for percutaneous passage of the catheter (Andrews, 1976). A similar reaction has been observed during the injection of contrast material for IV urography (Andrews, 1976; Witten, 1975), cholangiography (Andrews, 1976; Stanley and Pfister, 1976), and cerebral angiography (Tornell, 1968). The bradycardia-hypotensive response is due to a sudden increase in vagal tone and may be identified clinically as a marked slowing of the pulse; pallor; occasionally, nausea, vomiting, and intestinal cramping; dulling of the sensorium; or frank syncope. The vasovagal response may be reversed within minutes by the IV administration of 0.6 mg atropine. If there is no response within two to three minutes, additional aliquots of 0.3 mg atropine should be given every three minutes, not to exceed a total dose of 1.5 mg. On occasion, atropine will not counteract the hypotension despite the correction of the bradycardia. Under these circumstances, fluid infusion and elevation of the legs should correct the hypotension. A history of glaucoma or urinary retention is a relative contraindication for the use of atropine, but obviously the seriousness of the patient's status should dictate its use.

The most common radiologic procedure that may produce cardiac arrhythmias is pulmonary angiography. A discussion of the rhythm disturbances produced by left ventriculography and coronary angiography is beyond the scope of this chapter, but these disturbances should be well known to anyone performing these procedures.

Patients who have sustained a pulmonary embolus are prone to develop atrial arrhythmias, such as atrial fibrillation, atrial flutter, or atrial tachycardia, as a natural consequence of their acute disease. Therefore, they may arrive in the angiographic laboratory with an ongoing arrhythmia. Consultation with and the presence of an internist or cardiologist are helpful under these circumstances.

Atrial Arrhythmias

As the catheter is introduced into the right atrium and contacts the wall, atrial premature beats are frequently produced (Fig. 10–1A). These are usually of no clinical significance, and the procedure may be continued. On occasion, however, these premature beats may lead to atrial arrhythmias such as atrial fibrillation, atrial flutter, or atrial tachycardia (Fig. 10–2). These rhythm disturbances may be brief and self-limited; however, when sustained with a rapid ventricular response they may lead to palpitations, hypotension, or congestive heart failure (CHF). Under these circumstances, the procedure should be discontinued and immediate consultation with an internist or cardiologist sought. Frequently, techniques such as carotid sinus massage, edrophonium chloride administration, synchronized cardioversion, or atrial overdrive pacing may be utilized successfully on the scene, and the procedure may then be continued. These therapeutic modalities should be conducted only by those experienced in their application, since each intervention may be accompanied by its own complication. If a sustained atrial arrhythmia is initiated, the catheter should be withdrawn into either of the cavae but not removed from the venous system, since the catheter entry site may be used to insert a pacing electrode.

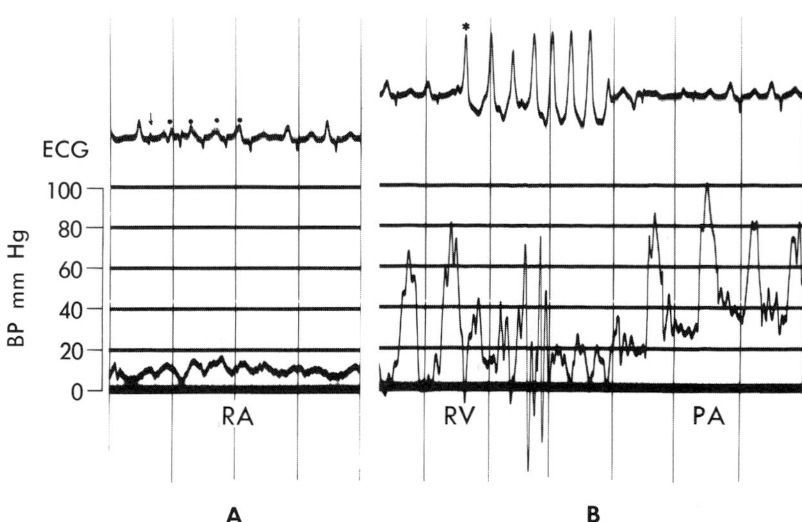

Figure 10–1. Right atrial (*RA*), right ventricular (*RV*), and pulmonary arterial (*PA*) pressures and ECG in a patient with chronic obstructive pulmonary disease (COPD) and severe pulmonary hypertension who was suspected of having a pulmonary embolus. This record was obtained as the catheter was advanced from the right atrium, through the right ventricle, and into the pulmonary artery. *A*, Patient's usual sinus P wave is very tall and peaked and is followed by a low-amplitude QRS (↓). A run of four premature atrial beats (·) follows this sinus beat. Premature atrial beats are commonly produced as the catheter is manipulated within the right atrium. *B*, Catheter manipulation in the right ventricle produces a run of ventricular tachycardia (*), which is abolished as soon as the catheter tip enters the pulmonary artery. Note the profound drop in right ventricular pressure during the burst of ventricular tachycardia. The time lines occur at intervals of one second. *BP* = blood pressure.

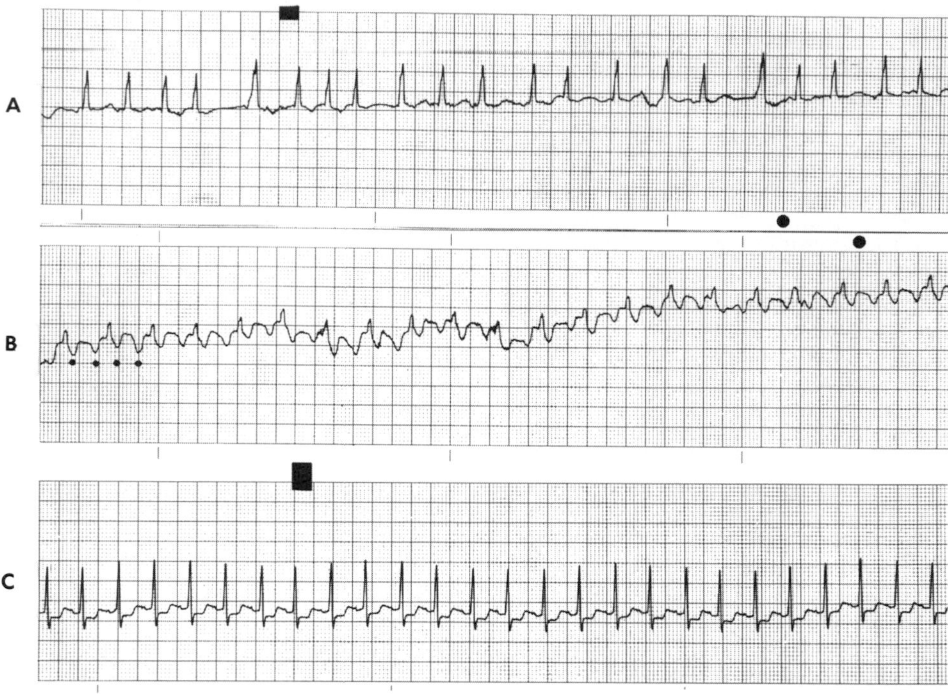

Figure 10–2. *A*, Atrial fibrillation. Note the irregular undulations of the baseline and the completely irregular intervals between each of the QRS complexes. *B*, Atrial flutter with 2:1 atrioventricular (AV) conduction. Note the regular appearance of flutter waves (·) at exactly twice the rate of the QRS complexes. The atrial rate is 290 and the ventricular rate is 145. *C*, Atrial tachycardia. Both atrial and ventricular rates are 175. The P waves are small and the PR interval is short (0.10 sec). Although this may resemble sinus tachycardia, the rate is faster than what would be expected in any condition other than that following maximal exercise.

Ventricular Arrhythmias

As the angiographic catheter traverses the right ventricle, premature ventricular contractions (PVCs) are invariably produced, as well as short runs of ventricular tachycardia (Fig. 10–1*B*). Sustained ventricular tachycardia seldom occurs; the ventricular irritability stops with the cessation of catheter manipulation. If the catheter is directed properly toward the right ventricular outflow tract, the ventricular ectopy will cease as the catheter enters the pulmonary artery. Ectopy persists when the catheter is entrapped in a papillary muscle or heads inferiorly to the patient's left, toward the right ventricular apex. At this time, it is best to withdraw the catheter to the right atrium and initiate right ventricular passage once again. An occasional patient will have profound ventricular ectopy. The best solution to this problem is a quick, accurate passage from the right atrium to the pulmonary artery; this minimizes the time the catheter tip spends in the easily irritated ventricle. Sustained ventricular tachycardia is rarely produced by this manipulation (Fig. 10–3), but if it occurs the catheter should be withdrawn to the right atrium and a bolus of lidocaine hydrochloride, 1 mg/kg, injected intravenously; this is followed immediately by an infusion of 2 to 4 mg/min. If the ventricular tachycardia is not aborted by the first 100 mg of lidocaine, additional injections using 50-mg aliquots should be used to a total dose of 225 mg. When this complication occurs, cardiology consultation should be sought. If the ventricular tachycardia is rapid to the point of hypotension and unconsciousness, the patient should be initially countershocked at 300 watt sec in the nonsynchronized mode.

Ventricular fibrillation is discussed in the appendix.

Conduction Defects

Patients who have pre-existent complete left bundle branch block (LBBB) (Fig. 10–4) should have a temporary transvenous right ventricular

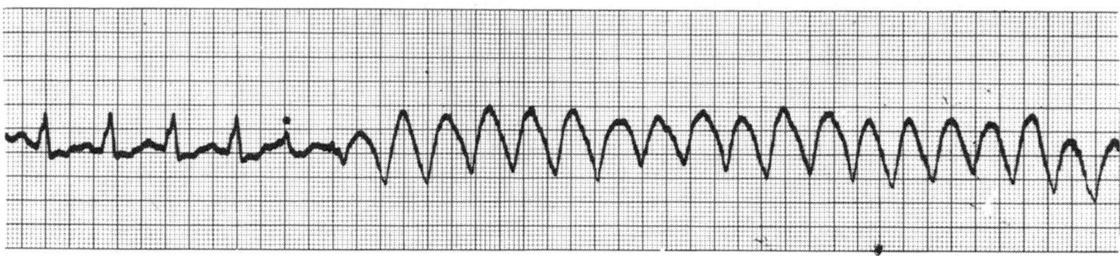

Figure 10–3. Sustained ventricular tachycardia. The fourth beat of sinus tachycardia is followed by a premature ventricular contraction (•), which initiates a sustained run of ventricular tachycardia.

pacing electrode inserted before pulmonary angiography is conducted. This is because the passage of the catheter across the tricuspid valve may produce complete heart block, leading to ventricular asystole. The anatomic basis for the occurrence of complete heart block under these circumstances is that the proximal portion of the right bundle branch passes just below the insertion of the medial leaflet of the tricuspid valve on the right side of the ventricular septum (Lev and Bharat, 1975). Therefore, the mild trauma of catheter contact in this area may produce transient right bundle branch block (RBBB). This is of no clinical consequence in a patient with normal intraventricular conduction, but in a patient with complete LBBB the addition of RBBB produces complete heart block. Temporary transvenous demand pacing will protect against this problem. When the angiographic procedure is completed, the pacing catheter may be removed.

SYSTEMIC EFFECTS AND COMPLICATIONS OF CONTRAST MEDIA

Radiographic contrast media have achieved a high degree of safety; severe complications from use of these agents occur only rarely. Contrast material is a powerful *pharmacologic* agent that has significant effects on numerous organ systems. Some of these effects are direct, druglike actions and may be expected to occur in almost every patient. These

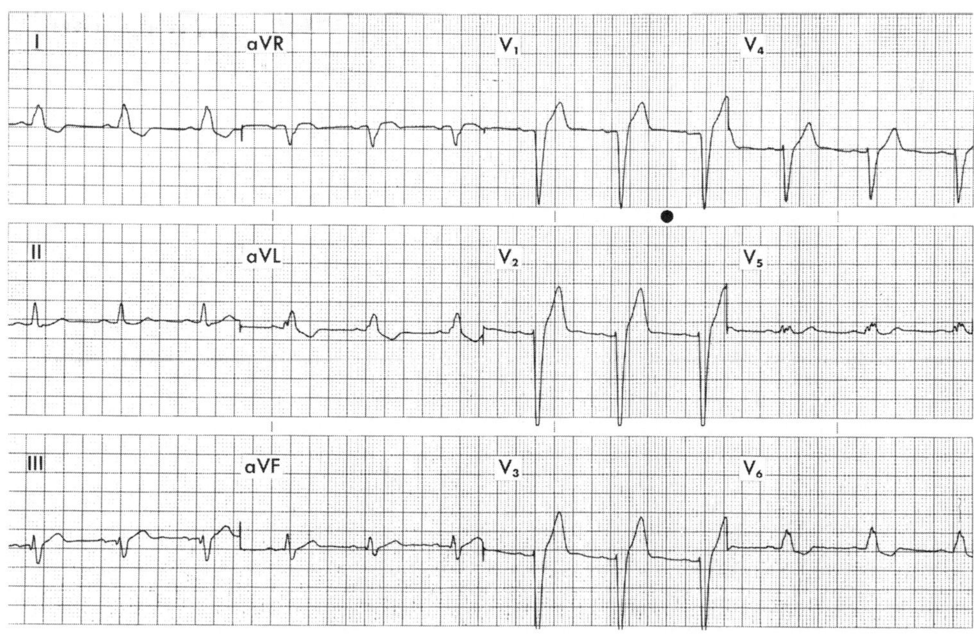

Figure 10–4. Left bundle branch block (LBBB). Note the wide, slurred QRS complexes, 0.12 sec in duration. Typically, the QRS complexes are upright in leads I, aVL, and V_6.

actions become significant only when they represent an exaggeration of the expected pharmacologic response or when they produce severe allergic or idiosyncratic reactions. Precise classification of contrast media reactions is difficult, because signs and symptoms may overlap. However, these reactions may be divided into two basic categories: pharmacologic and idiosyncratic.

In a biologic system, pharmacologic effects produce expected results that are based on physiologic and chemical principles. These reactions to contrast media are usually dose-related, although some of the more common ones (nausea and vomiting) are unrelated to the primary drug action. The most important pharmacologic property of contrast material is the powerful osmotic effect it produces in the vascular system. This initially causes rapid transfer of water into the intravascular space, producing hemodilution and volume expansion. Later, a large diuresis occurs and may produce significant depletion of intravascular volume.

The idiosyncratic or allergic response is more difficult to predict and is not well understood. It usually is not dose-related and cannot be explained by pharmacologic mechanisms.

This section deals primarily with the pharmacologic responses of the cardiovascular, renal, hematologic, and pulmonary systems to contrast media. The recognition and treatment of idiosyncratic or allergic reactions is not discussed at length, although reference is made to some of the proposed mechanisms and atypical reactions.

Cardiovascular System

The currently used ionic contrast material is hypertonic; such material has four to seven times the osmolality of blood (White, 1976), and therefore has the ability to cause a rapid increase in the intravascular volume because of a shift of water into the intravascular space. Contrast material also has a vasodilator effect on vascular smooth muscle. When a large dose of contrast material, such as may be used in pulmonary angiography with main and selective injections, is delivered over a short period of time into the right or left side of the circulatory system in a patient with a normal cardiovascular system, transient hypotension and tachycardia occur and cardiac output increases by as much as 50 per cent (Brown et al., 1965; Friesinger et al., 1965). Peripheral blood flow may increase by as much as 100 per cent because of vasodilatation caused by the hyperosmotic effect on vascular smooth muscle. The left ventricular filling pressure and stroke work index (the product of the cardiac index and systemic blood pressure) also increase. Systemic vascular resistance is reduced and muscle blood flow is enhanced. The increase in cardiac output is due to a combination of the peripheral vasodilatation and the induced hypervolemia, and their subsequent effects on ventricular function. These hemodynamic changes revert to normal within 20 minutes in most patients. Individuals who have normal cardiovascular systems can usually withstand this burden on their circulation without difficulty.

In patients with abnormal left ventricular function and borderline compensation, rapid expansion of the intravascular volume may cause the development of overt signs and symptoms of pulmonary edema. Since the degree of expansion of the intravascular space is proportional to the volume and osmolality of the contrast material, one must be prudent with regard to the amount of a contrast agent administered to patients with a history of CHF. If possible, such patients should be maximally compensated before angiographic or urographic procedures are performed. If it is not feasible to wait, because of the critical state of the illness and the importance of the diagnostic study for acute management, the patient may be diuresed with furosemide or ethacrynic acid during or after the study. Care must be taken following the study to ensure that the patient does not become fluid-depleted by the diuresis caused by the contrast agent.

ECG Changes

Invasive contrast studies that do not involve direct catheter manipulation within the heart rarely produce clinically significant changes in the ECG or in cardiac rhythm, although minor rhythm changes are frequently observed. In a group of 154 patients undergoing IV pyelography, 13 had a mild arrhythmia, two had a marked arrhythmia, and one showed changes compatible with ischemia (Small and Glenn, 1968). Thirty per cent of the total group had slight changes in the heart rate but no ECG changes. None of the patients had complications as a consequence of the ECG change. Unfortunately, the presence or absence of previous clinically detectable heart disease was not specified in this study.

In a group of 20 patients receiving IV infusion pyelograms of 300 ml and 10 patients receiving injections of 50 ml, there were 10 instances of ECG abnormalities (Berg et al., 1973). Six patients developed major ECG changes, ischemia, serious ventricular ectopy, or bundle branch block; all of these changes occurred in the infusion group. In the injection group, one patient developed a minor ECG abnormality. Three of the six patients showing a major ECG change had had a recent myocardial ischemic event preceding the contrast material administration.

A total of 275 patients were evaluated in a prospective study of the ECG responses to intravenous urography. An increase in heart rate of ten beats or more per minute was seen in half of the patients receiving the contrast agent as a bolus. S-T depression, Q-T prolongation, and premature ventricular contractions were observed in a minority of individuals. Three patients developed sustained ventricular tachycardia that responded to intravenous lidocaine administration; two of these received the contrast agent by bolus injection, and one by infusion. The investigators concluded that arrhythmias were more common in patients who received the contrast material by bolus injection than in those who received continuous infusion, especially in those with an antecedent history of an abnormal ECG, arteriosclerotic heart disease, or CHF (Stadalnik et al., 1977).

The mechanism by which contrast media produce arrhythmias has not been elucidated, although factors such as the sudden introduction of a hyperosmolar load, direct myocardial toxicity, and neurogenic stimulation have all been suggested (Stadalnik et al., 1974).

In summary, serious ECG changes are rarely encountered in patients undergoing IV pyelography. The highest-risk candidate is the elderly patient with a history of ischemic heart disease or CHF, especially one with a preexistent arrhythmia. Such patients should receive the lowest dose of contrast material needed to produce an adequate study, and their ECGs should be monitored during and for 30 minutes after the completion of the injection. The crash cart and defibrillator should be readily accessible.

Although not usually performed in the setting of an intensive care unit (ICU), a barium enema may be indicated in a patient housed in a critical care area. ECG changes that may occur are due to the discomfort of the procedure, to the distention of the bowel, and to the ensuing vagal effects on heart rate and atrioventricular (AV) conduction; they are not caused by any special property of the barium.

Minor, clinically insignificant rhythm changes were observed in 46 per cent of 95 patients undergoing a barium enema (Eastwood, 1972). However, serious arrhythmias or ischemic changes developed in 17 per cent of the entire group. Of these, ten had a history of heart disease and four were over 60 years of age. Although none of the patients in this series developed complications as a result of the barium enema, a severe vasovagal reaction responsive to atropine administration and rectal decompression has been reported (Andrews, 1976). This procedure should be used with discretion in elderly patients who have a history of heart disease or in ICU patients who have had unstable angina or myocardial infarction within the previous three weeks.

Hematologic System

Hemodilution, with a fall in the hemoglobin level and hematocrit value, occurs maximally within three to ten minutes following the bolus injection of contrast material (Brown et al., 1965; Friesinger et al., 1965; Rosenthal et al., 1973). The drop in the hematocrit value is proportionately greater than the drop in the hemoglobin level and is due to the hyperosmolality of the contrast material. The increase in intravascular tonicity causes water to pass out of the red blood cell, thereby shrinking its mass, and accounts for the greater proportional decrease in the hematocrit value (Rosenthal et al., 1973). This change in red blood cell contour may also be responsible for the microcirculatory sludging that may be seen following contrast material administration (Lasser et al., 1962).

A shift to the left in the oxyhemoglobin dissociation curve at the cellular level has also been demonstrated following the administration of contrast material. This occurs as a primary effect and is not related to a change in 2,3-diphosphoglyceric acid (2,3-DPG) concentrations (Rosenthal et al., 1973). When such a shift occurs, oxygen is more tightly bound to hemoglobin and is less readily released at the cellular level. Hypothetically, this could have a deleterious effect in patients who have a marginal cardiac reserve and who cannot respond with a compensatory increase in cardiac output following contrast material administration. In such patients, the lowering of tissue oxygen tension (Po_2) by this mechanism could produce clinical manifestations of ischemia. Thus far, this mechanism has not been proved clinically significant, although it may contribute theoretically to the observed ECG changes.

No significant changes in blood pH or arterial carbon dioxide (Pa_{CO_2}) or oxygen tension (Pa_{O_2}) values were noted following the intravascular injection of contrast material in studies by Becker and associates (1972) and Rosenthal and associates (1973). Measurable electrolyte alteration rarely occurs even with sodium-containing agents (White, 1976). Following selective and subselective pancreatic and hepatic arteriography using doses of contrast material totaling 3 ml/kg, there was no significant elevation in transaminase, amylase, alkaline phosphatase, or bilirubin levels (Goldstein and Bookstein, 1974). In the same study, following repeated hepatic venography by the wedge injection technique, several patients had transient elevations in the transaminase level, although single wedge injections produced no significant changes. Such transient enzyme level elevations are to be expected and are of no clinical significance. Increased sickling may occur in patients with SS or SA hemoglobinopathy following contrast studies (Richards and Nulsen, 1971). These patients should be well hydrated before and after undergoing such procedures.

Renal System

Since most contrast media, which by their composition are hypertonic, are excreted by the kidney, an osmotic diuresis is induced soon after the completion of a contrast agent injection (Hall and Childs, 1966). Despite this situation, renal insufficiency rarely occurs as a result of IV urographic procedures. In close to 116,000 excretory urograms performed at the Mayo Clinic, no instance of acute renal failure was documented in nondiabetic patients (Diaz-Buxo et al., 1975). However, renal failure following IV urography is a recognized but uncommon complication in patients who have diabetes or multiple myeloma, especially if dehydration or pre-existent renal disease with azotemia is present. In a series of over 4600 diabetic patients undergoing excretory urography, only eight developed acute oliguric renal failure, and all of these had clinical evidence of diabetic nephropathy, retinopathy, and neuropathy (Diaz-Buxo et al., 1975).

Acute renal failure following angiography is said to be very rare, although mild, reversible, and clinically insignificant elevation of creatinine may occur in 15 per cent of patients with normal or mildly impaired renal function (Teruel et al., 1981). In a retrospective study of 7400 patients undergoing angiography, only eight developed acute renal failure following the procedure (Port et al., 1974). Most of these patients had mild-to-moderate renal functional impairment, although many others with equally compromised renal function tolerated angiography without developing deterioration in their renal status.

Numerous other studies, as noted by Older and associates (1976), have documented a 0 to 5.3 per cent frequency of renal failure following angiography. However, in a study of 90 patients undergoing arteriography, nine developed renal failure following the procedure (Older et al., 1976). All these complications developed in patients with pre-existing renal disease and/or cardiovascular disease severe enough to require the chronic administration of digitalis, diuretics, or nitroglycerin. Hypotension was not present in any of these patients during the study and therefore could not be implicated in the genesis of the renal failure. It thus appears that this complication may be more common than was previously suspected.

The pathogenesis of renal failure following intravascular contrast material injection has been attributed to a number of mechanisms. Among these are increased blood viscosity due to aggregation and clumping of red blood cells, uricosuric effects, precipitation of Tamm-Horsfall urinary mucoprotein, tissue hypoxia due to the shift in the oxyhemoglobin dissociation curve, a direct toxic effect on the renal tubules, and possibly an allergic-like reaction to the contrast material (Diaz-Buxo et al., 1975). Contrast media, which have potent osmotic diuretic properties, may also compromise renal function by further depletion of the intravascular volume in a patient who is already dehydrated. The relative importance of each of the above mechanisms in producing renal failure has not been clearly elucidated.

Prevention of acute renal failure in patients undergoing intravascular contrast studies is best accomplished by first identifying the high-risk patient. Such individuals are those with pre-existing renal disease of any form, diabetes, multiple myeloma, severe cardiovascular disease with a history of CHF, and severe dehydration of any cause. Fluid should not be restricted and should be administered if dehydration is present. Patients with CHF should be in optimal fluid balance before undergoing study. Urinary output and the serum creatinine level should be monitored closely for the first 24 hours following the procedure. A sensitive indicator of impending renal failure may be the presence of a persistent nephrogram from 10 minutes to 24 hours following the injection (Robbins et al., 1975). A persistent nephrogram may indicate other renal problems, but should alert the clinician that renal insufficiency may be developing. Should this be true, fluid infusions and diuretics may reverse the impending problem.

Pulmonary System

The lungs are a common target organ for an allergic-like response; wheezing is a common symptom with hypersensitivity-like reactions and frequently responds quickly to antiallergic therapy. A decrease in respiratory function as measured by flow-volume curves has been reported in patients undergoing excretory urography (Rosenfield et al., 1976); this occurred regardless of whether they had a previous history of allergy. Patients with such a history did not have a more severe change than other patients. No patient developed any clinically significant symptoms. The mechanism and importance of this observation have yet to be determined.

Severe pulmonary edema may occur following the accidental aspiration of liquid, water-soluble contrast media (Chiu and Gambach, 1974). The hyperosmotic properties of these agents are responsible for drawing water from the pulmonary capillaries into the alveoli, thereby producing the pulmonary edema.

Hypersensitivity-like (Idiosyncratic) Reactions

For many years, direct evidence of a serologic or cellular immunologic response causing idiosyncratic reactions to contrast media has been suspected, but difficult to prove. Histamine has been shown to be released in response to contrast material administration both in vitro (Rockoff et al., 1970) and in vivo (Lasser et al., 1971), but by itself it does not prove to be an immunologic mechanism. In recent years there has been evidence that certain idiosyncratic reactions may be mediated through the immunologic system. Positive lymphocyte blast transformation reactions (McClennan et al., 1976) and specific antibody formation (Brasch and Caldwell, 1976) have been demonstrated in patients who experienced a severe idiosyncratic reaction following injection of a contrast agent. These data, although not proving a cause-and-effect relationship, do strongly suggest that some idiosyncratic reactions occurring with the use of contrast material may be mediated by immunologic mechanisms.

All radiologists should be familiar with the diagnosis and treatment of hypersensitivity-like contrast media reactions. Most of these reactions involve more than one organ system. For example, a mild reaction consisting of pallor, slight cough, and nausea is commonly observed. Table 10–2 summarizes the most common signs and symptoms of contrast media reactions in each organ system in increasing order of severity. The division of these reactions into mild, moderate, severe, and acute (life-threatening) is somewhat arbitrary, since the clinical implication of a moderate skin reaction may not have the same clinical seriousness as a moderate cardiovascular reaction.

Mild reactions usually need no specific therapy and will subside spontaneously. Moderate reactions should be cause to halt the study and may require immediate treatment. These signs and symptoms usually respond immediately to the IV injection of 25 to 50 mg diphenhydramine hydrochloride or the subcutaneous injection of 0.3 to 0.5 ml 1:1000 epinephrine, or both. Such patients should be observed closely until all signs and symptoms are relieved, to ensure that the condition does not recur.

Severe reactions must be treated more specifically and usually require continued observation of the patient in a critical care area. Severe bronchospasm may be treated by the IV administration of aminophylline in addition to epinephrine and diphenhydramine hydrochloride. Most of the severe cardiovascular reactions need to be evaluated immediately by an internist or cardiologist, but as a first line of treatment, hypotension caused by marked bradycardia should be treated with atropine, as discussed previously. Hypotension or shock unaccompanied by bradycardia is probably related to a sudden increase in the effective vascular space and should be initially treated by increasing the venous return. This is most quickly achieved by raising the legs and by increasing the rate of fluid infusion (preferably normal saline or Ringer's lactate solution). Any patient manifesting a severe cardiorespiratory reaction

TABLE 10–2. Signs and Symptoms of Contrast Media Reactions*

System	Mild	Moderate	Severe	Acute, Life-threatening
Cardiovascular	Pallor Diaphoresis	Vasospasm Cyanosis	Ischemic cardiac pain Hypotension Arrhythmias Acute pulmonary edema Shock	Cardiac arrest
Respiratory	Cough	Cough Dyspnea Wheezing (bronchospasm)	Acute asthma attack Cyanosis	Laryngospasm Laryngeal edema Apnea
Central nervous system	Anxiety Headache Fever†	Dizziness Agitation Vertigo Slurred speech Visual disturbance	Stupor Coma Convulsion	
Digestive	Nausea Vomiting Abdominal cramps Diarrhea	Salivary gland swelling†		
Skin	Erythema Conjunctival hyperemia	Urticaria Pruritus Angioneurotic edema	Cellulitis Lymphangitis†	
Urinary			Acute renal failure†	

*Modified from Pfister, R. C., Stanley, R. J., Thornbury, J. R., et al.: Management of adverse reactions to contrast media. The International Society of Radiology Committee on Contrast Media; Subcommittee on Treatment of Adverse Reactions, 1976.

†Usually delayed four to 36 hours before becoming apparent.

should be given high-flow oxygen by mask as the other diagnostic and therapeutic modalities are mobilized.

Laryngospasm is a life-threatening reaction and is treated by the subcutaneous administration of 0.3 to 0.5 ml 1:1000 epinephrine. Apnea may be due to oversedation or to airway obstruction caused by a relaxed tongue, and is best treated by inserting an oropharyngeal airway and extending the neck. Cardiac arrest and CPR are discussed in the appendix.

Corticosteroids are not useful in reversing the acute phase of a hypersensitivity-like reaction, since the onset of their action is delayed (Goodman and Gilman, 1975). These agents are useful as adjunct therapy once emergency drug therapy and supportive care have been delivered. Drugs used to treat these reactions should be kept readily available in the crash cart.

Several comprehensive reviews of contrast media reactions are available (Barnhard and Barnhard, 1968; Shehadi and Toniolo, 1980; Witten, 1975), including a survey of adverse reactions in over 300,000 patients (Shehadi and Toniolo, 1980) and a survey dealing with the emergency treatment of reactions to contrast media (Barnhard and Barnhard, 1968).

Hypotension as a contrast material reaction unresponsive to the usual mode of therapy, although unusual, is discussed in depth because of the need to recognize the problem quickly and because specific therapy may rapidly reverse this severe complication.

Five patients developed severe vascular collapse following contrast media studies (Obeid et al., 1975; Viner and Rhamy, 1975). They became suffused and cyanotic, complained of itching, and developed shock. Wheezing and shortness of breath were not present. They failed to respond to several IV doses of epinephrine, hydrocortisone, or diphenhydramine hydrochloride. Right atrial pressure was noted to be markedly reduced at this time, compared with control values, in two of the patients, indicating a sudden increase in intravascular space. All five patients were rapidly infused with saline solution and showed a prompt improvement in clinical status. Their reactions resembled an anaphylactic type of response, but were manifested primarily as circulatory collapse.

Any patient who becomes markedly hypotensive without striking bronchospasmic or cutaneous components following a contrast study should be rapidly volume-expanded if the usual therapy with epinephrine and diphenhydramine hydrochloride does not improve the clinical state. Under these circumstances, fluid therapy can be guided best by following left-sided cardiac filling pressures with the use of a balloon-tipped, flow-directed pulmonary arterial catheter.

A frequent dilemma is whether a contrast study should be performed in a patient with a history of a previous adverse reaction to a contrast agent. Although most authorities consider pretreatment of a high-risk patient to be of little value (Witten, 1975), one group has achieved a significant decrease in the frequency and severity of such reactions by pretreating high-risk patients with high doses of steroids (150 mg prednisone a day in divided doses, starting 18 hours before the procedure and continuing for 12 hours after completion of the procedure) (Zweiman et al., 1975). Most authorities do not recommend routine pretesting of a subject with small doses of contrast material, since this procedure identifies only a minority of patients who will sustain an adverse reaction (Pfister et al., 1976; Witten, 1975), and serious reactions can occur from the test dose alone.

REFERENCES

Andrews, E. J.: The vagus reaction as a possible cause of severe complications of radiological procedures. Radiology 121:1, 1976.

Barnhard, F. M., and Barnhard, H. J.: The emergency treatment of reactions to contrast media; updated 1968. Radiology 91:74, 1968.

Becker, J. A., Kinkhabwala, M., and Zolan, S.: Urography in renal failure. Radiology 105:505, 1972.

Berg, G. R., Hutter, A. M., and Pfister, R. C.: Electrocardiographic abnormalities associated with intravenous urography. N. Engl. J. Med. 289:87, 1973.

Brasch, R. C., and Caldwell, J. L.: The allergic theory of radiocontrast agent toxicity. Invest. Radiol. 11:347, 1976.

Brown, R., Rahimtoola, S. H., Davis, G. D., et al.: The effect of angiographic contrast medium on circulatory dynamics. Circulation 31:234, 1965.

Chiu, C. L., and Gambach, R. R.: Hypaque pulmonary edema; a case report. Radiology 111:91, 1974.

Diaz-Buxo, J. A., Wagoner, R. D., Hattery, R. R., et al.: Acute renal failure after excretory urography in diabetic patients. Ann. Int. Med. 83:155, 1975.

Eastwood, G. L.: ECG abnormalities associated with the barium enema. J.A.M.A. 219:719, 1972.

Friesinger, G. C., Schaffer, J., Criley, J. M., et al.: Hemodynamic consequences of the injection of radiopaque material. Circulation 31:730, 1965.

Goldstein, H. M., and Bookstein, J. J.: Biochemical evaluation of liver and pancreas following selective and subselective angiography. Radiology 111:293, 1974.

Goodman, L. S., and Gilman, A., (eds.): The Pharmacological Basis of Therapeutics, 5th ed. New York, 1975, Macmillan, p. 1500.

Gould, J. D. M., and Lingon, S.: Hazards of intra-arterial diazepam. Br. Med. J. 2:298, 1977.

Hall, J. W., and Childs, D. S.: The effects of diagnostic and therapeutic roentgenologic procedures on renal function. Med. Clin. North Am. 50:969, 1966.

Klatte, E. C., Brooks, A. C., and Rhamy, R. K.: Toxicity of intra-arterial barbiturates and tranquilizing drugs. Radiology 92:700, 1969.

Lasser, E. C., Farr, R. S., Fujimagaii, T., et al.: The significance of protein binding of contrast media in roentgen diagnosis. Am. J. Roentgenol. 87:338, 1962.

Lasser, E. C., Walters, A., Reuter, S. R., et al.: Histamine release by contrast media. Radiology 100:683, 1971.

Lev, M., and Bharat, S.: Anatomic basis for impulse generation and atrioventricular transmission. *In* Narula, O. S. (ed.): HIS Bundle Electrocardiography and Clinical Electrophysiology. Philadelphia, 1975, F. A. Davis Co., p. 6.

McClennan, B. L., Periman, P. O., and Rockoff, S. D.: Positive immunologic responses to contrast media. Invest. Radiol. 11:240, 1976.

McIntyre, K. M., and Sarahara, A. A.: Hemodynamic and ventricular responses to pulmonary embolism. Prog. Cardiovasc. Dis. 17:175, 1974.

Obeid, A. I., Johnson, L., Potts, J., et al.: Fluid therapy in severe systemic reaction to radiopaque dye. Ann. Intern. Med. 83:317, 1975.

Older, R. A., Miller, J. P., Jackson, D. C., et al.: Angiographically induced renal failure and its radiographic detection. Am. J. Roentgenol. 126:1039, 1976.

Pfister, R. C., Stanley, R. J., Thornbury, J. R., et al.: Management of adverse reactions to contrast media. The International Society of Radiology Committee on Contrast Media; Subcommittee on Treatment of Adverse Reactions, 1976.

Port, F. K., Wagoner, R. D., and Fulton, R. E.: Acute renal failure after angiography. Am. J. Roentgenol. 121:544, 1974.

Richards, D., and Nulsen, F. E.: Angiographic media and the sickling phenomenon. Surg. Forum 22:403, 1971.

Robbins, J. S., Mittemeyer, B. T., and Neiman, H. L.: The persistent nephrogram; a sentinel sign of contrast reactions. J. Urol. 114:758, 1975.

Rockoff, S. D., Brasch, R. C., Kuhn, L., et al.: Contrast media as histamine liberators. 1. Mast cell histamine release in vitro by sodium salts of contrast media. Invest. Radiol. 5:503, 1970.

Rosenfield, A. T., Littner, M. R., and Ulreich, S.: Respiratory effects of excretory urography. Invest. Radiol. 11:398, 1976.

Rosenthal, A., Litwin, S. B., and Laver, M. B.: Effect of contrast media used in angiocardiography on hemoglobin-oxygen equilibrium. Invest. Radiol. 8:191, 1973.

Shehadi, W. H., and Toniolo, G.: Adverse reactions to contrast media. Radiology 137:299, 1980.

Small, M. P., and Glenn, J. F.: Comparative evaluation of intravenous pyelographic contrast media and assessment of associated electrocardiographic alterations. J. Urol. 99:223, 1968.

Stadalnik, R., Davies, P., Vera, Z., et al.: Ventricular tachycardia during intravenous urography; report of two cases. J.A.M.A. 229:686, 1974.

Stadalnik, R. C., Vera, Z., DaSilva, O., et al.: Electrocardiographic response to intravenous urography: prospective evaluation of 275 patients. Am. J. Roentgenol. 129:825, 1977.

Stanley, R. J., and Pfister, R. C.: Bradycardia and hypotension following use of intravenous contrast media. Radiology 121:5, 1976.

Teruel, J. L., Marćen, R., Onaindia, J. M., et al.: Renal functional impairment caused by intravenous urography. A prospective study. Arch. Intern. Med. 141:1271, 1981.

Tornell, G.: Bradycardial reactions in cerebral angiography induced by sodium and methylglucamine iothalamate (Conray); comparison with urografin in a controlled study in man. Acta Radiol. 7:489, 1968.

Viner, N. A., and Rhamy, R. K.: Anaphylaxis manifested by hypotension alone. J. Urol. 113:108, 1975.

White, R. I.: Fundamentals of Vascular Radiology. Philadelphia, 1976, Lea & Febiger, pp. 27–41.

Witten, D. M.: Reactions to urographic contrast media. J.A.M.A. 231:974, 1975.

Zweiman, B., Mishkin, M., and Hildreth, E. A.: An approach to the performance of contrast studies in contrast material–reactive persons. Ann. Intern. Med. 83:159, 1975.

Chapter 11

CARDIOVASCULAR NUCLEAR MEDICINE AND ULTRASONOGRAPHY

by Harvey J. Berger, Arthur L. Riba, Alexander Gottschalk, and Barry L. Zaret

INTRODUCTION

During the past ten years, noninvasive imaging techniques have been applied broadly to the study of patients with cardiopulmonary disease. Developments in nuclear cardiology and echocardiography have made it possible to visualize the entire heart noninvasively. The clinical utility of these techniques is based on their relative ease of performance, safety, wide range of diagnostic applications, and reproducibility for serial studies. A fact of major importance is that these studies can be performed easily and rapidly at the bedside of the acutely ill patient; thus, they are ideally suited for use in the intensive care unit (ICU) environment. In the past, these techniques generally were limited to the stable patient, who could be brought to either the nuclear medicine or the ultrasound laboratory. Technologic development has contributed significantly to the recent expansion of these imaging approaches. Specialized computer systems have been coupled to more advanced scintillation cameras, thereby providing enhanced resolution, portability, and on-site data-processing capabilities. Cameras and computers now can be brought directly to the patient's bedside. High-count rate data acquisition can be obtained with commercially available instruments to improve markedly the statistical certainty of radionuclide data. In addition, the development of new radionuclides has contributed to the growth of this field. In a similar fashion, echocardiography has evolved from a limited M-mode examination alone to the two-dimensional technique, which provides detailed spatial information.

Detailed assessment of most forms of acquired heart disease can be achieved by the complementary use of plain-chest radiography and the newer, noninvasive cardiac imaging modalities. This chapter will emphasize uses of nuclear cardiology and echocardiography that are relevant to the radiologist involved in imaging of the critically ill. The basic principles and techniques will be reviewed first, followed by a discussion of the clinical applications of each technique.

NUCLEAR CARDIOLOGY

Cardiovascular nuclear imaging techniques suitable for the study of patients in the ICU can be divided into two general categories (Berger and Zaret, 1981). In the first, myocardial distributions of intracellular tracers are used to assess the adequacy of myocardial perfusion and the presence of necrosis. This approach, which allows evaluation of the patient with myocardial infarction or ischemia, can be performed in two distinct ways. In "cold-spot" imaging, radionuclide accumulation is maximal in areas of normal myocardium and minimal in the infarcted or ischemic zone; this procedure is performed with the potassium analogues, of which thallium-201 is the current radionuclide of choice. In contrast, in "hot-spot" imaging, uptake occurs in regions of acute necrosis; the technetium-99m (^{99m}Tc)-labeled phosphates (bone-scanning agents) are the current tracers employed. In the second category, intravascular tracers are used to assess cardiovascular performance. This also can be performed in two ways. In the first, gated cardiac blood pool imaging, the electrocardiogram (ECG) is introduced into the imaging process to control the temporal sequence of imaging of the entire equilibrium blood pool. In the alternative technique, first-pass radionuclide angiocardiography, only the first transit of the radionuclide bolus through the central circulation is analyzed. Since the introduction of these radionuclide techniques, they have progressed from the investigational stage to one of broad clinical application, particularly in the ICU setting.

Assessment of Myocardial Perfusion and Viability: Thallium-201 Imaging

The predominant factors governing thallium-201 distribution in the myocardium are regional myocardial perfusion and cellular viability. The distribution of thallium-201 in the myocardium is closely proportional to the regional myocardial blood flow over most of the flow range encountered clinically (DiCola et al., 1977; Strauss et al., 1975). The extraction of thallium-201 from the blood stream is extremely rapid and effective. Myocardial uptake of thallium-201 from the extracellular space represents the net result of both continuous extraction and release of thallium-201 by myocardial cells (Pohost et al., 1977).

Since thallium-201 has a low-energy primary photo peak and a relatively low target-to-background ratio, imaging with this radiotracer requires meticulous attention to technical details. The injected dose usually is 1.5 to 2 millicuries. High-count density images should be obtained in a minimum of three positions (Johnstone et al., 1979) Several computer methods have been proposed for image enhancement and quantification (Burow et al., 1971; Garcia et al., 1981; Watson et al., 1981). These techniques may be employed in data analysis in addition to interpretation of standardized analogue images. In normal hearts, the thallium-201 myocardial perfusion image demonstrates a homogeneous distribution of radioactivity in the left ventricular myocardium. There is a central zone of decreased radiotracer accumulation, corresponding to the left ventricular cavity. Small apical defects may be noted in normal hearts, because of relative thinning of the left ventricular myocardium at the apex. The right ventricle is not normally visualized when thallium-201 is injected at rest, but is visualized in the presence of either increased right ventricular mass or increased coronary blood flow. This may occur in right ventricular hypertrophy or in acute volume or pressure loading of the right ventricle (Wackers et al., 1981).

Clinical Applications of Thallium-201 at Rest

Resting studies have been used predominantly to evaluate patients with myocardial infarction (Berger et al., 1978a; Wackers et al., 1976). Infarcts are visualized as zones of relatively decreased radionuclide uptake that correspond to regions of necrosis (Figs. 11–1, 11–2). Early studies established a clear relationship between the frequency of resting perfusion de-

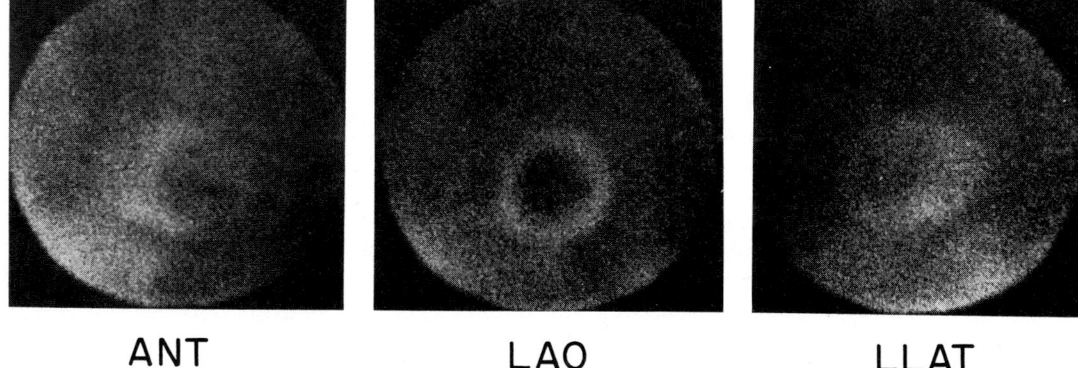

Figure 11–1. Resting thallium-201 images obtained in the anterior (*ANT*), 45° left anterior oblique (*LAO*), and left lateral (*LLAT*) positions in a patient with a large anterior wall myocardial infarction. Note the decreased perfusion in the anterior wall and the dilated cavity, particularly on the LAO image.

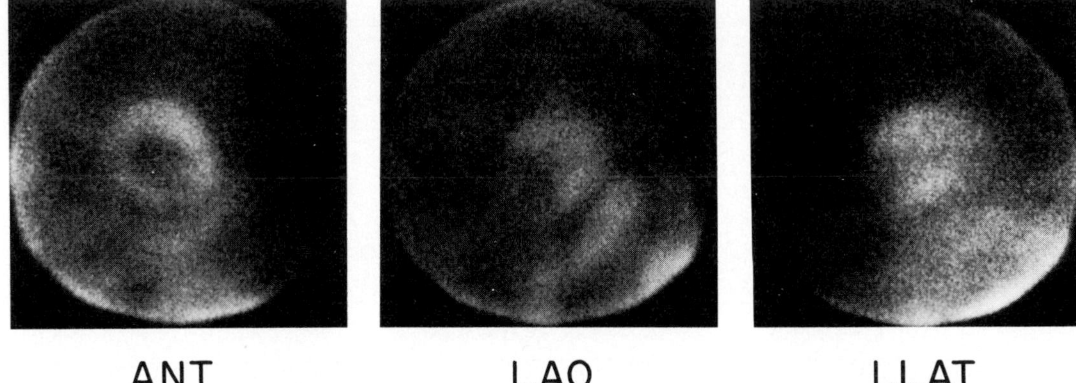

Figure 11–2. Resting thallium-201 images in a patient with an acute anteroseptal myocardial infarction and a history of a previous nontransmural myocardial infarction. Note the extensive perfusion defect involving the anteroseptal segment. The apex also is involved, possibly reflecting the previous infarct. Abbreviations as in Figure 11–1.

fects after infarction and the time interval between the onset of chest pain and imaging. The diagnosis of myocardial infarction can be made with the highest reliability during the initial 24 hours of infarction. Furthermore, patients with acute transmural myocardial infarction are more likely to have positive images than are patients with nontransmural infarction or smaller infarcts. Furthermore, the size of thallium-201 perfusion defects during the acute phase of infarction may have major prognostic importance (Silverman et al., 1980). Patients with large defects based on quantitative analysis have significantly higher postinfarction mortality than those with small defects. In addition, because of the relatively high sensitivity of thallium-201 imaging in the early hours of myocardial infarction, this approach has been suggested as a potential means of screening patients for admission to the coronary care unit (CCU) (Wackers et al., 1979).

Differentiation between acute and previous myocardial infarction cannot be made from a single thallium-201 study, unless a previous study is available for comparison. Transient myocardial ischemia also may be apparent on thallium-201 images obtained at rest, such as in patients with coronary artery spasm or unstable angina, especially when imaged during or soon after a period of pain (Wackers et al., 1978). In addition, studies have demonstrated that patients with severe critical coronary artery stenosis may have reversible perfusion abnormalities at rest in the absence of infarction or unstable angina (Berger et al., 1979). These data demonstrate the potential application of radionuclide techniques to clinical decision-making in the acutely ill patient.

Myocardial perfusion imaging is not limited to the study of acute ischemic heart disease. When combined with exercise stress, thallium-201 imaging is a highly sensitive technique for detection of reversible myocardial ischemia (Figs. 11–3, 11–4) (Berger and Zaret, 1981; Okada et al., 1980; Zaret et al., 1973). This is of particular importance in the follow-up of patients after acute myocardial infarction, or in the diagnostic assessment of patients with atypical symptoms or of those who are admitted to the CCU but show no objective evidence of infarction. Thallium-201 imaging combined with gated cardiac blood pool imaging also has been used to distinguish ischemic from idiopathic congestive cardiomyopathies. As noted previously, the presence of right ventricular thallium-201 visualization at rest is associated with increased right ventricular mass or coronary blood flow. Such findings have been demonstrated in patients with primary pulmonary hypertension, pulmonary embolism, and severe chronic obstructive pulmonary disease (COPD) (such as in cor pulmonale) (Figs. 11–5, 11–6) (Berger and Matthay, 1981; Cohen et al., 1976).

Infarct-Avid Imaging

An alternative imaging approach to the patient with acute myocardial infarction is the use of infarct-avid radiopharmaceuticals. Initial studies in humans were performed with radiolabeled tetracycline (Holman et al., 1974). However, the radionuclide most often employed at present is ^{99m}Tc stannous pyrophosphate, a commonly used bone-scanning agent. With this radionuclide, areas of infarction are visualized

Text continued on page 243

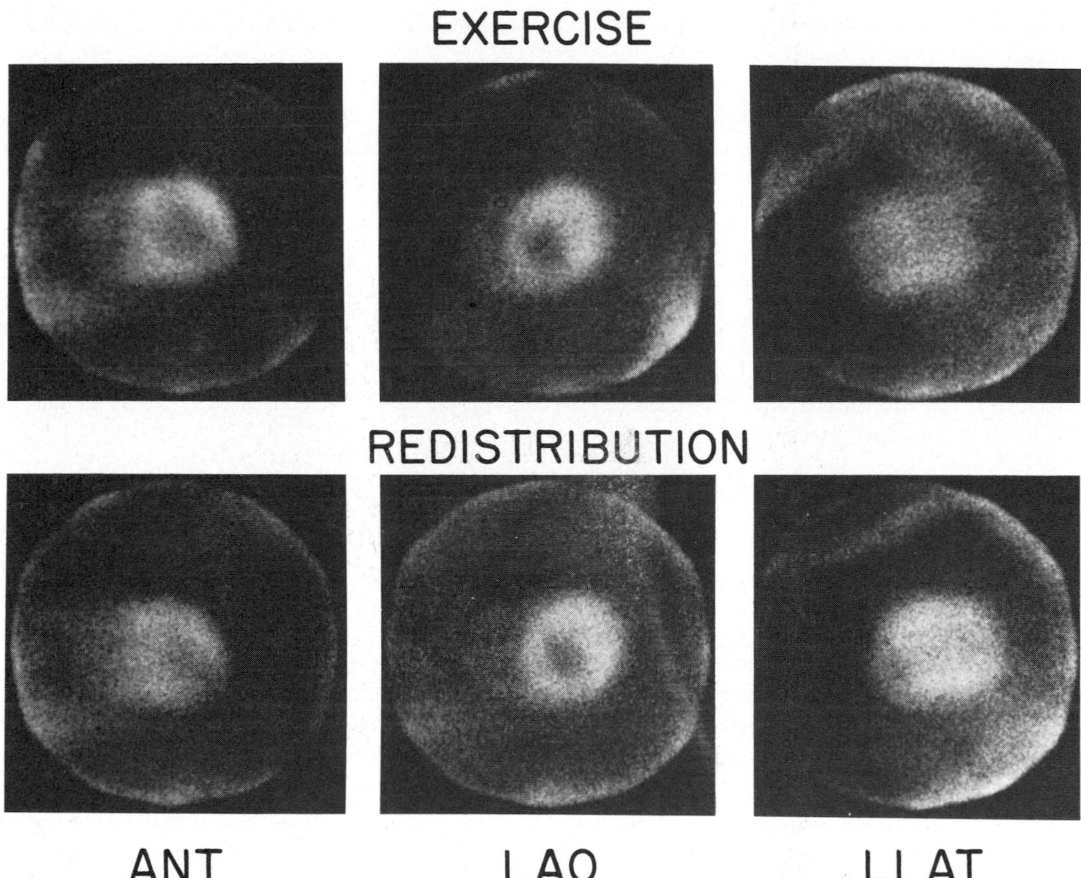

Figure 11–3. Thallium-201 images obtained immediately following exercise and four hours later at the time of redistribution in a patient with coronary artery disease. The exercise images demonstrate perfusion defects involving the septum and inferoapical region. At delayed imaging, there is redistribution predominantly in the septum. An apical perfusion defect persists. This study is consistent with exercise-induced myocardial ischemia superimposed upon previous myocardial infarction. This represents a high-risk finding post myocardial infarction. Abbreviations as in Figure 11–1.

EXERCISE

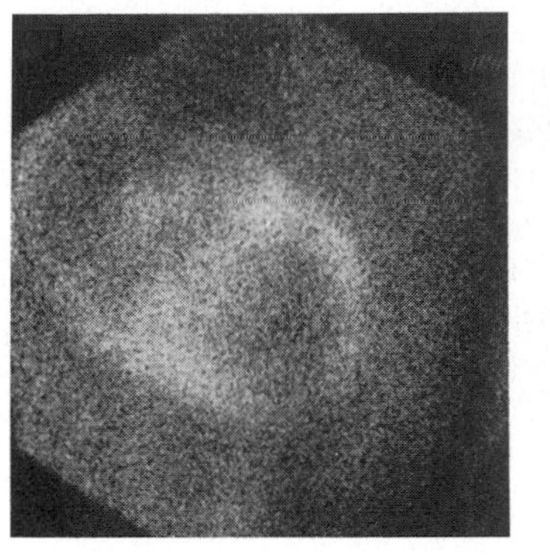

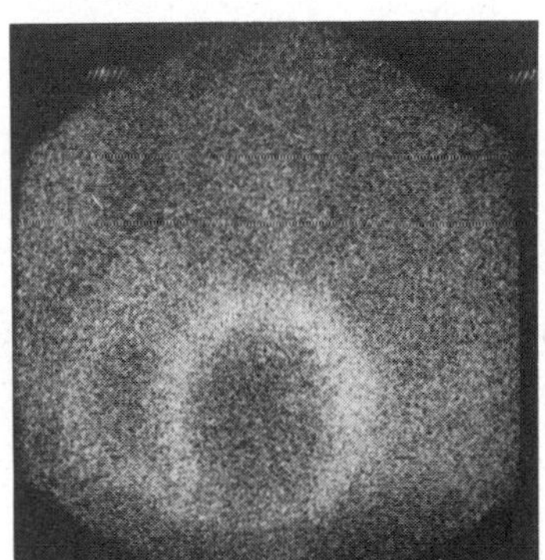

REDISTRIBUTION

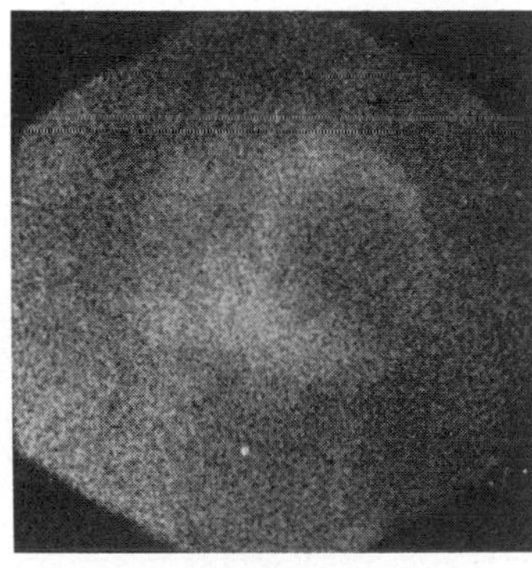

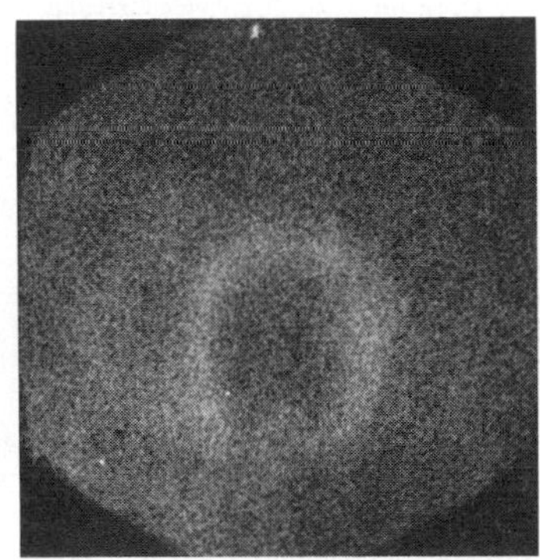

ANT LAO

Figure 11–4. Thallium-201 images obtained immediately following exercise and four hours later at delayed imaging in a patient with extensive anterior and inferior myocardial infarctions. Note the markedly dilated cavity and thin left ventricular walls. There is no significant difference between the exercise and redistribution images, consistent with myocardial infarction in the absence of exercise-induced myocardial ischemia. Abbreviations as in Figure 11–1.

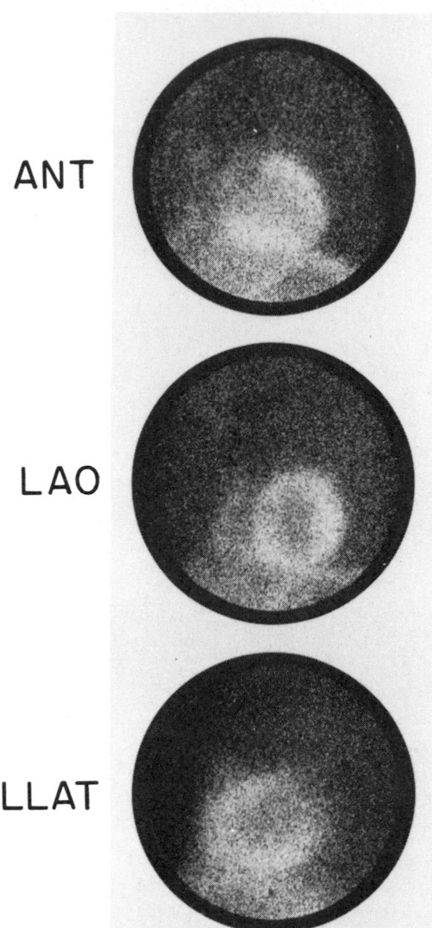

Figure 11–5. Resting thallium-201 images in a patient with previous apical myocardial infarction and cor pulmonale. Note the prominent visualization of the right ventricle at rest, consistent with right ventricular hypertrophy. An apical perfusion defect is demonstrated. At rest, the right ventricle usually is not visualized. Abbreviations as in Figure 11–1.

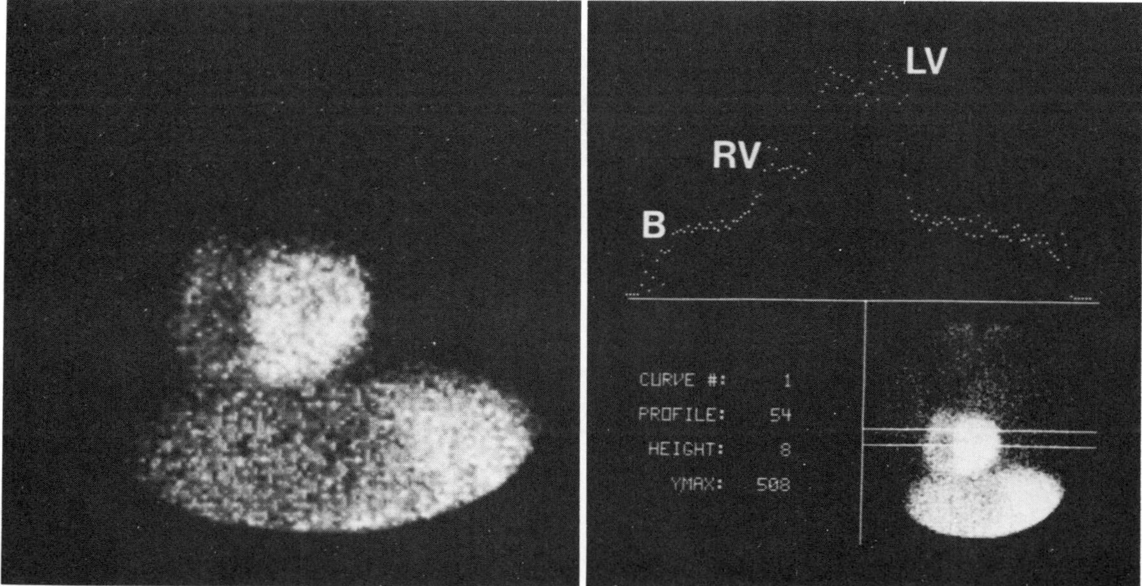

Figure 11–6. Computer method for quantifying the degree of right ventricular visualization. A resting, background-subtracted digital thallium-201 image in a patient with COPD is shown on the left. A computer-generated profile is shown on the right. The relative count rates for the background (*B*), right ventricle (*RV*), and left ventricle (*LV*) are depicted by the histogram. Note that right ventricular activity is approximately twice that in the background, but still less than in the left ventricle. This approach allows objective quantification of right ventricular visualization.

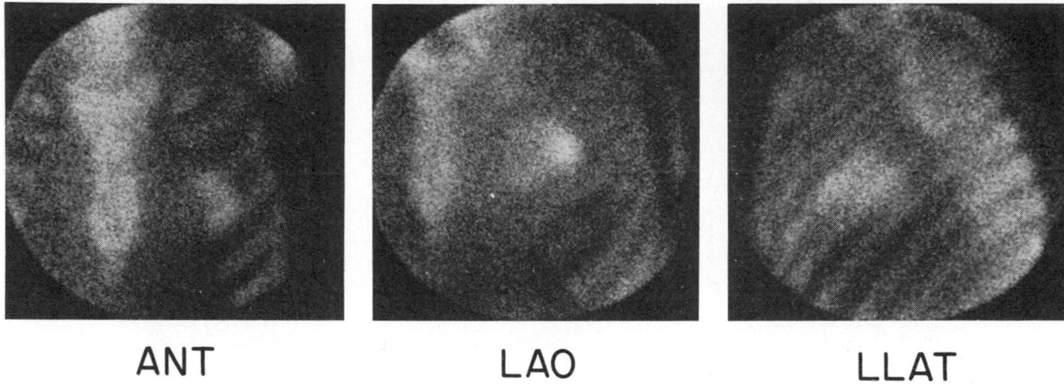

Figure 11–7. Technetium-99m stannous pyrophosphate images in a patient with acute lateral wall myocardial infarction. There is pyrophosphate deposition in the bony structures, as well as in the focal area of acute myocardial infarction. The activity in the area of infarction is greater than that in the ribs, almost comparable with that in the sternum. This finding is highly specific for acute transmural myocardial infarction. Abbreviations as in Figure 11–1.

as zones of increased tracer accumulation (Parkey et al., 1974). At this time, there are a limited number of instances in which pyrophosphate infarct imaging has major diagnostic value, and infarct-avid imaging therefore is the least frequently employed clinical technique in nuclear cardiology.

In acute myocardial infarction, pyrophosphate accumulation appears to temporally parallel calcium deposition. However, factors other than calcium deposition are involved in determining pyrophosphate uptake at the cellular level. Pyrophosphate binding to denatured proteins or other macromolecules that become accessible to radionuclides during the necrotic process appears to play a major role (Buja et al., 1977; Dewanjee and Kahn, 1976). Pyrophosphate accumulation also is dependent on regional myocardial blood flow, with peak accumulation occurring in myocardial regions where blood flow is approximately 30 to 40 per cent of normal. In regions with flow below this level, pyrophosphate uptake falls, although the degree of myocardial necrosis increases (Zaret et al., 1976).

Technetium-99m stannous pyrophosphate imaging is routinely performed in three positions one to three hours after intravenous (IV) administration of 15 millicuries of the tracer. The normal pyrophosphate image shows activity limited to bony structures, no activity being seen in the region of the heart. Interpretation of pyrophosphate images generally involves a grading system that takes into account both the site of abnormal pyrophosphate accumulation and its intensity (Fig. 11–7). Pyrophosphate imaging should be performed approximately 36 to 72 hours after the onset of chest pain. Images taken before that time generally do not show abnormalities, and they subsequently become normal approximately seven to ten days after the infarct appears.

Clinical Applications of Infarct-Avid Imaging

Initial studies with this approach were encouraging, demonstrating that pyrophosphate imaging was sensitive and specific for acute myocardial infarction. Based on studies published between 1974 and 1979, the sensitivity of the technique was approximately 89 per cent, with a specificity of 86 per cent (Holman and Wynne, 1980). However, there was a high incidence of abnormal scans (41 per cent) in patients with unstable angina in the absence of acute infarction. As with thallium-201 imaging, the sensitivity appears to be substantially lower in patients with relatively small or nontransmural myocardial infarcts.

It is clear that the majority of patients presenting to the CCU with acute myocardial infarction do not need pyrophosphate imaging for clinical diagnostic purposes; in most cases, the diagnosis has been established before the optimal time of pyrophosphate imaging. However, the technique appears to be useful in documenting acute infarction in patients who present several days after the acute event or after cardioversion, when conventional indices of myocardial infarction often are nondiagnostic. An important potential application of this imaging approach is in the surgical ICU following cardiac surgery, when routine enzymatic and electro-

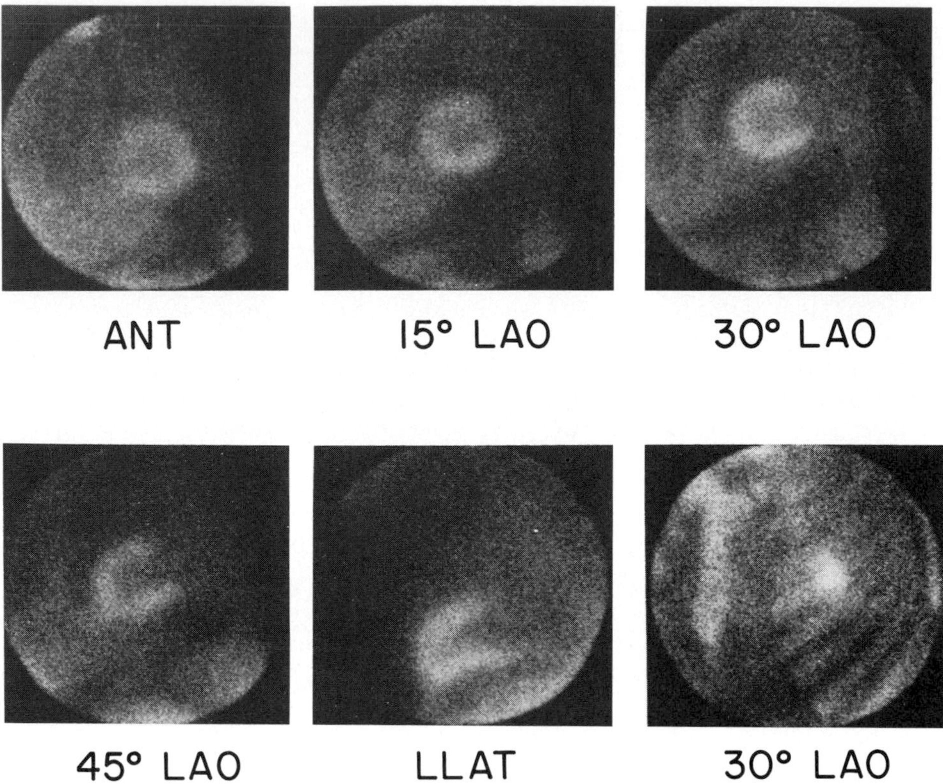

Figure 11–8. Resting thallium-201 images obtained in multiple positions and technetium-99m stannous pyrophosphate image obtained in the 30° LAO position (lower right image) in a patient with a small acute posterolateral myocardial infarction. Note the focal posterolateral perfusion defect demonstrated on the LAO thallium-201 images. This is most clearly defined on the 30° LAO thallium-201 image, corresponding to the area of pyrophosphate uptake. At time, multiple obliquities are required with thallium-201 imaging to differentiate perfusion defects from normal valvular structures. Abbreviations as in Figure 11–1.

cardiographic assessment often is unreliable (Platt et al., 1976). In a patient with previous myocardial infarction and superimposed acute ischemia or infarction, dual myocardial imaging with thallium-201 and ^{99m}Tc pyrophosphate often provides clinically meaningful complementary data (Figs. 11–8, 11–9) (Berger et al., 1978a).

The major applicability of pyrophosphate imaging may be in terms of defining prognosis (Holman et al., 1978; Olson et al., 1977). Studies have demonstrated that the "doughnut" imaging pattern (maximal uptake at the periphery of a large infarct) and the persistently abnormal image after infarction are associated with substantially higher complication rates and death either in the hospital or following discharge, than in remaining patients (Fig. 11–10). A similar situation may be present in patients with unstable angina, in whom abnormal pyrophosphate images in the absence of electrocardiographic and enzymatic evidence of infarction are associated with a higher incidence of subsequent infarction and death in the ensuing year.

Assessment of Cardiac Performance: Multiple-Gated Cardiac Blood Pool Imaging

This approach provides a means of imaging the entire equilibrium blood pool at various times during cardiac contraction by synchronizing the collection of scintillation data with a physiologic marker suitable for temporally identifying the sequence of the cardiac cycle (Strauss et al., 1971; Zaret et al., 1971). Since electrocardiographic events generally have a relatively fixed relationship to mechanical activity, repetitive sampling of specific phases of the cardiac cycle from each of many beats can be performed until the cardiac image has an adequate count density. In order to ensure the validity of the

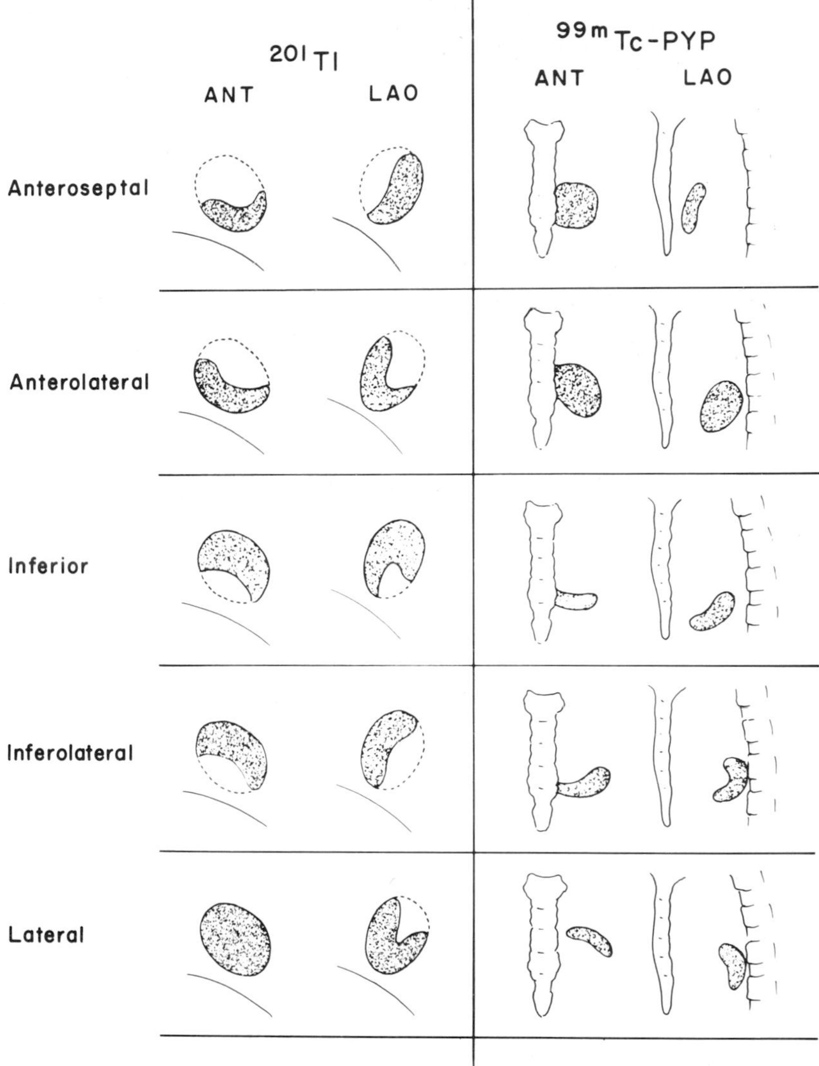

Figure 11–9. Schematic representation of various infarct patterns obtained with thallium-201, (*^{201}Tl*) and technetium-99m stannous pyrophosphate (*^{99m}Tc-PYP*). The areas of uptake are indicated by the shaded zones. For the pyrophosphate images, the bony structures are shown in white. Dual imaging with these two tracers allows differentiation of acute and remote myocardial infarction. Abbreviations as in Figure 11–1. (From Berger, H. J., Gottschalk, A., and Zaret, B. L.: Ann. Intern. Med. 88:145, 1978a.)

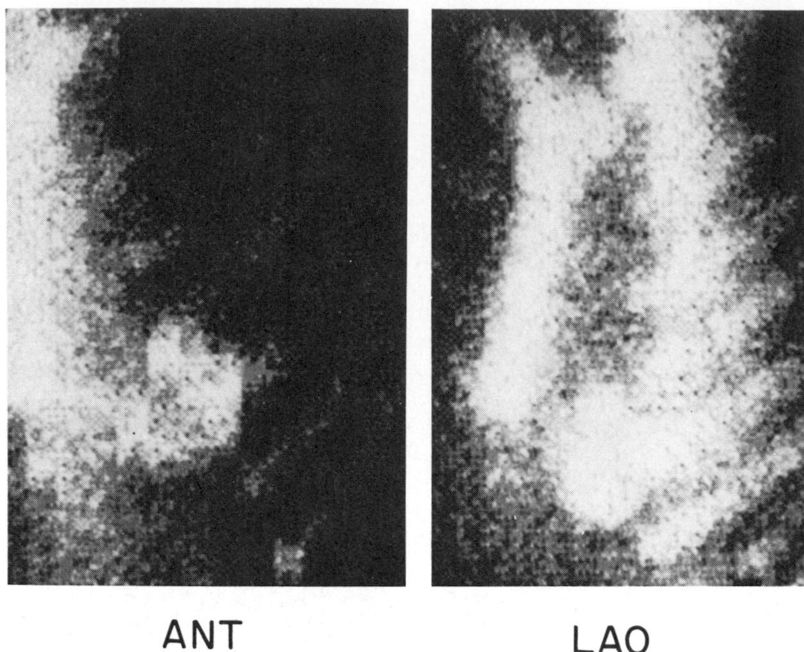

Figure 11–10. Technetium-99m stannous pyrophosphate images obtained in a patient with a larger anterior wall myocardial infarction. On the anterior position image, note the doughnut appearance with greater uptake at the periphery of the infarct. This has been associated with a high mortality and morbidity post infarction. Abbreviations as in Figure 11–1.

multiple-gated data, cardiac function must be relatively stable during the period of data acquisition.

The patient's autologous red blood cells are labeled with 20 to 30 millicuries of ^{99m}Tc pertechnetate. Scintillation data are collected temporally in synchrony with the ECG R wave. Depending on the heart rate, the R–R interval usually is divided into approximately 20 equal divisions (Fig. 11–11). Data occurring during consecutive intervals are sorted into the computer image, whose specific location in the

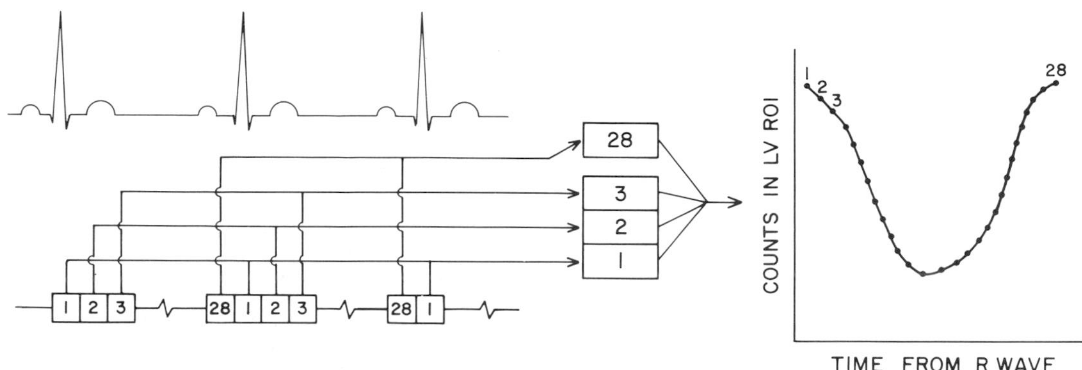

Figure 11–11. Schematic representation of the data processing involved in generation of a summed left ventricular time activity curve with multiple-gated equilibrium cardiac blood pool imaging. In this example, the cardiac cycle (R–R interval) has been subdivided into 28 equal segments. Data acquired during each of the specific time intervals shown below are stored in a computer memory for several hundred individual cardiac cycles. Following correction for noncardiac background activity, these individual frames are displayed as a relative left ventricular volume curve, as noted on the right. *LV ROI* = left ventricular region of interest. (From Zaret, B., and Berger, H.: Techniques of nuclear cardiology. *In* Hurst, J. W. (ed.): The Heart, 5th ed. New York, 1981, McGraw-Hill Book Co., pp. 1803–1843.)

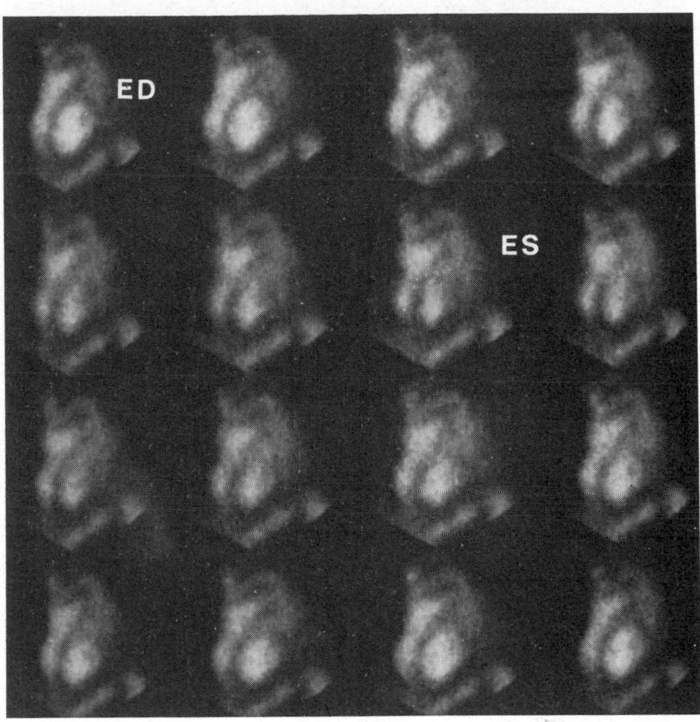

Figure 11–12. Sequential frames obtained from a multiple-gated cardiac blood pool study in the LAO position. The first frame represents end-diastole (*ED*) and the seventh frame end-systole (*ES*). The cardiac cycle has been divided into 16 equal frames. Note the good separation between the right and left ventricles, thickening of the interventricular septum during systole, and apical akinesis. (From Berger, H. J., Gottschalk, A., and Zaret, B. L.: Radiol. Clin. North Am. 18:441, 1980.)

temporal sequence is determined by the time elapsed from the onset of the R wave. The result is a single-image sequence spanning the entire cardiac cycle that is made up of data from several hundred individual cardiac beats (Burow et al., 1977; Green et al., 1975). Routine clinical studies require approximately eight to ten minutes of data acquisition for each position. Imaging should be performed in at least three positions, especially for analysis of regional wall motion. Quantitative assessment of global left ventricular performance must be performed in an obliquity that gives the clearest separation of the two ventricles, usually a 45-degree left anterior oblique view. Each chamber should be analyzed carefully in terms of relative position, size, synchrony of contraction, and symmetry of contraction. This is routinely performed with the endless-loop cine display (Fig. 11–12). A left ventricular time activity curve, analogous to a relative ventricular volume curve, allows assessment of the global ejection fraction and of the peak rates of filling and emptying. Left ventricular ejection fraction (LVEF) is determined from end-diastolic (EDC) and end-systolic (ESC) counts after background correction, using routine formulas:

$$\text{LVEF}(\%) = 100 \times (\text{EDC} - \text{ESC})/\text{EDC}$$

Recent studies also have shown that it may be possible to determine absolute left ventricular volumes using either conventional area-length methods or by quantification of the radioactivity emanating from the left ventricle (Dehmer et al., 1980; Slutsky et al., 1979).

An important modification of the technique of equilibrium blood pool imaging involves the use of a specially collimated nuclear probe and dedicated microprocessor (Bacharach et al., 1977; Berger et al., 1981; Wagner et al., 1976). Especially in the ICU environment, this computerized instrument has the major advantages of true portability, ease of operation, and augmented detector sensitivity (Figs. 11–13, 11–14). Data can be obtained, displayed, and analyzed on a beat-to-beat basis at high temporal resolution without the need for ECG gating. Since there are no images to guide the operator in determining the appropriate regions of interest, computerized algorithms and operator routines have been developed to aid in positioning the probe. A miniaturized semiconductor detector module, which can be affixed directly to the patient's chest, has recently been developed, potentially expanding further the clinical applicability of nonimaging probes (Hoffer et al., 1981). These techniques are particularly relevant to continuous monitoring of global left

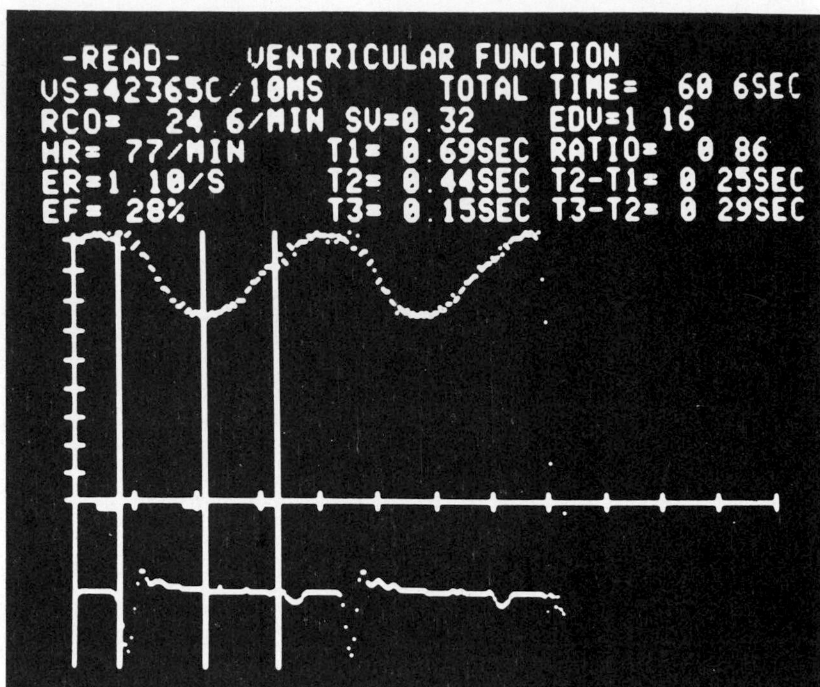

Figure 11–13. Left ventricular volume curve obtained over 60 seconds with the computerized nuclear probe. ECG is shown below. The left ventricular ejection fraction (*EF*) is 28 per cent, agreeing closely with the value obtained at contrast ventriculography.

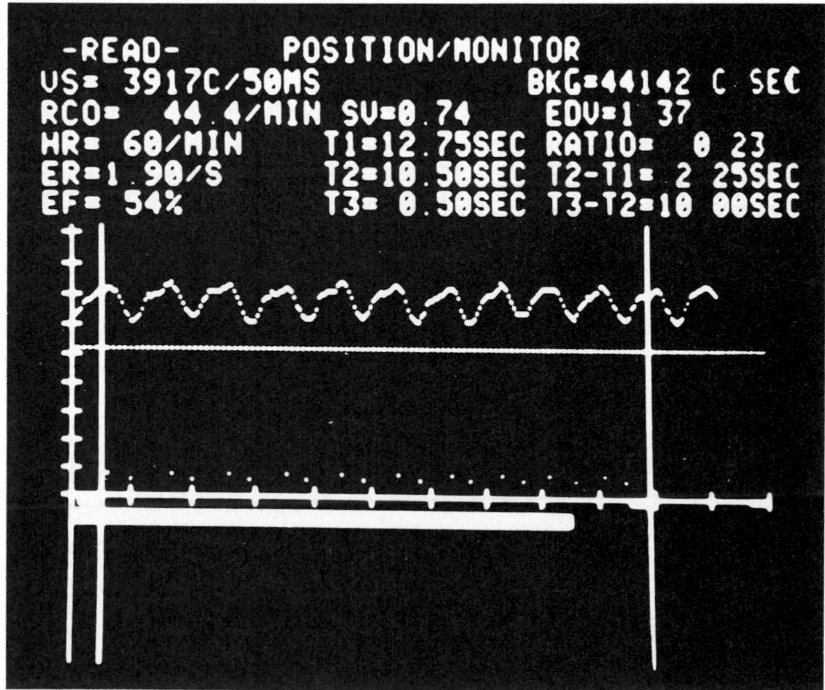

Figure 11–14. Beat-to-beat left ventricular time activity curve obtained with the computerized nuclear probe. Data are displayed at 20 points per second. The left ventricular ejection fraction (*EF*) is 54 per cent. Note the uniformity of beat-to-beat left ventricular function, as well as definition of the period of diastasis. This technique allows direct assessment of the effects of therapeutic interventions on left ventricular function, as well as definition of rapidly changing physiologic events.

ventricular performance or to assessment of acute therapeutic interventions.

Assessment of Cardiac Performance: First-Pass Radionuclide Angiocardiography

This technique differs from multiple-gated blood pool imaging in that analysis is limited to the initial transit of the radioactive bolus through the central circulation. Both right and left ventricular performance can be evaluated from the same study, because there is temporal and anatomic segregation of radioactivity within each of the cardiac chambers (Fig. 11–15) (Berger et al., 1979). This study can also be used to assess the presence and magnitude of left-to-right intracardiac shunting (Fig. 11–16).

Each study requires a separate radionuclide injection. This usually involves 10 to 20 millicuries of ^{99m}Tc pertechnetate or a renal scanning agent that is cleared more rapidly from the blood stream. Although ^{99m}Tc clearly is suitable for first-pass studies, it is preferable to have short half-lived tracers, allowing multiple sequential high-count rate studies. Several new tracers with these characteristics are undergoing investigation; the optimal one appears to be gold-195m with a half-life of 30.5 seconds (Wackers et al., in press). The choice of the scintillation camera for first-pass studies is an important factor in ensuring the reliability of the data. Since analysis is based on only a few cardiac cycles, the major limiting factor in this approach is the relatively low-count rates of the raw data when they are obtained on most conventional scintillation cameras. However, the use of a computerized multicrystal scintillation camera or of the newer single-crystal digital

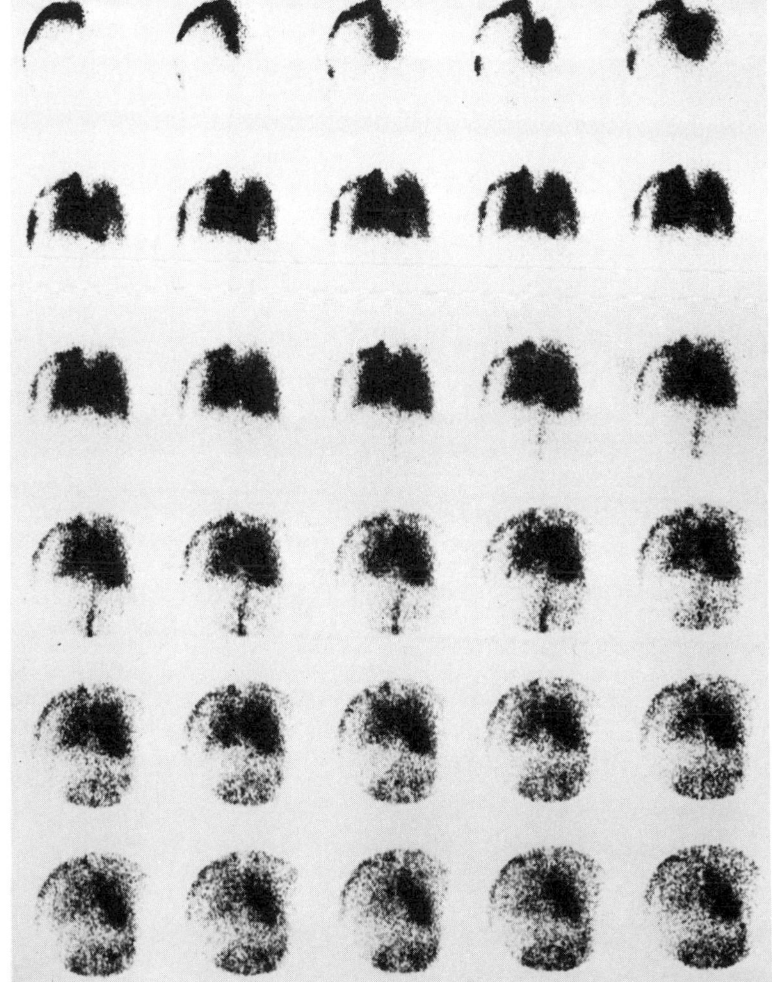

Figure 11–15. First-pass radionuclide angiocardiogram in a young adult with a small ventricular septal defect. Note the persistent pulmonary activity in the second and third rows. There is good visualization of the descending aorta, suggesting that the left-to-right shunt is relatively small. By computer analysis, the pulmonic to systemic flow ratio was 1.7 to 1. In the fourth and fifth rows, when there still is substantial pulmonary activity, the left ventricle also is visualized. (From Berger, H., Gottschalk, A., and Zaret B.: Nuclear medicine procedures. *In* Kelley, M. J., Jaffe, C. C., and Kleinman, C. S. (eds.): Cardiac Imaging in Infants and Children. Philadelphia, 1982, W. B. Saunders Co., pp. 112–154.)

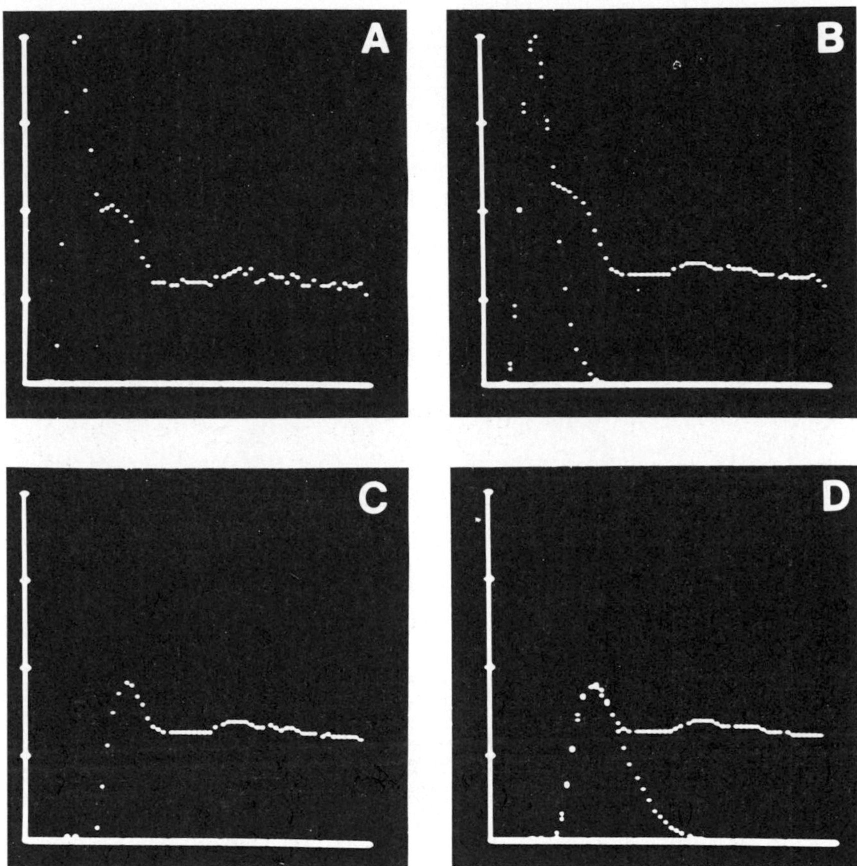

Figure 11–16. Computerized method for determining the pulmonic to systemic flow ratio as developed at Children's Hospital Medical Center, Boston, MA. A smooth pulmonary time activity curve is shown in panel *A*. The initial portion of the time activity curve is fit to a gamma variate in panel *B*. The area in the initially fit portion shown in panel *B* is proportional to the pulmonic flow. The derived histogram then is subtracted from the original curve, resulting in a second histogram that represents shunt and systemic recirculation (panel *C*). This remaining histogram also is fit to a gamma variate, as shown in panel *D*. The area of this new gamma variate fit is proportional to the shunt flow. The difference between the areas of the two fitted curves is proportional to systemic flow, allowing estimation of the pulmonic to systemic flow ratio. (From Berger, H., Gottschalk, A., and Zaret, B.: Nuclear medicine procedures. *In*: Kelley, M. J., Jaffe, C. C., and Kleinman, C. S. (eds.): Cardiac Imaging in Infants and Children. Philadelphia, 1982, W. B. Saunders Co., pp. 112–154.)

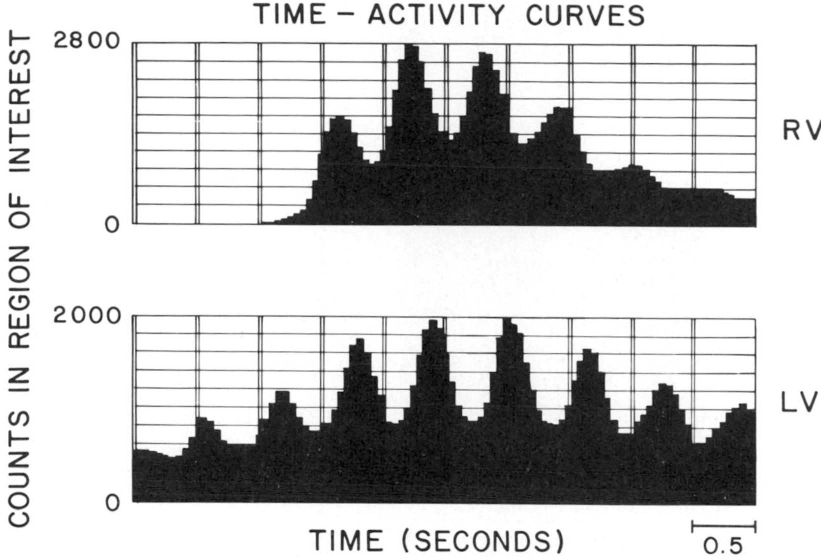

Figure 11–17. High-frequency, high-count rate time activity curves generated from right ventricular (*RV*) and left ventricular (*LV*) regions of interest, using the first-pass radionuclide angiocardiographic technique. The peaks represent end-diastole, and the valleys end-systole. This study was obtained using a computerized multicrystal scintillation camera, providing extremely high count rates. Either from the average of individual beats or from summation of several consecutive beats, ejection fraction and regional wall motion can be assessed. (From Berger et al.: Semin. Nucl. Med. 9:275, 1979.)

cameras allows accumulation of extremely high-count rates, minimizing this potential problem.

A representative cardiac cycle is created with either the R wave of the ECG or the peak of the volume curve to align end-diastoles of several serial beats (Fig. 11–17). Quantitative analysis can be obtained from data generated in any patient position. The left ventricular ejection fraction then is determined either as the average of several individual beats or from a summed cardiac cycle (Berger et al., 1978b; Marshall et al., 1977; Rerych et al., 1978). Images of relatively high-count density are derived from summed representative cycles obtained with higher-count rate cameras, and can be used for evaluation of regional wall motion. Through techniques analogous to those employed for analysis of the left ventricle, a high-frequency time-activity curve can be generated from a right ventricular region of interest, allowing determination of right ventricular ejection fraction (Berger et al., 1978b; Tobinick et al., 1978).

Clinical Applications of Ventricular Performance Studies

In patients with dyspnea, edema, or other evidence of possible heart failure, assessment of resting biventricular performance provides clinically useful information (Berger and Zaret, 1981; Berger et al., 1980). For example, cardiac and pulmonary etiologies for dyspnea can be distinguished. In addition, focal left ventricular dysfunction (such as an aneurysm) and diffuse left ventricular dysfunction (such as a cardiomyopathy) can be differentiated (Figs. 11–18, 11–19). Pseudoaneurysms that may require urgent surgical intervention can be identified, and the need for cardiac catheterization and aneurysmectomy can be defined. In terms of the cause of heart failure, there are specific patterns in congestive, hypertrophic, and ischemic cardiomyopathies (Bulkley et al., 1977; Nichols et al., 1978). For example, the presence of an enlarged left ventricle with relatively preserved left ventricular function suggests volume overload, as seen in valvular heart disease (Fig. 11–20). In patients with uremic cardiomyopathy, those with fluid overload and intrinsically normal left ventricular contractility can be differentiated from those with abnormal function (Hung et al., 1980). It is important to note that the ejection fraction alone may not directly define the presence of heart failure, since compensatory mechanisms may keep the ejection fraction within the normal range. In this setting, radionuclide techniques also may allow quantification of the degree of valvular regurgitation and ventricular enlargement, and evaluation of

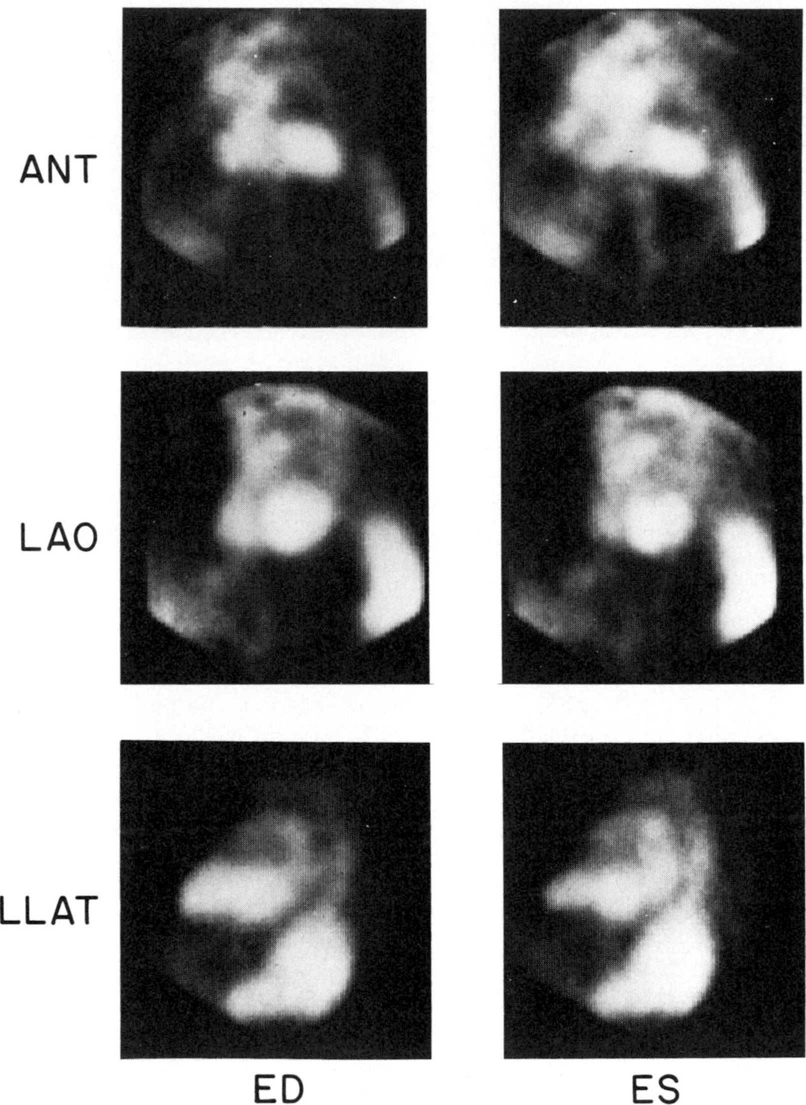

Figure 11–18. Multiple-gated equilibrium cardiac blood pool imaging in a patient with a posterobasal left ventricular aneurysm. Images are shown in multiple positions at end-diastole (*ED*) and at end-systole (*ES*). Note the discrete area of apical akinesis and left ventricular deformity on the left lateral position image. The remainder of the left ventricular myocardium contracts relatively well. The aneurysm is only positively defined on the lower images. For accurate assessment of regional left ventricular function, multiple-gated blood pool imaging should be performed in at least three positions. Other abbreviations as in Figure 11–1. (From Berger, H. J., Gottschalk, A., and Zaret, B. L.: Radiol. Clin. North Am. 18:441, 1980.)

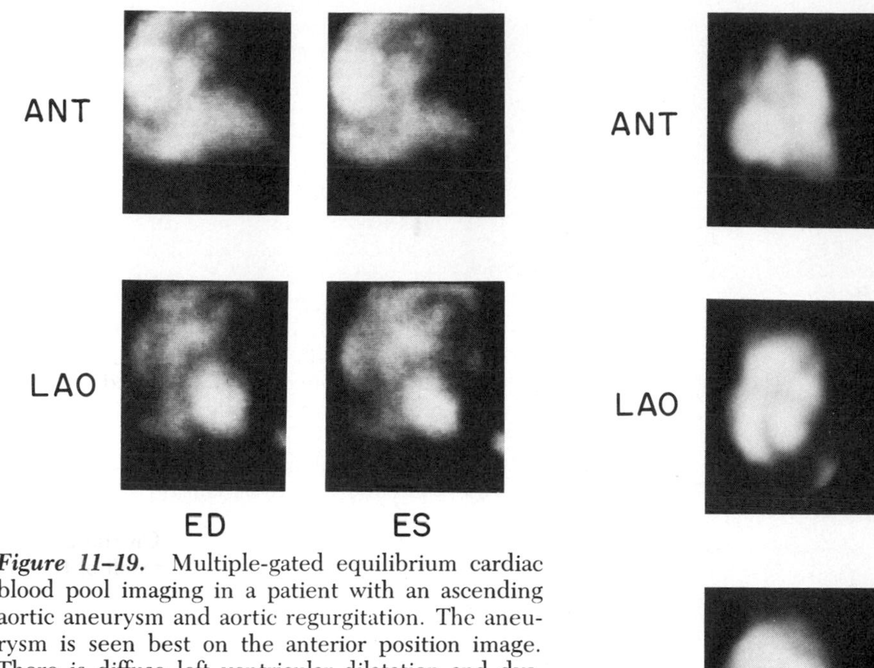

Figure 11–19. Multiple-gated equilibrium cardiac blood pool imaging in a patient with an ascending aortic aneurysm and aortic regurgitation. The aneurysm is seen best on the anterior position image. There is diffuse left ventricular dilatation and dysfunction. The global left ventricular ejection fraction is 31 per cent. Abbreviations as in Figure 11–18.

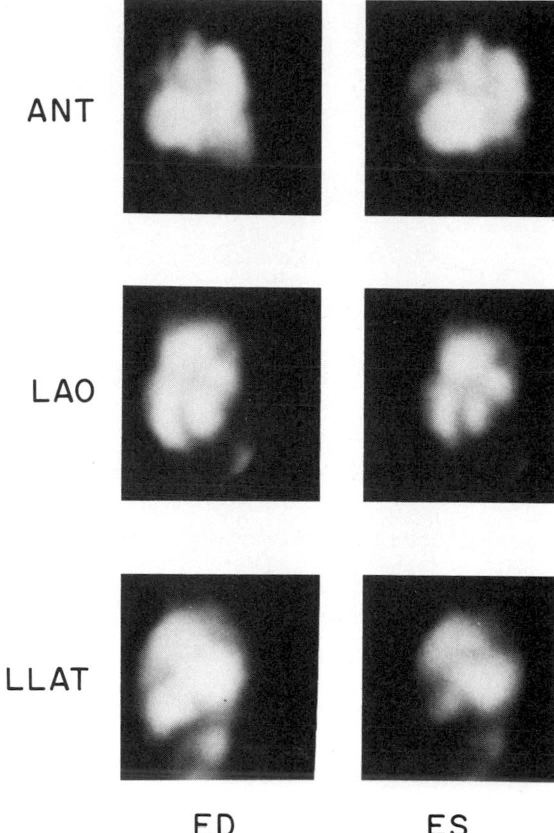

Figure 11–20. Multiple-gated equilibrium cardiac blood pool imaging in a patient with severe mitral stenosis and tricuspid stenosis. On both the left anterior oblique and left lateral images, a markedly dilated left atrium is seen. Similarly, a dilated right atrium is demonstrated on the anterior position image. Neither of the ventricles is dilated, making a volume overload lesion (such as regurgitation) unlikely. Global biventricular performance is preserved. This study demonstrates how the gated blood pool scan can help in defining the etiology of congestive heart failure. Abbreviations as in Figure 11–18.

the response to therapy. Radionuclide angiocardiography can be used to confirm the presence and magnitude of left ventricular dysfunction after infarction, even in patients with normal chest radiographs (Benge et al., 1980). Although the chest film provides indirect insights into pulmonary capillary wedge (PCW) pressure (by evaluation of pulmonary vascularity and heart size), there often is disparity, making direct measurement of left ventricular function particularly important.

In a patient with shock, determination of its cause is critical in order that the appropriate therapeutic intervention may be designed. Since the need for fluid and diuretic therapies differs in acute right and left ventricular myocardial infarction, identification of these two conditions may be of major clinical importance (Fig. 11–21). Radionuclide techniques also allow definition of other causes of shock, such as acute valvular regurgitation or acute ventricular septal rupture.

In terms of acute myocardial infarction, it is clear that the site of infarction affects the type and extent of ventricular dysfunction that occurs (Reduto et al., 1978). Anterior myocardial infarction causes a greater depression in left ventricular ejection fraction than does inferior infarction. In contrast, right ventricular dysfunction occurs almost exclusively in patients with inferior wall myocardial infarction. Several recent studies have also stressed the prognostic importance of the resting left ventricular ejection fraction as a predictor of early mortality following myocardial infarction, and the subsequent development of congestive heart failure (CHF) or death (Shah et al., 1980; Wackers et al., 1982).

In COPD, the major hemodynamic burden is on the right ventricle. Right ventricular function, especially as determined by ejection fraction, is highly dependent on right ventricular afterload (Berger et Matthay, 1981; Berger et al., 1978b; Brent et al., in press). In the pres-

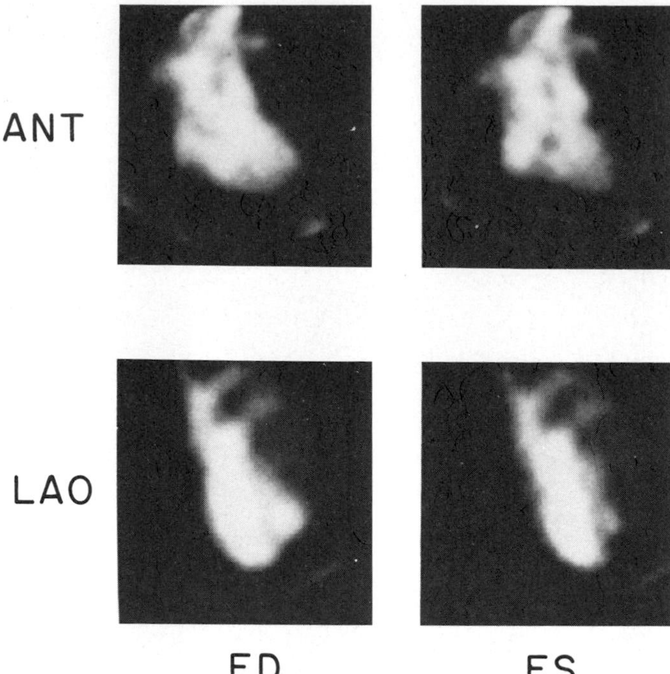

Figure 11–21. Multiple-gated cardiac blood pool imaging in a patient with right ventricular myocardial infarction and inferior wall left ventricular myocardial infarction. The right ventricle is markedly dilated and diffusely hypokinetic. On the anterior position image, the inferior wall of the left ventricle cannot be demonstrated because of overlap with the dilated right ventricle. Global left ventricular performance is normal. Similar findings would be expected in a patient with cor pulmonale. Abbreviations as in Figure 11–18.

ence of pulmonary arterial hypertension or pulmonary vasoconstriction, there are substantial abnormalities in right ventricular performance, and consequently the prognosis is poor. The degree of resting right ventricular dysfunction is related to the degree of arterial hypoxemia and ventilatory impairment. Abnormal right ventricular function is found to be a harbinger of subsequent cardiopulmonary decompensation. Left ventricular function usually is normal in COPD, except in the presence of concomitant valvular or coronary disease.

These radionuclide techniques have been used extensively to evaluate the effects of therapeutic interventions employed in the ICU. Studies can be used to answer questions specifically relating to general mechanisms of drug activity and efficacy, as well as to design and optimize therapy in a specific patient. A broad spectrum of therapeutic interventions, ranging from vasodilators to intracoronary thrombolysis, have already been evaluated, and this represents one of the most important clinical applications of radionuclide studies of ventricular performance.

ECHOCARDIOGRAPHY

The echocardiographic examination has become a routine part of the evaluation of many critically ill patients with heart disease because it is uniquely capable of simultaneously assessing ventricular size and function, the anatomy and motion of the cardiac valves, and the pericardium.

Basic Principles: M-Mode Technique

The basic principle of echocardiography is the creation of cardiac images by reflected ultrahigh-frequency sound waves (Feigenbaum, 1980; Popp, 1976; Popp et al., 1980). Bursts of sound waves are generated every microsecond by a transducer and propagated in a relatively linear fashion through the body. Whenever a sound pulse encounters a tissue interface of differing acoustic properties, part of its energy is reflected back to the transducer, which converts vibratory energy into an electrical signal. The elapsed time of one complete cycle from impulse generation to target reflection and reception back at the transducer is converted into a measured distance, based on the known constant velocity of sound waves in tissue. Thus, the reflected signal is displayed as a target on a calibrated line. Since the heart is moving, echo-producing interfaces interrogated by the one-dimensional sound beam are displayed as a series of moving dots. In M-mode echocardiography, incorporation of a sweep into the oscil-

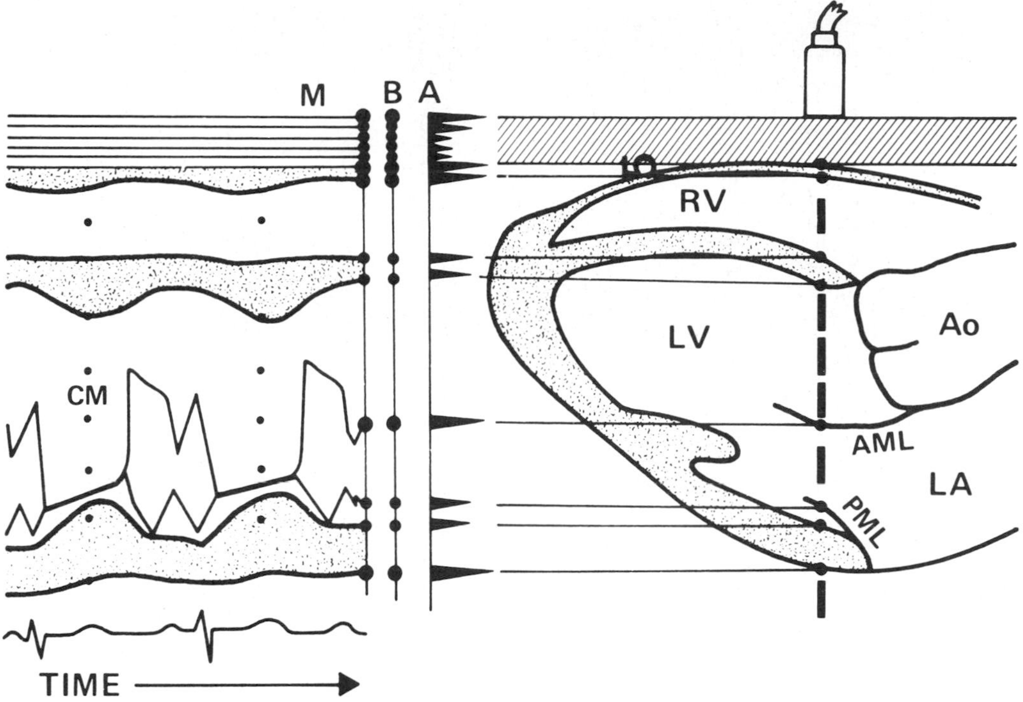

Figure 11–22. Schematic representation of an echocardiographic recording with the transducer positioned below the aortic valve at the level of the mitral valve. Three modes of operation are shown: *A* (amplitude), *B* (brightness), and *M* (motion). Clinical evaluation predominantly involves the M-mode technique. The depth of the echo signal is shown along the vertical axis, and time is represented along the horizontal axis. The intensity of the echo signal is proportional to its brightness, but dots now appear as thin wavy lines. To image other portions of the heart, the M-mode transducer is shifted and angulated to other positions. Note the characteristic pattern of the mitral valve as it opens and closes on the M-mode study. The interventricular septum and posterior wall are shown as shaded areas. *RV* = right ventricle; *LV* = left ventricle; *Ao* = aorta; *AML* = anterior mitral leaflet; *PML* = posterior mitral leaflet; *LA* = left atrium; *CM* = centimeters. (From Popp, R. L.: Circulation, 54:538, 1976.)

loscope display or a strip chart recorder with light-sensitive paper allows transcription of rapidly moving cardiac structures as continuous lines. Only targets moving within the path of the sound beam are recorded; adjacent structures are recorded by manual alteration of the direction of the transducer beam.

An M-mode echocardiographic examination is performed by placing the transducer along the left sternal border in the second to fourth intercostal space. This acoustic window permits recording of a series of one-dimensional sectors as the transducer is swept in an arc between the apex and base (Fig. 11–22). All four cardiac valves and chambers can be visualized by standardized tilting and angulating of the transducer (Fig. 11–23). Internal cavities of the ventricles are relatively free of echoes and appear as clear spaces. Air within lung tissue attenuates the echo beam and appears as dark shadows. Limitations of this technique include imaging of the heart in only a single dimension, an unfamiliar display format bearing little relationship to cardiac anatomy, and a lack of tomographic spatial information.

Basic Principles: Two-Dimensional Technique

Two-dimensional echocardiography provides spatial orientation of cardiac structures (Griffith and Henry, 1974; King, 1973; Kisslo et al., 1976; Von Ramm and Thurstone, 1976). The sound beam is either mechanically or electronically swept through a section of the heart, creating a two-dimensional imaging plane. The images are constructed from a series of discrete ultrasonic scan lines, at a rate of 30 frames per second. Viewing of sequential frames provides a real-time cine display of the heart and great vessels. These echoes correspond to the ana-

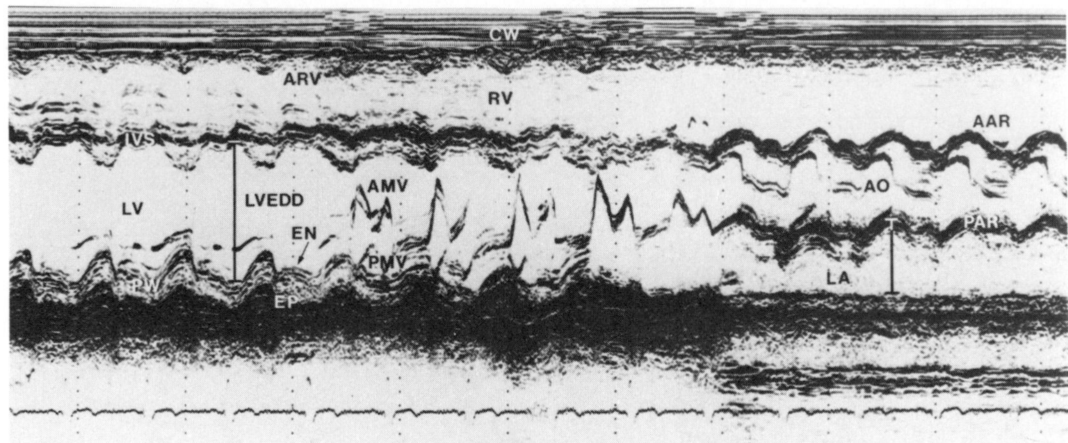

Figure 11–23. Standard parasternal M-mode sweep from the midventricular cavity to the base of the heart. *CW* = chest wall; *ARV* = anterior right ventricular wall; *RV* = right ventricular cavity; *IVS* = interventricular septum; *LV* = left ventricular cavity; *PW* = posterior wall; *LVEDD* = left ventricular end-diastolic dimension; *EN* = endocardium; *EP* = epicardium; *AMV* = anterior mitral valve; *PMV* = posterior mitral valve; *AO* = aortic valve; *AAR* = anterior aortic root; *PAR* = posterior aortic root; *LA* = left atrium.

tomic location of structures within the body, resulting in a tomographic image of the heart. Multiple tomographic planes are obtained by angulating and rotating the transducer, which permits detailed analysis of cardiac anatomy and function in different orientations.

The two-dimensional echocardiographic examination is performed in a manner similar to that for M-mode echocardiography. A series of cross-sectional planes are imaged, all referenced to three standardized orthogonal views: the long-axis, short-axis, and apical four-chamber (Fig. 11–24) (DeMaria et al., 1980b; Henry et al., 1980c). The long-axis view is obtained with the transducer in the parasternal position by sweeping the ultrasonic beam from the right shoulder to the left flank, traversing a plane from the base to the apex of the heart. Short-axis views also are obtained with the transducer in the parasternal position, but rotated 90 degrees so that the images are perpendicular to the long axis, traversing a plane from the left shoulder to the right iliac crest. With the transducer over the base of the heart, the aortic valve appears as individual leaflets within the central circular aorta. The right ventricular outflow tract appears superiorly as a crescent surrounding the aorta. The tricuspid valve is to the left of the aortic valve, the pulmonic valve is visualized superior and to the right of the aortic valve, and the two atria are below. As the transducer is arched inferiorly, the ultrasonic beam serially slices the left ventricular cavity, from the level of the mitral valve leaflets, to the papillary muscles, and then to the apex. The left ventricle appears as a circular structure surrounded by myocardium.

By moving the transducer to the apex and angulating the beam toward the base, the apical four-chamber view is obtained. The ultrasonic beam is perpendicular to the septum, and outlines the apex of the heart. Both ventricles and atria are shown. Subcostal and suprasternal approaches can also be employed for a more complete assessment of certain cardiac structures and vessels. Given the enhanced spatial orientation and wider view obtained with the two-dimensional technique, it is not surprising that this approach has broader applications in the critically ill patient than M-mode echocardiography, and this technique is stressed in this chapter.

Clinical Applications in Valvular Heart Disease

There are characteristic normal patterns on both the M-mode and two-dimensional echocardiographic studies for each of the cardiac valves (Kotler et al., 1980; Riba and Berger, in press). Furthermore, there are typical findings in several valvular lesions. Mitral stenosis results in predictable M-mode and two-dimensional echocardiographic findings. The leaflets are thickened and appear as parallel, dense echoes rather than as thin, rapidly moving lines.

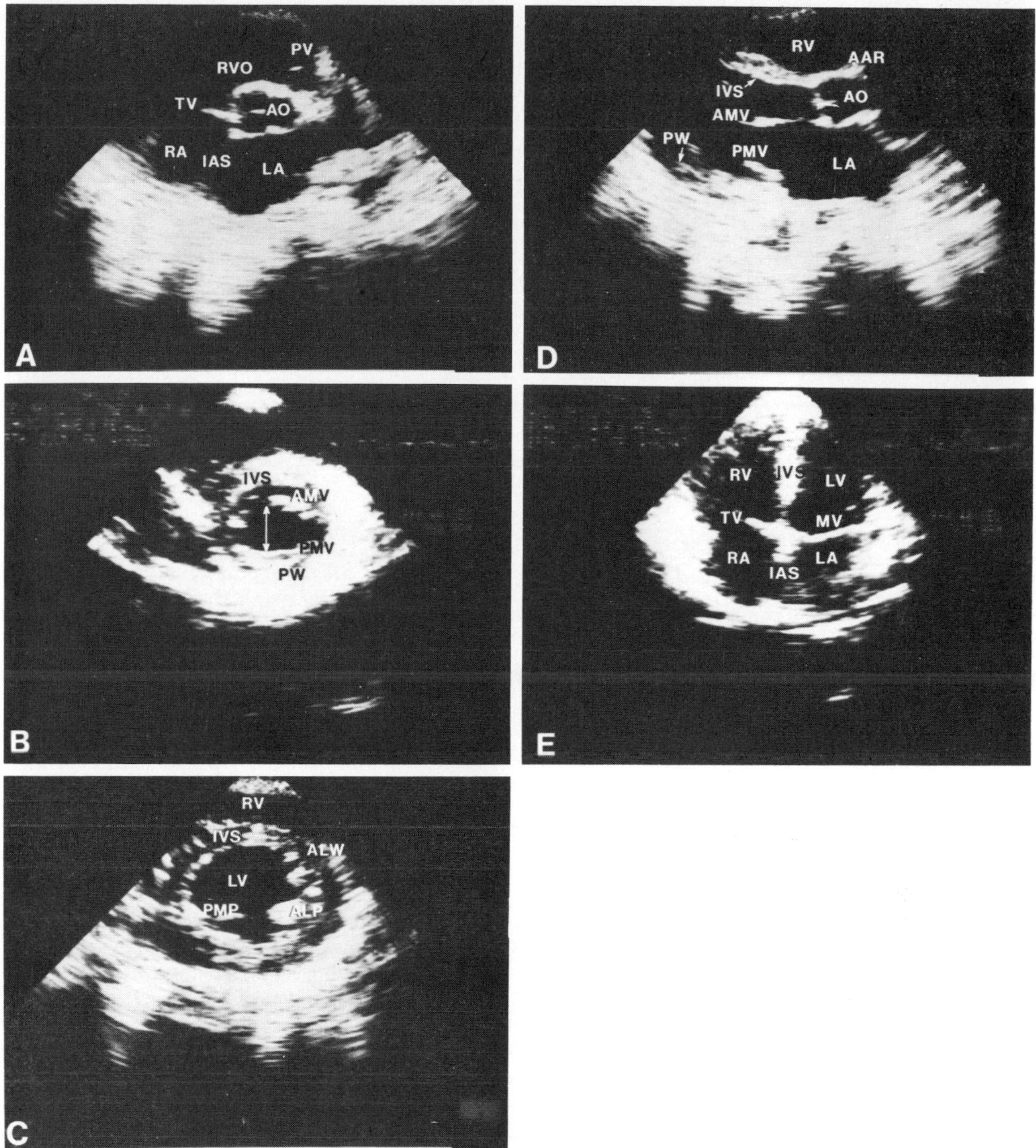

Figure 11–24. Standard two-dimensional views. *A*, Two-dimensional short-axis view obtained at the base of the heart. In diastole, the aortic valve appears as a tri-leaflet structure in a closed position. *B*, Short-axis view obtained at the level of the mitral valve leaflets. In diastole, the anterior and posterior leaflets are widely separated. *C*, Short-axis view of the left ventricle obtained at the level of the papillary muscles. *D*, Long-axis view of the left ventricle. At end-diastole, the mitral valve leaflets separate in the open position. The apex is not visualized. *E*, Apical four-chamber view. The apex is at the upper portion of the image. *RA* = right atrium; *LA* = left atrium; *IAS* = interatrial septum; *TV* = tricuspid valve; *PV* = pulmonic valve; *RVO* = right ventricular outflow tract; *PMP* = posteromedial papillary muscle; *ALP* = anterolateral papillary muscle; *ALW* = anterolateral wall. Other abbreviations as in Figure 11–23. (From Riba, A., and Berger, H. J.: Echocardiography in acquired heart disease. *In* Glenn et al. (eds.): Thoracic and Cardiovascular Surgery, 4th ed. New York, Appleton-Century-Crofts, in press.)

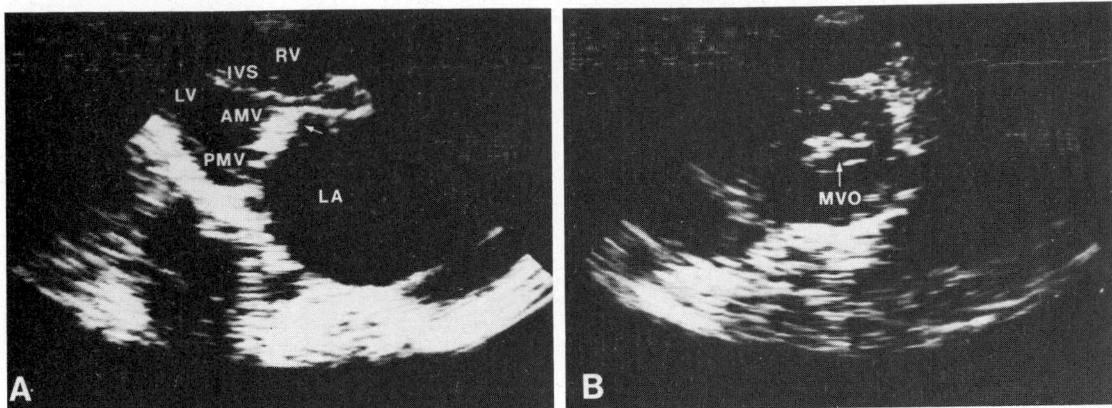

Figure 11–25. Two-dimensional long (*A*) and short-axis (*B*) views of the stenotic mitral valve in diastole. In the long-axis view the leaflets are thickened and domed (*arrow*) as the two leaflets bend toward each other, owing to commissural fusion. The short-axis view permits measurement of the actual mitral valve orifice (*MVO*). Other abbreviations as in Figure 11–23. (From Riba, A., and Berger, H. J.: Echocardiography in acquired heart disease. *In* Glenn et al. (eds.): Thoracic and Cardiovascular Surgery, 4th ed. New York, Appleton-Century-Crofts, in press.)

Fusion of the commissures results in parallel anterior motion of the posterior leaflet (Henry and Kastl, 1977). Using the two-dimensional technique, the entire mitral valve and its orifice can be visualized (Fig. 11–25) (Cope et al., 1975). There is a close correlation between the area of the mitral valve orifice as determined by two-dimensional imaging in the short-axis view and that measured directly at the time of operation or calculated from hemodynamic data (Henry et al., 1975; Martin et al., 1979; Nichol et al., 1977; Wann et al., 1978b).

The presence of mitral regurgitation cannot be identified directly by echocardiography, nor can it be assumed to be present if there is separation of the coapted mitral leaflets during systole. However, left ventricular dilatation and left atrial enlargement, which reflect the pathophysiologic consequences of volume overload, can be detected. There may be premature closure of the aortic valve, reflecting decreased forward cardiac output. At present, the severity of mitral regurgitation also cannot be predicted accurately by echocardiography. However, echocardiography can define anatomic abnormalities of the mitral valve which, in the proper clinical context, can help explain auscultatory findings (Mintz et al., 1979, 1980; Morganroth et al., 1980; Sweatman et al., 1972; Wann et al., 1978a). Characteristic mitral valve patterns occur in rheumatic mitral regurgitation, mitral valve prolapse, flail mitral valve leaflets, infective endocarditis, papillary muscle dysfunction, and mitral annular calcification (Fig. 11–26). However, it is important to stress that echocardiography often does not detect any abnormality

---

Figure 11–26. M-mode (*left*) and two-dimensional (*right*) echocardiograms in patients with mitral valve disease. (*A* and *E*,) Mitral valve prolapse. Characterisitc midsystolic posterior buckling of the coapted leaflets is demonstrated on the M-mode examination (*black arrow*). In systole, the long-axis view demonstrates superior and posterior arching of both mitral valve leaflets beyond the plane of the mitral annulus into the left atrium (*white arrow*). *B* and *F*, Flail posterior valve leaflet. The M-mode study demonstrates abnormal diastolic motion of the posterior leaflet (*large arrow*), coarse diastolic flutter (*open arrow*), and systolic prolapse (*thin arrow*). The systolic frame from the long-axis view shows whipping of the flail posterior leaflet into the left atrium (*arrow*) beyond the normal systolic coaptation. *C* and *G*, Mitral regurgitation secondary to papillary muscle dysfunction. Both studies show hypokinesia and scarring of the posterior wall. *D* and *H*, Mitral annular calcification. The M-mode study shows a dense band of echoes in the region adjacent and posterior to the posterior mitral valve leaflet (*black arrow*). The long-axis view shows a dense mass of echoes beneath the posterior mitral valve leaflet adjacent to the posterior left ventricular wall, extending into the submitral region (*closed white arrow*). Calcification also is present in the region of the anterior aortic annulus, extending into the base of the anterior aortic cusp (*open arrow*). *MA* = mitral annulus. Other abbreviations as in Figure 11–23.

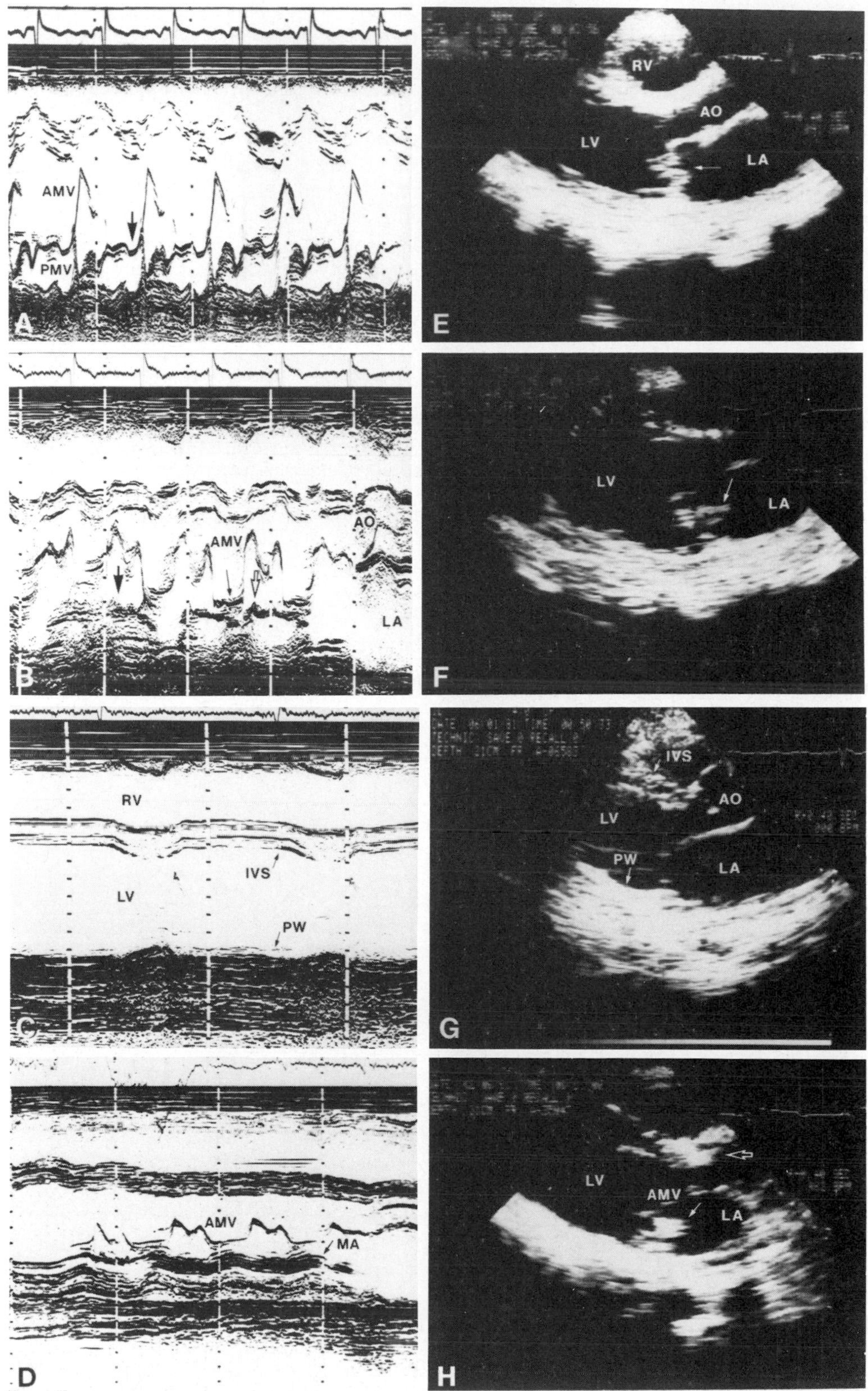

Figure 11–26. *See legend on opposite page.*

in patients with mitral regurgitation. Echocardiography may allow differentiation of primary mitral regurgitation due to valvular disease from that secondary to left ventricular dysfunction. Patients with papillary muscle dysfunction often have left ventricular wall motion abnormalities in the region of the affected papillary muscle. There is also inferior or apical displacement of the coapted mitral leaflets, as well as scarring of the papillary muscles.

Fibrocalcific degenerative changes of the aortic valve are characterized by increased echo density and a decrease in the extent of opening, but the findings may be variable depending on the orientation of the valve leaflets relative to the ultrasonic beam (DeMaria et al., 1980a; Schwartz et al., 1978; Weyman et al., 1975). Intense echoes from a calcified aortic valve may obscure leaflet definition and preclude identification of the actual aortic valve orifice (Fig. 11–27). The echocardiographic appearance of the aortic valve often is similar in patients with critical aortic stenosis and those with degenerative aortic sclerosis. The maximal aortic leaflet separation on the long-axis or short-axis views correlates qualitatively with the severity of aortic stenosis. However, in contrast to the mitral valve, planimetry of the aortic valve orifice is unreliable in estimating the degree of aortic stenosis, especially when the valve leaflets are unequally involved or when left ventricular function is depressed. The severity of aortic stenosis can best be assessed indirectly using echocardiographically-derived measurements of left ventricular dimensions and thickness.

In aortic regurgitation, the most notable M-mode finding is high-frequency diastolic fluttering of the anterior mitral valve leaflet, attributed to the regurgitant jet vibrating against the anterior leaflet (Skorton et al., 1980). In chronic

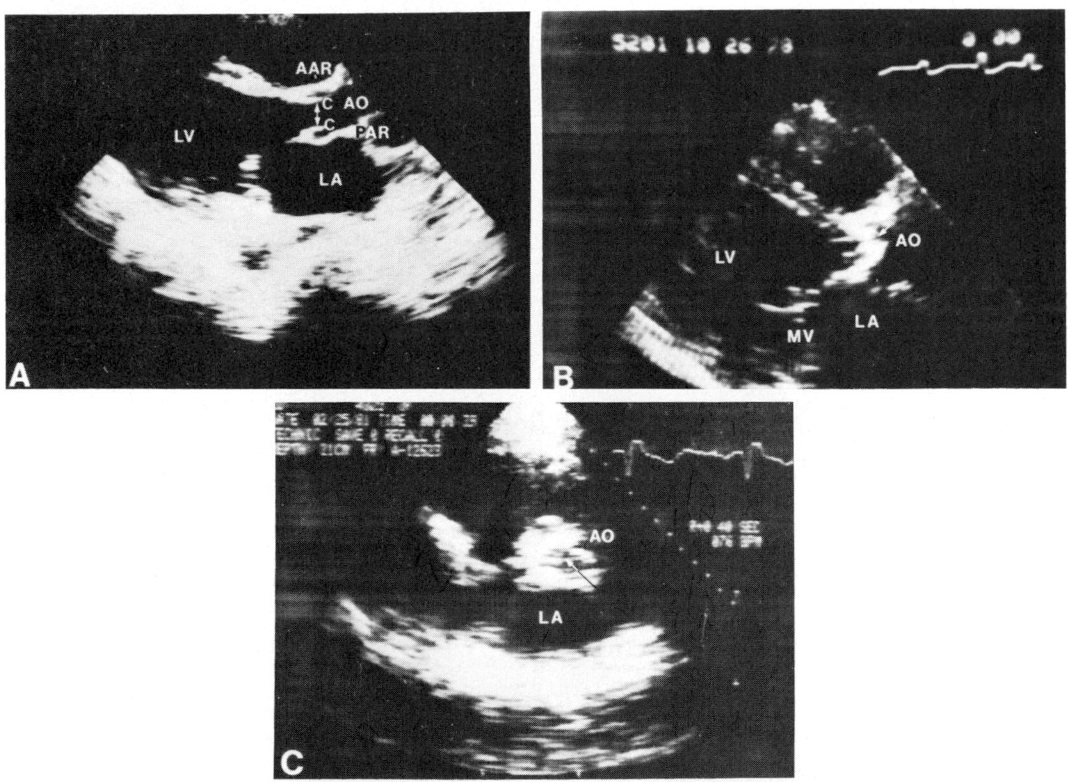

Figure 11–27. Two-dimensional echocardiogram of the normal aortic valve as depicted in the long-axis view in systole (*A*) compared with long-axis (*B*) and short-axis (*C*) views taken from a patient with aortic stenosis. The normal aortic valve appears as two thin cusp (C) echoes separating to the inner borders of the aortic root (*short arrow*). In contrast, patients with aortic stenosis display dense linear echoes with diminished intercusp separation during systole (*long arrow*). The aortic valve orifice is demonstrated (*arrow*). Abbreviations as in Figure 11–23. (From Riba, A., and Berger, H. J.: Echocardiography in acquired heart disease. *In* Glenn et al. (eds.): Thoracic and Cardiovascular Surgery, 4th ed. New York, Appleton-Century-Crofts, in press.)

aortic regurgitation, the left ventricular chamber usually is dilated and hypertrophied. In severe acute aortic regurgitation, such as may occur in endocarditis, there is preclosure of the mitral valve, reflecting the sudden increase in the left ventricular end-diastolic pressure (Botvinick et al., 1975; DeMaria et al., 1975). This finding may signal the need for urgent surgical intervention. In chronic aortic regurgitation, echocardiographic assessment of left ventricular end-diastolic and end-systolic dimensions is valuable in predicting the appropriate time for valve replacement, as well as the postoperative course (Henry et al., 1980a,b).

Echocardiographic evaluation of the pulmonic and tricuspid valves has relatively limited applications in acquired heart disease. However, the right ventricular dimension and area obtained from the four-chamber apical view have been employed to distinguish patients with right-sided volume overload due to valvular or congenital disorders from normals (Bommer et al., 1979). In addition, tricuspid regurgitation can be diagnosed by contrast echocardiography. In this approach, there is rapid injection of saline or indocyanine green dye into a peripheral vein, causing microcavitations that produce a cloud of echo reflections in the right atrium (Lieppe et al., 1978; Meltzer et al., 1981). Reflux of microcavitations into the inferior vena cava or hepatic veins is a relatively dependable indicator of tricuspid regurgitation.

Evaluation of Endocarditis and Prosthetic Valves

Echocardiography is invaluable in the evaluation of infective endocarditis (Davis et al., 1980; Gilbert et al., 1977; Stewart et al., 1980; Wann et al., 1976). The technique is capable of detecting valvular vegetations and delineating their complications, such as valvular disruption or ventricular dysfunction, in at least 80 per cent of patients with endocarditis. Vegetations are imaged as discrete irregular masses of shaggy or fuzzy echoes attached to a valve, not corresponding to a recognizable anatomic pattern. Vegetations usually do not alter the motion or overall appearance of the valve itself, unless the supportive structures are involved. Two-dimensional studies provide reliable information about the size, shape, and motion of vegetations (Fig. 11–28). In treated endocarditis, serial studies may show qualitative changes in the characteristics of the vegetations, as well as an increase in echo density suggestive of healing. Complications of endocarditis, such as flail mitral leaflets due to torn chords, ruptured sinus of Valsalva aneurysm, and intramyocardial abscess, can be documented reliably.

Before the advent of echocardiography, the noninvasive diagnosis of prosthetic valve dysfunction was based on definition of abnormal valve motion or restricted poppet motion on fluoroscopic examination. Two-dimensional

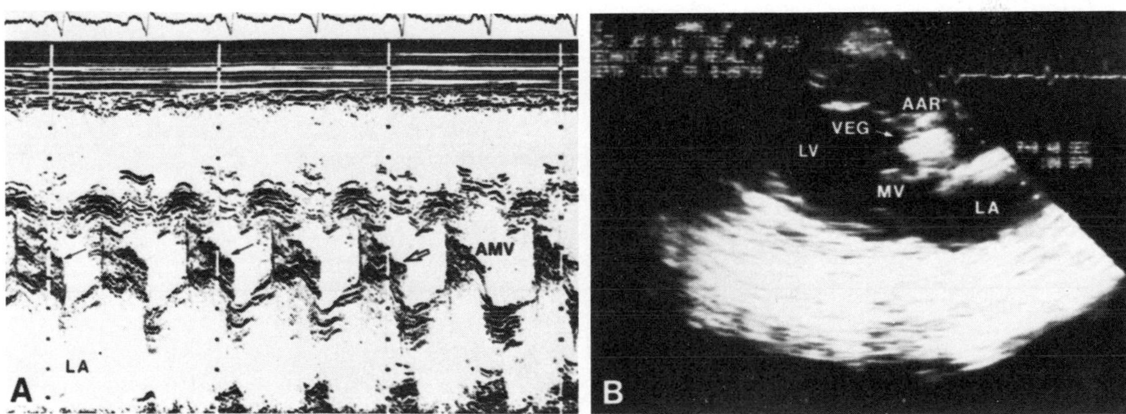

Figure 11–28. M-mode (*A*) and two-dimensional (*B*) echocardiograms in a patient with infective endocarditis of the aortic valve. The M-mode scan demonstrates a shaggy dense mass of echoes (*thin arrow*) attached to the aortic valve, prolapsing during diastole into the left ventricular outflow tract (*open arrow*). This finding is characteristic of a flail aortic valve cusp. On the two-dimensional study, there is a dense vegetation (*VEG*) destroying the aortic valve, partially prolapsing into the left ventricular outflow tract. *MV* = mitral valve. Other abbreviations as in Figure 11–23. (From Riba, A., and Berger, H. J.: Echocardiography in acquired heart disease. *In* Glenn et al. (eds.): Thoracic and Cardiovascular Surgery, 4th ed. New York, Appleton-Century-Crofts, in press.)

echocardiography has proved valuable in identifying porcine valve thickening or disruption, thrombosed or infected prosthetic valves, and dehiscence of the valve ring. It should be cautioned that materials used in the manufacture of prosthetic valves reflect echoes intensely, thereby making differentiation of some echo targets uncertain. (Popp et al., 1980; Riba and Berger, in press).

Evaluation of Left Ventricular Volume and Function

Echocardiography can provide a reliable assessment of left ventricular volume and function. This is best performed using two-dimensional techniques, although the one-dimensional views of the left ventricle obtained with M-mode echocardiography allow determination of the internal dimension of the left ventricle. From serial tomographic cross-sectional imaging, a detailed analysis can be derived of cardiac size and function, and of regional dynamic changes in circumference, thickness, and contractility (Fortuin and Pawsey, 1977; Mason and Fortuin, 1978).

The two-dimensional approach has been applied widely to patients with coronary artery disease, specifically acute myocardial infarction (Fig. 11–25). Diminished endocardial wall motion or reduced systolic thickening correlate well with regional ischemia or infarction (Fig. 11–29) (Eaton et al., 1979; Heger et al., 1979; Lieberman et al., 1981). The complications of myocardial infarction and the extent of regional asynergy can also be identified with two-dimensional echocardiography (Figs. 11–30, 11–31) (Asinger et al., 1981; Gibson et al., 1982; Katz et al., 1979; Weyman et al., 1976). Specifically, left ventricular aneurysms (true and pseudo-), mural thrombosis, and acute rupture of the interventricular septum can be reliably detected by means of this technique. Regional expansion of a myocardial segment on serial two-dimensional studies and asynergy at a distance from the acute infarct have been associated with a high mortality. (Eaton et al., 1979; Gibson et al., 1982). For demonstration of a

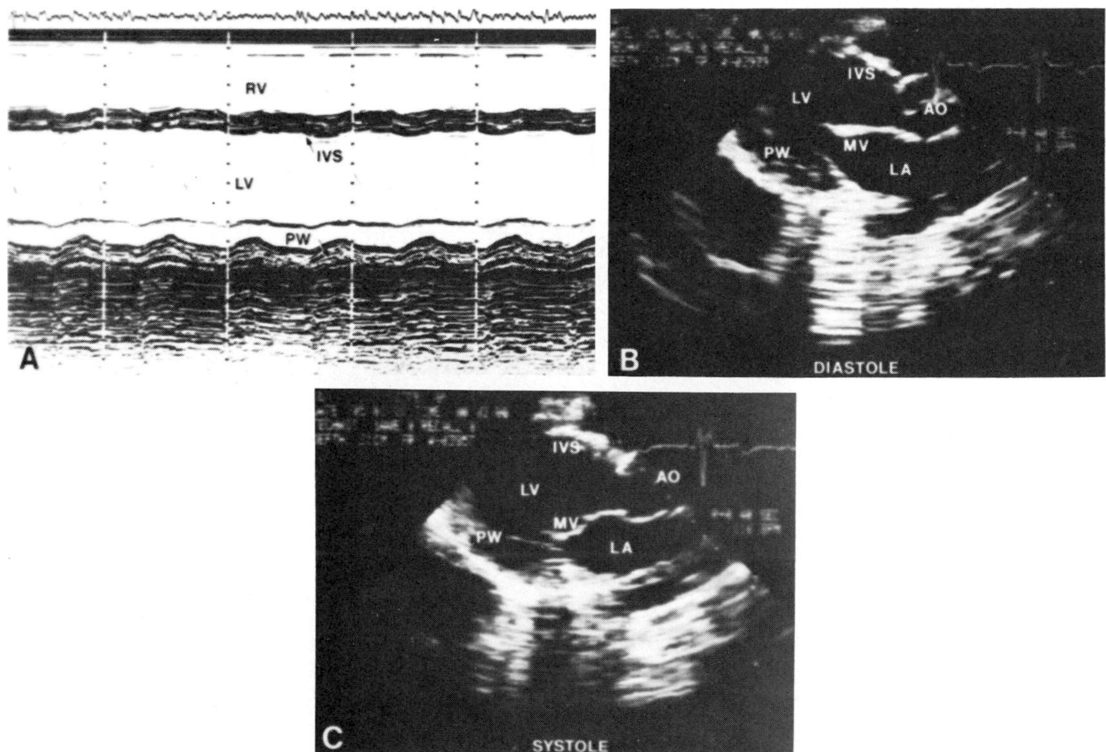

Figure 11–29. M-mode (*A*) and two-dimensional long-axis (*B*) echocardiograms from a patient with an anteroseptal myocardial infarction. The M-mode echocardiogram shows a thin echo-dense septum consistent with scarring. The septum also is scarred and akinetic on the two-dimensional study. *MV* = mitral valve. Other abbreviations as in Figure 11–23.

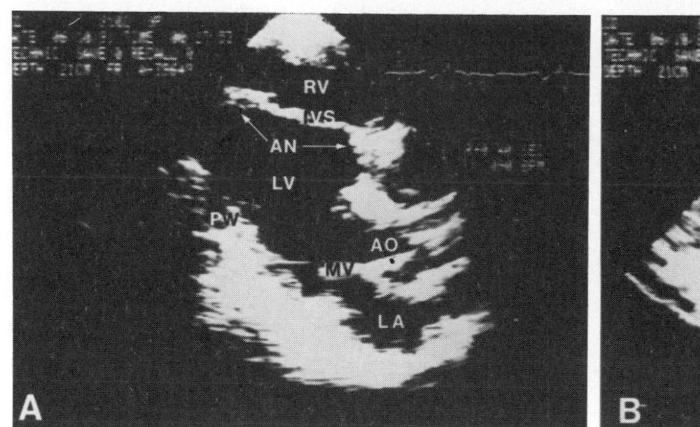

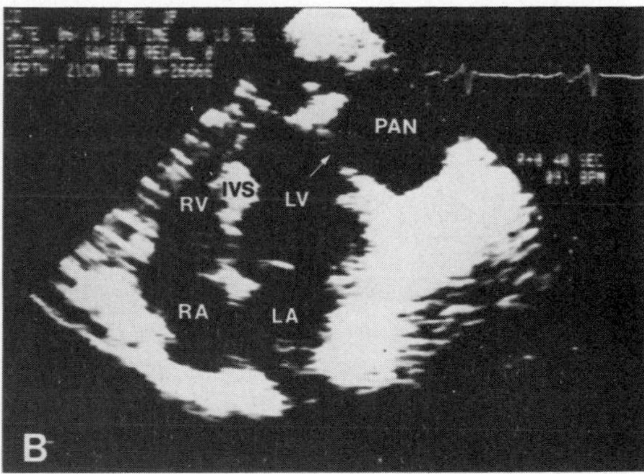

Figure 11–30. Two-dimensional echocardiograms demonstrating true (*A*) and false (*B*) left ventricular aneurysms. The true aneurysm appears on the long-axis view as a dyskinetic bulge arising from the mid and lower portions of the interventricular septum. The pseudoaneurysm, seen on the four-chamber apical view, appears as a contiguous echolucent chamber communicating with the left ventricular cavity through a relatively narrow orifice (*arrow*). *AN* = true aneurysm; *PAN* = pseudoaneurysm; *MV* = mitral valve; *RA* = right atrium. Other abbreviations as in Figure 11–23. (From Riba, A., and Berger, H. J.: Echocardiography in acquired heart disease. *In* Glenn et al. (eds.): Thoracic and Cardiovascular Surgery, 4th ed. New York, Appleton-Century-Crofts, in press.)

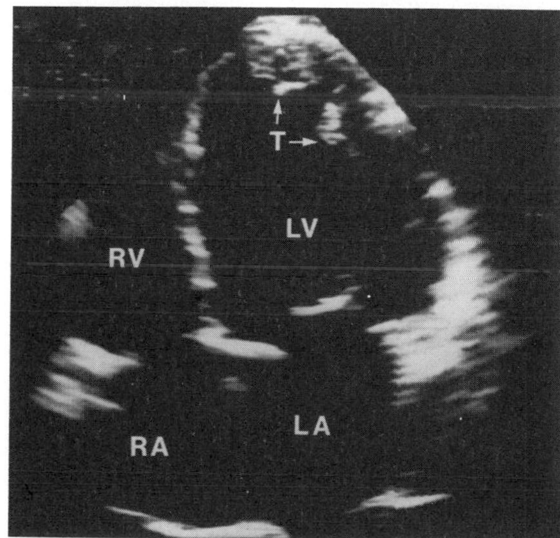

Figure 11–31. Apical four-chamber view of the left ventricle in a patient with an acute anteroapical myocardial infarction. This study demonstrates left ventricular thrombus. Note the distinct bright mass of echoes contiguous with the endocardium protruding into the left ventricular cavity. *T* = thrombus; *RA* = right atrium. Other abbreviations as in Figure 11–23.

ventricular septal defect, careful subcostal and apical views, as well as contrast material injection, may be needed. The defect appears as a discontinuity in a scarred septum that widens and protrudes toward the right ventricle during systole. Areas of negative contrast may be visualized in the right ventricle owing to left-to-right shunting of blood that does not contain microcavitations.

At this time, it is unclear whether echocardiographic or radionuclide assessment of regional function is preferable. For measurement of global performance, specifically ejection fraction, radionuclide angiocardiography appears optimal in terms of accuracy and reproducibility, particularly in the asymmetrically contracting ventricle. The characteristic findings in various cardiomyopathies can also be identified (DeMaria et al., 1980c). Congestive cardiomyopathy can be differentiated from myocardial infarction. There are distinct echocardiographic features of obstructive and nonobstructive hypertrophic cardiomyopathy, which is optimally assessed via echocardiography.

Evaluation of Pericardial Disease

Echocardiography is the preferred means of detecting pericardial effusion. Fluid within the pericardium appears as an echo-free space between the moving epicardium of the left ventricular posterior wall and the relatively flat pericardial-lung interface (Figs. 11–32, 11–33). During a transducer sweep from the apex to the base, the posterior pericardial free space usually obliterates at the atrioventricular junction (Teichholz, 1978). Large effusions may cause the heart to swing within the pericar-

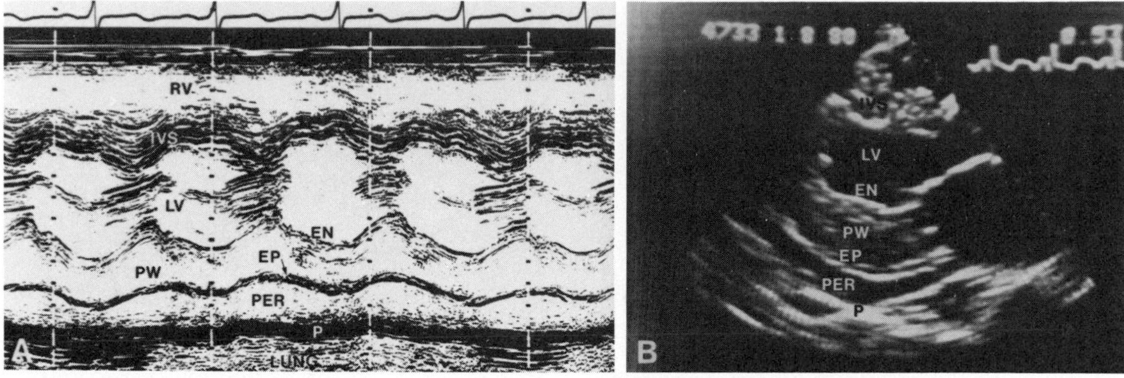

Figure 11–32. M-mode (*A*) and two-dimensional (*B*) echocardiograms from patients with large posterior pericardial effusions. There is an echo-free space present in both systole and diastole between the moving epicardium and stationary pericardial-lung interface. The long axis view (*B*) demonstrates that the effusion layers behind the entire posterior wall of the left ventricle and extends around the apex. *PER* = pericardial effusion; *P* = pericardium. Other abbreviations as in Figure 11–23. (From Riba, A., and Berger, H. J.: Echocardiography in acquired heart disease. *In* Glenn et al. (eds.): Thoracic and Cardiovascular Surgery, 4th ed. New York, Appleton-Century-Crofts, in press.)

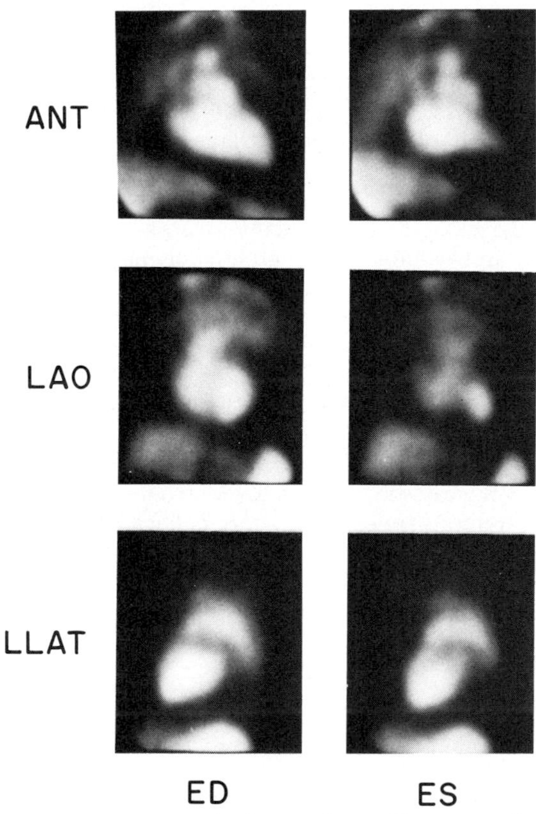

Figure 11–33. Multiple-gated equilibrium cardiac blood pool imaging in a patient with a large pericardial effusion. Note the large black halo surrounding the heart, with clear separation between the inferior surface of the heart and the liver. This is the classic finding in pericardial effusion. Although the echocardiographic examination clearly is preferred for assessment of pericardial fluid, this information can also be gained from the blood pool scan. Abbreviations as in Figure 11–18.

dium, which in turn makes the anterior and posterior walls of the heart move synchronously. Echocardiography in patients with cardiac tamponade usually shows a large effusion, with wide swings of the heart within the pericardium. There also are characteristic patterns in patients with constrictive pericarditis. Two-dimensional techniques allow definition of loculated pericardial effusions, as well as of malignant infiltration of the pericardium (Martin et al., 1978). Using the short-axis view, a pericardial effusion appears between the descending thoracic aorta and left ventricular epicardium, thereby allowing differentiation from a pleural effusion.

SUMMARY

In conclusion, cardiovascular imaging techniques have reached the point at which they can be applied clinically to the study of the critically ill patient. This chapter has focused on the applications of these techniques in the ICU. There certainly are instances in which radionuclide and echocardiographic techniques provide similar information, but they are inherently complementary and should be interpreted through the window provided by the plain chest radiograph. As the initial means of evaluation, the chest film provides insights into cardiac size, as well as pulmonary vascularity, particularly venous and arterial hypertension and shunt flow. In concert, this approach can provide detailed insights into cardiac pathophysiology and thus allow improvements in patient management.

REFERENCES

Asinger, R. W., Mikell, F. L., Sharma, B., and Hodges, M.: Observation on detecting left ventricular thrombus with two-dimensional echocardiography: emphasis on avoidance of false positive diagnoses. Am. J. Cardiol. 47:145, 1981.

Bacharach, S. L., Green, M. V., Borer, J. S., et al.: ECG-gated scintillation probe measurement of left ventricular function. J. Nucl. Med. 18:1176, 1977.

Benge, W., Litchfield, R. L., and Marcus, M. L.: Exercise capacity in patients with severe left ventricular dysfunction. Circulation 61:955, 1980.

Berger, B. C., Watson, D. D., Burwell, L. R., et al.: Redistribution of thallium at rest in patients with stable and unstable angina and the effect of coronary artery bypass surgery. Circulation 60:1114, 1979.

Berger, H. J., Davies, R. A., Batsford, W. P., et al.: Beat-to-beat left ventricular performance assessed from the equilibrium cardiac blood pool using a computerized nuclear probe. Circulation 63:133, 1981.

Berger, H. J., Gottschalk, A., and Zaret, B. L.: Dual radionuclide study of acute myocardial infarction: comparison of thallium-201 and technetium-99m stannous pyrophosphate imaging in man. Ann. Intern. Med. 88:145, 1978a.

Berger, H. J., Gottschalk, A., and Zaret, B. L.: Radionuclide assessment of left and right ventricular performance. Radiol. Clin. North Am. 18:441, 1980.

Berger, H. J., and Matthay, R. A.: Noninvasive radiographic assessment of cardiovascular function in acute and chronic respiratory failure. Am. J. Cardiol. 47:950, 1981.

Berger, H. J., Matthay, R. A., Loke, J., et al.: Assessment of cardiac performance with quantitative radionuclide angiocardiography: right ventricular ejection fraction with reference to findings in chronic obstructive pulmonary disease. Am. J. Cardiol. 41:897, 1978b.

Berger, H. J., Matthay, R. A., Pytlik, L. M.: First-pass radionuclide assessment of right and left ventricular performance in patients with cardiac and pulmonary disease. Semin. Nucl. Med. 9:275, 1979.

Berger, H. J., and Zaret, B. L.: Medical progress: nuclear cardiology. N. Engl. J. Med. 305:799, 855, 1981.

Bommer, W., Weinert, L., Neumann, A., et al.: Determination of right atrial and right ventricular size by two-dimensional echocardiography. Circulation 60:91, 1979.

Botvinick, E. H., Schiller, N. B., Wickramasekazan, R., et al.: Echocardiographic demonstration of early mitral valve closure in severe aortic insufficiency: its clinical implications. Circulation 51:836, 1975.

Brent, B. N., Berger, H. J., Matthay, R. A., et al.: Physiologic correlates of right ventricular ejection fraction in chronic obstructive pulmonary disease: a combined radionuclide and hemodynamic study. Am. J. Cardiol., in press, 1982.

Buja, L. M., Tofe, A. J., Kulkarni, P. V., et al.: Sites and mechanisms of localization of technetium-99m phosphorus radiopharmaceuticals in acute myocardial infarcts and other tissues. J. Clin. Invest. 60:724, 1977.

Bulkley, B. H., Hutchins, G. M., Bailey, I., et al.: Thallium-201 imaging and gated cardiac blood pool scans in patients with ischemic and congestive cardiomyopathy: a clinical and pathologic study. Circulation 55:753, 1977.

Burow, R. D., Pond, M., Schafer, A. W., and Becker, L.: "Circumferential profiles": a new method for computer analysis of thallium-201 myocardial perfusion images. J. Nucl. Med. 20:771, 1979.

Burow, R. D., Strauss, H. W., Singleton, R., et al.: Analysis of left ventricular function from multiple gated acquisition cardiac blood pool imaging: comparison to contrast angiography. Circulation 56:1024, 1977.

Cohen, H. A., Baird, M. G., Rouleau, J. R., et al.: Thallium-201 myocardial imaging in patients with pulmonary hypertension. Circulation 54:790, 1976.

Cope, G. D., Kisslo, J. A., Johnson, M. L., and Behar, V. S.: A reassessment of the echocardiogram in mitral stenosis. Circulation 52:664, 1975.

Davis, R. S., Strom, J. A., Frishman, W. H., et al.: The demonstration of vegetations by echocardiography in bacterial endocarditis: an indication for early surgical intervention. Am. J. Med. 69:57, 1980.

Dehmer, G. J., Lewis, S. E., Hillis, L. D., et al.: Nongeometric determination of left ventricular volumes from equilibrium blood pool scans. Am. J. Cardiol. 45:293, 1980.

DeMaria, A. N., Bommer, W., Joye, J., et al.: Value and limitations of cross-sectional echocardiography of the aortic valve in the diagnosis and quantification of valvular aortic stenosis. Circulation 62:304, 1980a.

DeMaria, A. N., Bommer, W., Joye, J. A., and Mason, D. T.: Cross-sectional echocardiography: physical principles, anatomic planes, limitations and pitfalls. Am. J. Cardiol. 46:1097, 1980b.

DeMaria, A. N., Bommer, W., Lee, G., and Mason, D. T.: Value and limitations of two-dimensional echocardiography in assessment of cardiomyopathy. Am. J. Cardiol. 46:1224, 1980c.

DeMaria, A. N., King, J. F., Salel, A. F., et al.: Echography and phonography of acute aortic regurgitation in bacterial endocarditis. Ann. Intern. Med. 82:329, 1975.

Dewanjee, M. K., and Kahn, P. C.: Mechanisms of localizations of ^{99m}Tc-labeled pyrophosphate and tetracycline in infarcted myocardium. J. Nucl. Med. 17:639, 1976.

DiCola, V. C., Downing, S. E., Donabedian, R. K., and Zaret, B. L.: Pathophysiological correlates of thallium-201 myocardial uptake in experimental infarction. Cardiovasc. Res. 11:141, 1977.

Eaton, L. W., Weiss, J. L., Bulkley, B. H., et al.: Regional cardiac dilatation after acute myocardial infarction: recognition by two-dimensional echocardiography. N. Engl. J. Med. 300:57, 1979.

Feigenbaum, H.: Echocardiography, 3rd ed. Philadelphia, 1980, Lea & Febiger.

Fortuin, N. J., and Pawsey, C. G. K.: The evaluation of left ventricular function by echocardiography. Am. J. Med. 63:1, 1977.

Garcia, E. V., Maddahi, J., Berman, D., and Waxman, A.: Space-time quantitation of thallium-201 myocardial scintigraphy. J. Nucl. Med. 22:309, 1981.

Gibson, R. S., Bishop, H. L., Stamm, R. B., et al.: Value of early two-dimensional echocardiography in patients with acute myocardial infarction. Am. J. Cardiol. 49:1110, 1982.

Gilbert, B. W., Haney, R. S., Crawford, F., et al.: Two-dimensional echocardiographic assessment of vegetative endocarditis. Circulation 55:346, 1977.

Green, M. V., Ostrow, H. G., Douglas, M. A., et al.: High temporal resolution ECG-gated scintigraphic angiocardiography. J. Nucl. Med. 16:95, 1975.

Griffith, J. M., and Henry, W. L.: A sector scanner for real-time two-dimensional echocardiography. Circulation 49:1147, 1974.

Heger, J. J., Weyman, A. E., Wann, L. S., et al.: Cross-sectional echocardiography in acute myocardial infarction: detection and localization of regional left ventricular asynergy. Circulation 60:531, 1979.

Henry, W. L., Bonow, R. O., Borer, S. S., et al.: Observations on the optimum time for operative intervention for aortic regurgitation. I. Evaluation of the results of aortic valve replacement in symptomatic patients. Circulation 61:471, 1980a.

Henry, W. L., Bonow, R. O., Rosing, D. R., and Epstein, S. E.: Observations on the optimum time for operative intervention for aortic regurgitation. II. Serial echocardiographic evaluation of asymptomatic patients. Circulation 61:484, 1980b.

Henry, W. L., DeMaria, A., Gramiak, R., et al.: Report of the American Society of Echocardiography Committee on nomenclature and standards in two-dimensional echocardiography. Circulation 62:212, 1980c.

Henry, W. L., Griffith, J. M., Michaelis, L. L., et al.: Measurement of mitral orifice area in patients with mitral valve disease by real-time, two-dimensional echocardiography. Circulation 51:827, 1975.

Henry, W. L., and Kastl, D. G.: Echocardiographic evaluation of patients with mitral stenosis. Am. J. Med. 62:813, 1977.

Hoffer, P. B., Berger, H. J., Steidley, J., et al.: A miniature cadmium telluride detector module for continuous monitoring of left-ventricular function. Radiology 138:477, 1981.

Holman, B. L., Chisholm, R. J., and Braumwald, E.: The prognostic implications of acute myocardial infarct scintigraphy with ^{99m}Tc-pyrophosphate. Circulation 57:320, 1978.

Holman, B. L., Lesch, M., Zweiman, F. G., et al.: Detection and sizing of acute myocardial infarcts with ^{99m}Tc (Sn) tetracycline. N. Engl. J. Med. 291:159, 1974.

Holman, B. L., and Wynne, J.: Infarct avid (hot spot) myocardial scintigraphy. Radiol. Clin. North Am. 18:487, 1980.

Hung, J., Harris, P. J., Uren, R. F., et al.: Uremic cardiomyopathy—effect of hemodialysis on left ventricular function in end-stage renal failure. N. Engl. J. Med. 302:547, 1980.

Johnstone, D. E., Wackers, F. J. T., Berger, H. J., et al.: Effect of patient positioning on left lateral thallium-201 myocardial images. J. Nucl. Med. 20:183, 1979.

Katz, R. J., Simpson, A., DiBianco, R., et al.: Noninvasive diagnosis of left ventricular pseudoaneurysm. Role of two-dimensional echocardiography and radionuclide gated pool imaging. Am. J. Cardiol. 44:372, 1979.

King, D. L.: Cardiac ultrasonography. Cross-sectional ultrasonic imaging of the heart. Circulation 47:843, 1973.

Kisslo, J., von Ramm, O. T., and Thurstone, F. L.: Cardiac imaging using a phased array ultrasound system. II. Clinical technique and application. Circulation 53:262, 1976.

Kotler, M. N., Mintz, G. S., Segal, B. L., and Parry, W. R.: Clinical uses of two-dimensional echocardiography. Am. J. Cardiol. 45:1061, 1980.

Lieberman, A. N., Weiss, J. L., Jugdutt, B. I., et al.: Two-dimensional echocardiography and infarct size: relationship of regional wall motion and thickening to the extent of myocardial infarction in the dog. Circulation 63:739, 1981.

Lieppe, W., Behar, V. S., Scallion, R., and Kisslo, J. A.: Detection of tricuspid regurgitation with two-dimensional echocardiography and peripheral vein injections. Circulation 57:128, 1978.

Marshall, R. C., Berger, H. J., Costin, J. C., et al.: Assessment of cardiac performance with quantitative radionuclide angiocardiography: sequential left ventricular ejection fraction, normalized left ventricular ejection rate, and regional wall motion. Circulation 56:820, 1977.

Martin, R. P., Rakowski, H., French, J., and Popp, R. L.: Localization of pericardial effusion with wide angle phased array echocardiography. Am. J. Cardiol. 42:904, 1978.

Martin, R. P., Rakowski, H., Kleiman, J. H., et al.: Reliability and reproducibility of two-dimensional echocardiographic measurement of the stenotic mitral valve orifice area. Am. J. Cardiol. 43:560, 1979.

Mason, S. J., and Fortuin, N. J.: The use of echocardiography for quantitative evaluation of left ventricular function. Prog. Cardiovasc. Dis. 21:119, 1978.

Meltzer, R. S., Hoogenhuyze, D. V., Serruys, P. W., et al.: Diagnosis of tricuspid regurgitation by contrast echocardiography. Circulation 63:1093, 1981.

Mintz, G. S., Kotler, M. N., Parry, W. R., and Segal, B. L.: Statistical comparison of M-mode and two-dimensional echocardiographic diagnosis of flail mitral leaflets. Am. J. Cardiol. 45:253, 1980.

Mintz, G. S., Kotler, M. N., Segal, B. L., and Parry, W. R.: Two-dimensional echocardiographic evaluation of patients with mitral insufficiency. Am. J. Cardiol. 44:670, 1979.

Morganroth, J., Jones, R. H., Chen, C. C., and Naito, M.: Two-dimensional echocardiography in mitral, aortic, and tricuspid valve prolapse. The clinical problem, cardiac nuclear imaging considerations and a proposed standard for diagnosis. Am. J. Cardiol. 46:1164, 1980.

Nichol, P. M., Gilbert, B. W., and Kisslo, J. A.: Two-dimensional echocardiographic assessment of mitral stenosis. Circulation 55:120, 1977.

Nichols, A. B., McKusick, K. A., Strauss, H. W., et al.: Clinical utility of gated cardiac blood pool imaging in congestive left heart failure. Am. J. Med. 65:785, 1978.

Okada, R. D., Boucher, C. A., Strauss, H. W., and Pohost, G. M.: Exercise radionuclide imaging approaches to coronary artery disease. Am. J. Cardiol. 46:1188, 1980.

Olson, H., Lyons, K., Aronow, W., and Waters, H.: Identification of high risk unstable angina pectoris for mortality and myocardial infarction. Circulation 55 & 56:Suppl. 3:III-173 (abstr.), 1977.

Parkey, R. W., Bonte, F. J., Meyer, S. L., et al.: A new method for radionuclide imaging of acute myocardial infarction in humans. Circulation 50:540, 1974.

Platt, M. R., Parkey, R. W., Willerson, J. T., et al.: Technetium stannous pyrophosphate myocardial scintigrams in the recognition of myocardial infarction in patients undergoing coronary artery revascularization. Ann. Thorac. Surg. 21:311, 1976.

Pohost, G. M., Zir, L. M., Moore, R. H., et al.: Differentiation of transiently ischemic from infarcted myocardium by serial imaging after a single dose of thallium-201. Circulation 55:294, 1977.

Popp, R. L.: Echocardiographic assessment of cardiac disease. Circulation 54:538, 1976.

Popp, R. L., Rubenson, D. S., Tucker, C. R., and French, J. W.: Echocardiography: M-mode and two-dimensional methods. Ann. Intern. Med. 93:844, 1980.

Reduto, L. A., Berger, H. J., Cohen, L. S., et al.: Sequential radionuclide assessment of left and right ventricular performance after acute transmural myocardial infarction. Ann. Intern. Med. 89:441, 1978.

Rerych, S. K., Scholz, P. M., Newman, G. E., et al.: Cardiac function at rest and during exercise in normals and in patients with coronary heart disease: evaluation by radionuclide angiocardiography. Ann. Surg. 187:449, 1978.

Riba, A., and Berger, H. J.: Echocardiography in acquired heart disease. *In* Glenn, W., Baue, A., Geha, A., et al. (eds.): Thoracic and Cardiovascular Surgery, 4th ed. New York, Appleton-Century-Crofts, in press, 1982.

Schwartz, A., Vignola, P. A., Walker, M. J., et al.: Echocardiographic estimation of aortic valve gradient in aortic stenosis. Ann. Intern. Med. 89:329, 1978.

Shah, P. K., Pichler, M., Berman, D. S., et al.: Left ventricular ejection fraction determined by radionuclide ventriculography in early stages of first transmural myocardial infarction: relation to short-term prognosis. Am. J. Cardiol. 45:542, 1980.

Silverman, K. J., Becker, L. C., Bulkley, B. H., et al.: Value of early thallium-201 scintigraphy for predicting mortality in patients with acute myocardial infarction. Circulation 61:996, 1980.

Skorton, D. J., Child, J. S., and Perloff, J. K.: Accuracy of the echocardiographic diagnosis of aortic regurgitation. Am. J. Med. 69:377, 1980.

Slutsky, R., Karliner, J., Ricci, D., et al.: Ventricular volumes by gated equilibrium radionuclide angiography: a new method. Circulation 60:556, 1979.

Stewart, J. A., Silimperi, D., Harris, P., et al.: Echocardiographic documentation of vegetative lesions in infective endocarditis: clinical implications. Circulation 61:374, 1980.

Strauss, H. W., Harrison, K., Langan, J. K., et al.: Thallium-201 for myocardial imaging: relation of thallium-201 to regional myocardial perfusion. Circulation 51:641, 1975.

Strauss, H. W., Zaret, B. L., Hurley, P. J., et al.: A scintiphotographic method for measuring left ventricular ejection fraction in man without cardiac catheterization. Am. J. Cardiol. 28:575, 1971.

Sweatman, T., Selzer, A., Kamagaki, M., and Cohn, K.: Echocardiographic diagnosis of mitral regurgitation due to ruptured chordae tendineae. Circulation 46:580, 1972.

Teichholz, L. E.: Echocardiographic evaluation of pericardial diseases. Prog. Cardiovasc. Dis. 21:133, 1978.

Tobinick, E., Schelbert, H. R., Henning, H., et al.: Right ventricular ejection fraction in patients with acute anterior and inferior myocardial infarction assessed by radionuclide angiography. Circulation 57:1078, 1978.

Von Ramm, O. T., and Thurstone, F. L.: Cardiac imaging using a phased array ultrasound system. I. System design. Circulation 53:258, 1976.

Wackers, F. J., Berger, H. J., and Zaret, B. L.: Radionuclide ventriculography. *In* Wagner, G. (ed.): Myocardial Infarction: Measurement and Intervention. Hague, Martinus Nijhoff, 1982, pp. 199–233.

Wackers, F. J., Giles, R., Hoffer, P., et al.: Gold-195m, a new generator-produced short-lived radionuclide for sequential assessment of left ventricular performance. Am. J. Cardiol., in press, 1982.

Wackers, F. J., Klay, J. W., Laks, H., et al.: Pathophysiologic correlates of right ventricular thallium-201 uptake in a canine model. Circulation 64: 1256, 1981.

Wackers, F. J. T., Lie, K. I., Liem, K. L., et al.: Potential value of thallium-201 scintigraphy as a means of selecting patients for the coronary care unit. Br. Heart J. 41:111, 1979.

Wackers, F. J. T., Lie, K. I., Liem, K. L., et al.: Thallium-201 scintigraphy in unstable angina pectoris. Circulation 57:738, 1978.

Wackers, F. J. T., Sokole, E. B., Samson, G., et al.: Value and limitations of thallium-201 scintigraphy in the acute phase of myocardial infarction. N. Engl. J. Med. 295:1, 1976.

Wagner, H. N., Jr., Wake, R., Nickoloff, E., and Natarajan, T. K.: The nuclear stethoscope: a simple device for generation of left ventricular volume curves. Am. J. Cardiol. 38:747, 1976.

Wann, L. S., Dillon, J. C., Weyman, A. E., and Feigenbaum, H.: Echocardiography in bacterial endocarditis. N. Engl. J. Med. 295:135, 1976.

Wann, L. S., Feigenbaum, H., Weyman, A. E., and Dillon, J. C.: Cross-sectional echocardiographic detection of rheumatic mitral regurgitation. Am. J. Cardiol. 41:1258, 1978a.

Wann, L. S., Weyman, A. E., Feigenbaum, H., et al.: Determination of mitral valve area by cross-sectional echocardiography. Ann. Intern. Med. 88:337, 1978b.

Watson, D., Campbell, N., Read, E. K., et al.: Spatial and temporal quantitation of planar thallium myocardial images. J. Nucl. Med. 22:577, 1981.

Weyman, A. E., Feigenbaum, H., Dillon, J. C., and Chang, S.: Cross-sectional echocardiography in assessing the severity of aortic stenosis. Circulation 52:828, 1975.

Weyman, A. E., Peskoe, S. M., Williams, E. S., et al.: Detection of left ventricular aneurysms by cross-sectional echocardiography. Circulation 54:936, 1976.

Zaret, B. L., DiCola, V. C., Donabedian, R. K., et al.: Dual radionuclide study of myocardial infarction: relationship between myocardial uptake of potassium-43, technetium-99m stannous pyrophosphate, regional myocardial blood flow and creatine phosphokinase depletion. Circulation 53:422, 1976.

Zaret, B. L., Strauss, H. W., Hurley, P. J., et al.: A noninvasive scintiphotographic method for detecting regional ventricular dysfunction in man. N. Engl. J. Med. 284:1165, 1971.

Zaret, B. L., Strauss, H. W., Martin, N. D., et al.: Noninvasive regional myocardial perfusion with radioactive potassium: study of patients at rest, with exercise and during angina pectoris. N. Engl. J. Med. 288:809, 1973.

Chapter 12

NEONATAL INTENSIVE CARE RADIOLOGY

by Gerald A. Mandell

INTRODUCTION

There are many causes of respiratory distress in the newborn, both medical and surgical. The radiograph is extremely helpful in differentiating one cause of respiratory distress from another. The following discussion will dwell on the medical causes of respiratory distress and the iatrogenic complications of treatment with mechanical ventilation, tubes, and catheters.

Hyaline Membrane Disease (HMD)

Hyaline membrane disease, or idiopathic respiratory distress syndrome, is one of the most common causes of respiratory distress in the newborn. Prematurity, C-section delivery, and diabetic mothers are predisposing factors. Common to all infants with HMD is the lack of the surface tension–reducing substance surfactant. Without surfactant, the alveoli are not adequately distended and alveolar collapse ensues; hypoxia and acidosis result. Complications of severe hypoxia include intracranial hemorrhage, disseminated intravascular coagulation (DIC), pulmonary hemorrhage, and congestive heart failure (CHF) from a patent ductus arteriosus (PDA). Continuous positive pressure (CPAP) and positive end-expiratory pressure (PEEP) not only open up the alveoli but lead to other complications such as pneumothorax, pneumomediastinum, pulmonary interstitial emphysema (PIE), pneumoperitoneum, massive gas embolism, and bronchopulmonary dysplasia (BPD).

Clinically, infants with HMD show signs of respiratory distress in the first few hours of life. The disease is a spectrum, ranging from very mild to very severe. The symptoms consist of progressively increasing dyspnea, tachypnea, grunting, nasal flaring, and retractions (intercostal, suprasternal, and substernal). Radiographic changes are usually minimal in the mild forms of the disease. The classic roentgenographic findings in moderate-to-severe HMD consist of underaeration, finely granular appearance of pulmonary parenchyma (collapsed alveoli and alveolar ducts), and bilateral symmetric branching air bronchograms (Ellis and Nadelhaft, 1957; Petersen and Pendleton, 1955). Air bronchograms beyond the main stem right bronchus and the first bifurcation of the left bronchus are abnormal. Secondary air hunger signs include aeroesophagus and sternal retractions (Fig. 12–1). The aeroesophagus can also be seen in H-type tracheoesophageal fistula and gastroesophageal reflux. With mild-to-moderate HMD, emphysema of the distal airways may cause overaeration rather than the expected underventilation.

Sometimes, in moderate-to-severe disease, the lung may be overaerated as a result of mechanical ventilation. The lung density decreases markedly when mechanical ventilation is instituted (Giedion et al., 1973). There usually is clinical and radiologic improvement by 72 hours as surfactant develops and aeration improves. The initial differential diagnosis is mainly between HMD, sepsis, and severe wet lung disease.

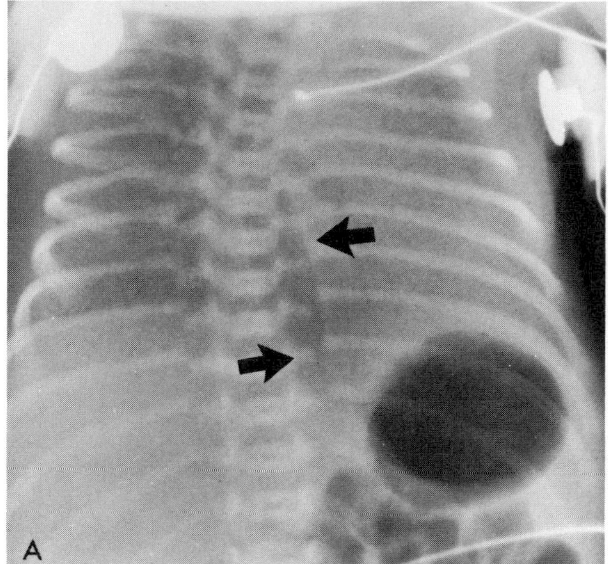

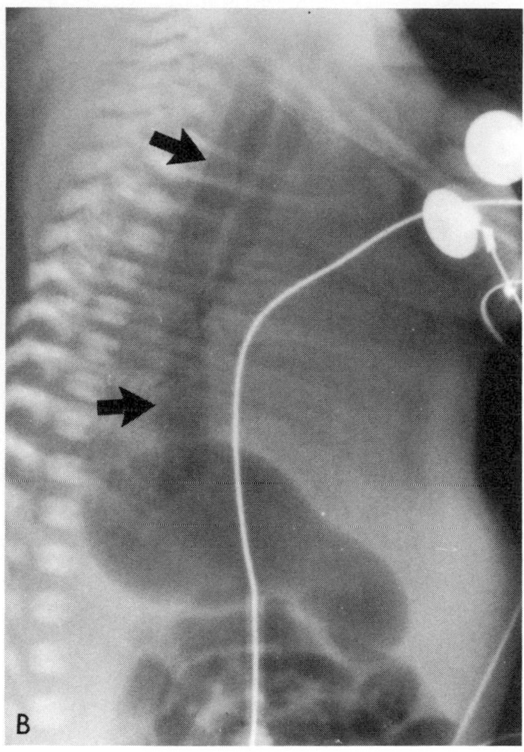

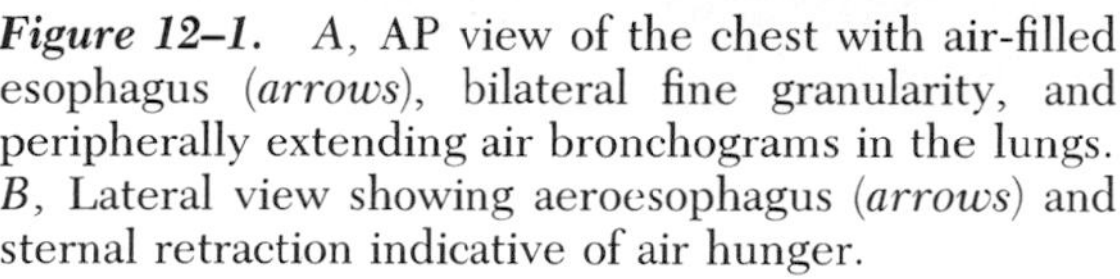
Figure 12–1. *A*, AP view of the chest with air-filled esophagus (*arrows*), bilateral fine granularity, and peripherally extending air bronchograms in the lungs. *B*, Lateral view showing aeroesophagus (*arrows*) and sternal retraction indicative of air hunger.

Transient Respiratory Distress of the Newborn (Transient Tachypnea, Wet Lung Disease)

Transient respiratory distress of the newborn (TRDN) is probably more common than HMD, and usually is present by 2 to 4 hours of age. Specific symptoms include tachypnea, nasal flaring, grunting, retractions, and, in some cases, cyanosis. Resolution in TRDN usually occurs between 24 and 72 hours, and these infants need minimal supportive oxygen therapy.

As the name "wet lung syndrome" implies, there is delayed clearance of fluid from the newborn infant's lung (Swischuk, 1970). Most fluid is cleared by lymphatics and veins. C-section infants commonly have TRDN because a substantial volume of fluid is not eliminated from their lungs by the usual uterine squeeze. Extra fluid can also be seen in vaginally delivered infants, especially those newborns who are relatively small in comparison with the uterine confines or who are delivered quite rapidly. Polycythemia from intrauterine placental transfusion or excessive milking of the cord, hypervolemia in infants of diabetic mothers, and hypoproteinemia (Steele and Copeland, 1972) with reduced oncotic pressure have been proposed as other predisposing factors. Aspiration of clear amniotic fluid secondary to fetal distress or breech delivery can cause clinical and radiographic conditions indistinguishable from wet lung.

The roentgenographic findings consist of symmetric parahilar patches or streaks, mild-to-moderate overaeration, and, occasionally, mild cardiomegaly or pleural effusions (Fig. 12–2) (Steele and Copeland, 1972). Interpretation is more difficult when the parahilar pattern is predominantly in the right lung, or with a localized alveolar patch (Wesenberg et al., 1971). The radiographic appearance in TRDN is almost always clear by 48 to 72 hours. If the wet lung pattern and cardiomegaly persist beyond 72 hours, hypoplastic left heart syndrome, cor triatriatum, and myocardial dysfunction must be considered. The initial radiographic appearances of sepsis and wet lung disease are similar.

Pulmonary Hemorrhage

Pulmonary hemorrhage is usually due to capillary damage in response to severe hypoxia. Pulmonary hemorrhage may accompany HMD, neonatal pneumonia, BPD, congenital heart

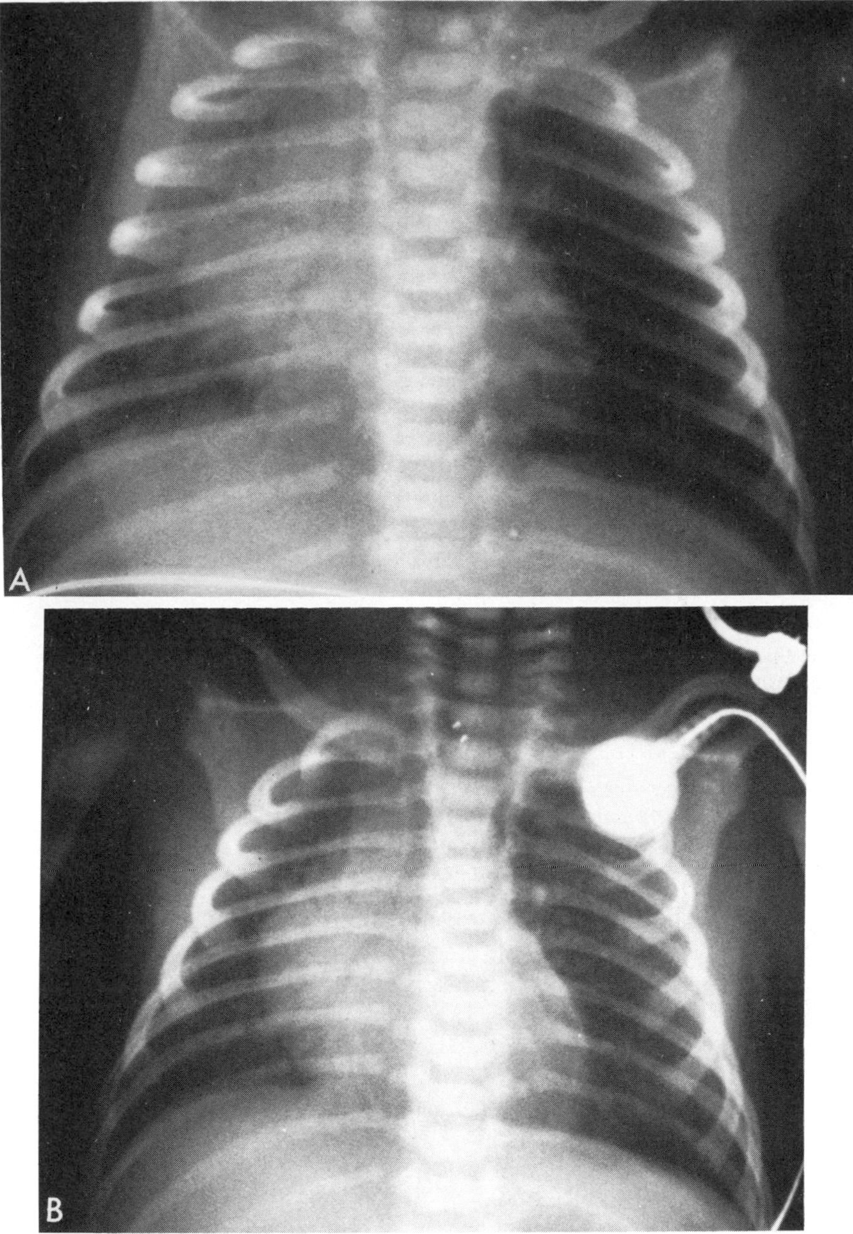

Figure 12–2. *A*, AP view of the chest of a 4-hour-old infant with increased markings in the right lung. *B*, A repeat radiograph two days later with remarkable clearing of wet lung.

disease, and hypoxia after a difficult or prolonged delivery. Small areas of hemorrhage are difficult to identify when superimposed on preexisting pulmonary disease. Massive pulmonary hemorrhage is characteristically homogeneous, opaque, and airless on the chest radiograph (Fig. 12–3). Differentiation from pneumonia is made by the rapid clearance of hemorrhage within 12 to 24 hours.

Neonatal Pneumonia

Neonatal pneumonia is predominantly bacterial in origin. The most common organisms are nonhemolytic *Streptococcus*, *Staphylococcus aureus*, and *Escherichia coli*. *Candida albicans* can also cause widespread pulmonary infection in the newborn (Kassner et al., 1981). Prolonged labor, premature rupture

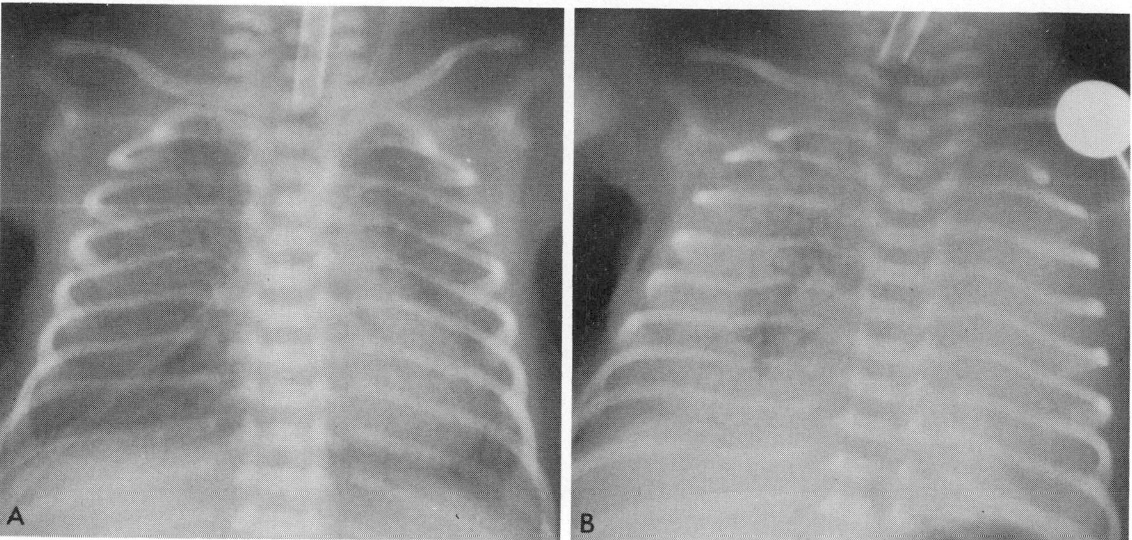

Figure 12–3. *A*, Initial radiograph of hyaline membrane disease. *B*, One day later the increased opacity is due to pulmonary hemorrhage.

of membranes, vaginal infection, placental infection, and contamination with maternal fecal material or bacteria from the improperly cleansed perineum are the predisposing factors. Diagnosis of sepsis depends greatly on radiographic demonstration of infiltrates together with a clinical suspicion. The infants are often afebrile and occasionally hypothermic. Shortly after birth, tachypnea, retractions, and cyanosis may be evident. Neutropenia has been reported in group B streptococcal infections.

The radiograph may show a diffusely granular pattern with air bronchograms mimicking HMD, or parahilar haziness and streaks mimicking wet lung syndrome or heart failure. Coarse, patchy, or diffusely nodular lesions may also be seen. Lobar consolidation is an infrequent roentgenographic manifestation.

Group B streptococcal neonatal infections appear to be the most common (Ablow et al., 1976). These infants initially may have clear lungs or segmental consolidations or may be roentgenographically indistinguishable from infants with HMD (Fig. 12–4). Premature infants with diffuse disease have the worst prognosis. Radiologically helpful signs include bilateral air bronchograms with *hyper*aeration in contrast with the *hypo*aeration with air bronchograms seen in HMD (Ablow et al., 1977). The subtle aeration sign can only be used when ventilation has not been altered by mechanical means. The immediate postnatal radiographs are extremely helpful. Small pleural effusions and worsening consolidations also lend support to the diagnosis of group B streptococcal infection; empyema, pneumtoceles, and abscesses are not common

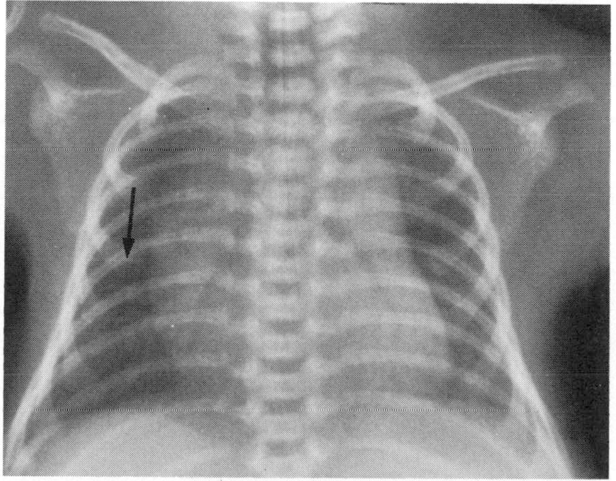

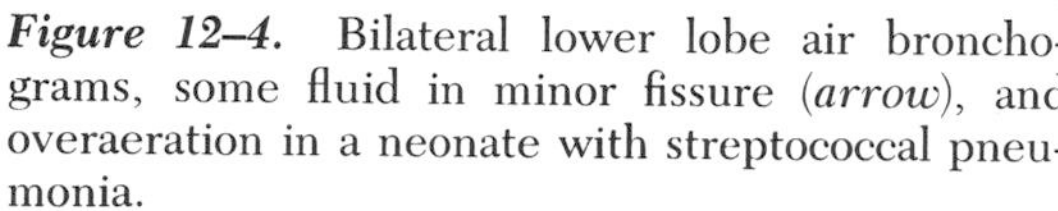

Figure 12–4. Bilateral lower lobe air bronchograms, some fluid in minor fissure (*arrow*), and overaeration in a neonate with streptococcal pneumonia.

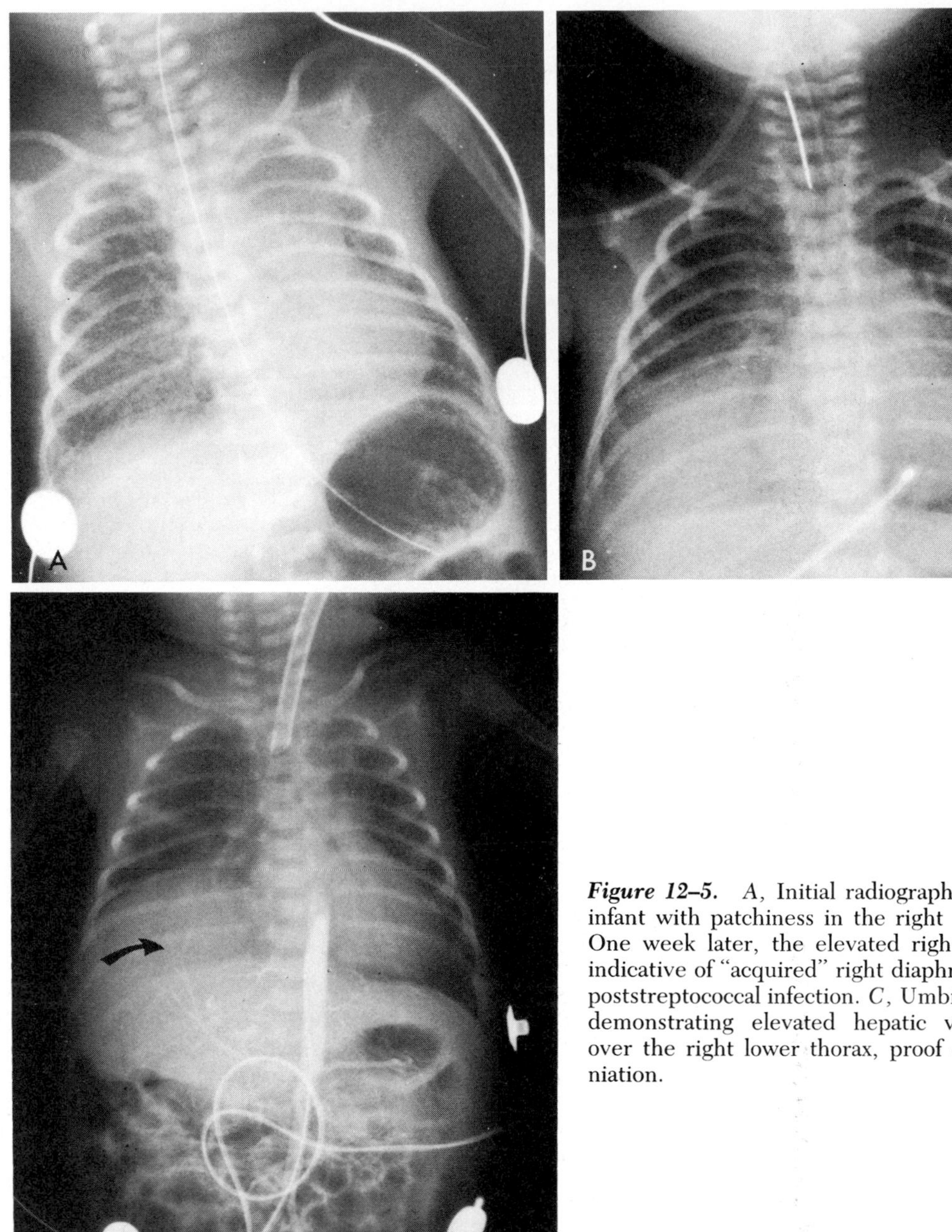

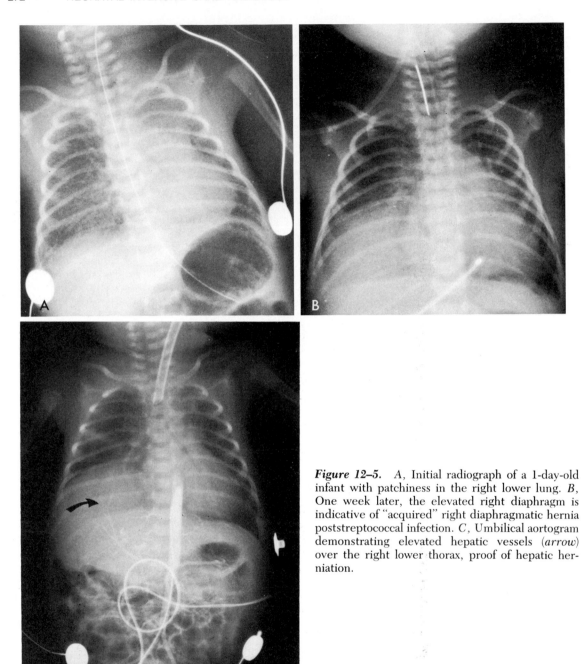

Figure 12–5. *A*, Initial radiograph of a 1-day-old infant with patchiness in the right lower lung. *B*, One week later, the elevated right diaphragm is indicative of "acquired" right diaphragmatic hernia poststreptococcal infection. *C*, Umbilical aortogram demonstrating elevated hepatic vessels (*arrow*) over the right lower thorax, proof of hepatic herniation.

in neonatal pneumonias. Infants with gradually elevating right diaphragms should be suspected of having "acquired" diaphragmatic hernia, which has been reported recently in association with group B streptococcal infections (Fig. 12–5) (McCarten et al., 1981).

Meconium Aspiration

Intrauterine fetal distress is probably caused by hypoxemia, which induces rapid respirations and defecation. Meconium in the amniotic fluid is inhaled, leading to respiratory distress. These

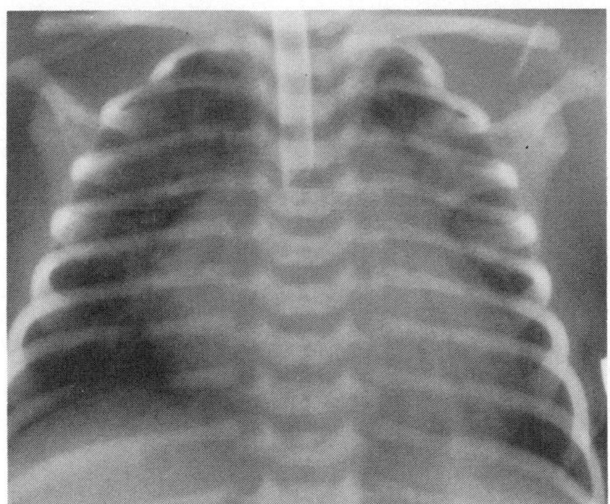

Figure 12–6. Multiple patches of disease and an enlarged heart in a patient with anoxia and meconium aspiration syndrome.

neonates are usually postmature and may have central nervous system (CNS) damage. Depending on the severity of aspiration, the symptoms are variable and may include tachypnea, grunting, retractions, or even cyanosis. Roentgenographically, hyperaeration is an expression of air trapping secondary to particles of meconium in the smaller bronchi. Coarse, bilateral patchy or nodular infiltrates representing atelectasis are most common. Occasionally, "cystic" changes representing streaky disease interspersed with areas of compensatory overaeration can be seen (Fig. 12–6) (Gooding et al., 1971). Mild cases may simply manifest overaeration with minor streaks or patches. Pleural effusions are sometimes evident. Pneumothorax and pneumomediastinum may result from sudden attempts to clear bronchi of meconium. The roentgen appearance of proximal humeral ossification centers (38 weeks of gestation) is a sign of postmaturity.

Suction of the tracheobronchial passages is necessary to remove as much debris as possible. Oxygen support together with humidity and body temperature maintenance is necessary. Intermittent gastric suction prevents additional aspiration in a neurologically compromised newborn. Right-to-left shunting with increased pulmonary vascular resistance (persistent fetal circulation, PFC) may occur. Anoxic sequelae include "bell-shaped" chest configuration secondary to poor intercostal muscle movement (Fig. 12–7*A*), hydrocephalus secondary to intracranial bleed and tissue damage, and even pylorospasm mimicking pyloric stenosis (Fig. 12–7*B*).

The lungs take weeks to clear and a "dirty" chest radiograph persists long after clinical recovery.

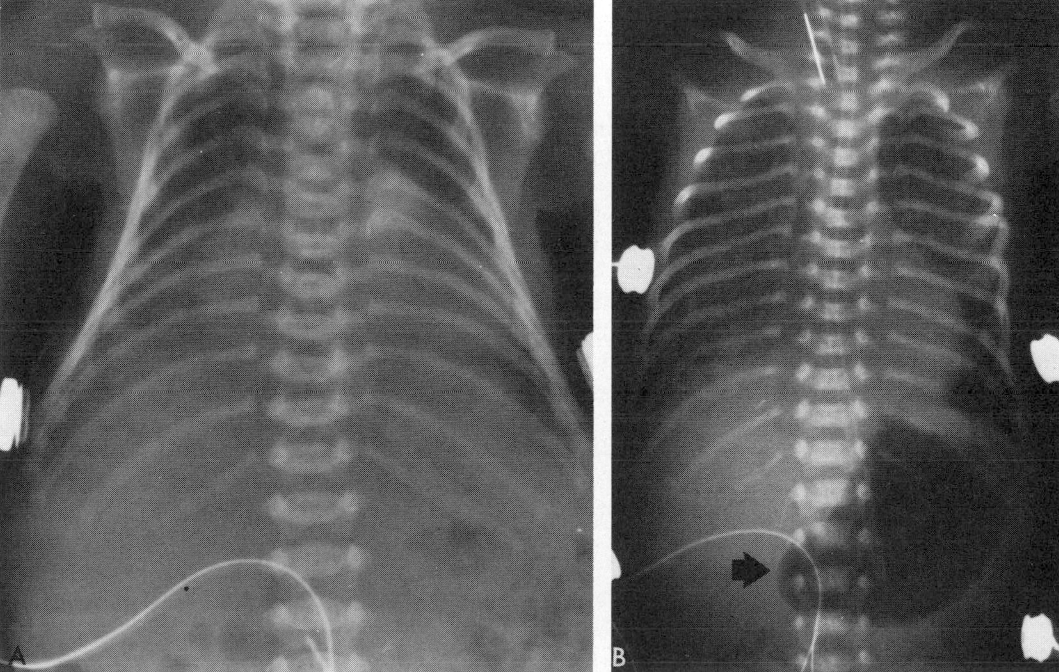

Figure 12–7. *A*, AP view of a chest with bell-shape configuration in an anoxic neonate. *B*, In another neonate, the stomach is distended by air (*arrow*) secondary to pylorospasm.

Persistent Fetal Circulation Syndrome (PFC)

Sometimes an abnormal persistent elevation of pulmonary vascular resistance results in right-to-left shunting via the patent foramen ovale or the PDA in full-term infants. This produces severe cyanosis in the first 24 hours of life. In most cases (Silverstein et al., 1981) perinatal hypoxia is the stimulus for the pulmonary vasoconstriction in the infant. Other factors influencing the development of PFC are hypoglycemia, acidemia, and hyperviscosity.

Roentgenographically the lungs are usually clear, which helps to differentiate PFC from pulmonary disease. However, venous congestion, patchy infiltrates, pleural effusions, hepatomegaly, or even mild HMD may be present (Neilson et al., 1976). Mild-to-moderate cardiomegaly is usually seen (Bauer et al., 1974), and differentiation of PFC from cyanotic heart disease may be difficult. Angiography may be necessary to exclude the diagnoses of transposition of the great vessels, hypoplastic left heart syndrome, or right ventricular outflow tract obstruction as the cause of the cyanosis. Treatment usually consists of oxygen therapy, correction of acidosis, and vasodilators such as tolazoline. The patient generally improves in two to six days, with lung clearance and disappearance of the cardiomegaly.

Patent Ductus Arteriosus (PDA)

Nineteen per cent of patients with HMD develop PDA (Thieboult et al., 1975). Sequential radiographs of infants with HMD are often helpful in early diagnosis of PDA (Slovis et al., 1980). The increased perfusion causes an engorgement of the pulmonary vascular bed, which diminishes compliance and ventilation; ventilatory pressures then usually have to be elevated. Indomethacin therapy or surgical intervention may be necessary to prevent the progression of lung disease to BPD.

Early radiographic signs of PDA (Fig. 12–8*A*) include preferential shunting to the right lung, sometimes with unilateral edema, perihilar haze, overaeration, and a slight increase in the cardiothoracic ratio. Elevation of the left bronchus signifies left atrial enlargement. Chest radiographs may detect the patent ductus 24 to 48 hours before its clinical presentation. Echocardiography, or umbilical arteriography with 1 to 2 ml of contrast medium, can substantiate the diagnosis (Fig. 12–7*B*). After surgical or medical closure there is reduction of the pulse pressure and disappearance of the murmur. Radiographs show clearance of the edema within 48 hours of closure.

Bronchopulmonary Dysplasia (Oxygen Toxicity, Ventilator Lung)

Bronchopulmonary dysplasia (BPD) is usually the end result of therapy for HMD with elevated concentrations of oxygen, mechanical ventilation, and endotracheal intubation. Its frequency is estimated at 17 to 68 per cent (Oppermann et al., 1977). There is a difference of opinion regarding the relative contributions of high oxygen exposure and mechanical ventilator injury toward the development of BPD (Edwards et al., 1977; Stocks et al., 1978). In these studies the neonates with HMD who developed BPD tended to be more premature than the group without evidence of BPD, and those succumbing to BPD had the most severe prematurity. Stiffening of the lungs by the increased perfusion via a PDA and/or by diffuse pulmonary interstitial emphysema requires increased ventilatory pressures and increased oxygen concentrations, which predispose the patient to BPD. Stage I, as described by Northway and Rosan (1968), consists radiologically of the classic HMD picture with bilateral fine granular changes and air bronchograms in the lungs (Fig. 12–9*A*). Pathologically, hyaline membranes, hyperemia, atelectasis, and lymphatic dilatation are present. Stage II of the disease develops four to ten days postnatally. The chest radiograph (Fig. 12–9*B*) becomes more diffusely opaque, sometimes obscuring the cardiomediastinal silhouette. Interstitial edema, intraluminal eosinophilic exudate, some hyaline membranes, and patchy bronchiolar necrosis are noted pathologically. There is pulmonary edema, probably secondary to vascular damage, with seepage of fluid into the interstitium and alveoli. Between the 10th and 20th days of life, Stage III appears with cystlike changes. These bubbles collapse during expiration, differentiating them from pulmonary interstitial emphysema. Pathologically, bronchial and bronchiolar mucosal metaplasia and hyperplasia with macrophagic and histiocytic exudate are seen. Areas of alveolar collapse and emphysematous alveoli alternate, giving the bubbly appearance to the lungs (Fig. 12–9*C*). In Stage IV, the radiograph shows multiple strands that radiate from the hila and diffuse hyperaeration. Stage IV usually coincides with the patient's discharge from the

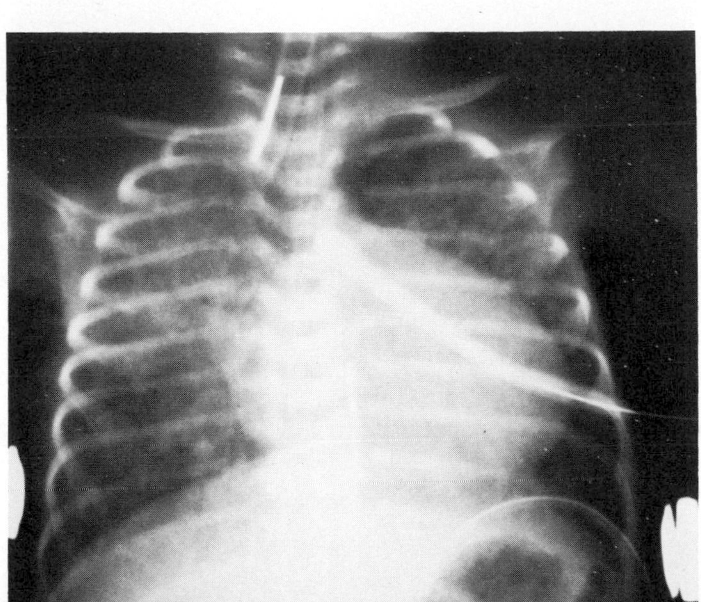

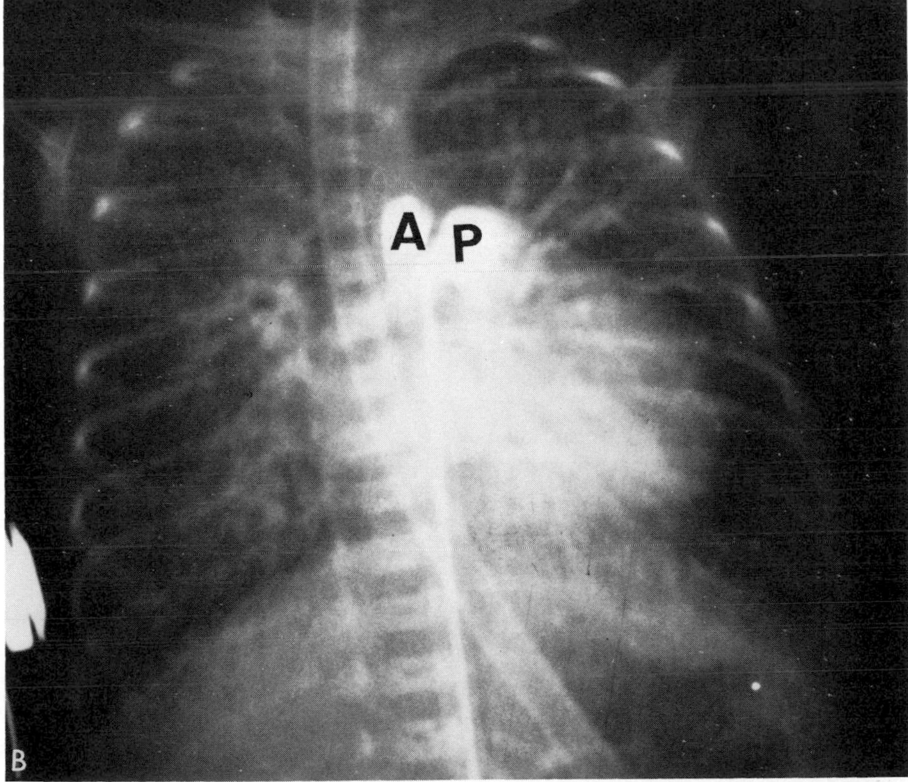

Figure 12–8. *A*, Preferential perfusion of patent ductus arteriosus demonstrated by increased markings in the right lung. *B*, Umbilical aortogram confirming the left-to-right shunt at the ductus level. P = pulmonary artery; *A* = aorta.

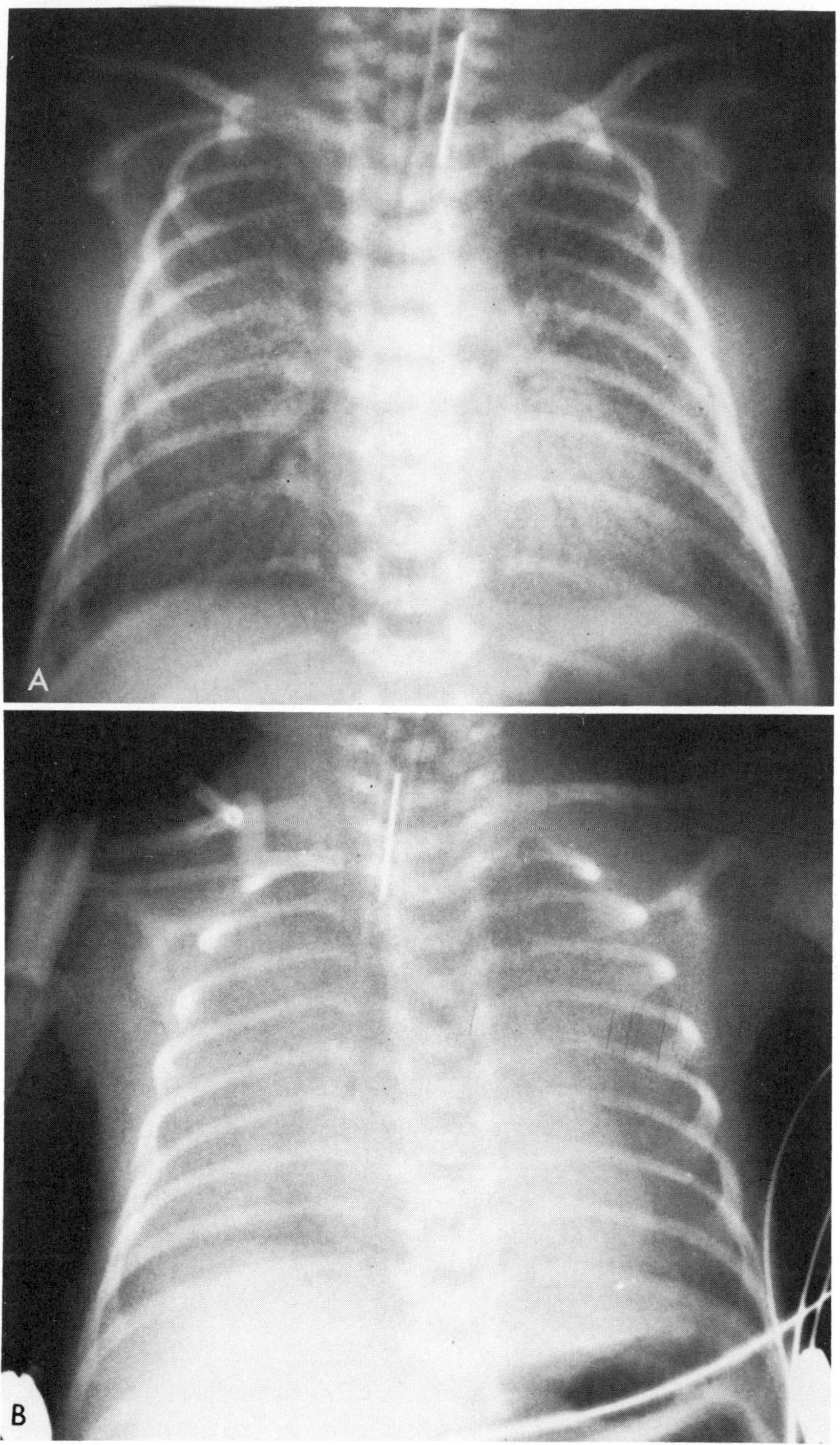

Figure 12–9. *A,* Initial radiograph demonstrates typical granularity of hyaline membrane disease. *B,* Seven days later, increasing density of lungs indicates the second stage of bronchopulmonary dysplasia.

Figure continued on opposite page

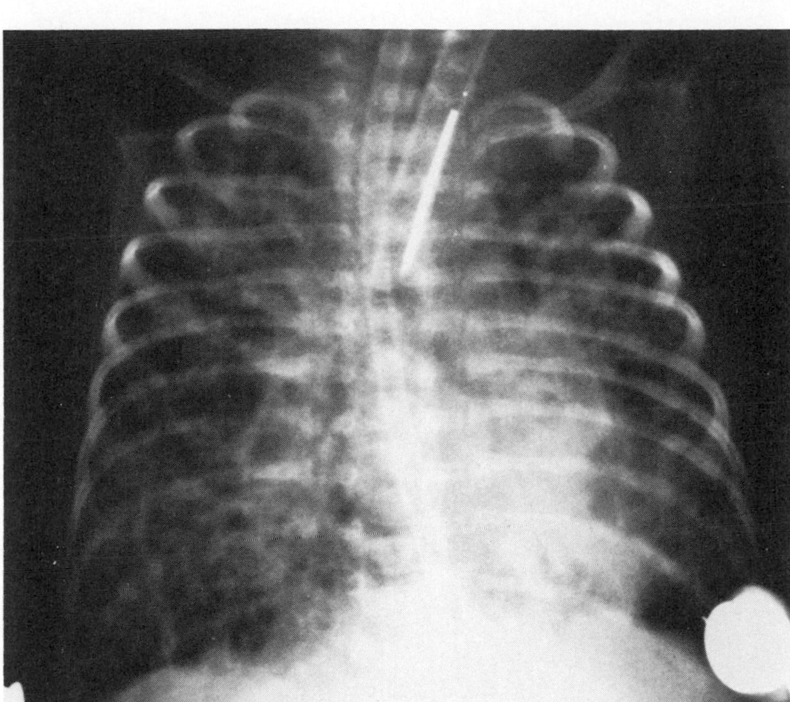

Figure 12–9. *(Continued)* *C*, Finally, the advanced stage III disease of BPD is shown, with a diffuse cystic pattern.

hospital, generally after the first month of life. This stage may gradually clear or may progress to cor pulmonale and death. The classic stages and disease patterns of BPD are described above. When atelectasis protects a portion of the lung, the disease may be asymmetric (Sickler and Gooding, 1976). Sometimes the diffuse hazy or bubbly pattern characteristic of stages II and III does not appear and the lungs have larger areas of atelectasis alternating with areas of emphysema. Trauma secondary to tracheal intubation and suctioning may cause endobronchial granulation tissue that may obstruct a bronchus, giving the picture of acquired lobar emphysema (Miller et al., 1981). These infants are usually malnourished and chronically debilitated. Gastroesophageal reflux may lead to aspiration pneumonitis. The supine, premature, debilitated infant with an immature esophageal sphincter is a prime candidate for chronic aspiration.

COMPLICATIONS OF MECHANICAL VENTILATION

Following mechanical ventilation and positive end-expiratory pressure (PEEP), there usually is a dramatic diminution in the degree of respiratory distress. The effects of PEEP are to increase arterial oxygenation and lower the requirements for supplemental oxygen (McCloud and Ravin, 1977). The lung volume is increased to functional residual capacity. The elevated pressure is transmitted to the small airways and alveoli to prevent atelectasis, to reduce shunting during the expiratory phase, and to press alveolar fluid against the alveolar walls. In theory, the elevation of the pressure gradient between the alveolus and pulmonary capillary results in the water entering the capillaries from the alveoli and interstitial spaces.

However, alveolar hyperinflation may rupture the alveoli. This may result in interstitial emphysema, pneumomediastinum, pneumothorax, pneumopericardium, pneumoperitoneum, and even intravascular air embolism (Giedion et al., 1973). Extra-alveolar collections of air may occur singly or in combination. HMD is the most common underlying condition associated with extra-alveolar dissection of air. Meconium aspiration, neonatal pneumonia, and BPD also predispose the patient to develop extra-alveolar air collections.

Pulmonary Interstitial Emphysema (PIE)

With alveolar rupture, air travels initially along the perivascular sheaths toward the

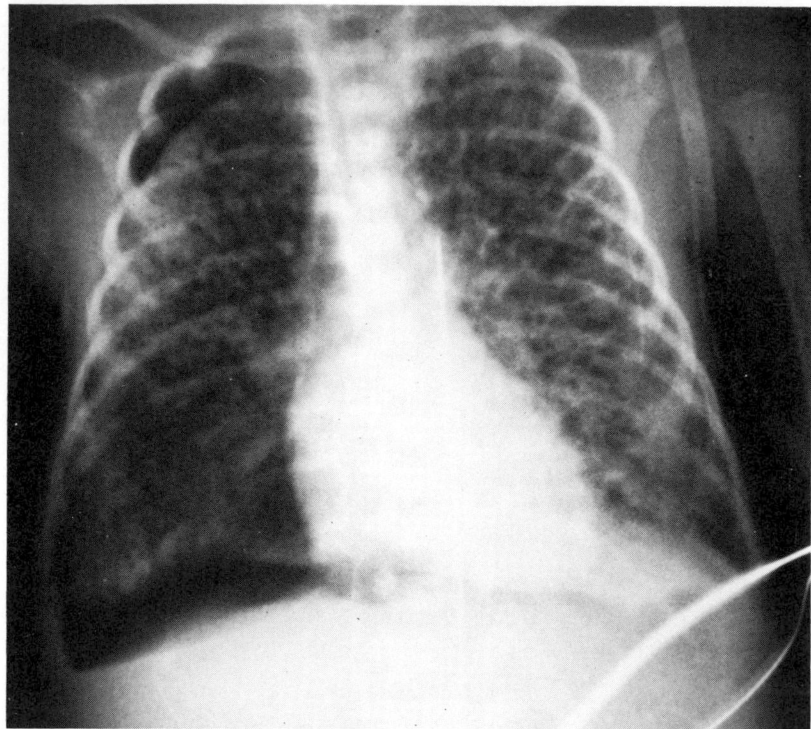

Figure 12–10. Diffuse lenticular air collections of pulmonary interstitial emphysema throughout both lungs. An associated right pneumothorax and pneumoperitoneum are also present.

pleura, mediastinum, or pericardium. When the air is trapped in the interstitium of the lung, the radiograph may show bubbles of air in the lung that may be unilateral or bilateral, localized or diffuse. The lenticular chaotic pattern of interstitial air helps to differentiate PIE from the air bronchograms characteristic of respiratory distress syndrome and pneumonia. The diffuse air bubbles in the interstitium (Fig. 12–10) (Swischuk, 1970), some localized in dilated lymphatics, stiffen the lungs and make ventilation more difficult. Pneumomediastinum or pneumothorax usually follows. Localized air collections can be small, ovoid, or round and are sometimes referred to as pseudocysts (Clark and Edwards, 1979). These may decompress with pneumothorax or pneumomediastinum or just spontaneously disappear, usually in three to 18 days (Fig. 12–11). Areas of PIE can coalesce with the emergence of larger extra-alveolar interstitial collections (Fig. 12–12). With the emergence of a check valve mechanism because of damaged lung tissue, the localized interstitial emphysema can continue to increase in size. Sometimes the abnormal emphysematous region is of such magnitude that it compresses ipsilateral and contralateral normal portions of the lungs and leads to worsening respiratory distress (Magilner et al., 1974). After conservative therapy, perhaps with selective bronchial intubation, emphysematous areas may have to be decompressed by a chest tube (Brooks et al., 1977) or removed by surgical means (Bauer et al., 1978). Lung perfusion scanning has been reported to aid in the selection of patients for surgical intervention (Leonidas et al., 1978). A large perfusion defect in areas of emphysema is suggestive of a lung with permanent dysfunction.

Pneumomediastinum

The pneumomediastinum, usually of no clinical significance per se, may be the first indicator of barotrauma. It is characteristically recognized in the superior mediastinum by its uplifting of the lobes of the thymus gland, producing the "spinnaker sail sign" (Fig. 12–13). Mediastinal air can dissect under tension to deep cervical regions, subcutaneous tissues, and extraperitoneal spaces. A crescentic epiphrenic collection of air that outlines the muscle bundles of the diaphragm is either extrapleural or extraperitoneal (Christensen and Landay, 1980). It is important to distinguish between subpulmonic pneumothorax needing pleural drainage and pneumoperitoneum possibly secondary to a ruptured viscus. Extraperitoneal air remains quite fixed on decubitus films, whereas intraperitoneal or intrapleural air moves. Mediastinal air may dissect in linear streaks along the descending aorta to the extraperitoneum and peritoneum (Fig. 12–14). The inferior pulmonary ligament, a double layer of visceral pleura extending from the hilum to the diaphragm and anchoring the lung, is a potential space. Mediastinal air may dissect into the inferior pulmonary ligament and appear as an oval-to-triangular infrahilar lucency (Fig. 12–15) (Volberg et al., 1979).

Pneumothorax

The incidence of pneumothorax may be as high as 33 per cent in patients receiving mechanical ventilatory assistance and PEEP for treatment of HMD (Ogata et al., 1976). The commonly recognized pneumothorax in the supine neonate is lateral in position. In the supine neonate, air most commonly accumulates in the lateral pleural space. However, in approximately 75 per cent of cases, air may be seen medial to the lung (Mandell and Chawla, 1981). The appearance of the medial pneumothorax is well described by Moskowitz and Griscom (1976). In the supine neonate it rises anterior to the stationary lung, which is anchored by pulmonary vessels and the pulmonary ligament. The pleural air causes a hyperlucent hemithorax (Fig. 12–16). With further accumulation, the air in the pleural space may cross the midline in the upper or lower portions of the mediastinum (Fig. 12–17) (Fletcher, 1978). Anterior pneumothoraces may be under tension and require immediate insertion of a pleural chest tube to relieve dyspnea. A posterolaterally positioned chest tube may not relieve the pneumothorax. Anterior placement of chest tubes in the herniated pleural space (Fig. 12–18) has been demonstrated by Mandell and Chawla (1981) to clear the pneumothorax rapidly, usually within one half-hour of insertion. Subsequently the chest tube can be withdrawn more proximally.

Pneumopericardium

The pneumopericardium usually occurs in preterm infants with respiratory distress syndrome. The collection of air in the pericardial cavity can be sufficient to compromise the pulmonary venous return to the heart and cause cardiac tamponade. With tension pneumopericardium there is abrupt onset of bradycardia, hypotension, and cyanosis. Radiographically a lucent halo surrounds the heart (Fig. 12–19).

Text continued on page 282

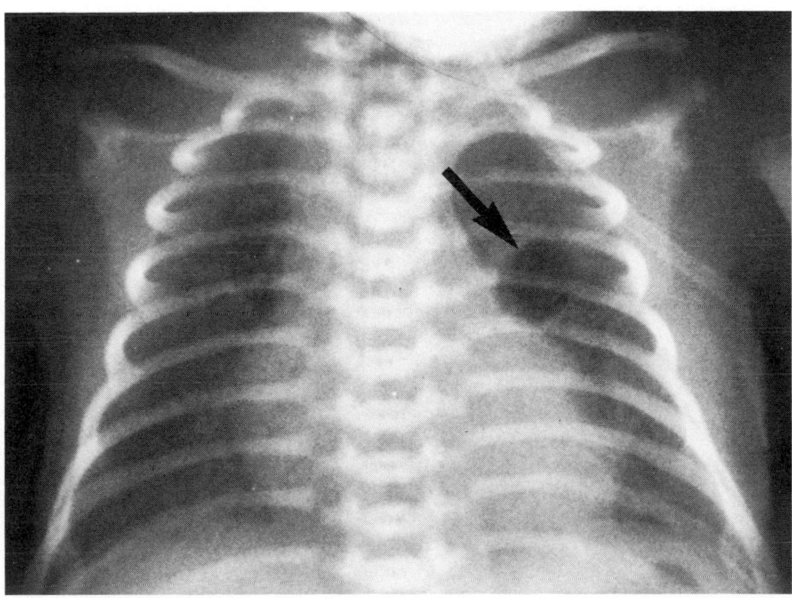

Figure 12–11. In the left upper lung is a small pseudocyst, a localized interstitial extra-alveolar collection (*arrow*).

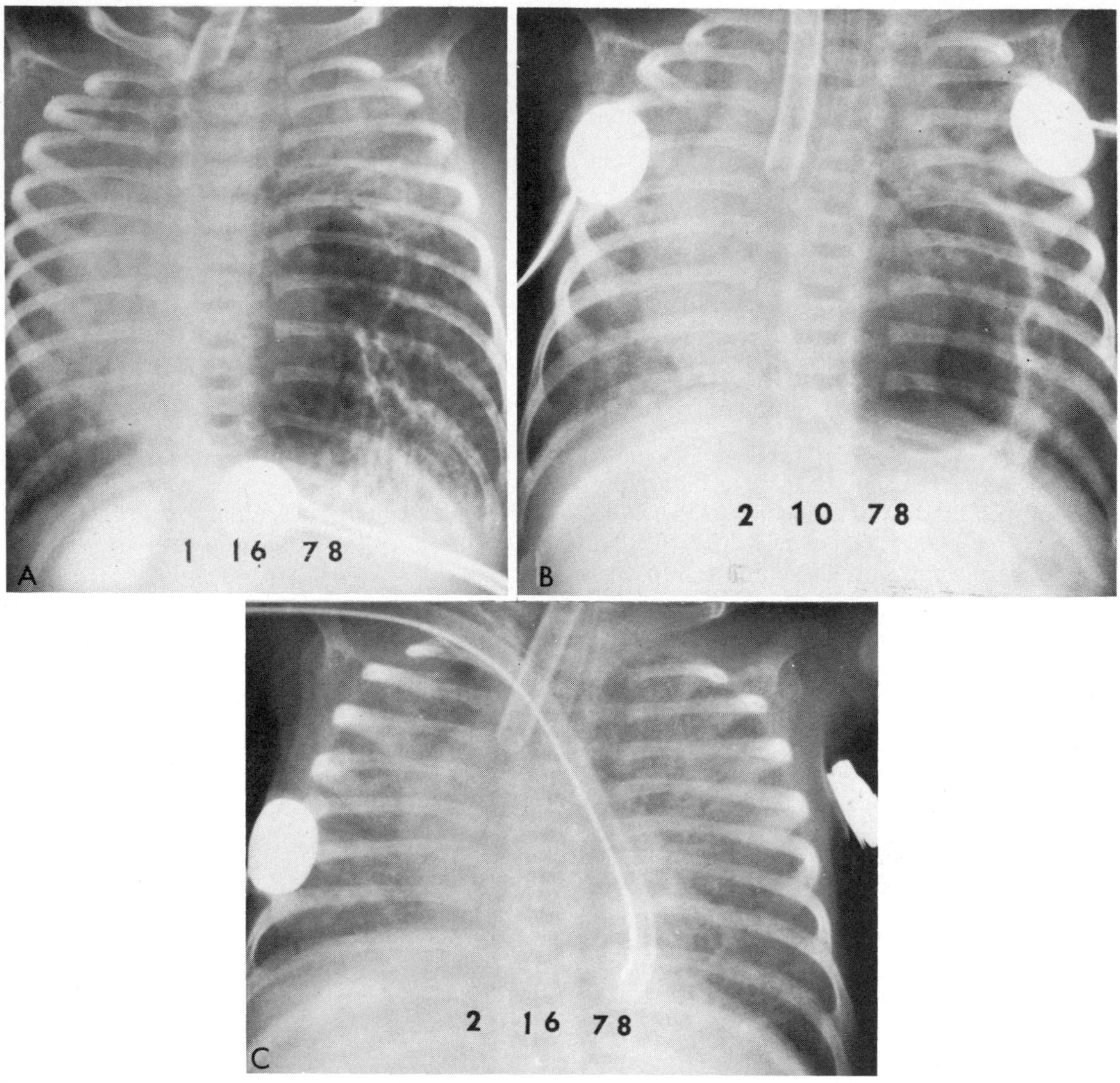

Figure 12–12. *A*, Stage 3 BPD with diffuse interstitial emphysema and a large cyst lateral to the hilum. *B*, Over the next three weeks the cyst enlarged. *C*, Subsequently, a chest tube was inserted to drain the cyst. (Courtesy of A. E. O'Hara, M.D., Philadelphia, PA)

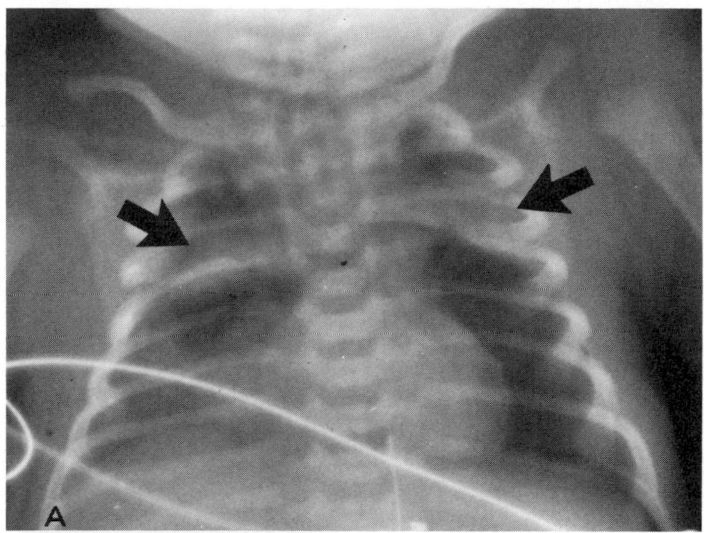

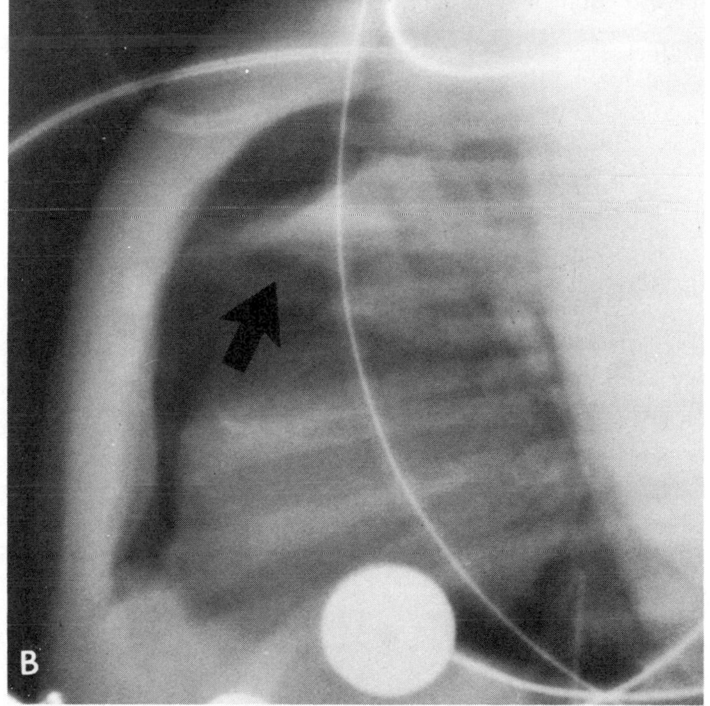

Figure 12–13. Thymic lobes uplifted by anterior pneumomediastinum on AP (*A*) and lateral (*B*) views, so-called "spinnaker sails" (*arrows*).

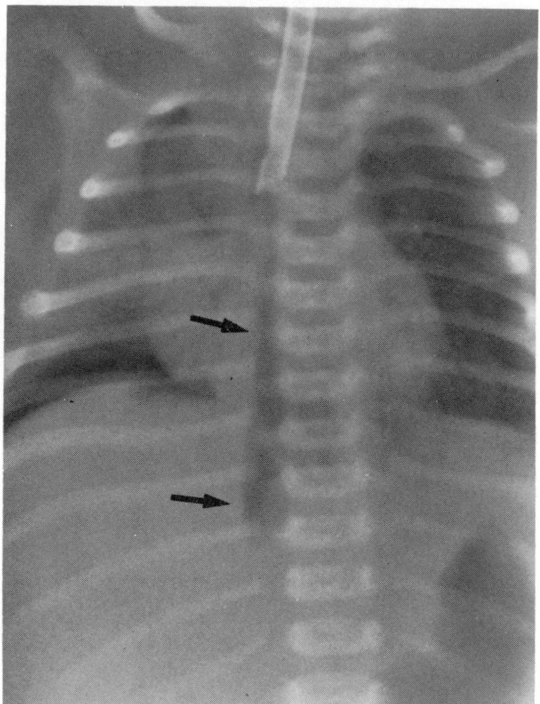

Figure 12–14. A linear streak of air dissecting from the mediastinum toward the peritoneum (*arrows*).

Differentiation from pneumomediastinum is usually made by visualization of the halo continuous below the inferior cardiac surface. If the location of the extra-alveolar air is in question, a lateral decubitus projection will move the air to the nondependent side in the freely communicating pericardial cavity. Mediastinal air does not mobilize readily. In cardiac tamponade the heart size becomes markedly reduced secondary to the diminished blood return (Higgins et al., 1979). Mortality from untreated neonatal pneumopericardium is 86 per cent (Lawson et al., 1980), and rapid needle aspiration of the pericardium is necessary to prevent sudden death. Smaller collections of pericardial air may be treated conservatively. If symptoms recur after pericardiocentesis, a catheter may be required to drain the pericardial cavity. As reported by Brans et al., (1976), patients with pneumopericardium treated by pericardiocentesis had a 79 per cent survival; those treated conservatively had a 32 per cent survival.

Pneumoperitoneum

Mechanical ventilators may drive mediastinal air along vascular sheaths across the diaphragm, with a resultant pneumoperitoneum (Campbell et al., 1975). The classic pneumoperitoneum consists of a "football sign" (Fig. 12–20), distended flanks, and the ligamentum teres outlined by the free peritoneal air. It is of utmost importance to differentiate between ventilator-induced pneumoperitoneum and enteric perforation. Cross-table supine lateral views are sometimes helpful. If a large air fluid level is seen, this implies peritonitis secondary to bowel perforation. Pneumoperitoneum secondary to mediastinal dissection, however, lacks a fluid component. Nonetheless, the absence of a fluid level does not exclude the possibility of a perforated viscus: Kaufman et al. (1976) found that only 43 per cent of neonatal gastrointestinal perforations had a demonstrable air fluid level. If the amount of intraperitoneal air is small, even a large amount of peritoneal fluid will not be easily detected.

Neonatal gastric ulcerations and perforations, usually secondary to anoxia or stress, result in the largest intraperitoneal air collections from enteric sources (James et al., 1976; Lloyd, 1969). A large pneumoperitoneum, absence of gastric air, and (usually) absence of ventilator support help to confirm the diagnosis of gastric perforation. A nasogastric tube extending beyond the contour of the stomach is definite evidence of perforation (Coopersmith and Rabinowitz, 1973). The other major cause of peritonitis in the neonate is necrotizing enterocolitis, with perforations usually occurring in the distal ileum or proximal colon. Pneumatosis intestinalis, bowel distention, and portal venous air are clues to the diagnosis of necrotizing enterocolitis (Fig. 12–21) (Daneman et al., 1978). Prematurity, anoxia, PDA, and umbilical catheterization are some of the factors predisposing the infant to this ischemic bowel disease.

When there is a large pneumoperitoneum and a pneumomediastinum in an infant with ventilator-assisted peak inspiration of over 30 cm H_2O, the lung is usually the source of the abdominal air (Knight and Abdenour, 1981). If a ventilated infant has less than 28 cm H_2O peak inspiratory pressure, gastric perforation should be excluded with an aqueous contrast agent instilled via the feeding tube (Fig. 12–20). Usually there is no time to study the entire GI tract, and laparotomy is performed. Paracentesis can be done to measure the oxygen concentration in the peritoneal gas and to sample any intra-abdominal fluid present.

Systemic Air Embolism

Systemic intravascular air embolism secondary to respirator therapy, a rare occurrence,

Text continued on page 288

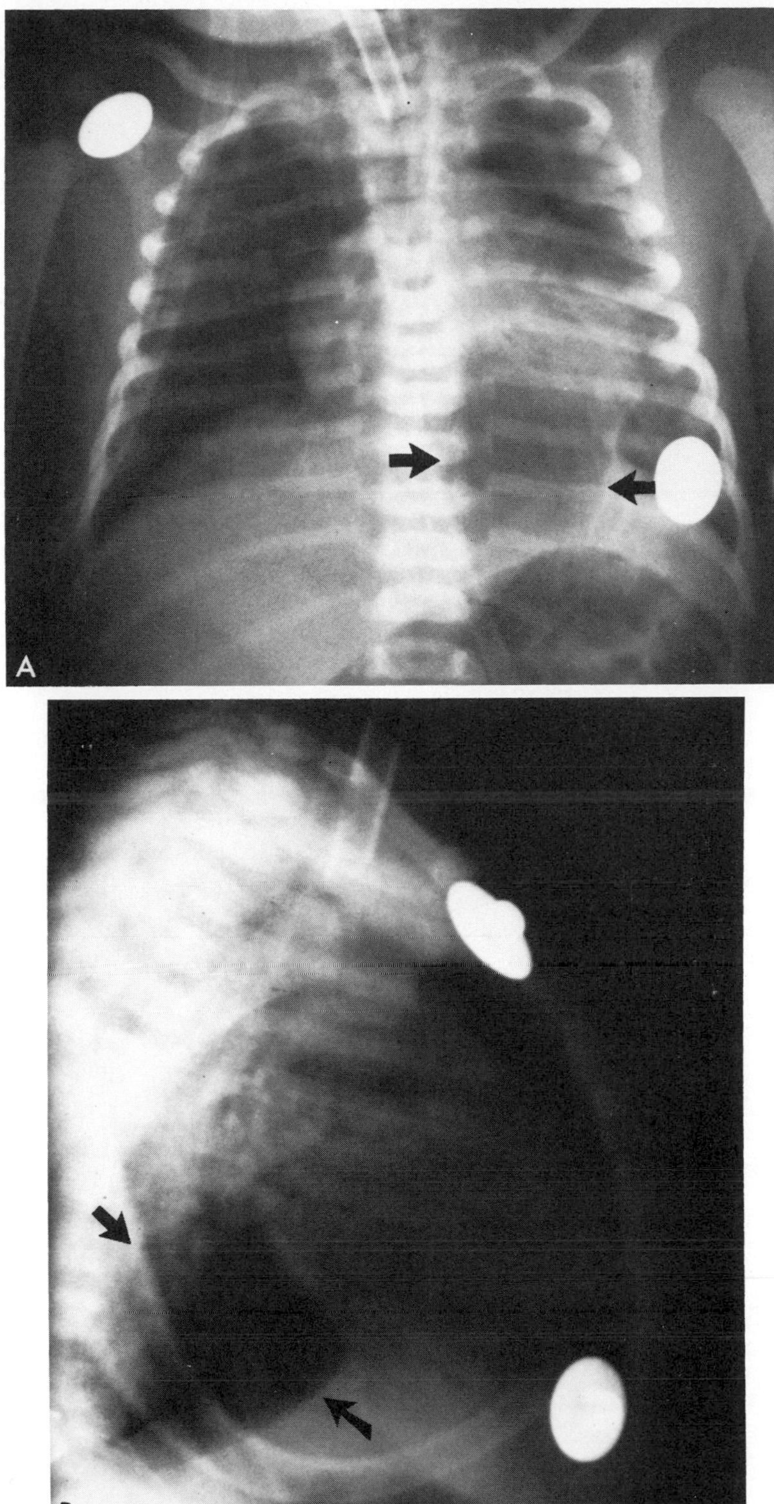

Figure 12–15. A large medial inferior collection of air in the left pulmonary ligament on the AP view (*A*) (*arrows*) and posteriorly placed on the lateral view (*B*) (*arrows*).

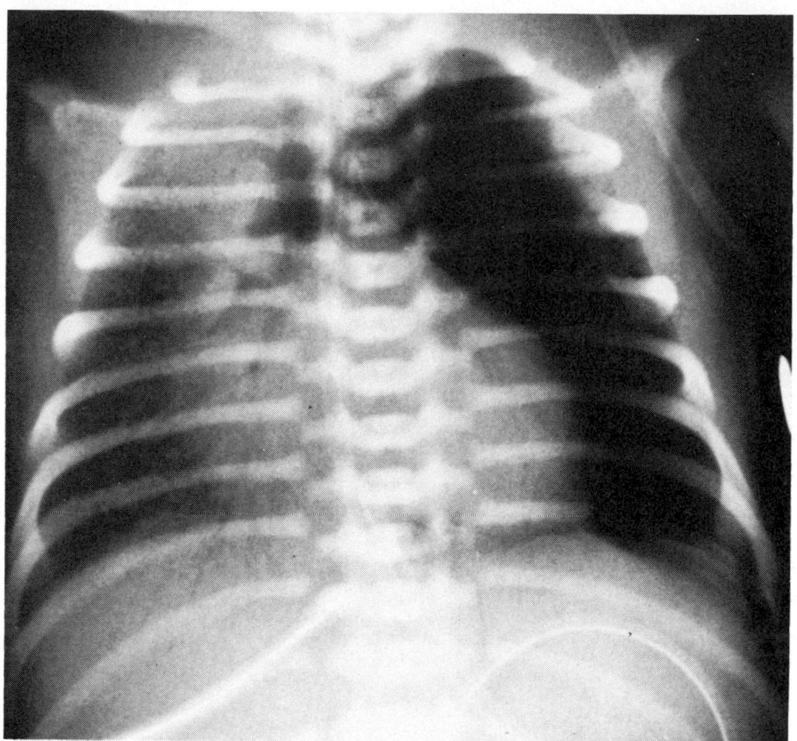

Figure 12–16. Hyperlucent left hemithorax secondary to air accumulating in the pleural space anterior to the lung.

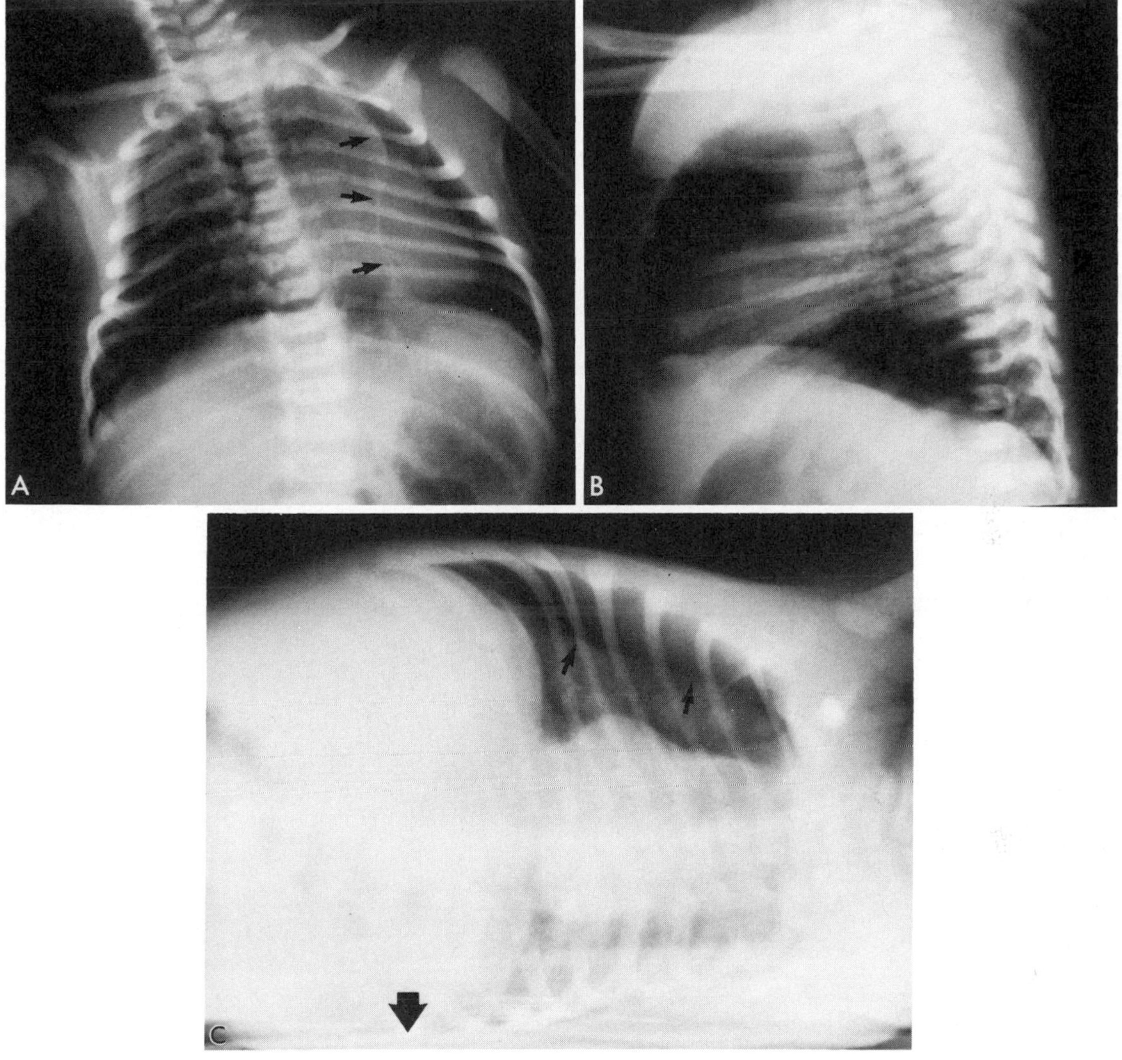

Figure 12–17. *A*, on the AP view the pleural space distended with air has herniated from right to left, in a retrosternal potential location (*arrows*). *B*, The lateral view shows the hyperlucent retrosternal space. *C*, The left lateral decubitus demonstrates that the air in the freely communicating pleural space moves from medial to lateral (*arrows*).

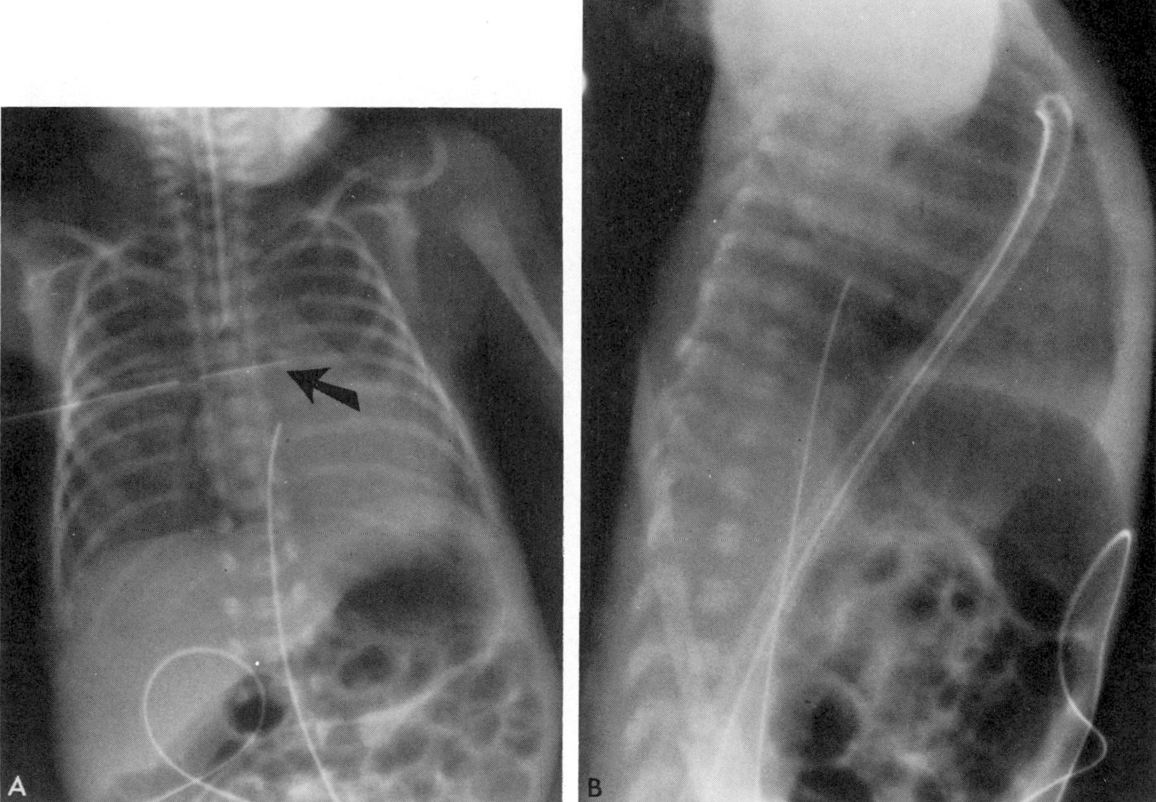

Figure 12–18. *A*, A medially herniated chest tube (*arrow*) on an AP view of the chest. *B*, The retrosternal location is confirmed on the lateral view.

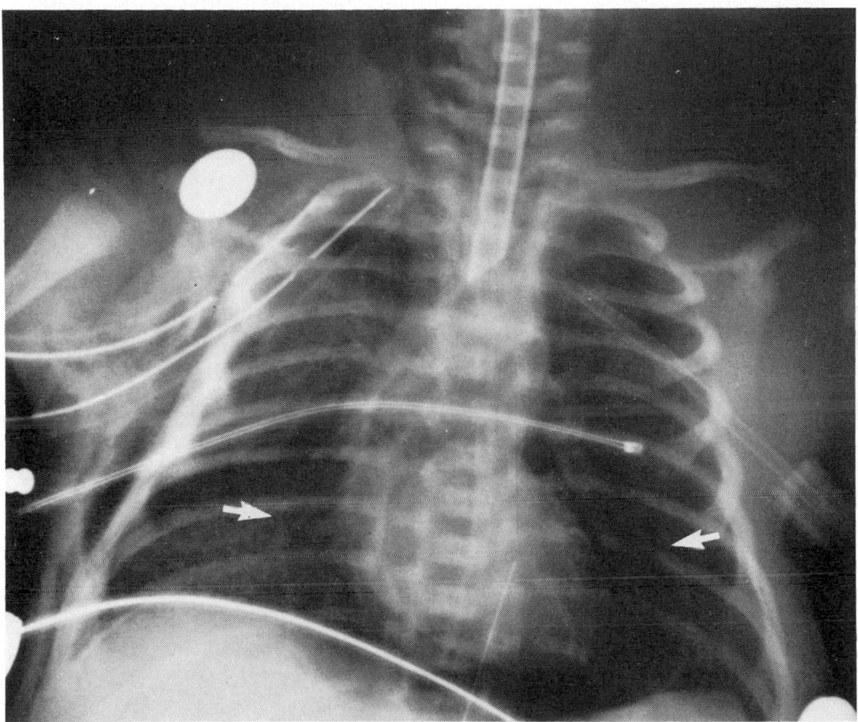

Figure 12–19. A halo of lucency representing pneumopericardium outlines a small heart and thin pericardium (*arrows*). The small heart is indicative of cardiac tamponade. Of note is the cervical and right lateral wall emphysema.

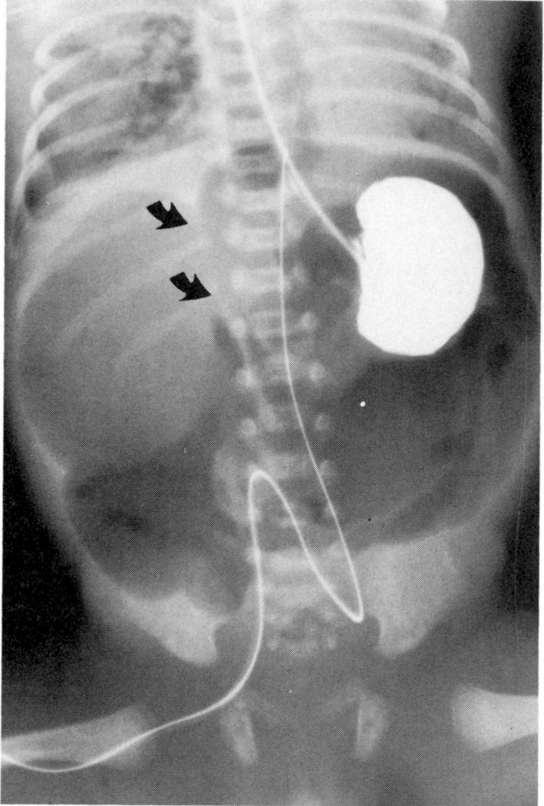

Figure 12–20. "Football sign" with large pneumoperitoneum. The ligamentum teres (*arrows*) is outlined by air. Water-soluble contrast material in the stomach shows no evidence of gastric perforation.

is incompatible with life. Air in the vascular system most likely results from formation of either alveolar-capillary or bronchovenous fistulas following alveolar rupture. When the intra-alveolar pressure exceeds the left atrial pressure, air enters the pulmonary veins and travels to the heart and then into the systemic circulation. The radiologic diagnosis is made by visualization of air within the systemic vascular circulation (Fig. 12–22). Air is simultaneously present in both arterial and venous circulations. Intracardiac air is a consistent finding. The air can also be seen in the cerebral ventricles, apparently having crossed the blood-brain barrier. Only one infant has been reported to have survived this insult (Oppermann et al., 1979).

COMPLICATIONS OF TUBES AND CATHETERS

Life support in intensive care units (ICUs) frequently involves the use of endotracheal tubes, intravascular catheters, pleural drainage tubes, and feeding tubes. Malposition of these tubes can be readily detected by radiography. Improper placement of these conduits can lead to rapid deterioration of the neonate.

Endotracheal Tube Position

The polyvinylchloride orotracheal tube is usually identified by a radiopaque lead line at its tip. The tip should be located between the first thoracic vertebra and the carina. Adequate securing of the tube at the mouth with adhesive tape prevents proximal movement. A cadaver study (Donn and Kuhns, 1980) noted movement of the tube on flexion, extension, and rotation of the head. Most of the head and neck motion occurs primarily at the level of the first four cervical vertebrae. The tube tip moves caudad with flexion and cephalad with extension on the radiographs for endotracheal tube placement.

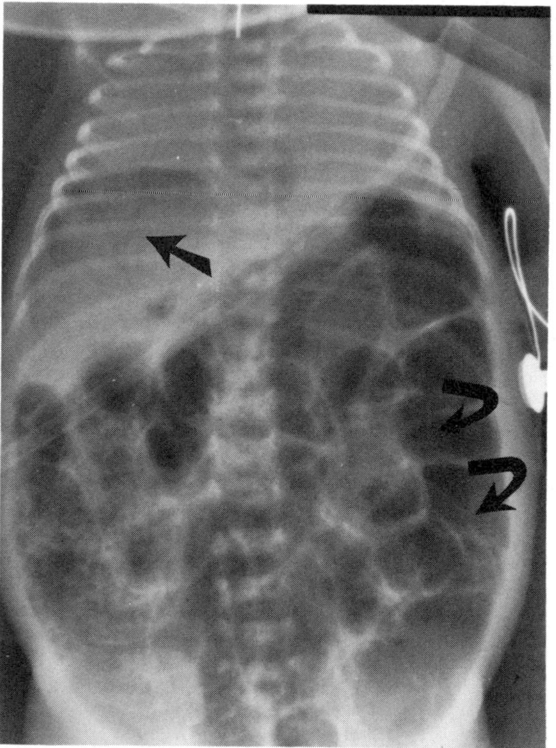

Figure 12–21. Abdominal radiograph with branching lucent shadows in the hepatic region (*arrow*); distended loops of bowel with a bubbly, streaky pattern of pneumatosis intestinalis on the right side of the abdomen; and evidence of free air, sharply defined serosal surface of loops of bowel (*curved arrows*).

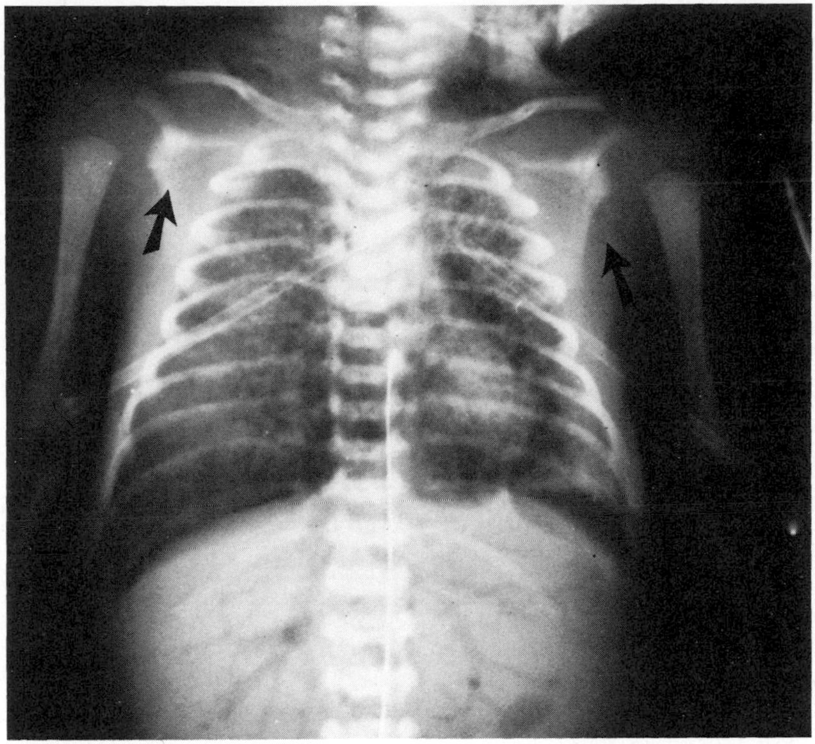

Figure 12–22. Evidence of systemic air embolism with air in the hepatic, splenic, and brachial vessels (*arrows*) and in the heart.

Therefore, when assessing tube position on the radiograph, the position of the head and neck should also be evaluated. (Todres et al., 1976).

Most endotracheal tube mishaps are due to placement in the larynx or right bronchus (Fig. 12–23*A*,*B*). Occasionally the esophagus or stomach is intubated, reducing the aeration of the lungs (Fig. 12–23*C*).

Endotracheal Tube Complications

Complications of intubation include perforation of the pharynx, usually the posterior pharyngeal wall or piriform sinuses (Fig. 12–24) (Clarke et al., 1980). Immediate problems include cervical emphysema, pneumomediastinum, and pneumothorax. These usually heal spontaneously after seven to ten days. Rarely, vigorous intubations can result in tracheal perforation, an often lethal occurrence (Serlin and Daily, 1975). Suctioning catheters introduced through the endotracheal tube can be threaded too far, rupturing a bronchus and causing a pneumothorax. This usually occurs on the right, because the right bronchus is in more direct continuity with the trachea (Fig. 12–25). The therapeutic results are variable (Anderson and Chandra, 1976). In some infants with conservative pleural tube drainage, these lesions heal in a few weeks. Others require surgery to close the bronchopleural fistula.

Complications of traumatic or prolonged intubation in the neonate can result in subglottic granulomas and membranes or cartilaginous stenoses. Some stenoses have been reported after as little as 72 hours' intubation (Holinger et al., 1976). Other factors influencing formation of a postintubation tracheal narrowing are the size of the tube in relation to the size of the lumen of the airway, the number of tube changes, the tube material (rubber or plastic), and the type of sterilization (gas or chemical). Acquired subglottic stenoses are becoming more common with the aggressive use of PEEP and endotracheal intubation in the neonate. In Holinger's series of subglottic stenoses, approximately one third were acquired and 86 per cent of these were from endotracheal intubations. The acquired lesions were usually more severe than their congenital counterparts. Circumferential subglottic stenosis with a concomitant glottic web or stenosis was the most common endoscopic finding (Fig. 12–26) (Holinger et al., 1976). Tracheotomies have been utilized in a large percentage of acquired subglottic

Text continued on page 292

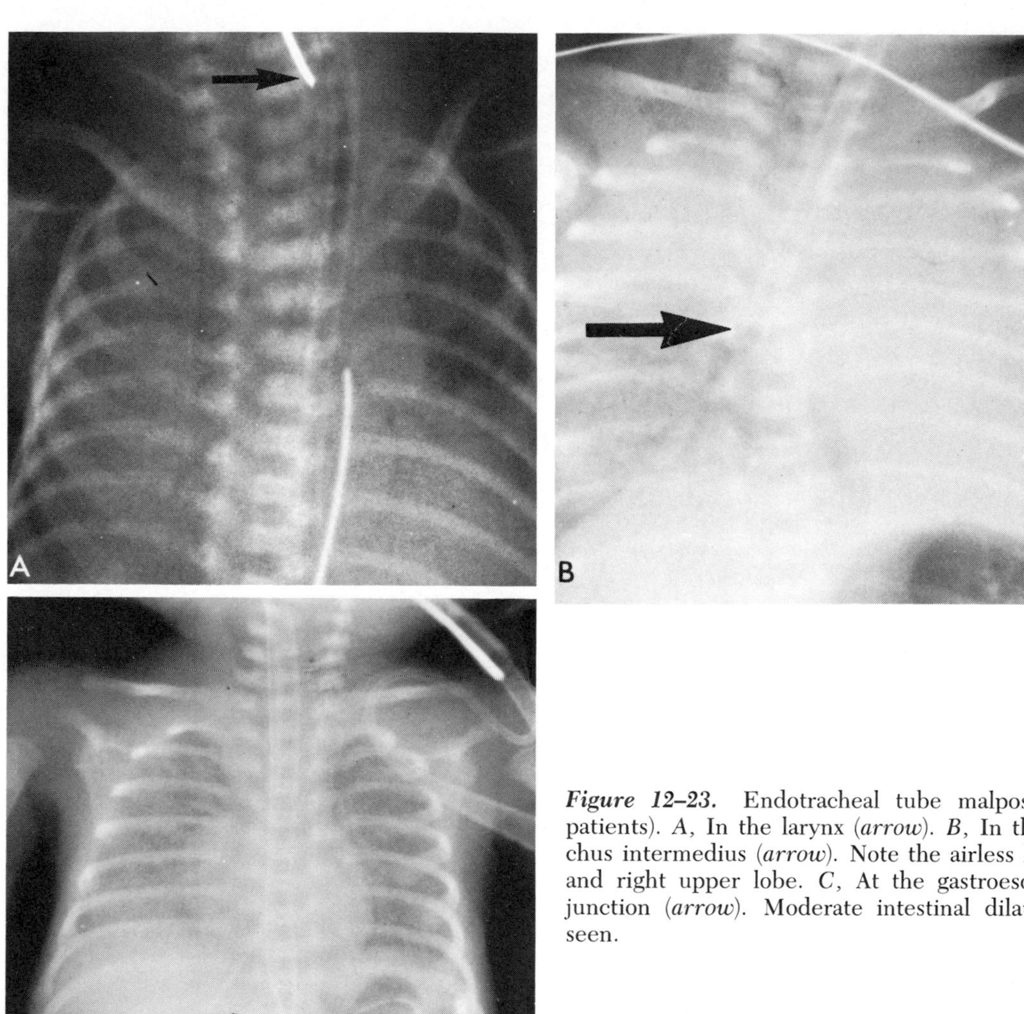

Figure 12–23. Endotracheal tube malposition (3 patients). *A*, In the larynx (*arrow*). *B*, In the bronchus intermedius (*arrow*). Note the airless left lung and right upper lobe. *C*, At the gastroesophageal junction (*arrow*). Moderate intestinal dilatation is seen.

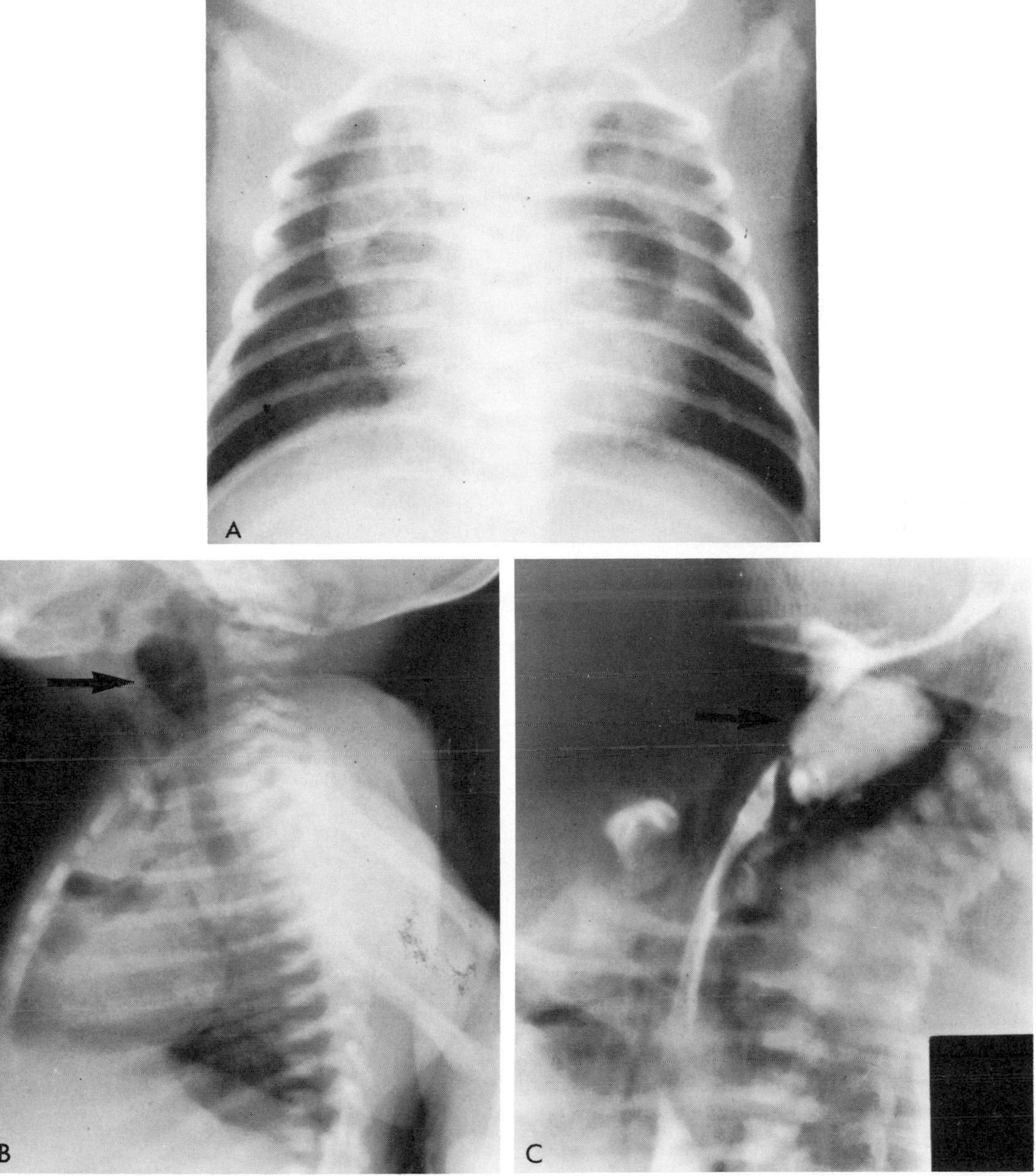

Figure 12–24. *A*, AP view of the chest demonstrates pneumomediastinum from endotracheal tube perforation of the pharynx. *B*, On the lateral view, air is visible in the retropharyngeal and mediastinal spaces, and a large air collection is seen in the neck (*arrow*). *C*, Lateral view with dilute barium solution showing pseudodiverticulum (*arrow*).

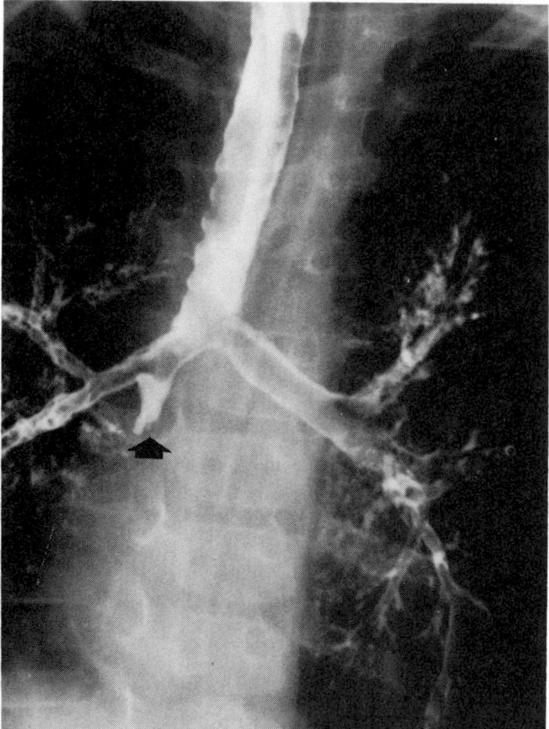

Figure 12–25. Bronchogram shows a ruptured bronchus from excessive suctioning through an endotracheal tube (*arrow*). (Courtesy of Marie Capitanio, M.D., St. Christopher's Hospital for Children, Philadelphia, PA.)

stenoses as a temporizing procedure pending adequate growth of the airway.

Feeding Catheters

Feeding catheters in neonates are usually threaded through the mouth and ultimately land in either the stomach, duodenum, or jejunum, depending on their proposed functions. These polyvinyl tubes are frequently malpositioned in the pharynx or esophagus and can result in traumatic perforation of either, with concurrent pneumomediastinum, cervical emphysema, and pneumothorax. The perforation is usually on the right because the esophagus in the posterior mediastinum contacts the right parietal pleura just below the bifurcation of the trachea (Kassner et al., 1977). Clark et al. (1980) proposed that the rightward deviation and inadequate extramural support of the esophagus on the right predisposed the infant to perforation of the right wall of the esophagus. Most pharyngeal perforations occur on the posterior wall or piriform sinus. Traumatic pharyngeal and cervical esophageal pseudodiverticulum can mimic esophageal atresia and fistula (Lynch et al., 1974). Differentiation can sometimes be made by the associated extra-alveolar collection of air, the absence of a posterior impression on the trachea, and an increased distance between the trachea and esophagus (Lucaya et al., 1979).

The most common indication of perforation is difficulty in passing a feeding tube. The most common symptoms are respiratory distress, excessive salivation, choking, coughing, stridor, and increased oral secretions. There is usually a delay in diagnosis because the radiographic signs and clinical symptoms are not recognized. The false passage sometimes may be submucosal or retroesophageal. It can be localized to the neck or occasionally may extend below the diaphragm into the retroperitoneal space (Fig. 12–27). A small amount of water-soluble contrast material injected via the tube can identify the location of the perforation. Surgery is not usually required once the tube has been repositioned in the esophagus, and the patient placed on antibiotics and maintained on intravenous hyperalimentation for ten days. A repeat contrast material examination should be performed after ten days to two weeks. Occasionally the patient may develop a post-traumatic abscess

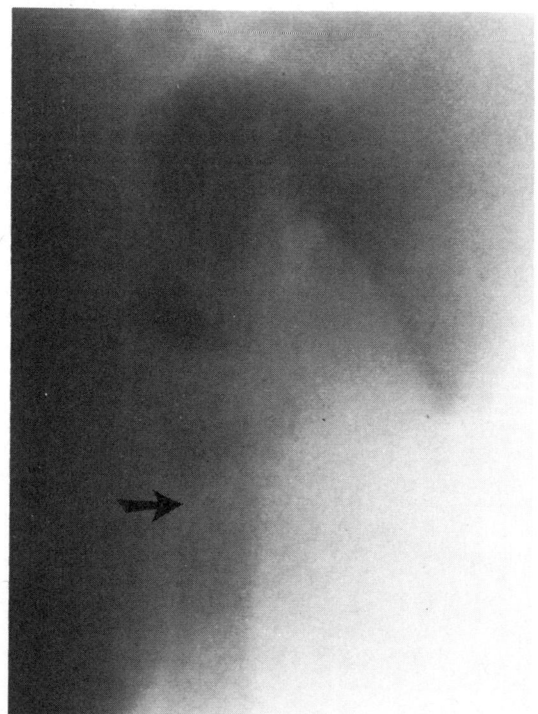

Figure 12–26. Lateral view of upper airway showing circumferential web (*arrow*) below the cords.

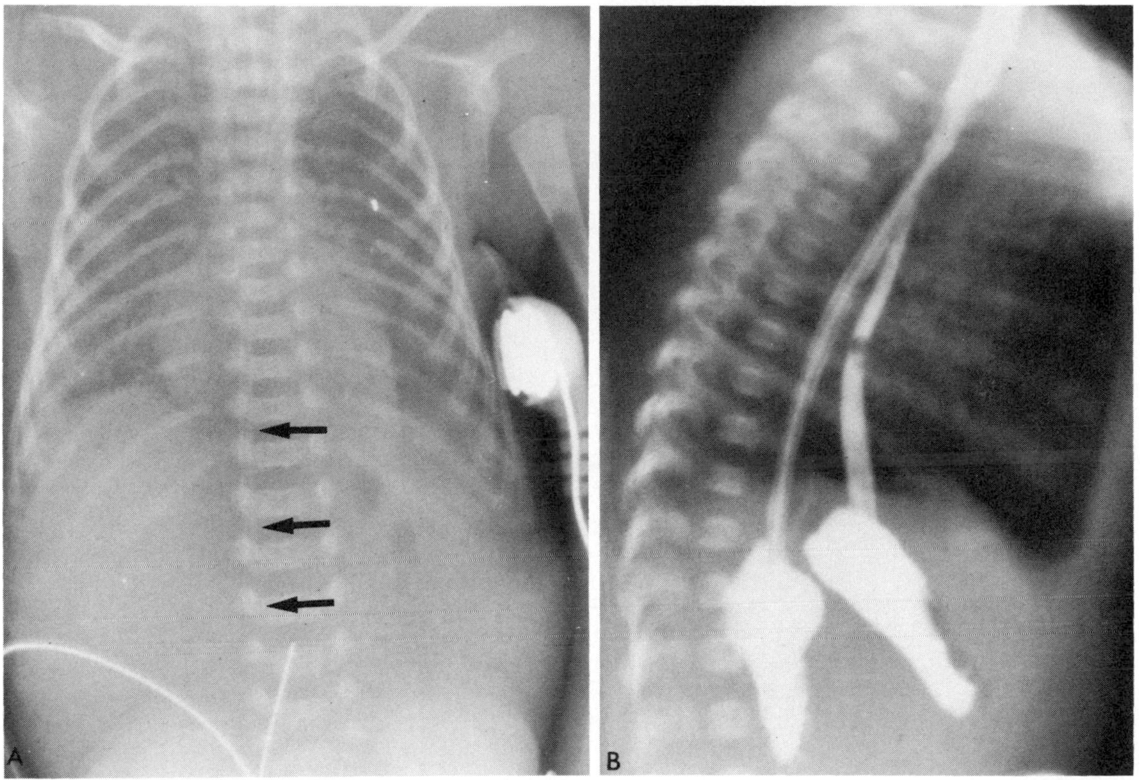

Figure 12–27. *A*, AP view showing feeding catheter (*arrows*) with a straight atypical course below the diaphragm. *B*, Lateral view with aqueous contrast material placed through the feeding tube shows the retroperitoneal catheter. Contrast material is also seen anteriorly in the stomach and esophagus.

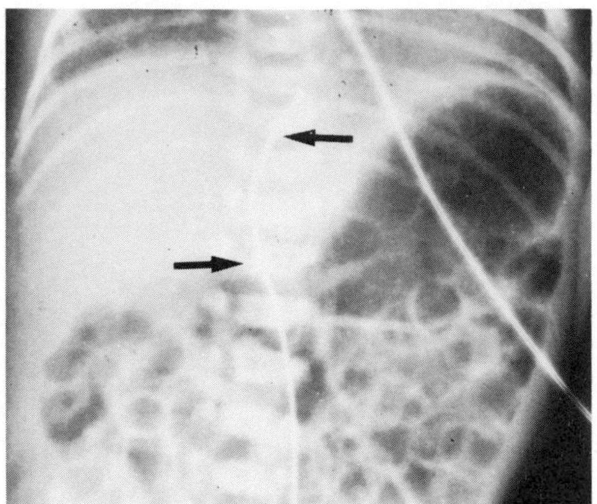

Figure 12–28. Shallow reverse "S" configuration of the umbilical venous line through the ductus venosus to the inferior vena cava (*arrows*).

that has to be surgically drained. Included in the differential diagnosis are spontaneous esophageal rupture, esophageal tracheal fistula with or without atresia, and congenital diverticula.

Transpyloric polyvinyl tubes are used for feeding low-birth-weight infants in the intensive care nursery, to prevent aspiration pneumonitis and avoid the need for parenteral alimentation (Pereira and Lemons, 1981). Merten et al. (1980) reported five infants with perforation of the duodenum from this procedure. Altered radiographic configuration of the tube in the region of the superior or inferior flexure, associated with clinical deterioration, pneumoperitoneum, peritonitis, or a retroperitoneal fistula, is diagnostic of duodenal perforation. Tubes should be positioned beyond the inferior flexure in the distal duodenum, avoiding the fixed portions of duodenum and consequent possible perforation (Siegle et al., 1976).

Pleural Drainage Tubes

Pleural drainage tubes are usually placed to relieve a respirator-induced tension pneumothorax. The most frequent complication is lung perforation. A review of autopsies of newborn infants (Moessinger et al., 1978) showed that 25 per cent of percutaneous pleural drainages for relief of a pneumothorax have perforated the lung. The clinical diagnosis of lung perforation is extremely difficult. Recovery of blood from the tracheostomy tube or the persistence of a large air leak suggest the diagnosis.

Umbilical Catheters

Umbilical intravascular catheters are routinely used for exchange transfusions, monitoring of blood gases, hyperalimentation, and pressure estimation, and as a source of blood samples. Nos. 3.5 to 5 French radiopaque polyvinyl catheters with end-holes to prevent clot formation are used for umbilical catheterization. The vessels usually remain patent for the first four days of life, but in hypoxic infants they may remain patent for longer. Fluoroscopy or anteroposterior and lateral radiographs should be used to verify proper catheter position (Baker et al., 1969).

The umbilical venous line is seldom utilized because of the risk of hepatic fibrosis, portal hypertension, and portal vein thromboembolism. The tip of the umbilical venous line should be positioned in the inferior vena cava near the right atrium after traversing a mild reverse "S" through the ductus venosus (Fig. 12–28). Liver necrosis and clot formation can result from improper positioning and infusion of hypertonic solutions and bicarbonate into the hepatic bed. Ultimately, hepatic calcifications may form (Ablow and Effman, 1972). Perforation and hemorrhage can also occur with umbilical vein catheterization (Fig. 12–29) (Kanto and Parrish, 1977). Intracardiac catheters may produce cardiac arrhythmias, damage the cardiac valves, cause endocarditis, and perforate the myocardium (Fig. 12–30) (Symchych et al., 1977). Other less frequent complications include pulmonary emboli, infection, and colonic perforation following exchange transfusions (Sommerschild, 1971). Scott (1965) reported a 20 per

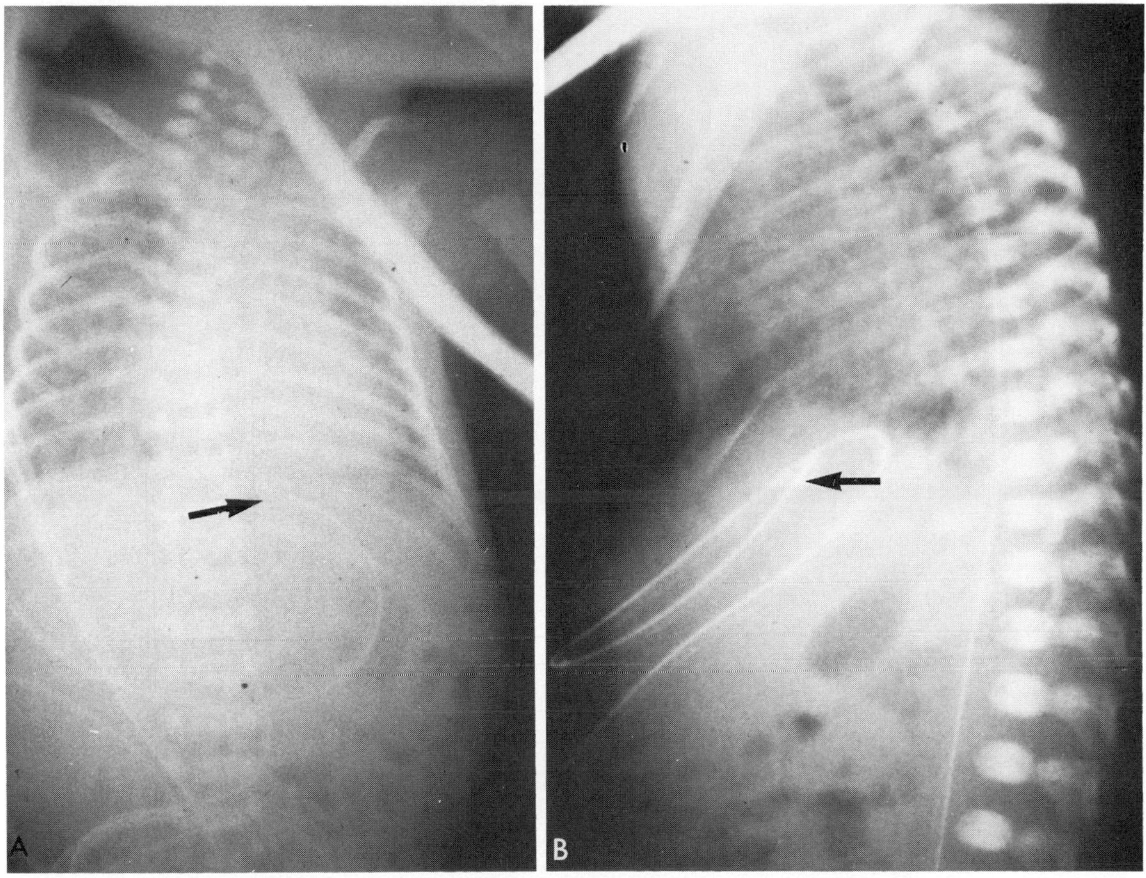

Figure 12–29 AP (*A*) and lateral (*B*) views of the umbilical venous line in abnormal course, probably in the peritoneal cavity (*arrow*).

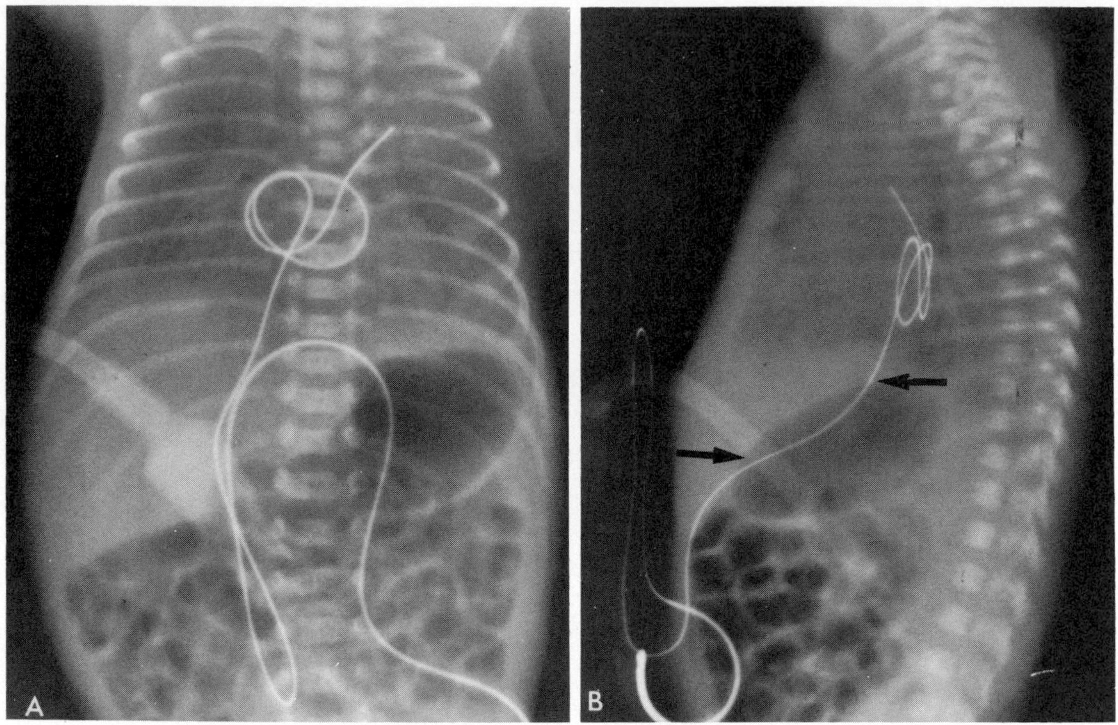

Figure 12–30. A coiled umbilical venous line in the left atrium, ending in the left superior pulmonary vein on AP (*A*) and lateral (*B*) views. A shallow "S" configuration coursing through the liver is seen on the lateral view (*arrows*). The venous line traveled through the right atrium and foramen ovale to get to the left atrium and left pulmonary vein.

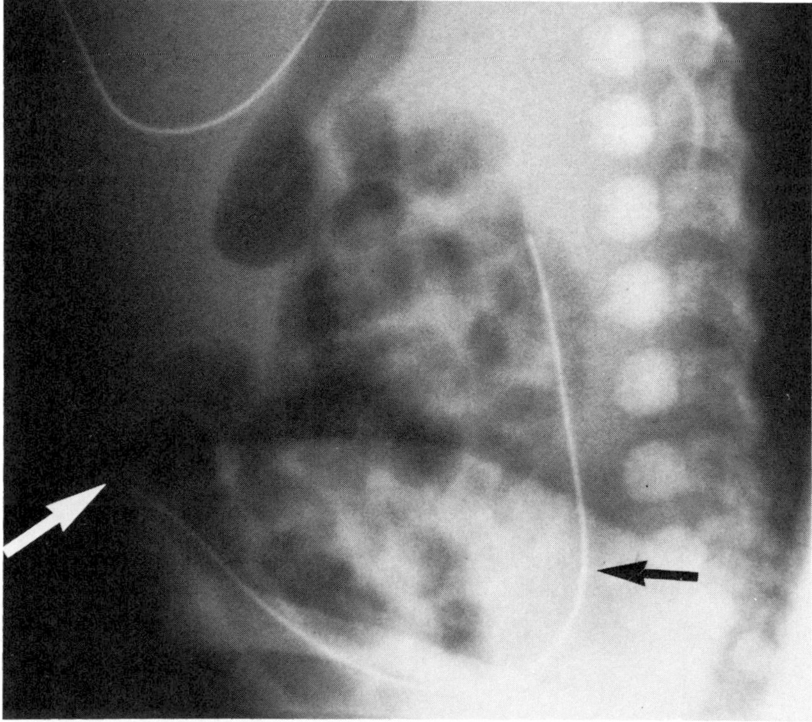

Figure 12–31. Lateral view depicting the umbilical artery catheter going from anterior (umbilicus) (*white arrow*) via the umbilical artery through the hypogastric-iliac artery complex to the aorta (*black arrow*). The tip of the catheter is placed too high.

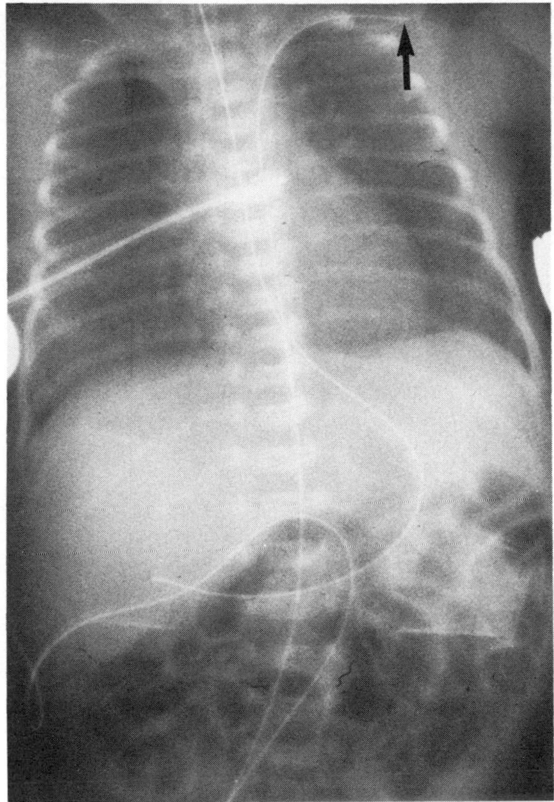

Figure 12–32. An umbilical artery line malpositioned in the left subclavian artery (*arrow*).

cent overall incidence of complications with the use of venous catheterization.

Umbilical arterial catheters ideally should be positioned between the upper vertebral plate of L3 and the lower plate of L4, avoiding the origins of the major abdominal arteries and the bifurcation of the aorta (Fig. 12–31). The catheter loops through the hypogastric-internal iliac arteries to reach the abdominal aorta. The alternative position is the sixth and seventh thoracic vertebral level in the descending aorta. The longer tubing probably increases the propensity toward thromboembolism. One should carefully avoid placing arterial lines in the left common carotid artery, innominate artery, external iliac artery, femoral artery, or pulmonary artery via the ductus arteriosus (Fig. 12–32). Thrombotic complications following umbilical artery catheterization ranged from 3.5 per cent (Gupta et al., 1968) and 16 per cent (Cochran et al., 1968) in clinical series. In an autopsy series, Goetzman et al. (1974) found thrombotic complications in 24 per cent of their patients. Although angiography shows an even higher incidence (Williams et al., 1972), most of the arteriographically demonstrated lesions are without clinical manifestations. Thromboses of the aorta and iliac, renal, celiac, splenic, and pulmonary arteries have been reported. Other complications of umbilical arterial catheterization include perforation of vessels with or without massive bleeding, peritoneal cavity perforation (Miller et al., 1979), umbilical arteriovenous fistulas, false aneurysms of the aorta (Spangler et al., 1977), infection and thromboembolic disease such as renal artery thrombosis with hypertension (Merten et al., 1978), gangrene of the buttock, spinal cord damage with paraplegia (Aziz and Robertson, 1973), and complete obstruction of the aorta.

REFERENCES

Ablow, R. C., Driscoll, S. G., Effman, E. L., et al.: Comparison of early onset group-B streptococcal neonatal infection and the respiratory distress syndrome of the newborn. N. Engl. J. Med. 294:65, 1976.

Ablow, R. C., and Effman, E. L.: Hepatic calcifications associated with umbilical vein catheterization in the newborn infant. AJR 114:380, 1972.

Ablow, R. C., Gross, I., Effman, E. L., et al.: The radiographic features of early onset group-B streptococcal neonatal sepsis. Radiology 124:771, 1977.

Anderson, K. D., and Chandra, R.: Pneumothorax secondary to perforation of sequential bronchi by suction catheters. J. Pediatr. Surg. 11:687, 1976.

Aziz, E. M., and Robertson, A. F.: Paraplegia: a complication of umbilical arterial catheterization. J. Pediatr. 82:1051, 1973.

Baker, D. H., Berdon, W. E., and James, L. S.: Proper localization of umbilical arterial and venous catheters by lateral roentgenograms. Pediatrics 43:34, 1969.

Bauer, C. R., Brennan, M. J., Doyle, C., and Poole, C. A.: Surgical resection for pulmonary interstitial emphysema in the newborn infant. J. Pediatr. 93:656, 1978.

Bauer, C. R., Tsipuras, D., and Fletcher, B. D.: Syndrome of persistent pulmonary vascular obstruction of the newborn: roentgen findings. AJR 120:285, 1974.

Bomsel, F., Gouchard, M., Larroche, J. C., and Magder, L.: Radiologic diagnosis of massive pulmonary hemorrhage of the newborn. Ann. Radiol. 18:419, 1975.

Brans, Y. W., Pitts, M., and Cassady, G.: Neonatal pneumopericardium. Am. J. Dis. Child. 130:393, 1976.

Brooks, J. G., Bustamante, S. A., Koops, B. L., et al.: Selective bronchial intubation for the treatment of severe localized pulmonary interstitial emphysema in newborn infants. J. Pediatr. 91:648, 1977.

Campbell, R. E., Boggs, T. R., Jr., and Kirkpatrick, J. A., Jr.: Early neonatal pneumoperitoneum from progressive massive pneumomediastinum. Radiology 114:121, 1975.

Christensen, E. E., and Landay, M. J.: Visible muscle of the diaphragm: sign of extraperitoneal air. AJR 135:521, 1980.

Clarke, T. A., Coen, R. W., Feldman, B., and Papile, L.: Esophageal perforations in premature infants and comments on the diagnosis. Am. J. Dis. Child. 134:367, 1980.

Clarke, T. A., and Edwards, D. R.: Pulmonary pseudocysts in newborn infants with respiratory distress syndrome. AJR 133:417, 1979.

Cochran, W. D., Davis, H. T., and Smith, C. A.: Advantages and complications of umbilical artery catheterization in the newborn. Pediatrics 42:769, 1968.

Coopersmith, H., and Rabinowitz, J. G.: A specific sign for neonatal gastric perforation. J. Can. Assoc. Radiol. 24:141, 1973.

Daneman, A., Woodward, S., and deSilva, M.: The radiology of neonatal necrotizing enterocolitis (NEC). A review of 47 cases and the literature. Pediatr. Radiol. 7:70, 1978.

Donn, S. M., and Kuhns, L. R.: Mechanism of endotracheal tube movement with change of head position in the neonate. Pediatric Radiol. 9:37, 1980.

Edwards, D. K., Dyer, W. M., and Northway, W. H., Jr.: Twelve years' experience with bronchopulmonary dysplasia. Pediatrics 59:839, 1977.

Edwards, D. K., Higgins, C. B., Meritt, A., et al.: Radiographic and echocardiographic evaluation of newborns treated with indomethacin for patent ductus arteriosus. AJR 131:1009, 1978.

Ellis, K., and Nadelhaft, J.: Roentgenographic findings in hyaline membrane disease in infants weighing 2000 grams and over. AJR 78:444, 1957.

Fletcher, B. D.: Medial herniation of the parietal pleura: useful sign of pneumothorax in supine neonates. AJR 130:469, 1978.

Giedion, A., Hoefliger, H., and Dangel, P.: Acute pulmonary x-ray changes in hyaline membrane disease treated with artificial ventilation and positive end-expiratory pressure (PEEP). Pediatr. Radiol. 1:145, 1973.

Goetzman, B. W., Stadalnik, R. C., Bogren, H. G., et al.: Thrombotic complications of umbilical artery catheters: a clinical and radiographic study. Pediatrics 56:374, 1975.

Gooding, C. A., and Gregory, G. A.: Roentgenographic analysis of meconium aspiration of the newborn. Radiology 100:131, 1971.

Gooding, C. A., Gregory, G. A., Tabor, P., et al.: Clinical and experimental studies of meconium aspiration of the newborn. Ann. Radiol. 14:162, 1971.

Gupta, J. M., Robertson, N. R., and Wigglesworth, J. S.: Umbilical artery catheterization in the newborn. Arch Dis. Child. 43:382, 1968.

Higgins, C. B., Broderick, T. W., Edwards, D. K., and Shumaker, A.: The hemodynamic significance of massive pneumopericardium in preterm infants with respiratory distress syndrome. Radiology 133:363, 1979.

Hoffman, R. R., Jr., Campbell, R. E., and Decker, J. P.: Fetal aspiration syndrome: clinical roentgenologic and pathologic features. AJR 122:90, 1974.

Holinger, P. H., Kutnick, S. L., Schild, J. A., and Holinger, L. D.: Subglottic stenosis in infants and children. Ann. Otol. 85:591, 1976.

James, A. E., Heller, R. M., White, J. J., et al.: Spontaneous rupture of the stomach in the newborn: clinical and experimental evaluation. Pediatr. Res. 10:79, 1976.

Kanto, W. P., Jr., and Parrish, R. A., Jr.: Perforation of the peritoneum and intra-abdominal hemorrhage: a complication of umbilical vein catheterizations. Am. J. Dis. Child. 131:1102, 1977.

Kassner, E. G., Baumstark, A. E., Balsam, D., and Haller, J. O.: Passage of feeding catheters into the pleural space: radiographic sign of trauma to the pharynx and esophagus in the newborn. AJR 128:19, 1977.

Kassner, E. G., Kauffman, S. L., Yoon, J. J., et al.: Pulmonary candidiasis in infants: clinical, radiologic and pathologic features. AJR 137:707, 1981.

Kaufman, R. A., Kuhns, L. R., Poznanski, A. K., and Holt, J. F.: Gastrointestinal perforation without intraperitoneal air-fluid level in neonatal pneumoperitoneum. AJR 127:915, 1976.

Knight, P. J., and Abdenour, G.: Pneumoperitoneum in the ventilated neonate: respiratory or gastrointestinal origin? J. Pediatr. 98:972, 1981.

Lawson, E. E., Gould, J. B., and Taeusch, H. W., Jr.: Neonatal pneumopericardium: current management. J. Pediatr. Surg. 15:181, 1980.

Leonidas, J. C., Fergus, M. B., Moylan, B., et al.: Ventilation-perfusion scans in neonatal regional pulmonary emphysema complicating ventilatory assistance. AJR 131:243, 1978.

Lloyd, J. R.: The etiology of gastrointestinal perforations in the newborn. J. Pediatr. Surg. 4:77, 1969.

Lucaya, J., Herrera, M., and Salcedo, S.: Traumatic pharyngeal pseudodiverticulum in neonates and infants: two case reports and review of the literature. Pediatr. Radiol. 8:65, 1979.

Lynch, E. P., Coran, A. G., Cohen, S. R., and Lee, F. A.: Traumatic esophageal pseudodiverticula in the newborn. J. Pediatr. Surg. 9:675, 1974.

Magilner, A. D., Capitanio, M. A., Wertheimer, I., et al.: Persistent localized intrapulmonary interstitial emphysema: an observation in three infants. Radiology 111:379, 1974.

Mandell, G. A., and Chawla, M. S.: Chest tube positioning in neonatal pleural herniation. AJR 137:1029, 1981.

McCarten, K. M., Rosenberg, H. K., Borden, S., IV, and Mandell, G. A.: Delayed appearance of right diaphragmatic hernia associated with group-B streptococcal infection in newborns. Radiology 139:385, 1981.

McCloud, T. C., and Ravin, C. E.: PEEP: radiographic features and associated complications. AJR 129:209, 1977.

Merten, D. F., and Goetzman, B. W.: Persistent fetal circulation; a commentary. AJR 128:1067, 1977.

Merten, D. F., Goetzman, B. W., and Wennberg, R. P.: Persistent fetal circulation; an evolving clinical and radiographic concept of pulmonary hypertension of the newborn. Pediatr. Radiol. 6:74, 1977.

Merten, D. F., Mumford, L., Filston, H. C., et al.: Radiological observations during transpyloric tube feeding in infants of low birth weight. Radiology 136:67, 1980.

Merten, D. F., Vogel, M. M., Adelman, R. D., et al.: Renovascular hypertension as a complication of umbilical arterial catheterization. Radiology 126:751, 1978.

Miller, D., Kirkpatrick, B. U., Kodroff, M., et al.: Pelvic exsanguination following umbilical artery catheterization in neonates. J. Pediatr. Surg. 14:264, 1979.

Miller, K. E., Edwards, D. K., Hilton, S., et al.: Acquired lobar emphysema in premature infants with bronchopulmonary dysplasia: an iatrogenic disease? Radiology 138:589, 1981.

Moessinger, A. C., Driscoll, J. M., Jr., and Wigger, H. J.: High incidence of lung perforation by chest tube in neonatal pneumothorax. J. Pediatr. 92:635, 1978.

Moskowitz, P. S., and Griscom, N. T.: The medial pneumothorax. Radiology 120:143, 1976.

Neilson, H. C., Riemenschneider, T. A., and Jaffe, R. B.: Persistent transitional circulation. Radiology 120:649, 1976.

Northway, W. H., Jr., and Rosan, R. C.: Radiographic features of pulmonary oxygen toxicity in the newborn: bronchopulmonary dysplasia. Radiology 91:49, 1968.

Ogata, E. S., Gregory, G. A., Kitterman, J. A., et al.: Pneumothorax in respiratory distress syndrome: incidence and effect on vital signs, blood gases and pH. Pediatrics 58:177, 1976.

Oppermann, H. C., Wille, L., Bleyl, V., and Obladen, M.: Bronchopulmonary dysplasia in premature infants: a radiological and pathological correlation. Pediatr. Radiol. 5:137, 1977.

Oppermann, H. C., Wille, L., Obladen, M., and Richter, E.: Systemic air embolism in respiratory distress syndrome of the newborn. Pediatr. Radiol. 8:139, 1979.

Pereira, G. R., and Lemons, J. A.: Controlled study of transpyloric and intermittent gavage feeding in small preterm infants. Pediatrics 67:68, 1981.

Peterson, H. G., Jr., and Pendleton, M. E.: Contrasting roentgenographic pulmonary patterns of hyaline membrane and fetal aspiration syndromes. AJR 74:800, 1955.

Scott, J. M.: Iatrogenic lesions in babies following umbilical vein catheterization. Arch. Dis. Child. 40:426, 1965.

Serlin, S. P., and Daily, W. J. R.: Tracheal perforation in the neonate: complication of endotracheal intubation. J. Pediatr. 86:596, 1975.

Sickler, E. A., and Gooding, C. A.: Asymmetric lung involvement in bronchopulmonary dysplasia. Radiology 118:379, 1976.

Siegle, R. L., Rabinowitz, J. G., and Sarasohn, C.: Intestinal perforation secondary to nasojejunal feeding tubes. AJR 126:1229, 1976.

Silverstein, E. F., Ellis, K., Casarella, W. J., et al.: Persistence of the fetal circulation: radiologic considerations. AJR 137:497, 1981.

Slovis, T. L., and Shankaran, S.: Patent ductus arteriosus in hyaline membrane disease; chest radiography. AJR 135:307, 1980.

Sommerschild, H. C.: Intestinal perforation in the newborn infant as a complication in umbilical vein infusion or exchange transfusion. Surgery 70:609, 1971.

Spangler, J. G., Kleinberg, F., Fulton, R. E., et al.: False aneurysm of the descending aorta; complication of umbilical artery catheterization. Am. J. Dis. Child. 131:1258, 1977.

Steele, R. W., and Copeland, G. A.: Delayed resorption of pulmonary alveolar fluid in the neonate. Radiology 103:637, 1972.

Stocks, J., Godfrey, S., and Reynolds, E. O. R.: Airway resistance in infants after various treatment for hyaline membrane disease; special emphasis on prolonged high levels of inspired oxygen. Pediatrics 61:178, 1978.

Swischuk, L. E.: Transient respiratory distress of the newborn—TRDN; a temporary disturbance of a normal phenomenon. AJR 108:557, 1970.

Symchych, P. S., Krauss, A. N., and Winchester, P.: Endocarditis following intracardiac placement of umbilical venous catheters in neonates. J. Pediatr. 90:287, 1977.

Thieboult, D. W., Emmanouilides, G. C., Nelson, R. T., et al.: Patent ductus arteriosus complicating the respiratory distress syndrome in preterm infants. J. Pediatr. 86:120, 1975.

Todres, I. D., deBros, F., Kramer, S. S., et al.: Endotracheal tube placement in the newborn infant. J. Pediatr. 89:126, 1976.

Volberg, F. M., Jr., Everett, C. J., and Brill, P. W.: Radiologic features of inferior pulmonary ligament air collections in neonates with respiratory distress. Radiology 130:357, 1979.

Weber, A. L., DeLuca, S., and Shannon, D. C.: Normal and abnormal position of the umbilical artery and venous catheter on roentgenogram and review of complications. AJR 120:361, 1974.

Wesenberg, R. L., Graven, S. N., and McCabe, E. B.: Radiological findings in wet lung disease. Radiology 98:69, 1971.

Williams, H. J., Jarvis, C. W., Neal, W. A., and Reynolds, J. W.: Vascular thromboembolism complicating umbilical artery catheterization. AJR 116:475, 1972.

Wolfson, S. L., Frech, R., Hewitt, C., and Shenklin, D. R.: Radiographic diagnosis of hyaline membrane disease. Radiology 93:339, 1969.

Chapter 13

PHYSICAL ASPECTS OF THE PORTABLE RADIOGRAPH

by Kenneth E. Weaver and David J. Goodenough

The portable radiograph presents a challenging problem for radiographic imaging systems in that one must often use less than optimal conditions to generate a useful radiographic image. This chapter discusses in four sections the physical and psychophysical aspects of the portable radiographic imaging task. The first section considers practical factors that arise in portable radiographic imaging, including contrast factors, resolution factors, and noise factors; the second section describes the generating apparatus that is used in portable radiographic procedures; the third section considers aspects of radiation safety involving exposure to personnel; and the concluding section offers a practical approach to the selection of a screen/film system for portable radiography.

PRACTICAL CONSIDERATIONS

Factors known classically to affect our ability to perceive the presence or absence of an abnormality or "signal" in a radiographic image include contrast, "noise," and boundary sharpness.

Contrast is a measure of the relative difference in brightness between the signal and the background. The overall perceived contrast is dependent on the inherent "subject contrast," the radiographic imaging system, the size of the signal, and the strength of the viewbox luminance.

Noise, which is random or patterned background density, is a major problem in portable radiography. On each exposure, one is limited to a finite number of x-ray photons, based on patient dosage considerations and the radiographic imaging system employed. The noise is largely due to the finite number of photons used in making up the image (Rossmann, 1963, 1968). Both the character and amplitude of these fluctuations influence the ability to perceive the signal.

The sharpness of the perceived boundaries of the signal is determined by the shape of the signal itself, the intrinsic resolution properties of the radiographic imaging system, and motion unsharpness, which is determined by exposure time.

In this section each of these factors is discussed in detail. It should be kept in mind that the overall assessment of radiographic image quality reflects a complicated interrelationship of these factors.

Contrast Factors

Several factors determine the overall perception of contrast. Subject contrast is due to the inherent properties of the signal. It is the ratio of the x-ray intensities transmitted by two selected portions of the subject. It depends on the physical composition of the subject, the x-radiation quality, and the intensity of scattered radiation. Subject contrast is modified by the screen/film combination into radiographic contrast, which is defined as the difference in optical density between two selected portions of the radiograph.

The relationship between subject contrast

and radiographic contrast is probably best understood by consideration of the well-known characteristic curve of a medical radiographic film (the H and D curve). The characteristic curve of the screen/film depends on the type of film and the processing conditions, and is usually independent of the quality and distribution of the x-radiation reaching the fluorescent screen. An H and D curve is characterized by the relationship between density (D) and the logarithm of the x-ray exposure (E) reaching the screen/film combination:

$$D = G \log_{10} E + K \qquad (1)$$

where G is the slope of the approximately straight-line portion of the curve between densities of 0.25 and 2.0 above the base plus fog (G is referred to as the average film gradient), and K is a constant.

This equation may be reduced to a convenient working form; for an average x-ray exposure ($\overline{E}$), it is found that

$$\Delta D = 0.43G \, \Delta E/\overline{E} \qquad (2)$$

where small changes in density (ΔD) may be related to small changes in x-ray exposure (ΔE). Moreover, the relationship between density and the transmitted light (T) coming through the radiograph (when placed on the viewbox) is given by:

$$D = -\log_{10} T \qquad (3)$$

The radiographic contrast (C_R) is approximately equal to:

$$C_R = G(\mu_s - \mu_B)d \, \frac{E_B}{E_B + E_\emptyset} \qquad (4)$$

where d is the diameter of the signal, $E_\emptyset$ is the exposure due to scattered radiation, and E_B is the exposure due to primary radiation. Equation 4 indicates that increased radiographic contrast can be obtained by increasing the film gradient (G), by increasing the difference between the attenuation coefficient of the signal and background ($\mu_S - \mu_B$) (that is, subject contrast), by increasing the diameter of the signal (d), or by reducing scattered radiation.

One should keep in mind the contrast-latitude trade-off found in radiographic systems. The higher the slope (G) of an H and D curve, the greater the radiographic contrast, as can be seen from equation 2. On the other hand, the latitude (that is, the range of exposures, and thus, densities) that may be adequately imaged on a single film is reduced as the slope is increased. As the slope increases, the finite exposure range that may be recorded between the toe region and the shoulder region decreases.

The average gradient, the relative speed, and the fog level of the film are all dependent on the relative development time, the temperature of the developer, and the developer replenishment rate; thus, these processor parameters must be strictly controlled in a quality assurance sense. Without processor quality control, even meticulous radiographic techniques will not yield uniform-quality radiographs.

Radiographic Contrast and Kilovoltage Selection

Several considerations must be taken into account in the choice of kilovoltage for portable radiography: (1) the lower the kilovoltage, the more subject contrast one may hope to transfer to the recording system; (2) the lower the kilovoltage, the less adequate the penetration (thus, exposure time and motion unsharpness are increased); and (3) the scatter contribution is itself a function of energy.

When a beam of x-rays passes through a patient, portions of the beam are transmitted, absorbed, and scattered. Scattered radiation basically tends to irradiate the whole area of the film more or less uniformly, thus producing a general fogging of the film. The net effect is a reduction in contrast.

The relative abundance of scattered radiation as compared with the primary radiation reaching the screen/film increases with the volume or area of the patient irradiated and as the kilovoltage or photon energy is increased. The contribution from scattered radiation in radiography can approach as much as 90 per cent for the abdomen, 50 per cent for the chest, and 25 per cent for extremities such as the knee.

The amount of scattered radiation reaching the film can be reduced by the use of collimation to limit the useful beam to the area of radiographic interest. Another means of reducing radiographic scatter is by using a lower kilovoltage beam, since the ratio of scattered to nonscattered radiation increases with increasing photon energy. However, this is not always practical, because of the thickness of the body parts and the higher patient exposure occurring at lower kilovoltages. Use of an air gap or x-ray grid are other means of reducing scattered

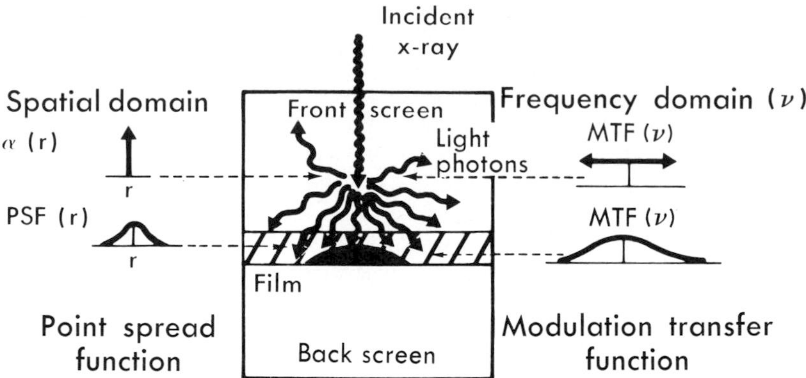

Figure 13–1. Screen/film system: schematic illustration of conversion of x-ray energy to light photons and accompanying loss of resolution (*see text*).

radiation. However, an air gap cannot be used in portable radiography, and a grid is rarely used in portable chest radiography. In radiography of the abdomen, where a grid would be used, a linear parallel grid with a ratio of 6:1 to 8:1 is recommended.

One may ask why, if scattered radiation increases with increasing kilovoltage, there is a trend toward tube potentials in excess of 100 kilovolt peaks (kVp) in chest radiography (Jacobsen et al., 1970). With the use of grids or an air gap, one can reduce scatter substantially to maintain radiographic contrast. The higher kilovoltages reduce exposure time (and thus, motion unsharpness) and increase that latitude of the system. For example, with the high-kilovoltage technique, mediastinal and retrocardiac structures are rendered visible on the radiograph because the relative x-ray intensities reaching the screen/film are now both within the working range (that is, latitude) of the H and D curve of the film. Unfortunately, the difficulty of eliminating scatter in portable chest radiography has limited the useful kilovoltage potentials to the neighborhood of 80 to 85 kVp.

Resolution Factors

As previously mentioned, lower kilovoltage techniques require increased exposure times for adequate patient penetration, and therefore result in increased motion unsharpness. In addition to motion unsharpness, there are two other sources of resolution degradation or unsharpness in screen/film radiography: (1) receptor unsharpness—the inherent blurring operation caused by the transducing or conversion of x-rays into light within the intensifying screen; and (2) geometric unsharpness (focal spot unsharpness)—the blurring due to the finite size and x-ray intensity distribution of the x-ray focal spot. Combinations of the above sources of unsharpness generally lead to an overall blurring or defocusing effect.

This blurring or unsharpness may be characterized by its spatial extent, which is generally the blur size or "point spread function," or it may be characterized in the spatial frequency domain by the modulation transfer function (MTF), which describes how the spatial frequencies making up an object are transferred by the image-recording system (Rossmann, 1969). Thus, high spatial frequency components, for example, which generally make up the important edge structures in radiography, are generally poorly relayed through the radiographic system. The schematic diagram shown in Figure 13–1 reveals how the incident x-ray photons are transduced or converted in an intensifying screen to a burst of light photons that then produce the latent image within the film. The transducing operation is itself a blurring operation. Each incident x-ray photon confined essentially to a point dimension causes a burst of light photons that, before reaching the film, spread over a considerable spatial area and degrade the information concerning the exact spatial origin of the x-ray photon. Instead of a sharp, one-to-one correspondence between the incident x-ray and the developed image point, we have a point source imaged on the film as a blur or point spread function. The overall system point spread function might be considered a gaussian-shaped function. This is convenient in that a rotationally symmetric gaussian distribution may be fully described by a single parameter, namely, its standard deviation (σ), which is a measure of the width of the distribution and the extent of the blurring. A specification of σ for each of the three blurring sources mentioned previously may be used to describe the relative blurring effect of each source of unsharpness: σ_m, σ_r, and σ_g. In addition, by assuming that the individual blur functions are gaussian, one may determine the overall unsharpness or blurring function by the root mean square (rms) of the individual blur contributions:

$$\sigma = \sqrt{\sigma_m^2 + \sigma_r^2 + \sigma_g^2}$$

Table 13–1 indicates the ways in which various blur sources combine in an overall blur or degradation function. For example, one may generally consider that a good estimate of the overall blur width is given by 4σ or 95 per cent of the area of the gaussian distribution. From this table, one may note that at a magnification of 1 (that is, no magnification), as one goes from slow screens *(A, D)* to fast screens *(H, K)*, time and total motion unsharpness are reduced; the total unsharpness is also reduced. One may also note that at a magnification of 1 for a thin object, total unsharpness is independent of focal spot size.

If the magnification study is carefully performed with selected focal spots and image receptors, overall unsharpness may actually be reduced. For example, at a magnification of 1.5 with a fast screen *(I, L)*, total unsharpness is approximately equal to or less than that on nonmagnification studies using slow screens *(A, D)*. Unfortunately, portable radiography rarely lends itself to magnification that, when combined with an air gap, can reduce the overall blur function and scatter contribution. It is also apparent from Table 13–1 that the x-ray generator output and the focal spot size are important in determining the limits of magnification. This is discussed more fully in the article by Weaver and associates (1975).

Noise Factors

The blurring or unsharpness that accompanies the transducing operation shown in Figure 13–1 also introduces changes in the appearance and amplitude of the statistical x-ray fluctuations that constitute noise in the x-ray beam. In a sense, these fluctuations are also "imaged" by the screen. Sharply varying (uncorrelated point to point) noise fluctuations in the image are not found; instead, the noise (or density fluctuations) takes on a characteristic mottled (or correlated) appearance. Instead of "salt and pepper," sharply varying density values across a uniformly exposed film, relatively larger areas of "quantum mottle" (high- and low-density patches) are found. In some ways, the blurring operation can be considered as a "noise smoothing" effect.

As mentioned previously, there are certain fundamental limitations imposed on image quality by the constraint of having to use a finite radiation dose in most radiographic procedures. A finite radiation dose implies an upper limit to the number of x-ray photons that will be stopped by the recording system (the image

TABLE 13–1. Factors Combining to Cause an Overall Blur

		Magnification	Relative Exposure Time (sec)	Focal Spot Unsharpness (mm)	Screen/Film Unsharpness (mm)	Motion Unsharpness (mm/sec)	Total Unsharpness (mm)
		M	t	$4\sigma_g$	$4\sigma_r$	$4\sigma_m$	$4\sigma_T$*
←Slow Screen→	A	1.0	0.2	1	0.33	5	1.053
	B	1.5	0.3	1	0.33	5	1.552
	C	2.0	0.4	1	0.33	5	2.068
	D	1.0	0.2	2	0.33	5	1.053
	E	1.5	0.3	2	0.33	5	1.656
	F	2.0	0.4	2	0.33	5	2.242
←Fast Screen→	H	1.0	0.1	1	0.66	5	0.828
	I	1.5	0.15	1	0.66	5	0.931
	J	2.0	0.2	1	0.66	5	1.166
	K	1.0	0.1	2	0.66	5	0.828
	L	1.5	0.15	2	0.66	5	1.096
	M	2.0	0.2	2	0.66	5	1.452

$$*\sigma_T = \left(\frac{\sigma_r^2}{M^2} + \sigma_m^2 t^2 + \sigma_g^2\left(\frac{M-1}{M}\right)^2\right)^{1/2}$$

receptor). As is well known, in most photon-limited imaging systems the resulting uncertainty in information is described by Poisson statistics. A mean number of absorbed counts per unit area (N) results in an expected standard deviation (S) in the number of counts around that mean value, given by the square root of N; thus, $S = N^{1/2}$.

In terms of the light transmission reaching the eye, the relative (noise) fluctuations around the mean transmission value ($\sigma(T)/T$) are given by the following (Goodenough et al., 1973):

$$\frac{\sigma(T)}{T} \cong \frac{G}{\bar{n}^{1/2}a^{1/2}} F$$

It can be noted that, as in the equation for radiographic contrast, the G factor and a factor related to the size of the signal (in this case, the area of the signal being searched [a]) are found. In addition, the expected number of absorbed photons per unit area ($\bar{n}$) enters into the equation, as well as a factor, F, which is related to the inherent resolution properties of the recording system (Rossmann, 1963). In fact, a system with high spatial frequency transfer capability tends to transfer the Poisson noise fluctuations a little better, because such noise has a significantly high spatial frequency component. However, the F factor also introduces a complication into the evaluation of noise in radiographic imaging. That is, the modulation of the noise statistics by the MTF gives the characteristic shape or appearance to the noise fluctuations, which, as mentioned previously, is often described as quantum mottle (Rossmann, 1963, 1968). Quantum mottle is important because the perception of noise is influenced not only by the amplitude or excursions of the noise around the mean value, but also by the characteristic mottled appearance or pattern of this noise. Certain noise patterns seem to be more objectionable in certain viewing tasks than other types of noise.

The question arises as to why noise is important in portable radiographic procedures. The answer is found in the fact that portable procedures are often attempted on systems with limited x-ray generator output. The use of faster screen or faster film, to reduce the effect of patient motion and/or to lower the kilovoltage while keeping the imaging task within the finite generator output of the x-ray system, may be contemplated. For a given film density, the faster the speed of the recording film, the fewer the number of x-ray photons that will be absorbed in the screen. Therefore, the noise amplitude will tend to increase.

The question also arises as to how to decide whether the increased contrast or decreased motion unsharpness (or both) is of more importance than the increased noise. In the consideration of "white noise" (that is, noise that varies sharply from point to point), it can be assumed that increased noise amplitude reduces image detail at about the same rate at which a corresponding increase in contrast enhances image detail. This fact is usually considered as the "signal-to-noise ratio" approach. In this approach, it is assumed that a figure of merit in a system is the relative ratio of the contrast of the signal divided by the relative noise amplitude of the surrounding (competing) background. As a gross approximation, it is assumed that the noise amplitude in an image will increase as the square root of the film speed. For every increase in speed by a factor of 4, twice as much contrast in the signal will be needed to detect a given signal on the 4X system as on the image obtained from the conventional speed system. Although this approach is probably oversimplified, it does show that contrast gains obtained from increased speed may be lessened by the effect of increased noise. As the signal size becomes small and looks more and more like typical noise excursions, the preceding signal-to-noise ratio approach should become more and more correct. It should be noted that, in the case of large signals (on the order of 1 cm or larger), the real influence of the finite photon flux becomes smaller and smaller. In particular, the relative noise fluctuations for 1 cm-diameter signals for present medium speed screen/medium speed film combinations are less than one part in 1000 (this results from stopping about 10^7 x-ray photons per square centimeter of screen).

Another problem with noise is that the human eye is looking essentially for borders or edges (high frequencies); thus, even a large signal having a low-contrast, unsharp edge may have important edge information obscured by noise fluctuations.

Figure 13–2 illustrates the complicated interrelationship between resolution and noise in radiographic imaging systems. The radiographs shown were obtained by using two different screen/film combinations of relative screen and film speeds that were matched so that the overall system speed (and thus motion unsharpness) would be equal. Calcium tungstate intensifying screens were used in both systems. It

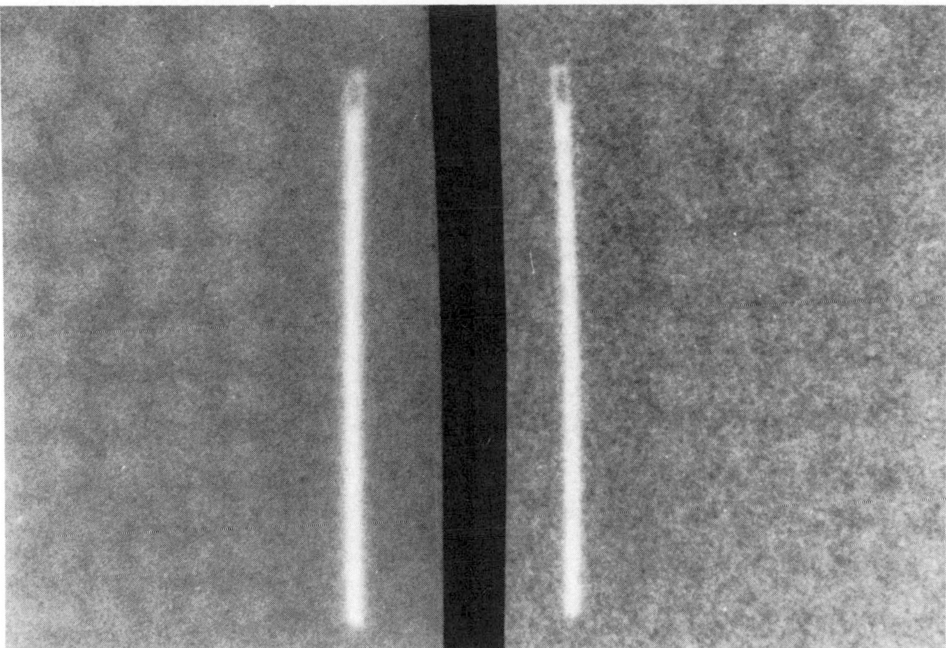

Figure 13–2. Radiographs of a steel needle and plastic beads taken with medium-speed screens and fast film *(right)* and with fast screens and normal-speed film *(left)*. The needle is seen best on the high-resolution system.

was found that the image of contrast-filled, vessel-type objects (needles) is essentially resolution-limited. This type of object is imaged better with the system with the higher resolution properties, that is, with the sharper system. The low-contrast, tumor-type objects (plastic spheres), which are essentially noise-limited, are actually detected better when radiographed with the system that shows poorer sharpness and more smoothly varying noise. Thus, the system with a higher intrinsic sharpness does not always afford the best detection for low-contrast, noise-limited detail. This subject has been discussed at length in other sources (Goodenough et al., 1973, 1974). Thus, as a general rule, for high-contrast vessels, where sharp border information is necessary, resolution is a key factor; for small, low-contrast nodules with diffuse borders, on the other hand, reduced noise becomes increasingly more important even at the expense (and somewhat as a consequence) of less sharpness.

MOBILE DIAGNOSTIC X-RAY EQUIPMENT

Mobile x-ray systems are classified by the type of power supply and by the high voltage waveform utilized to energize the x-ray tube. These power supply types are conventional single-phase, full wave rectified, battery-operated constant potential, and capacitor discharge systems. The constant potential and capacitor discharge systems can be operated from a conventional or typical hospital power supply (110 V, 3 kilovolt-amperes [kVA]), in contrast to the single-phase, full wave rectified system, which requires the installation of a special power line similar to that for conventional stationary equipment. For example, to operate at 100 kVp and 300 milliamperes (mA) would require a power demand of approximately 30 kVA. This power requirement severely limits the practicality and usefulness of this particular system, since special wiring is necessary in each of the rooms and at various locations where use is intended.

Principle of Operation

CONVENTIONAL SINGLE-PHASE SYSTEM. The conventional x-ray generator utilizes the hospital power supply directly (that is, it requires a simultaneous input equivalent to the output), is stepped up by the high-voltage transformer, and is rectified to produce the waveform shown in Figure 13–3. If operated from the conventional 100-V line, the maximum tube current is about 15 mA at 100 kVp.

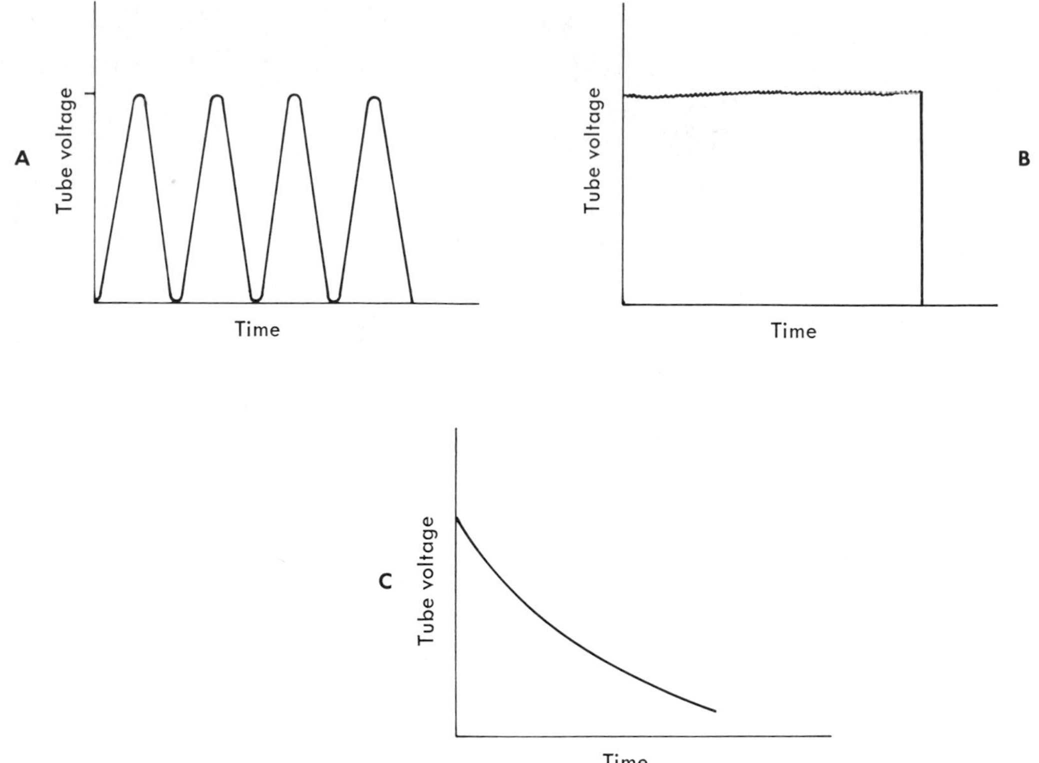

Figure 13–3. Tube voltage waveform for a conventional single-phase, full-wave rectified x-ray unit, *A*, a constant potential unit, *B*, and a capacitor discharge unit, *C*.

CONSTANT POTENTIAL SYSTEM. The constant potential system operates from a power supply consisting of a rechargeable battery pack. The direct-current (DC) voltage from this battery is converted to a 500-Hz alternating-current (AC) voltage source by an inverter, and is stepped up by the high-voltage transformer and rectifier to give a near-constant potential waveform (very similar to a three-phase system). However, in a practical sense (at the image receptor), a constant potential output makes the 100-mA rating roughly comparable with a 200-mA output of a traditional single-phase generator (Barone, 1971). The rechargeable battery pack has an exposure capacity of approximately 10,000 mA at 100 kVp; the capacity is proportionately higher at lower kilovoltage levels. The system contains an integrated battery that can be recharged in approximately eight hours from a conventional 110-V supply.

CAPACITOR DISCHARGE SYSTEM. With the capacitor discharge system, the voltage from a standard 110-V outlet is stepped up by the high-voltage transformer to the selected kilovoltage, and the charge is stored on two capacitors. This type of approach is practical, since a charge sufficient to produce an x-ray exposure at high tube currents (200 to 400 mA) is accumulated on the capacitors in a charging time of such a reasonable duration (five to 20 seconds) that it is not necessary to exceed the typical hospital power supply of 110 V at 3 kVA. The capacitors become the high-voltage supply, and the x-ray tube is connected across them. A grid bias of several kilovolts is applied to prevent the tube from conducting. This bias prevents the electrons emitted by the cathode from being accelerated and striking the anode. Once the grid bias is removed (exposure switch initiated t_0), the tube will conduct and the charge (electrons) stored on the capacitors will discharge through the x-ray tube. If at a later time (t_1) the grid bias is reapplied to the x-ray tube, it will no longer conduct and the exposure will be terminated (see Fig. 13–4). This mode of operation is referred to as "wave tail cut-off." If the capacitors are allowed to discharge completely, the exponential waveform shown in Figure 13–3 will be produced (Weaver et al., 1978).

Comparison of the voltage waveforms for the various generators shows distinct differences (Fig. 13–3), which will result in differences in the x-ray beam quality and quantity between the systems. Predicting the effect produced by capacitor discharge systems becomes much more complex, however, since the overall voltage waveform is a function of the milliamperage selected. For the capacitance used in x-ray equipment currently marketed in the United States, the tube voltage will drop by 1 kV for each milliampere-second of charge selected. For example, if a technique of 60 kV and 15 mAs is selected on initiation of the exposure (t_0), the voltage will fall from 60 kV to 45 kV on termination (Fig. 13–4*A*). Production of x-rays at the lower voltages is very inefficient; it is also of little use diagnostically and produces unnecessary patient exposure.

Beam Quality Comparison

The major difference in beam quality between the three systems is the dependency of kilovoltage on the milliamperage selected in the capacitor system. For the single-phase and constant potential systems, the kilovoltage waveform remains essentially constant regardless of milliampere-seconds. However, with the capacitor system, the effective penetrating energy of the primary beam for a 30-mAs technique (Fig. 13–4*B*) will be significantly less than for a 15-mAs technique (Fig. 13–4*A*) because of the difference in the average voltage.*

Figure 13–5 depicts the energy spectra of x-ray beams impinging on a 20-cm Masonite phantom for a single-phase, full wave rectified system and a capacitor discharge system, respectively (Fewell and Weaver, 1976). Each system was operated at a tube voltage of 60 kVp, and the spectra were taken at exposures of 15 and 30 mAs. It can be noted that, for the single-phase unit, doubling the exposure produced the well-known increase in all parts of the energy spectrum shown in Figure 13–5*A*. However, in the case of the eapacitor discharge unit operating at an initial tube potential of 60 kVp (Fig. 13–5*B*), the increase in exposure from 15 to 30 mAs contributed additional photons only to that portion of the spectrum below approximately 40 kiloelectron volts (keV); thus, effective beam quality was reduced.

An example of the practical implications of these observations is shown in skull phantom radiographs made at 70 kVp with the capacitor discharge unit (Fig. 13–6). Note that the density in the region of the sella turcica changes from a density of 0.84 at a 15-mAs exposure to 0.96 at a 25-mAs exposure, whereas increasing the exposure to 50 mAs only raises the density to 1.0. The incident exposures for these techniques were 140 milliroentgens (mR), 190 mR, and 240 mR, respectively. The 70-kV, 50-mAs exposure was recommended by the "suggested technique" chart supplied with the capacitor discharge unit; following this suggested technique would lead to an unnecessary patient exposure of at least 25 per cent.

In summary, although the capacitor energy storage principle serves a very useful role in providing mobile diagnostic systems with higher tube currents than those of other mobile equipment, a lack of understanding of the nature of the operation can lead to unnecessary patient exposure through inappropriate selection of technique factors. A good rule of thumb (for the thicker body parts) is to keep the tube

*It should be noted, however, that when portable chest radiography is being performed, the capacitor unit may have a beam quality and output similar to the constant potential systems if the technique utilizes only several milliampere-seconds.

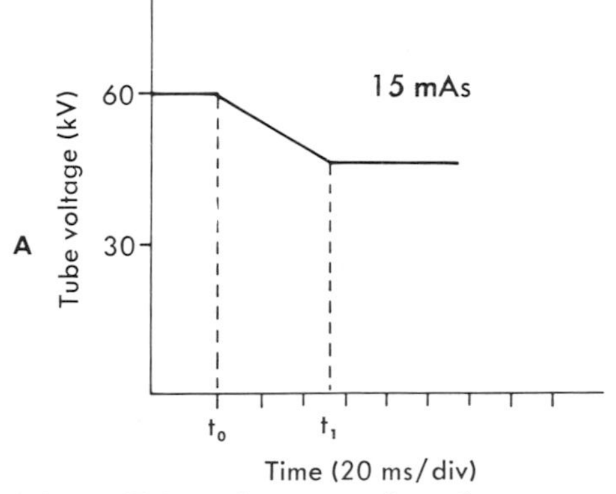

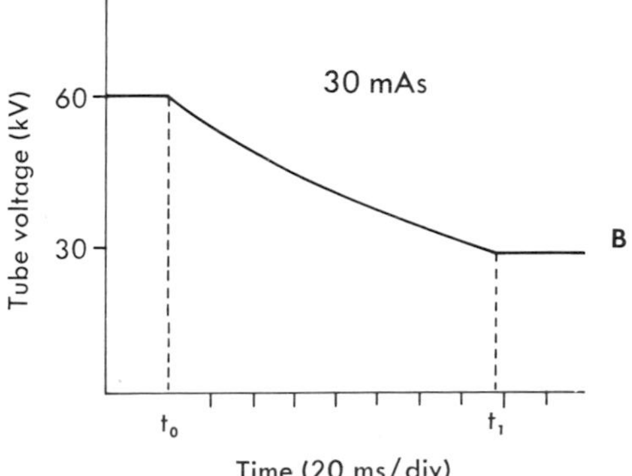

Figure 13–4. Tube voltage waveform for a capacitor discharge unit at a 15-mAs discharge, *A*, and at a 30-mAs discharge, *B*.

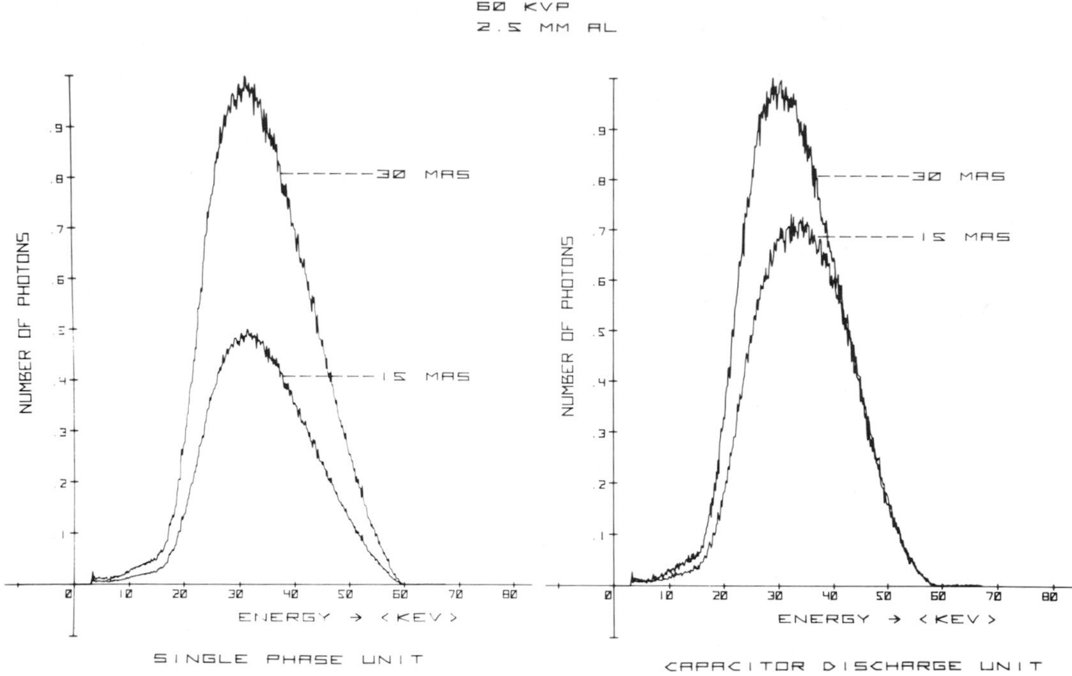

Figure 13–5. Primary entrance spectra at 15 and 20 mAs for a single-phase, full-wave rectified unit, *A*, and a capacitor discharge unit, *B*.

current–time (mAs) selected equal to or less than 30 per cent of the starting tube voltage.

Field Emission X-ray Systems

In conventional x-ray tubes the source of electrons is produced by thermionic emission. The cathode is simply heated by passing a current through it, and electrons in the conduction band are supplied with an energy equal to or greater than the work function of the emitting material; that is, the electrons are provided with enough energy to escape from the material.

Field emission is a cold cathode process that occurs when a sufficient electronic field is applied to reduce the potential barrier at the metal (cathode) surface to the extent that there is an appreciable probability that electrons in the conduction band will be able to tunnel through the barrier and out of the metal. To obtain the large electric field strength necessary for field emission production (in excess of 10^7 V/cm), the emitter cathodes are sharpened points (see Fig. 13–7). In field emission a large fraction of the conduction electrons that strike the barrier have a chance of being emitted. The current density of the field emitter is of the order of 10^8 amperes per square centimeter of emitting surface. This is approximately 10^6 times greater than the current densities in thermionic tubes. However, anode heat loading considerations necessitate the use of very short pulses (on the order of 30 nanoseconds). Present equipment utilizes 1000 pulses per second. The instantaneous tube current may be as high as 1000 to 2000 *amperes,* the average current 30 to 50 *milliamperes.*

The sole manufacturer of diagnostic field emission x-ray equipment is Hewlett-Packard, McMinnville Division, who is currently producing a 240-kVp mobile unit for chest radiography. The use of high kVp helps to compensate for the relatively low tube current associated with the system.

The field emission x-ray tubes are relatively small and utilize sharpened points, as mentioned earlier. The electron beam discharges from a number of these fine, needle-sharp metal points onto a truncated conical tungsten target. The tube construction is shown in Figure 13–7. Owing to the conical shape of the anode, the focal spot will be somewhat rotationally symmetric with a depression in the center. The manufacturer specifies the focal spot size as 2.5 mm equivalent.

The field emission tube life on the chest unit is reported (Hallembeck) as being between 1200 and 3900 exposures (these tubes are leased on a per-exposure basis). Because of the extremely short time duration of high voltage, the tube does not require a great bulk of insulation; it therefore does not have to be insulated with oil, and changing of the tube becomes a relatively simple task.

This unit is provided with a phototimed cassette. Our experience with this device confirms that reported by Tabrisky et al. (1980): the system is very reliable and reduces the retake

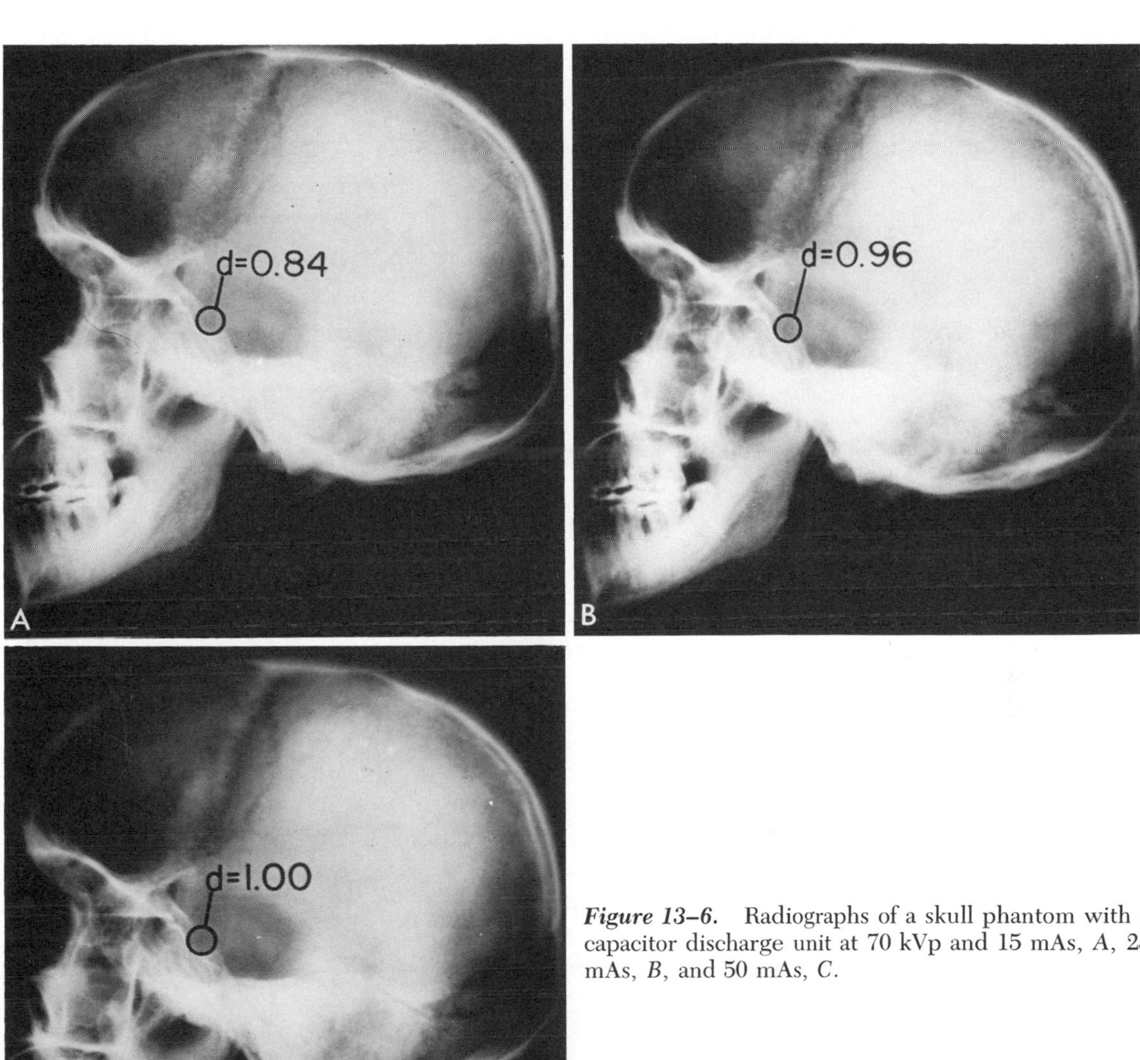

Figure 13–6. Radiographs of a skull phantom with a capacitor discharge unit at 70 kVp and 15 mAs, *A*, 25 mAs, *B*, and 50 mAs, *C*.

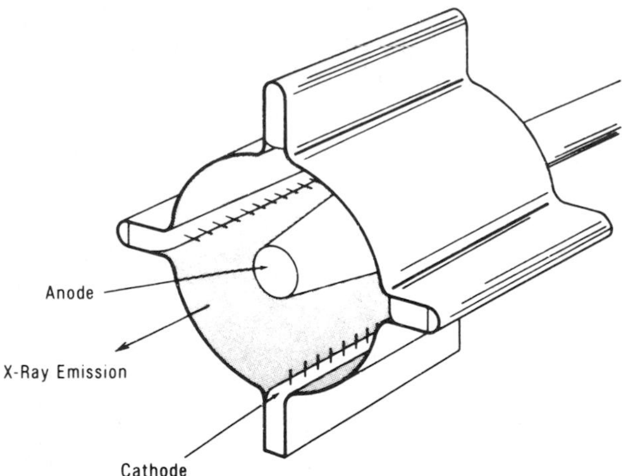

Figure 13–7. Schematic diagram of a field emission x-ray tube.

rate significantly. The only drawback is that the cassette holder is somewhat heavy, so that a second person is sometimes needed to help with positioning.

In a comparison of the 240 kVp with a conventional unit operated between 80 and 95 kVp, Tabrisky et al. (1980) reported the following:

> The 240 kVp demonstrated consistently good visualization of central air passages, hilar contours, and pulmonary detail. It was superior to the conventional portables in eliminating respiratory motion, defining lung infiltrates and localizing the endotracheal tube relation to the carina. The 240 kVp system had noticeable deficiencies in depicting calcification, bone detail and fat planes. These were not of clinical significance.*

RADIATION PROTECTION IN MOBILE RADIOGRAPHY

For an operator of mobile diagnostic x-ray equipment, the source of exposure comes primarily from radiation scattered from the patient. Several factors influence the magnitude of this exposure: exposure time, the distance from the patient to the operator, and shielding.

Reduction of the exposure time for a particular technique will correspondingly reduce operator exposure. Exposure time can be minimized by use of the fastest screen/film combination commensurate with necessary image quality.

Distance is probably the easiest and most effective way of reducing unnecessary exposure. The greater the distance from the scattering source (the patient), the less will be the exposure by approximately the inverse square of the distance. In the diagnostic x-ray energy range, the ratio of scattered to incident exposure at 1 m is on the order of 1:1000. With a medium-speed screen/film system, the incident exposure for a chest radiograph is about 10 to 20 mR per film, whereas that for a spine radiograph (lumbar lateral) is around 1300 mR per film. Therefore, at 1 m from the patient, the exposure from scattered radiation would be on the order of 0.02 mR per film for a chest radiograph and 1.3 mR per film for a radiograph of the spine. At 2 m from the patient, these levels would be approximately 0.005 mR and 0.3 mR, respectively. Therefore, if the operator simply maximizes his distance from the patient, he can significantly reduce the exposure level. It has been found that if a distance of at least 1.5 to 2.0 m is used in intensive care radiography, the exposure for the operator will be almost insignificant (Vogel and Lohr, 1976).

As regards the exposure to nonoccupational workers, Herman et al. (1980) found that the maximum *weekly* exposure at the nurses' station in an ICU with four beds was approximately 0.05 mR (based on 20 exposures per week per bed) when the equipment was operating at 80 kVp. The nearest bed was 11 feet, and the furthest 17 feet, from the point of measurement. This level is well below the maximal permissible whole body exposure of 10 mR per week for a nonoccupational worker.

Another mechanism that can be used to reduce operator exposure is shielding. This can take the form of structural shielding (positioning oneself so that there is a wall or barrier intercepting scattered radiation) or a lead apron worn by the operator. The use of the lead apron will reduce the exposure by a factor of *at least* 100 to the *trunk* of the body. The exact amount

*This unit is no longer manufactured.

depends on the x-ray beam quality and on the thickness of the lead apron.

In summary, use of the fastest screen/film combination adequate for diagnostic information, the maximum operator-patient distance, and a lead apron will reduce the total body exposure of the operator to levels that can be considered almost insignificant.

SCREEN/FILM SELECTION

The choice of a screen/film system for portable chest radiographic procedures is often difficult. In particular, the advent of fast screen/film systems, many of them using rare-earth phosphors, has complicated the task facing the physician who must make a decision based on the diagnostic trade-offs between motion unsharpness, spatial resolution (including geometric unsharpness), contrast, noise, and patient exposure. Although the faster systems may offer advantages for reduced motion unsharpness (particularly for the limited radiation output of certain portable chest units), their use may also be accompanied by decreased spatial resolution and increased noise.

Analytic techniques introduced into the field by Rossman (1962), Doi (1964), Morgan et al. (1964), and others in the early 1960s have not provided a simple predictive methodology of assessing diagnostic screen/film quality when they are used in a general diagnostic imaging task. On the other hand, in those cases in which a particular diagnostic signal could be defined and localized, such as a vessel in angiography, bone detail in skeletal radiography, and punctate calcifications in mammography, excellent results have been obtained (Doi, 1977; Doi et al., 1977; Genant et al., 1977). One problem of more general extension is that most analytic image evaluation techniques involve application of two-dimensional optical measurements to an image of a three-dimensional object. Thus, one has a complicated perceptual task of unfolding information from superimposed planes of differing radiographic magnification (Doi and Rossman, 1975; Takahashi and Sakuma, 1975). Moreover, the complicated anatomic patterns are enhanced or diminished by the use of different screen/film systems to the point at which they may actually constitute "structure noise." Then, too, there is a lack of published data on physiologic motion and how it enters into the final "diagnostic" evaluation.

The Quality Assurance Committee of the Department of Radiology at The George Washington University Medical Center, composed of physicians, physicists, engineers, and technologists, decided to obtain empirical data from a selection of screen/film systems on the relationship between judgments of diagnostic quality and perceived physical attributes of radiographs (Vucich et al., 1979). This correlation (or its lack) is of fundamental importance in the choice of an imaging system.

Members of the Quality Assurance Committee devised a test protocol to examine diagnostic and physical quality of different radiographic screen/film systems. These systems included the conventional system used in the department (Dupont High Plus/Cronex 4) and four other systems, which offered relative system speeds that are a factor of two or more faster or slower than the conventional system. The investigation arose from discussions on the optimal choice of a screen/film combination for portable chest procedures, an application where system speed could be of major importance.

In this section we will illustrate methodology, on the understanding that much of the work is still developmental. Wherever possible, we retrospectively point out possibilities for improvement in design or statistical analysis. In our studies we also have investigated whether an anthropomorphic, static phantom could be related to actual patient data, and sought useful relationships between an evaluation of clinical diagnostic image quality and analytic image measurements made on the screen/film systems.

Data Collection

Sample radiographs. Radiographs were made of patients and of the modified 3M chest phantom shown in Figure 13–8. An improved vascular system and lung parenchyma were introduced into the phantom, the appearance of which was deemed reasonable by participating radiologists.

The phantom was radiographed twice with each screen/film system under consideration. Eight patients were involved in the evaluation, and each was radiographed by the department's conventional system plus one other screen/film system. Only those patient radiographs judged to have equal optical density (O.D.) in the lung parenchyma were included in the evaluation. Phantom radiographs were required to differ in optical density by less than 0.10 at selected sites in the intercostal spaces. The optical density of patient radiographs was, of course, more

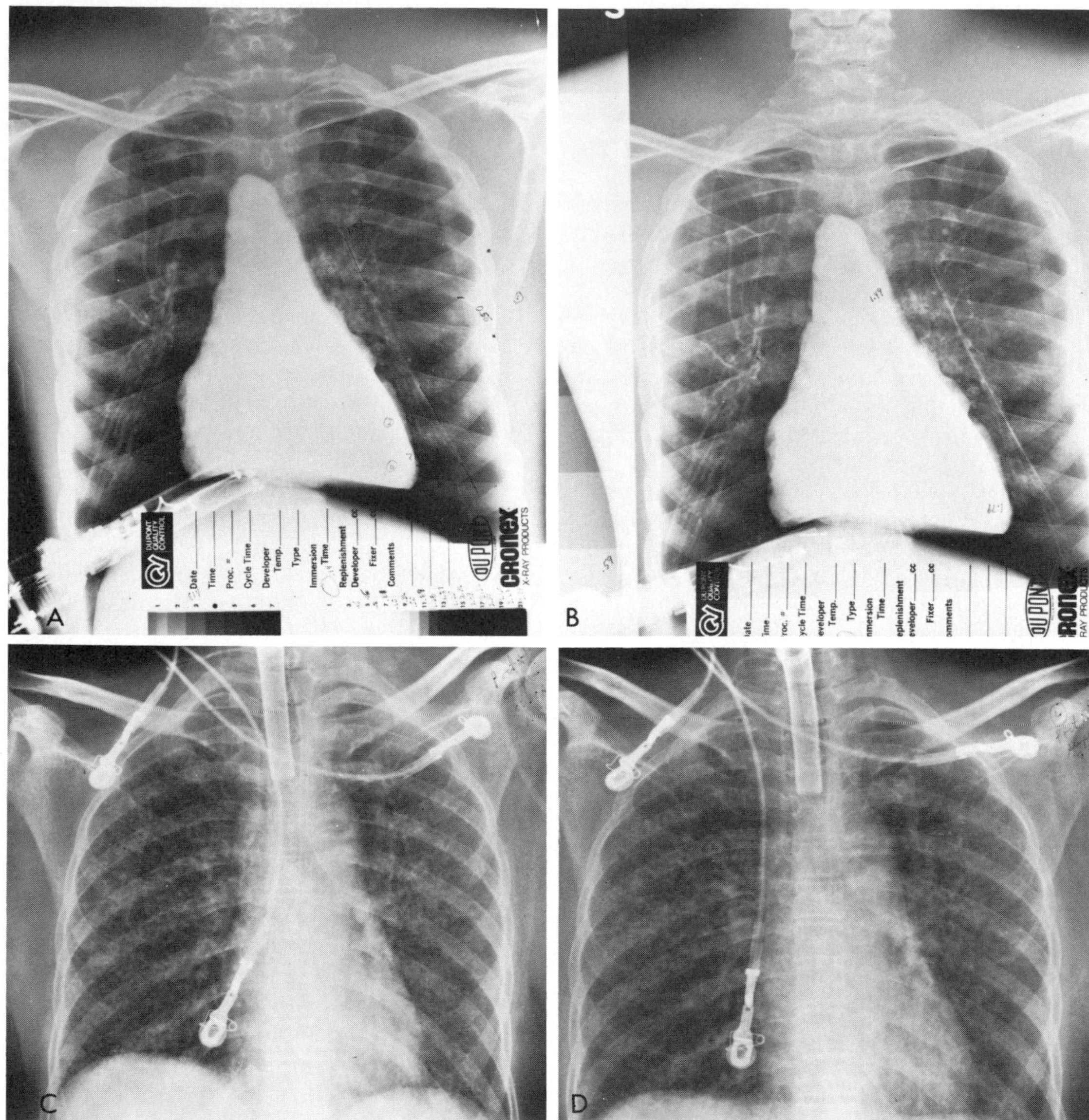

Figure 13–8. *A*, Radiograph of a phantom using a medium-speed screen/film combination (System B). *B*, Radiograph of a phantom using a rare-earth screen/film combination with a speed approximately double that of the system used in *A* (system D). *C*, Radiograph of a patient utilizing System B. *D*, Radiograph of a patient utilizing System D.

TABLE 13–2. Description of Screen/Film Systems

System	Relative Speed	Screen	Film	Resolution at a Contrast Response of 40%
A	0.55	calcium tungstate	conventional, wide latitude	1.6 l.p./mm*
B	1.00	calcium tungstate	conventional	1.6 l.p./mm*
C	1.60	rare earth	conventional	1.6 l.p./mm**
D	1.90	rare earth	green-sensitive	1.2 l.p./mm*
E	2.50	rare earth	conventional, wide latitude	1.9 l.p./mm*

*From Operational Health Physics. Proceedings of the Ninth Mid-Year Topical Symposium of the Health Physics Society, Denver, CO, 1976.
**Manufacturer's data.

difficult to control than that of the phantom radiographs.

All systems were mounted in the same type of cassette, and uniform processor performance was assured by sensitometric control. Fixed mA (mAs changed by varying time) was used so that the focal spot size would not be expected to change. System speed, screen/film characteristics, and an indication of resolution appear in Table 13–2.

EVALUATION OF RADIOGRAPHS. Radiologists were asked to choose, on the basis of their clinical experience, anatomic landmarks appearing in posterior/anterior (P/A) chest radiographs whose visualization is related to the visualization of significant radiologic findings. These anatomic landmarks were then incorporated into an evaluation form, shown in Table 13–3. In addition, physical parameters defined and interpreted by radiologists were assembled into a second evaluation form, shown in Table 13–4.

Three radiologists were asked to evaluate

TABLE 13–3. Subjective Assessment of Anatomic Landmarks*

Bony Thorax (Ribs and Clavicles) (10)	Retrocardiac Area (30)
Cortical Margins (5)	***Left Diaphragm (15)***
( ) optimally visualized (5)	( ) totally visualized (15)
( ) adequately visualized (4)	( ) partially visualized (7)
( ) poorly visualized (2)	( ) not visualized (0)
( ) not visualized (0)	( ) disease precludes evaluation (N)
( ) disease precludes evaluation (N)	
Trabeculae (5)	***Spine (15)***
( ) optimal detail (5)	( ) too well visualized (7)
( ) adequate detail (4)	( ) optimally visualized (15)
( ) poor detail (2)	( ) acceptably visualized (7)
( ) not visualized (0)	( ) poorly visualized (3)
( ) disease precludes evaluation (N)	( ) not visualized (0)
	( ) disease precludes evaluation (N)

Trachea (15)	Diaphragm (15)	Pulmonary Vasculature (30)
Visible To: (15)	***Diaphragm Outline (15)***	***Maximum Measurable To: (30)***
( ) left main stem bronchus (15)	( ) both visualized (15)	( ) right costophrenic angle (30)
( ) carina (10)	( ) right only (7)	( ) right midlung (20)
( ) neck and upper mediastinum (5)	( ) left only (7)	( ) right descending pulmonary artery (10)
( ) not visible (0)	( ) not visualized (0)	( ) none (0)
( ) disease precludes evaluation (N)	( ) disease precludes evaluation (N)	( ) disease precludes evaluation (N)

*Maximal total score = 100.

TABLE 13–4. Subjective Assessment of Physical Parameters*

Contrast (35)	Density (15)
( ) optimal (35)	( ) optimal (15)
( ) good (23)	( ) good (10)
poor, but diagnostic	poor, but diagnostic
( ) too gray (11)	( ) too dark (5)
( ) too black/white (11)	( ) too light (5)
unacceptable, not diagnostic	( ) unacceptable (0)
( ) too gray (0)	
( ) too black/white (0)	
Graininess (20)	**Detail (30)**
( ) no grain visible (20)	( ) optimal (30)
( ) minimal grain (13)	( ) good (20)
( ) grainy, but does not interfere with diagnosis (6)	( ) poor detail, but does not interfere with diagnosis (10)
( ) grain interferes with diagnosis (0)	( ) lack of detail interferes with diagnosis (0)

*Maximal total score = 100.

each radiograph, using only one type of form at a session. Consistent viewing conditions were maintained. The radiographs were presented to the radiologists one at a time in an arbitrary, but consistent, order. The visibility of each anatomic landmark was rated by marking the appropriate box on the evaluation form. The weighting factors used to calculate a score are shown in parentheses in Tables 13–3 and 13–4, although these were not displayed on the evaluation forms actually used by the radiologists. These weighting factors reflect the relative importance placed upon each anatomic landmark or physical parameter by the radiologists.

Data Analysis

Scoring. The weighting factors assigned to each major parameter were divided among the response choices for each subparameter, as illustrated in Tables 13–3 and 13–4. The assigned point scores for the response choices were used to develop total percentage possible scores for each screen/film system, for each sample radiograph, and for each radiologist. Scores were adjusted, as illustrated in Table 13–5, for the case in which an anatomic landmark could not be visualized because it was obscured by pathology. The percentage possible scores were then averaged over the appropriate radiographs to produce a mean score for each radiologist's rating of each screen/film system.

A rank was assigned to each system for each radiologist and each parameter by ordering the systems according to their mean scores. If two or more systems received an equal mean score, the average of the two ranks was assigned to both. The results for each radiologist were averaged to yield a mean rank for each system and parameter. These mean ranks were calculated separately for the scores from patient radiographs and from phantom radiographs. Table 13–6 shows the ranks assigned for the total of anatomic landmarks, which includes the scores for all anatomic landmarks in Table 13–3.

Discussion of Ranked Data. In this preliminary experiment the curves for total anatomic and physical parameters (Fig. 13–9*A*, *E*) agree closely for phantom radiographs. Figure 13–9*B*, *C*, *D* shows the ranking preference for the subjective assessment of certain physical parameters that were the constituents for Figure 13–9*E*. Figure 13–9*B*, the curves for the detail parameters, shows that slow-speed systems score higher when used with phantoms, and fast-speed systems score better when used with patients. In Figure 13–9*C*, the phantom curve shows perceived system quantum mottle increasing with system speed, as is usually observed. The patient curve in Figure 13–9*C* shows the same trend, with the important exception that System D was ranked highest (best). Figure 13–9*D* indicates that the radiologists seemed to show a preference for the contrast of System D in the patient radiographs, as opposed to the phantom radiographs. The performance of System D appears to be the result of optimizing the combination of motion unsharpness, intrinsic resolution, and noise. The data should be considered as "hypothesis suggesting" rather than "hypothesis proving";

TABLE 13–5. Calculation of Percentage Possible Anatomic Score for One Radiograph*

Bony Thorax (Ribs and Clavicles) (10)

Cortical Margins (5)

( ) optimally visualized (5)
(X) ADEQUATELY VISUALIZED (4)
( ) poorly visualized (2)
( ) not visualized (0)
( ) disease precludes evaluation (N)

Trabeculae (5)

( ) optimal detail (5)
(X) ADEQUATE DETAIL (4)
( ) poor detail (2)
( ) not visualized (0)
( ) disease precludes evaluation (N)

Retrocardiac Area (30)

Left Diaphragm (15)

( ) totally visualized (15)
( ) partially visualized (7)
( ) not visualized (0)
(X) DISEASE PRECLUDES EVALUATION (N)

Spine (15)

(X) TOO WELL VISUALIZED (7)
( ) optimally visualized (15)
( ) acceptably visualized (7)
( ) poorly visualized (3)
( ) not visualized (0)
( ) disease precludes evaluation (N)

$$\text{\% Possible Anatomic Score} = \frac{4 + 4 + 0 + 0 + 20 + 0 + 7}{5 + 5 + 15 + 0 + 30 + 0 + 15} = \frac{35}{70} = 50\%$$

Trachea (15)

Visible To: (15)

( ) left main stem bronchus (15)
( ) carina (10)
( ) neck and upper mediastinum (5)
(X) NOT VISIBLE (0)
( ) disease precludes evaluation (N)

Diaphragm (15)

Diaphragm Outline (15)

( ) both visualized (15)
( ) right only (7)
( ) left only (7)
( ) not visualized (0)
(X) DISEASE PRECLUDES EVALUATION (0)

Pulmonary Vasculature (30)

Maximum Measurable To: (30)

( ) right costophrenic angle (30)
(X) RIGHT MIDLUNG (20)
( ) right descending pulmonary artery (10)
( ) none (0)
( ) disease precludes evaluation (N)

*As evaluated by one radiologist.

TABLE 13–6. Mean Scores for Total of Anatomic Landmarks (for Patient Radiographs) with Ranks Assigned

	Radiologist I		**Radiologist II**		**Radiologist III**		**All Radiologists**
System	***Mean Score***	***Rank***	***Mean Score***	***Rank***	***Mean Score***	***Rank***	***Mean Rank***
A	76.4	(2)	83.6	(2)	79.0	(2)	(2.0)
B	74.6	(3)	73.7	(3)	65.6	(3)	(3.0)
C	60.1	(4)	70.6	(4)	43.5	(5)	(4.3)
D	94.3	(1)	85.8	(1)	82.0	(1)	(1.0)
E	49.6	(5)	56.1	(5)	60.0	(4)	(4.7)

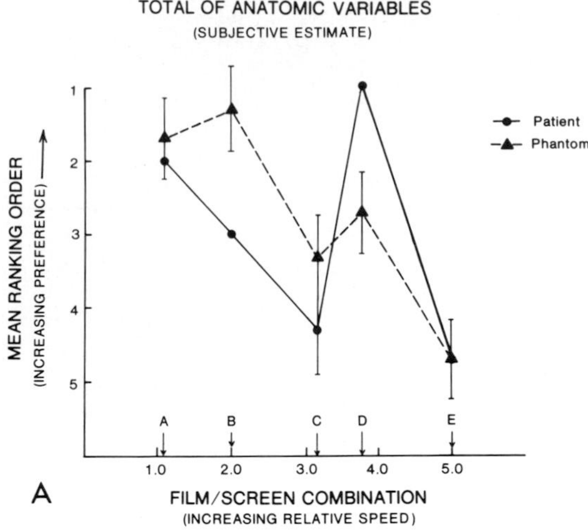

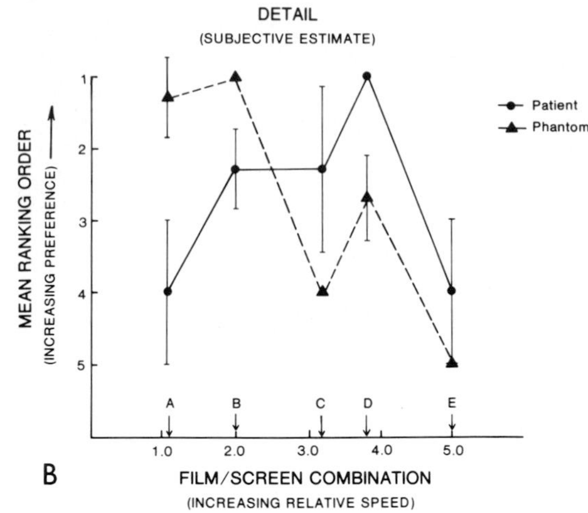

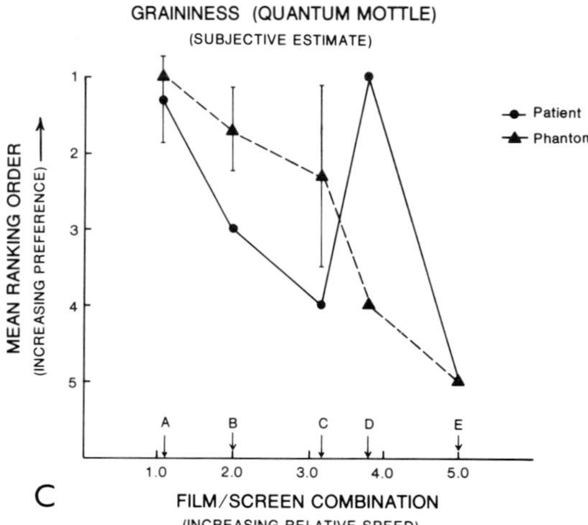

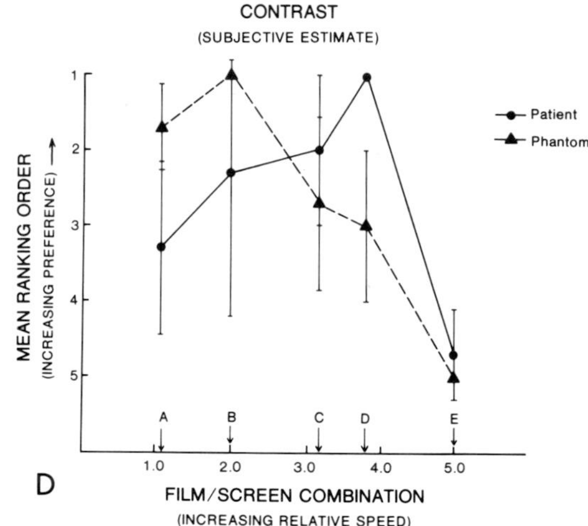

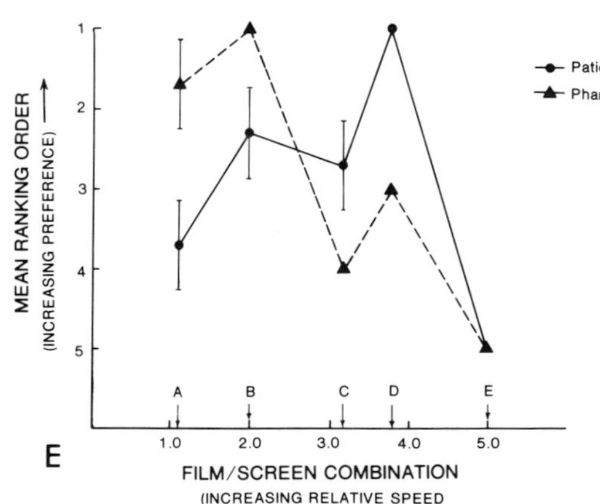

Figure 13–9. Results of subjective assessment of film/screen systems using anatomic variables shown in Table 13–3. *B* to *E*, Results of subjective assessment of film/screen systems using the scores from Table 13–4 for: *B* the detail category; *C* the graininess category; *D* the contrast category; and *E* all four of the categories of physical variables shown in Table 13–4.

however, it is felt that further study is warranted.

One of the more interesting results of this preliminary work is the fact that one finds a statistically significant reversal of ranking preference on the total physical score (Fig. 13–9*E*) when comparing phantom radiographs with patient radiographs. Note especially the ranking for System B (the conventional system) and System D (more than twice as fast). It is concluded that either motion or other, as yet unidentified sources of difference between static phantoms and patients should be carefully borne in mind in subsequent attempts at evaluation.

Summary

There probably is no screen/film system that can offer all things to all diagnostic tasks, particularly in light of variable kVp and exposure time requirements, nor is there one system that can perform optimally with the wide range of radiographic conditions present in radiology departments today. In addition, the physical data currently available on screen/film systems are insufficient to be used as the sole determinants of the system of choice. The selection of a screen/film system is ultimately a clinical decision and must be made by the radiologists.

The authors are aware of more formal approaches to screen/film selection, such as ROC analysis. The method of selection presented in this chapter is suggested neither as a counterargument to, nor as a replacement for, such approaches, but as a method more easily implemented in a clinical setting. The method presented here removes some of the subjectivity inherent in a radiologist's simply choosing one system over another, and also allows analysis of the results. It is expected that, at a later date, further application of the use of anatomic landmarks for evaluations of screen/film systems will lead to better definition of the potential signals to be studied.

REFERENCES

Barone, G. J.: A comparative study of the dose distribution for three-phase and single-phase x-ray equipment. Ph.D. thesis, Oregon State University, June, 1971.

Blackwell, H. R.: Contrast thresholds of the human eye. J. Opt. Soc. Am. 36:624, 1946.

Cleare, H. M., Splettstosser, H. R., and Seemann, H. F.: An experimental study of the mottle produced by x-ray intensifying screens. Am. J. Roentgenol. 88:168, 1962.

Doi, K.: Measurement of optical transfer functions of x-ray intensifying screens. Oyo Buturi 33:50, 1964.

Doi, K.: Wiener spectrum analysis of quantum in radiology. *In* Moseley, R. D., and Rust, J. H. (eds.): Television in Diagnostic Radiology. Birmingham, AL, 1969, Aesculapius Publishing Co., pp. 313–333.

Doi, K.: Advantages of magnification radiography. Proceedings of the Symposium on Breast Carcinoma, The Radiologist's Expanded Role, Buffalo, NY, Oct. 1976. New York, 1977, John Wiley & Sons, pp. 13–92.

Doi, K., and Rossmann, K.: Longitudinal magnification in radiologic images of thick objects: a new concept in magnification radiography. Radiology 114:443, 1975.

Doi, K., Rossmann, K., and Duda, E. E.: Application of longitudinal magnification effect to magnification stereoscopic angiography: a new method of cerebral angiography. Radiology 124:395, 1977.

Fewell, T. R., and Weaver, K. E.: The measurement of diagnostic x-ray spectra with a high purity germanium spectrometer. Proceedings of the 1974 BRH/SPIE Symposium—Medical X-ray Photo-optical Systems Evaluation, S.P.I.E. 56:9, 1976.

Genant, H. K., Doi, K., Mall, J. C., and Sickles, E. A.: Direct radiographic magnification for skeletal radiology: an assessment of image quality and clinical application. Radiology 123:47, 1977.

Goodenough, D. J., Rossmann, K., and Lusted, L. B.: Factors affecting the detectability of a simulated radiographic signal. Invest. Radiol. 8:339, 1973.

Goodenough, D. J., Rossman, K., and Lusted, L. B.: Radiographic applications of receiver operating characteristic curves. Radiology 110:89, 1974.

Hallembeck, G. S.: Clinical evaluation of the 240 kV chest radiography system. Department of Radiology, Oak Park Hospital, Oak Park, IL. Available from Hewlett-Packard, McMinnville, OR.

Herman, M. W., Patrick, J., and Tabrisky, J.: A comparative study of scattered radiation levels from 80 kVp and 240 kVp x-rays in the surgical intensive care unit. Radiology 137:552, 1980.

Hewlett-Packard: Technical Bulletin—350 kV chest x-ray technique. Hewlett-Packard, McMinnville, OR, 1974.

Jacobsen, G., Bohlig, H., and Kiviluoto, R.: Essentials of chest radiography. Radiology 95:445, 1970.

Morgan, R. H., Bates, L. M., Gopalarao, U. V., and Marinaro, A.: Frequency response characteristics of x-ray films and screens. Am. J. Roentgenol. 92:426, 1964.

Rossmann, K.: Modulation transfer function of radiographic systems using fluorescent screens. J. Opt. Soc. Am. 52:774, 1962.

Rossmann, K.: Spatial fluctuations of x-ray quanta and the recording of radiographic mottle, Am. J. Roentgenol. 90:863, 1963.

Rossmann, K.: Effect of quantum mottle and modulation transfer on measurement of radiographic image quality. *In* Moseley, R. D., and Rust, J. H. (eds.): Diagnostic Radiologic Instrumentation. Springfield, IL, 1968, Charles C Thomas.

Rossmann, K.: Point spread function, line spread function, and modulation transfer function; tools for the study of imaging systems. Radiology 93:257, 1969.

Tabrisky, J., Herman, M. W., Torrance, D. J., and Hieshima, G. B.: Mobile 240 kVp phototimed chest radiography. Am. J. Roentgenol. 135:295, 1980.

Takahashi, S., and Sakuma, S.: Magnification Radiography. Berlin, 1975, Springer-Verlag.

Vogel, H., and Löhr, H.: X-ray protection zones during x-ray examens in intensive care. Roentgenblaetter 29:459, 1976.

Vucich, J. J., Goodenough, D. J., Lewicki, A. M., et al.: Use of anatomical criteria in screen/film selection for portable chest procedures. Proceedings from Symposium on Optimization of Chest Radiography, The University of Wisconsin, Madison, WI, 1979. HHS Publication (FDA) 80–8124.

Weaver, K. E., Barone, G. J., and Fewell, T. R.: Selection of technique factors for mobile capacitor energy storage equipment. Radiology 128:223, 1978.

Weaver, K. E., Wagner, R. F., and Goodenough, D. J.: Performance considerations of x-ray tube focal spots. Proceedings of the 1974 BRH/SPIE Symposium—Medical X-ray Photo-optical Systems Evaluation, S.P.I.E. 56:150, 1975.

APPENDIX

CARDIOPULMONARY RESUSCITATION

by H. Joel Gorfinkel

Cardiopulmonary resuscitation (CPR) is conducted whenever cardiopulmonary arrest occurs. In recent years the American Heart Association, in conjunction with its local affiliates, has standardized the methods for conducting CPR—basic life support (BLS) and advanced life support (ALS). ALS techniques usually fall into the domain of the intensive care specialist after BLS has been successfully conducted at the scene of the arrest, and is not covered in this appendix. Since BLS has now been standardized and refined as to the most efficient means of conducting CPR, it behooves at least one member of a radiology department, as well as any angiographer, to take the BLS-CPR course currently being offered in most communities. There is definitely a correct way to conduct CPR and, obviously, many wrong ways. CPR performed incorrectly may not only be inefficient, but may actually be harmful to the patient, causing fractured ribs and lacerations of the lungs, liver, or spleen. Information concerning these courses is available from local American Heart Association affiliates.

The most common cause of cardiopulmonary arrest is ventricular fibrillation, which may occur as an angiographic catheter is being manipulated in the ventricle. Complete heart block as a cause of arrest is much less common, but may occur in specific conditions (see Chapter 10).

Excellent monographs dealing with the techniques of CPR are available from the American Heart Association; details of these techniques may also be found in a supplement to the Journal of the American Medical Association (Standards, 1980). A basic outline of CPR of the adult is presented here:

A. Identify that cardiopulmonary arrest has occurred.
   1. The patient is unresponsive.
   2. Respirations have stopped.
   3. No carotid or femoral pulse is palpable, and no identifiable pressure waveform is present on the monitor if the catheter has been introduced beyond the right atrium or if an intra-arterial line is in place.
   4. The electrocardiogram (ECG) shows ventricular fibrillation or ventricular asystole (Fig. A–1). Be sure that the ECG electrodes are properly connected and that the arrhythmia is not due to a loose connection.

B. Have a technician alert the hospital cardiac arrest team.

C. Start an intravenous (IV) line in a large vein if one has not been inserted previously.

D. If the onset of ventricular fibrillation has been witnessed, rap the patient sharply with the fist over the middle third of the sternum. This form of "thump" cardioversion may be effective in reverting ventricular fibrillation if it is performed in the first 15 to 20 seconds.

E. Using an oropharyngeal tube, establish an airway. Do not attempt endotracheal intubation unless you are experienced in this technique.

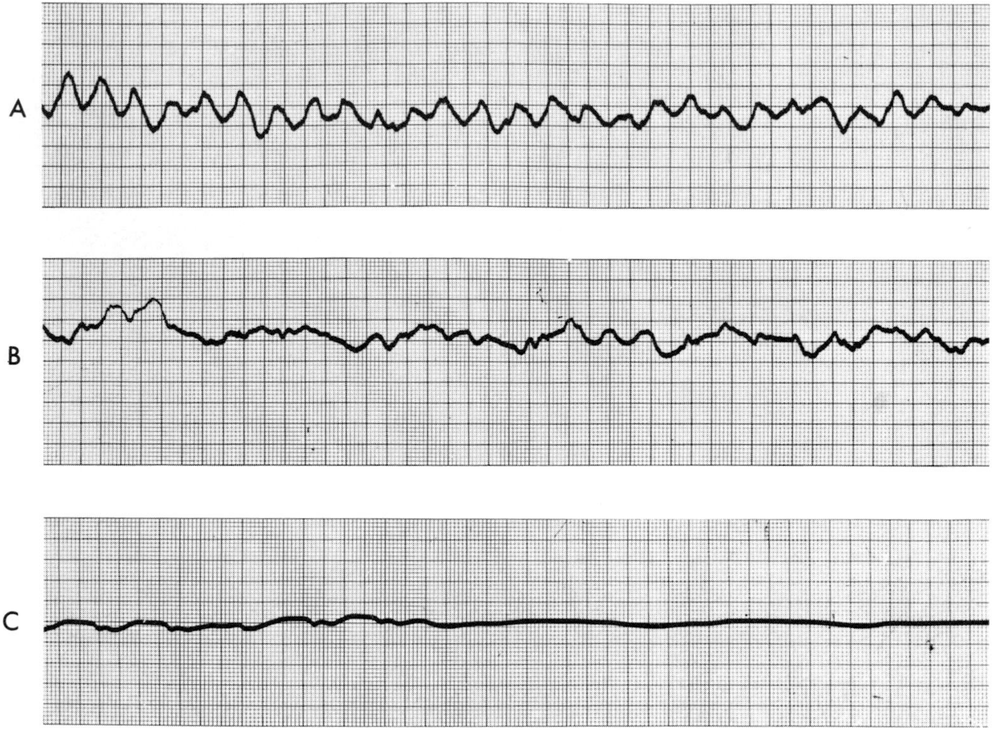

Figure A–1. A, Coarse ventricular fibrillation. This form usually responds immediately to electrical countershock. B, Fine ventricular fibrillation. This form needs treatment with epinephrine to convert it to the coarse form before electrical defibrillation will be successful (*see text*). C, Complete cardiac asystole. The baseline is flat with no evidence of atrial or ventricular activity. This usually signifies a far-advanced arrest status (*see text*).

F. With a second operator, start CPR. One operator conducts closed chest massage at a rate of 60 chest depressions a minute, and the other administers artificial ventilation via a mask attached to high-flow oxygen, utilizing a ventilation bag or pressure valve. Ventilation should be administered at a rate of one breath for every five cardiac compressions.

G. Administer 1 mEq/kg of sodium bicarbonate (1 to 2 ampules) intravenously as a bolus immediately to counteract the rapidly developing acidosis. Bicarbonate administration is repeated at one half the initial dose every ten minutes; however, the exact dose should be governed by frequent determinations of arterial blood gas values. Have a technician or nurse keep an accurate record of the types, doses, and sequence of all drugs administered.

H. Coincident with identification of ventricular fibrillation and the initiation of CPR, apply the defibrillator paddles to the chest (Fig. A–2), either in an anterior precordial-to-back orientation or in a cardiac base-to-apex orientation for two handheld paddles, and apply one 300-watt sec nonsynchronized countershock. (Remember to energize the paddles.) Be sure that the electrode jelly does not bridge the gap between the two electrodes, because this will short-circuit the effective energy that should be delivered to the patient; this most commonly occurs with the use of handheld paddles. All personnel must be free from contact with the patient or the table at this moment in order to avoid serious electrical injuries.

After the countershock has been applied, resume CPR immediately, pausing only momentarily to observe if the arrhythmia has been converted.

Ventricular fibrillation is usually converted with one shock if the onset is appreciated and CPR is started immediately. Inadequate CPR techniques and inadequate treatment of the acidosis with bicarbonate and ventilation are the most common causes of resistant ventricular fibrillation.

I. If, at this point, ventricular fibrillation has not been reverted, continue CPR and bicarbonate treatment. The ventricular fibrillation must now be re-evaluated.

1. If, following countershock, a rhythm that was transiently restored rapidly deteriorates into ventricular fibrillation once again, intravenously inject a bolus of lidocaine hydrochloride (1 mg/kg—75 to 100 mg for an adult), and again defibrillate the patient. Lidocaine may be repeated every three to five minutes; 50-mg boluses to a total dose of 225 mg are used. If this successfully terminates the arrhythmia, continue the lidocaine infusion at a rate of 2 to 4 mg/min (1 to 2 ml/min of a solution containing 1 gm of lidocaine in 500 ml of 5 per cent dextrose and water).

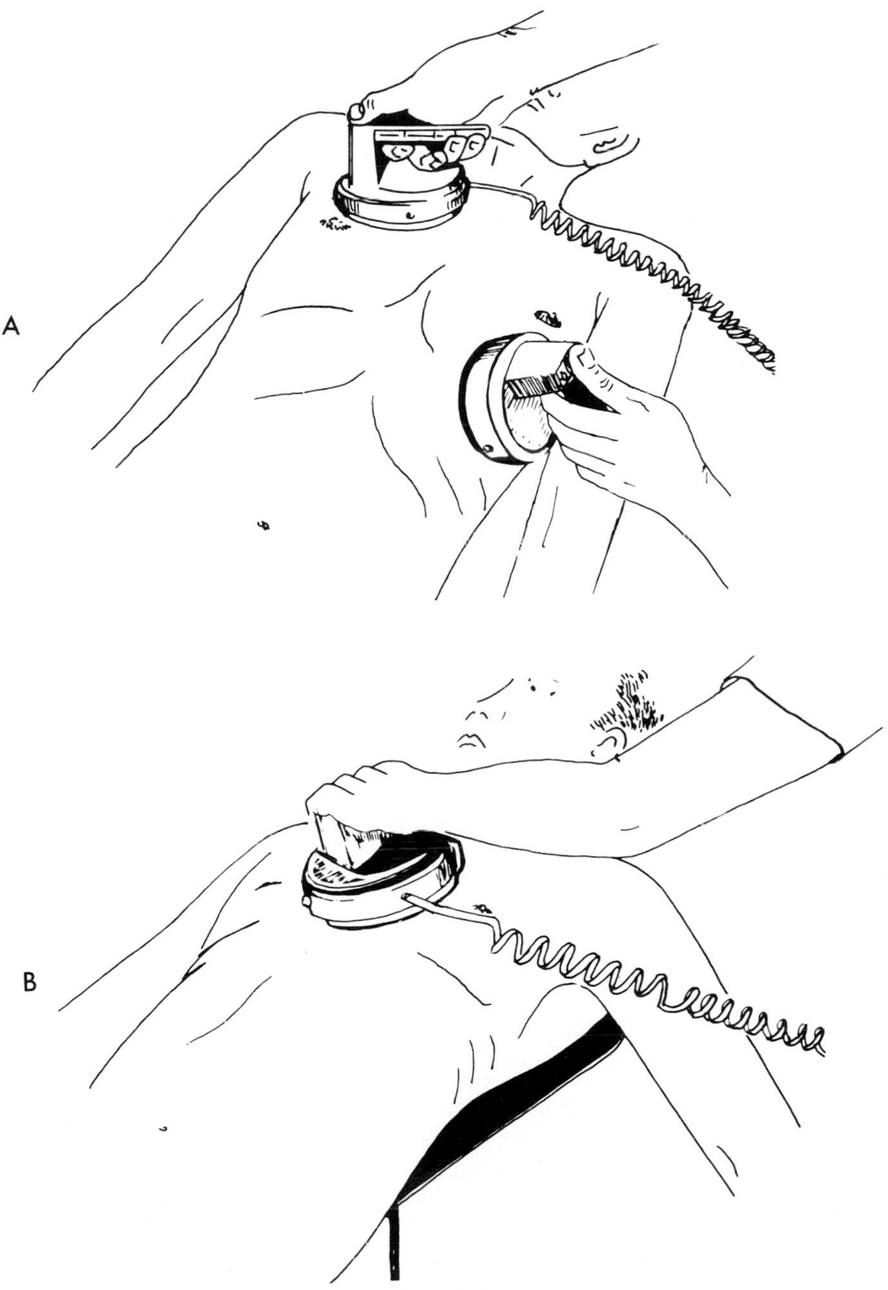

Figure A–2. Proper chest positions for defibrillator paddles. *A*, Position for two handheld paddles. *B*, Position for unit using one handheld paddle and back plate. (By permission of the American Heart Association, Inc.)

2. If the ventricular fibrillation was not even temporarily reverted and the fibrillatory waves appear fine rather than coarse (Fig. A–1*B*), inject 5 ml of a 1 to 10,000 epinephrine solution through the pulmonary arterial catheter, or IV if the catheter has not been inserted. Continue CPR for another 30 seconds and apply another 400-watt sec countershock. This sequence may be repeated in five minutes.

J. If reversion has still not been successful, continue CPR and bicarbonate treatment, inject 5 ml of 10 per cent calcium chloride (or 10 ml of 10 per cent calcium gluconate) solution IV, and again attempt defibrillation. This regimen may be repeated every ten minutes.

Calcium and sodium bicarbonate solutions must not be injected sequentially through the same IV line, since this will produce a calcium carbonate precipitate. This problem may be averted by flushing the line with normal saline solution or with dextrose and water between infusions of these two solutions.

Should ventricular fibrillation deteriorate to complete cardiac asystole (Fig. A–1*C*), continue calcium chloride and epinephrine administration and optimize the acid-base balance in an effort to convert the rhythm pattern back to ventricular fibrillation. In doing so, it may be possible to countershock the fibrillation back to an electrically functional rhythm and thereby produce the return of an effective pulse. All the while, continue CPR. Discontinue the resuscitative effort only after every conceivable mode of therapy has been tried and has failed. It is impossible to give an arbitrary time limit after which resuscitation should be stopped. Some patients have responded after an hour of vigorous resuscitative efforts; usually, such patients continue to show some electrical responsiveness to therapy. Continued total cardiac asystole is a very grave situation and usually indicates irreversible cardiac death. By the time such a state has developed, the radiologic team will have been joined by the hospital's cardiac arrest team. Other therapeutic modalities, such as transthoracic pacemaker electrode placement, may be attempted in consultation with them. Unfortunately, this procedure is rarely effective in this clinical setting.

K. Once the patient has been successfully resuscitated, follow the blood pressure, pulse, rhythm, adequacy of ventilation, and level of consciousness closely. Do not assume that all is now well just because an adequate-appearing rhythm has been established.

REFERENCE

Standards and Guidelines for Cardiopulmonary Resuscitation (CPR) and Emergency Cardiac Care (ECC). J.A.M.A. (Suppl.) 244:453, 1980.

INDEX

Page numbers in *italics* refer to illustrations. Page numbers followed by (t) refer to tables.